CARDIAC ADAPTATION

Proceedings of the Eighth International Meeting of the
International Study Group for Research
in Cardiac Metabolism
[now the International Society for Heart Research]
26–29 May, 1976
Tokyo, Japan

Organized by the
Japanese Study Group for Research in Cardiac Metabolism,
the Japanese Circulation Society, and
the Japan Heart Foundation

Officers of the Organization Committee:
Mikamo, Y. (Tokyo), Honorary Chairman
Kobayashi, T. (Tokyo), Chairman
Yamamura, Y. (Osaka), Vice Chairman
Ito, Y. (Tokyo), Congress Secretary

Recent Advances in Studies on Cardiac Structure and Metabolism

Series Editor: G. Rona (*formerly with the late E. Bajusz*)

Volume 1: **MYOCARDIOLOGY** (edited by E. Bajusz and G. Rona)
Volume 2: **CARDIOMYOPATHIES** (edited by E. Bajusz and G. Rona, with A. J. Brink and A. Lochner)
Volume 3: **MYOCARDIAL METABOLISM** (edited by N. S. Dhalla)
Volume 4: **MYOCARDIAL BIOLOGY** (edited by N. S. Dhalla)
Volume 5: **MYOCARDIAL CELL DAMAGE** (edited by A. Fleckenstein and N. S. Dhalla)
Volume 6: **PATHOPHYSIOLOGY AND MORPHOLOGY OF MYOCARDIAL CELL ALTERATIONS** (edited by A. Fleckenstein and G. Rona)
Volume 7: **BIOCHEMISTRY AND PHARMACOLOGY OF MYOCARDIAL HYPERTROPHY, HYPOXIA, AND INFARCTION** (edited by P. Harris, R. I. Bing, and A. Fleckenstein)
Volume 8: **THE CARDIAC SARCOPLASM** (edited by P.-E. Roy and P. Harris)
Volume 9: **THE SARCOLEMMA** (edited by P.-E. Roy and N. S. Dhalla)
Volume 10: **THE METABOLISM OF CONTRACTION** (edited by P.-E. Roy and G. Rona)
Volume 11: **HEART FUNCTION AND METABOLISM** (edited by T. Kobayashi, T. Sano, and N. S. Dhalla)
Volume 12: **CARDIAC ADAPTATION** (edited by T. Kobayashi, Y. Ito, and G. Rona)

Recent Advances in Studies on
Cardiac Structure and Metabolism, Volume 12

CARDIAC ADAPTATION

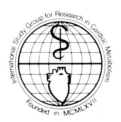

Edited by

Tachio Kobayashi, M.D., F.A.C.C.
Professor and Chairman, Showa University Fujigaoka Hospital
Honorary Professor of The University of Tokyo
Tokyo, Japan

Yoshio Ito, M.D.
Professor, Fourth Department of Internal Medicine
Faculty of Medicine
The University of Tokyo
Tokyo, Japan
and
George Rona, M.D., Ph.D., F.R.C.P. (C)
Professor of Pathology
McGill University
Montréal, Québec, Canada

UNIVERSITY PARK PRESS
Baltimore · London · Tokyo

UNIVERSITY PARK PRESS
International Publishers in Science and Medicine
233 East Redwood Street
Baltimore, Maryland 21202

Typeset by The Composing Room of Michigan, Inc.
Manufactured in the United States of America by
Universal Lithographers, Inc.,
and The Optic Bindery Incorporated.

Library of Congress Cataloging in Publication Data

International Society for Heart Research.
Cardiac adaptation.

(Recent advances in studies on cardiac structure and metabolism; v. 12)
"Proceedings of the eighth international meeting of the International Study
Group for Research in Cardiac Metabolism (now the International Society
for Heart Research) 26–29 May 1976, Tokyo, Japan."
Includes bibliographies and indexes.
1. Heart – Congresses. 2. Metabolism – Congresses.
I. Kobayashi, Tachio, 1912–   II. Ito, Yoshio, 1940–
III. Rona, George, 1924–   IV. Title. V. Series.
RC667.R4 Vol. 12 [RC681-A3-2] 616.1' 2'008s [599'.01' 16]
ISBN 0-8391-0672-6   77-25354

Contents

Heart Growth and Its Disturbances

Altered Myocardial Metabolism

Chemical Models

Myocardial Ischemia

Cardiomyopathies

Enzyme Changes in Myocardial Injury

Cardiac Protection

Reperfusion of Ischemic Myocardium

Tissue Culture of Cardiac Muscle Cells

Contributing Authors

Abiko, Y., *Asahikawa* (Japan)
Adelstein, R. S., *Bethesda, Md.* (USA)
Adler, C. P., *Freiburg* (Federal Republic of Germany)
Ageta, M., *Kurume* (Japan)
Ahmad, M., *Aligarh* (India)
Akagami, H., *Osaka* (Japan)
Alexander, C. S., *Minneapolis, Minn.* (USA)
Al-Janabi, N., *Baghdad* (Iraq)
Allison, T. B., *Newington, Conn.* (USA)
Ammerante, T., *London* (England)
Anazawa, S., *Tokyo* (Japan)
Aoyagi, R., *Niigata* (Japan)
Arai, T., *Sapporo* (Japan)
Arai, T., *Sendai* (Japan)
Asazuma, S., *Kyoto* (Japan)
Ashraf, M., *LaJolla, Cal.* (USA)
Athias, P., *Dijon* (France)
Badonnel, M.-C., *Montréal, Qué.* (Canada)
Ban, M., *Nagoya* (Japan)
Bannai, S., *Niigata* (Japan)
Barnhorst, D. A., *Rochester, Minn.* (USA)
Bhagat, B., *St. Louis, Mo.* (USA)
Bing, R. J., *Pasadena, Cal.* (USA)
Bitensky, L., *London* (England)
Bittar, N., *Madison, Wis.* (USA)
Blanchaer, M. C., *Winnipeg, Man.* (Canada)
Bloor, C. M., *LaJolla, Cal.* (USA)
Bos, G., *Leiden* (The Netherlands)
Boutet, M., *Québec, Qué.* (Canada)
Braimbridge, M. V., *London* (England)
Buja, L. M., *Dallas, Tex.* (USA)
Čanković-Darracott, S., *London* (England)
Charbonné, F., *Clermont-Ferrand* (France)
Chayen, J., *London* (England)
Crass, M. F., III, *Lubbock, Tex.* (USA)
Danielson, G. K., *Rochester, Minn.* (USA)
De Jong, J. W., *Rotterdam* (The Netherlands)
DeLuca, M., *LaJolla, Cal.* (USA)
Demaster, E. G., *Minneapolis, Minn.* (USA)
Dewey, J. D., *Rochester, Minn.* (USA)
Dhalla, N. S., *Winnipeg, Man.* (Canada)
Earl, C. A., *Nedlands* (Western Australia)
Eguchi, S., *Niigata* (Japan)
Everett, A. W., *Nedlands* (Western Australia)
Fenner, C., *Davis, Cal.* (USA)
Ferrans, V. J., *Bethesda, Md.* (USA)
Ferro, A. M., *San Francisco, Cal.* (USA)
Fink, G. C., *Dallas, Tex.* (USA)
Fischer, V. W., *Winnipeg, Man.* (Canada)
Flaherty, J. T., *Baltimore, Md.* (USA)
Flameng, W., *Giessen* (Federal Republic of Germany)

Folts, J. D., *Madison, Wis.* (USA)
Franc, F., *Prague* (Czechoslovakia)
Frelin, C., *Dijon* (France)
Fujita, T., *Osaka* (Japan)
Fukunaka, M., *Osaka* (Japan)
Fushimi, H., *Osaka* (Japan)
Goodman, M. F., *Los Angeles, Cal.* (USA)
Goon, D. J. W., *Minneapolis, Minn.* (USA)
Goshima, K., *Nagoya* (Japan)
Gott, V., *Baltimore, Md.* (USA)
Gottwick, M. G., *Boston, Mass.* (USA)
Grau, A., *London* (England)
Haneda, T., *Sendai* (Japan)
Hara, A., *Tokyo* (Japan)
Harary, I., *Los Angeles, Cal.* (USA)
Harrison, C. E., Jr., *Rochester, Minn.* (USA)
Hasegawa, M., *Tokyo* (Japan)
Hashimoto, I., *Kyoto* (Japan)
Hashimoto, S., *Osaka* (Japan)
Hatano, R., *Tokyo* (Japan)
Hatt, P. Y., *Limeil-Brevannes* (France)
Haze, K., *Tokyo* (Japan)
Hearse, D. J., *New York, N.Y.* (USA)
Hermens, W. Th., *Leiden* (The Netherlands)
Higuma, N., *Niigata* (Japan)
Hiroe, M., *Tokyo* (Japan)
Hirosawa, K., *Tokyo* (Japan)
Holsinger, J. W., Jr., *Newington, Conn.* (USA)
Honna, T., *Sendai* (Japan)
Hopkins, B. E., *Nedlands* (Western Australia)
Howe, B. B., *Morris Plains, N.J.* (USA)
Hüttner, J., *Montréal, Qué.* (Canada)
Ibukiyama, C., *Tokyo* (Japan)
Ichihara, K., *Asahikawa* (Japan)
Iimura, O., *Sapporo* (Japan)
Ingwall, J. S., *LaJolla, Cal.* (USA)
Inokawa, K., *Matsumoto* (Japan)
Inui, Y., *Osaka* (Japan)
Irisawa, H., *Hiroshima* (Japan)
Irmler, R., *Berlin* (German Democratic Republic)
Ishida, S., *Kurume* (Japan)
Ishizawa, K., *Kyoto* (Japan)
Ito, T., *Nagoya* (Japan)
Ito, T., *Tokyo* (Japan)
Ito, Y., *Tokyo* (Japan)
Iwane, H., *Tokyo* (Japan)
Izumi, T., *Niigata* (Japan)
James, T. N., *Birmingham, Ala.* (USA)
Jones, M., *Bethesda, Md.* (USA)
Kagawa, T., *Osaka* (Japan)
Kageyama, S., *Tokyo* (Japan)
Kakiuchi, Y., *Sapporo* (Japan)
Kakizawa, N., *Nagoya* (Japan)

xii

Kamikawa, T., *Hamamatsu* (Japan)
Kamiyama, A., *Tokyo* (Japan)
Kamiyama, T., *Davis, Cal.* (USA)
Kao, R. L., *Galveston, Tex.* (USA)
Kashahara, K., *Osaka* (Japan)
Kashiwakura, Y., *Tokyo* (Japan)
Katagiri, T., *Tokyo* (Japan)
Kato, M., *Osaka* (Japan)
Kawai, C., *Kyoto* (Japan)
Kawamura, K., *Birmingham, Ala.* (USA)
Kawamura, K., *Kyoto* (Japan)
Kawashima, Y., *Osaka* (Japan)
Kennett, F. F., *Richmond, Va.* (USA)
Khuri, S., *Baltimore, Md.* (USA)
Kikuchi, Y., *Fukuoka* (Japan)
Kimura, N., *Kurume* (Japan)
Kirk, E. S., *New York, N.Y.* (USA)
Kitamura, K., *Tokyo* (Japan)
Kobayashi, K., *Hershey, Pa.* (USA)
Kobayashi, K., *Sendai* (Japan)
Kobayashi, T., *Sapporo* (Japan)
Kogure, T., *Tokyo* (Japan)
Koiwaya, Y., *Fukuoka* (Japan)
Koizumi, T., *Tokyo* (Japan)
Koke, J. R., *Madison, Wis.* (USA)
Kölbel, F., *Prague* (Czechoslovakia)
Konno, S., *Tokyo* (Japan)
Kosuga, M., *Tokyo* (Japan)
Kotani, S., *Osaka* (Japan)
Koyama, T., *Sapporo* (Japan)
Kumazawa, T., *Tokyo* (Japan)
Kumudavalli-Reddy, M., *Chicago, Ill.*
   (USA)
Kun, E., *San Francisco, Cal.* (USA)
Kuroiwa, A., *Fukuoka* (Japan)
Lacktis, J. W., *Chicago, Ill.* (USA)
Laurent, G. L., *Nedlands* (Western
   Australia)
Lefer, A. M., *Philadelphia, Pa.* (USA)
Lentz, R. W., *Rochester, Minn.* (USA)
Lombardini, J. B., *Lubbock, Tex.* (USA)
McLean, M., *Charlottesville, Va.* (USA)
Malý, M., *Prague* (Czechoslovakia)
Manabe, H., *Osaka* (Japan)
Manasek, F. J., *Chicago, Ill.* (USA)
Maron, B. J., *Bethesda, Md.* (USA)
Martin, A. F., *Chicago, Ill.* (USA)
Mason, D. T., *Davis, Cal.* (USA)
Masuda, A., *Osaka* (Japan)
Matsuguchi, H., *Fukuoka* (Japan)
Matsumoto, S., *Tokyo* (Japan)
Matsuoka, M., *Niigata* (Japan)
Mitsui, H., *Kyoto* (Japan)
Mitsutake, A., *Fukuoka* (Japan)
Miura, Y., *Sendai* (Japan)
Miyahara, M., *Sapporo* (Japan)

Miyazawa, K., *Sendai* (Japan)
Mizuno, K., *Nagoya* (Japan)
Mizutani, K., *Nagoya* (Japan)
Mochizuki, S., *Hershey, Pa.* (USA)
Monma, Y., *Sapporo* (Japan)
Moravec, J., *Limeil-Brevannes* (France)
Moravec-Mochet, M., *Limeil-Brevannes*
   (France)
Morgan, H. E., *Hershey, Pa.* (USA)
Mori, M., *Fukuoka* (Japan)
Mori, T., *Osaka* (Japan)
Morimoto, M., *Matsumoto* (Japan)
Mukherjee, A., *Dallas, Tex.* (USA)
Murashige, H., *Kyoto* (Japan)
Murota, M., *Tokyo* (Japan)
Nadel, E. M., *Winnipeg, Man.* (Canada)
Nagano, M., *Tokyo* (Japan)
Nagasawa, H. T., *Minneapolis, Minn.* (USA)
Naito, T., *Kyoto* (Japan)
Nakagawa, M., *Tokyo* (Japan)
Nakai, Y., *Tokyo* (Japan)
Nakajima, T., *Sendai* (Japan)
Nakamura, M., *Fukuoka* (Japan)
Nakamura, T., *Nagoya* (Japan)
Nayler, W. G., *London* (England)
Neely, J. R., *Hershey, Pa.* (USA)
Niitami, H., *Tokyo* (Japan)
Nohara, Y., *Tokyo* (Japan)
Nonoyama, A., *Osaka* (Japan)
Nose, Y., *Fukuoka* (Japan)
Nylen, E., *Winnipeg, Man.* (Canada)
Ogawa, K., *Nagoya* (Japan)
Okada, R., *Tokyo* (Japan)
Okubo, M., *Nagoya* (Japan)
Okuda, M., *Saitama Prefecture* (Japan)
Olson, H. E., *London* (England)
Omae, M., *Kyoto* (Japan)
Onishi, S., *Osaka* (Japan)
Oratz, M., *New York, N.Y.* (USA)
O'Riordan, J., *Baltimore, Md.* (USA)
Ota, K., *Kurume* (Japan)
Ozawa, K., *Tokyo* (Japan)
Padieu, P., *Dijon* (France)
Patzer, B., *Chicago, Ill.* (USA)
Pinson, A., *Jerusalem* (Israel)
Platt, M. R., *Dallas, Tex.* (USA)
Raben, M. S., *Boston, Mass.* (USA)
Rabinowitz, M., *Chicago, Ill.* (USA)
Ramey, C. A., *Newington, Conn.* (USA)
Rannels, D. E., *Hershey, Pa.* (USA)
Remme, W. J., *Rotterdam* (The
   Netherlands)
Rona, G., *Montréal, Qué.* (Canada)
Ross, D. N., *London* (England)
Rothschild, M. A., *New York, N.Y.* (USA)
Russell, B. L., *Saskatoon* (Canada)

Saito, H., *Sapporo* (Japan)
Saito, N., *Tokyo* (Japan)
Sakuma, H., *Sendai* (Japan)
Salel, A. F., *Davis, Cal.* (USA)
Sandritter, W., *Freiburg* (Federal Republic of Germany)
Sasajima, T., *Sapporo* (Japan)
Sassa, H., *Ogaki* (Japan)
Sassa, S., *Kyoto* (Japan)
Sato, T., *Osaka* (Japan)
Sato, T., *Sendai* (Japan)
Scales, F. E., *Dallas, Tex.* (USA)
Schaper, J., *Sprudelhof* (Federal Republic of Germany)
Schreiber, S. S., *New York, N.Y.* (USA)
Schwarz, F., *Bad Nauheim* (Federal Republic of Germany)
Sekiguchi, M., *Tokyo* (Japan)
Seraydarian, M. W., *Los Angeles, Cal.* USA)
Shibata, N., *Osaka* (Japan)
Shida, H., *Nagano Prefecture* (Japan)
Shimizu, K., *Tokyo* (Japan)
Shimizu, M., *Tokyo* (Japan)
Shiozu, H., *Nagoya* (Japan)
Shirato, K., *Sendai* (Japan)
Shoji, T., *Sapporo* (Japan)
Shug, A. L., *Madison, Wis.* (USA)
Sims, J. M., *Chicago, Ill.* (USA)
Smith, S. J., *Leiden* (The Netherlands)
Smith, T. W., *Boston, Mass.* (USA)
Song, S. H., *London, Ont.* (Canada)
Song, W., *Lubbock, Tex.* (USA)
Sparrow, M. P., *Nedlands* (Western Australia)
Sperelakis, N., *Charlottesville, Va.* (USA)
Stam, H., *Rotterdam* (The Netherlands)
Su, K.-M., *Tokyo* (Japan)
Sulakhe, P. V., *Saskatoon* (Canada)
Sulakhe, S. J., *Saskatoon* (Canada)
Sullivan, J. M., *Winnipeg, Man.* (Canada)
Sunaga, T., *Tokyo* (Japan)
Sunamori, M., *Tokyo* (Japan)
Suzuki, T., *Tokyo* (Japan)
Suzuki, Y., *Hamamatsu* (Japan)
Sybers, H. D., *Houston, Tex.* (USA)
Tajuddin, M., *Aligarh* (India)
Takahashi, S., *Kyoto* (Japan)
Takano, H., *Osaka* (Japan)
Takeshita, A., *Fukuoka* (Japan)
Takishima, T., *Sendai* (Japan)
Tamura, K., *Niigata* (Japan)
Tanabe, T., *Sapporo* (Japan)

Tanaka, H., *Tokyo* (Japan)
Tariq, M., *Aligarh, Tex.* (USA)
Taylor, R. R., *Nedlands* (Western Australia)
Templeton, G. H., *Dallas, Tex.* (USA)
Thiedemann, K.-U., *Bethesda, Md.* (USA)
Tomizuka, S., *Tokyo* (Japan)
Tomlinson, C. W., *Winnipeg, Man.* (Canada)
Toshima, H., *Kurume* (Japan)
Toyama, S., *Osaka* (Japan)
Tsugane, J., *Matsumoto* (Japan)
Tsukuura, T., *Tokyo* (Japan)
Tsuzuku, A., *Tokyo* (Japan)
Urthaler, F., *Birmingham, Ala.* (USA)
Van Der Wiel, H. L., *Rotterdam* (The Netherlands)
Verdouw, P. D., *Rotterdam* (The Netherlands)
Veselý, P., *Prague* (Czechoslovakia)
Wada, A., *Osaka* (Japan)
Wakabayashi, C., *Sapporo* (Japan)
Wakamatsu, Y., *Nagoya* (Japan)
Wallace, G., *Los Angeles, Cal.* (USA)
Watanabe, T., *Kyoto* (Japan)
Weglicki, W. B., *Richmond, Va.* (USA)
Whitman, V., *Hershey, Pa.* (USA)
Wikman-Coffelt, J., *Davis, Cal.* (USA)
Wildenthal, K., *Dallas, Tex.* (USA)
Willerson, J. T., *Dallas, Tex.* (USA)
Winbury, M. M., *Morris Plains, N.J.* (USA)
Witteveen, S. A. G. J., *Leiden* (The Netherlands)
Wollenberger, A., *Berlin-Buch* (German Democratic Republic)
Wrogemann, K., *Winnipeg, Man.* (Canada)
Yabe, Y., *Tokyo* (Japan)
Yagi, T., *Sapporo* (Japan)
Yamada, T., *Tokyo* (Japan)
Yamagami, T., *Osaka* (Japan)
Yamamoto, M., *Nagoya* (Japan)
Yamamoto, N., *Tokyo* (Japan)
Yamasawa, I., *Tokyo* (Japan)
Yamazaki, N., *Hamamatsu* (Japan)
Yazaki, Y., *Tokyo* (Japan)
Yepez, C., *London* (England)
Yokota, H., *Osaka* (Japan)
Yokota, Y., *Kurume* (Japan)
Yoneda, S., *Osaka* (Japan)
Yoshida, F., *Tokyo* (Japan)
Yoshida, S., *Sapporo* (Japan)
Yoshida, Y., *Nagoya* (Japan)
Yoshimura, S., *Tokyo* (Japan)
Yoshinaga, K., *Sendai* (Japan)
Zak, R., *Chicago, Ill.* (USA)

Editorial Foreword

At the Third Annual Meeting of the International Study Group for Research in Cardiac Metabolism held at Stowe, Vermont in June 1970, in his introductory remarks, Dr. Richard J. Bing outlined the progress of cardiac metabolism studies and predicted that further application of biochemical and biophysical methods to the study of cardiac metabolism would contribute to more thorough understanding of the mechanisms underlying heart failure, myocardial infarction, and cardiomyopathies. The subsequent international meetings of the Study Group and the reports of their proceedings, published in *Recent Advances in Studies on Cardiac Structure and Metabolism,* clearly reflect the progress made in this field.

During the past few years, we have witnessed a remarkable explosion of new information in cardiology, made possible by the introduction of sophisticated investigative methods. Dr. Bing updates this progress in his special introductory lecture. The development of myocardial biopsy and, in particular, the introduction by Konno, Sekiguchi, and Sakakibara in 1961 of endomyocardial biopsy made possible biochemical, biophysical, immunological, and ultrastructural studies of human myocardium and led to a closer integration with animal experimental data. It was as a tribute to the Japanese cardiologists who pioneered the application of cardiac biopsy studies to human conditions that the Eighth International Meeting of the Study Group assembled in Tokyo.

Contributions in the second section help to explain how changes affecting myocardial protein and nucleoprotein metabolism, as well as modifications in structure of cardiac muscle cells, serve myocardial adaptation. These adaptive changes may be initiated during early embryonic life or during the development of cardiac hypertrophy. The third section gives an account of the neuromuscular interrelation in pacemaker activity and the fine structure and histochemistry of the sinoatrial node and conduction system.

The fourth section is a collection of papers on conditions that affect heart growth. It appears that alterations in synthesis, processing, or degradation of RNA play a key role in modification of heart size. In human hearts, the importance of polyploidization of cardiac muscle cells and formation of new sarcomeres is discussed in the development of cardiac hypertrophy. The fifth section deals with altered myocardial metabolism following myocardial ischemia and in various forms of experimentally induced and human cardiomyopathies. There is a good collection of papers discussing the significance of enzyme changes following ischemic myocardial injury (section six). The information supplied by these metabolic studies made possible the design of biologically supported interventions for cardiac protection. Particularly notable in these studies is the progress made in explaining the effect of reperfusion of the ischemic myocardium (sections seven and eight).

For the first time in this series, in the ninth section, there is an extensive documentation of information derived from the utilization of a new method—tissue culture of cardiac muscle cells. The history of this model is reviewed by Dr. A. Wollenberger. The work of internationally recognized experts, including Japanese cell biologists and cardiologists, clearly establishes the great practical value of this method.

It is hoped that Volume 12 with its rich fund of information will provide useful data for scientists working in this ever-expanding field and will stimulate further outstanding results related to cardiac structure and metabolism.

G. Rona

SPECIAL
LECTURE

Recent Advances in Studies on
Cardiac Structure and Metabolism, Volume 12
Cardiac Adaptation
Edited by T. Kobayashi, Y. Ito, and G. Rona
Copyright 1978 University Park Press Baltimore

CONTRIBUTION OF MYOCARDIAL METABOLISM TO THE KNOWLEDGE OF MYOCARDIAL FAILURE AND MYOCARDIAL INFARCTION

R. J. BING

Huntington Memorial Hospital and Huntington Institute of
Applied Medical Research, Pasadena, and the University of Southern
California, Los Angeles, California, USA

INTRODUCTION

As the introductory remarks for this volume, this chapter focuses on two topics: myocardial failure and myocardial infarction. Clinically, these topics represent the most frequent cardiac disorders seen at the bedside. But the more important reason for choosing these subjects is that knowledge of cardiac metabolism has permitted us to gain insight into these two conditions and has brought to the fore entirely different fundamental backgrounds. The biochemical basis for myocardial failure is in many respects different from that of myocardial infarction, although there is some overlapping; this difference expresses itself not only in different clinical symptomology but also in a different approach to treatment. While the metabolic causes of heart failure are diffuse, those of myocardial infarction are specific. And, in medicine, diseases with specific causes are more readily amenable to treatment, while diseases with diffuse, nonspecific mechanisms are difficult to approach therapeutically. In this respect, heart failure belongs to the group of conditions that are in line with atherosclerosis, that is, diseases of multiple origins; myocardial infarction, on the other hand, is synonymous with local ischemia of the heart muscle.

MYOCARDIAL FAILURE

The term myocardial failure is of relatively recent origin; the term was first used in the book, *Diseases of the Heart,* by James Mackenzie (1910). Mackenzie

---

Original work presented in this paper was supported by grants from the United States Public Health Service (#5 RO1 AA00304-05), The Margaret W. and Herbert Hoover, Jr. Foundation, and The Council for Tobacco Research.

speaks here of dilatation of the heart, a term that was used with frequency by his predecessors Austin Flint (Landis, 1912), Constantine Paul (1883), and, before them, by Hope (1831) and other clinicians of the 18th and early 19th centuries.

Mackenzie demonstrated the relationship between dilatation of the heart and clinical signs and symptoms of heart failure. He described the symptomology that we identify today with myocardial or congestive failure. He described subjective symptoms of breathlessness, palpitation, weakness, dropsy, diminished secretion of urine, enlargement of the liver, lividity of the face, and pulmonary congestion.

> So long as the contractile force of the heart is able to maintain a degree of arterial pressure sufficient to supply the organs and the tissues, the heart failure will be limited to those subjective symptoms involved in great reduction of reserve force. The patient is comfortable at rest, for the heart is then able to maintain the circulation, but is distressed by exertion, for the heart has so little reserve force that it is unable to meet the extra demands. When the force of the heart fails to maintain the arterial pressure at the height necessary for the tissues, then we get the symptoms in the remote organs and tissues, such as dropsy, ascites, enlarged liver (Mackenzie, 1910).

The terminology in this extract has a modern ring. The terms used by Mackenzie—contractile force of the heart, maintenence of circulation, cardiac reserve, extra demands on the heart, and force of the heart—are the subjects of recent inquiry.

In 1839, James Hope, an early English writer, published his book on diseases of the heart and great vessels (Hope, 1831). In the delightful book, *A Short History of Cardiology* (Herrick, 1942), Hope, who lived from 1801 to 1841, is described as a man who spent two years as resident physician and neurosurgeon of Laennec and who worked with Corvisart, Napoleon's physician. During his lifetime he was not one of the more popular physicians, having been accused of seeking position by use of influence and wire-pulling. He is said to "have worn religion on his sleeve, and just as he had begun to realize the folly of some of his foolish ways, he was tragically cut down in his prime by tuberculosis" (Herrick, 1942), an illness that ended many an illustrious career at that time. Hope's discussion in *A Treatise on the Diseases of the Heart and Great Vessels* of the anatomy and physiology of the heart strikes a modern note. Hope also speaks of cardiac dilatation and hypertrophy and discusses their diagnosis, but he never mentions heart failure. Nevertheless, he was way ahead of his time when he wrote of the mechanism of pulmonary edema, mentioning that "the blood, not being freely transmitted by the left ventricle, accumulates in the lung by retardation." Digitalis, which had been discovered 50 years earlier by Withering, was not one of his popular remedies. Indeed, it was not used for a long time after its discovery.

Constantine Paul published his book on diseases of the heart in 1883 and also speaks of cardiac hypertrophy and dilatation, defining the latter as a distension of the heart without the ability to return upon itself (Paul, 1883). Among many medical school teachers (including Rhomberg and Friedrich Muller), heart failure has not been a favorite term (Bing, personal observation). Even as late as 1930, "cardiac tonics" were in vogue, which included digitalis, caffeine, and strychnine.

Within this very brief description of the history of myocardial failure, there is no description of the basic mechanisms of heart failure, of cardiac dilatation, or of cardiac hypertrophy, and all the studies were purely clinical. It is to the merit of the science of cardiac metabolism that, today, myocardial failure is considered from a new and fresh point of view.

I do not claim that the history of cardiac metabolism began with our work on catheterization of the coronary sinus in 1957 (Bing *et al.*, 1947, 1949). But a beginning was made at that time to consider myocardial failure other than from a purely clinical point of view. We reported that, in myocardial failure in man, the myocardial O_2 extraction ratios of substrates remained unchanged (Blain *et al.,* 1956). We thought at that time that the *in vivo* study of cardiac metabolism was the wave of the future. However, it soon became apparent that this was only a beginning and that much could be gained from research on metabolism in isolated systems. As time progressed, we investigated the problem of myocardial failure from three different viewpoints: 1) that of contractility of the heart, more specifically contractile proteins in myocardial failure, 2) that of mechanisms responsible for coupling excitation with contraction introducing the element of calcium uptake and transfer, and 3) that of the role of mitochondria.

Contractility in Myocardial Failure

The measurement and definition of contractility have been one of the thorniest subjects in the history of cardiac metabolism. The reason is that, in the whole heart beating in its natural environment, contractility is difficult to define. Measurements that define the contractile state, be it at the papillary muscle or glycerinated fibers of the heart *in vitro,* can be made with accuracy only in *in vitro* preparations. We must not confuse or equate hemodynamic changes with contractility; although, for example, valuable estimations of contractility in the whole heart can be obtained by correlating end-diastolic pressure to the stroke volume or by determination of the ejection fraction.

The contractile state itself can only be defined with accuracy in isolated preparation. We made an effort to accomplish this in 1958, when we compressed actomyosin from heart muscle into bands and made these bands contract by adding ATP (Kako and Bing, 1958); we found diminished contraction of the failing heart. In these early days, contractility was difficult to measure and more difficult to define. We have now learned to measure contractility in *in vitro* preparation in which the muscle is maintained at a constant length and is made to contract isometrically; one can then quantitate contractility by the amount of isometric force or stress, i.e., the force per cross-sectional area of muscle developed (Julian, 1971; Maruyama *et al.*, in press). I emphasize *constant length*, because when one alters sarcomere length of the muscle, the amount of force developed increases together with the initial length at which the muscle is held (the Starling Frank mechanism). Changes in length do not adequately describe contractility, and much confusion has arisen over the interpretation of data on muscle mechanics obtained by interjecting effects resulting from changes in sarcomere length (Huxley, 1971; Julian, 1971; Maruyama *et al.*, in press).

We can determine maximal development of force P_0, dP/dt_{max}, and the time it takes for this force to develop (t_0). Our laboratory is using the glycerinated heart muscle fiber, a model first developed by Szent-Gyorgyi. These parameters define the contractile state. In addition, we also can measure the force-velocity relationship by determining the isotonic shortening of the muscle at a given force level beginning at P_0 (that is, at the maximal force obtained at zero velocity). This is usually accomplished by monitoring shortening with high-speed photographic recordings "during quick release," allowing the muscle to isotonically shorten as tension is reduced in a stepwise manner. A. V. Hill was the first to identify the relationship between velocity of shortening and force development as hyperbolic. The intercept at the velocity axis is called V_{max}, and the intercept on the force axis at zero velocity is P_0.

The Relationship between Calcium Transport and Uptake

We know now that there is an inward displacement of calcium ions across the cardiac cell membrane; this triggers release of additional calcium ions from intercellular storage sites (Nayler, 1967). Ca^{2+}, derived from sarcoplasmic reticulum or from the outside of the cell, combines with the regulatory proteins, troponin and tropomyosin. This binding results in the activation of myosin, ATPase, and the splitting of high energy phosphates. As a result contraction ensues. Binding of Ca^{2+} by regulatory proteins is inhibited when calcium ions are again removed to storage sites within and without the cell. Thus, Ca^{2+} binding to sarcoplasmic reticulum or other myocardial membrane fractions is of prime importance in the chain that links excitation with contraction and relaxation of cardiac muscle. Apparently, calcium uptake and binding by the sarcoplasmic reticulum and mitochondria are disturbed during myocardial failure.

What about contractility in failure? We have mentioned that the contractile state can be defined in two ways: by the isometric tension development and by the force-velocity relationship. Apparently, during myocardial failure, force development, as well as V_{max}, is reduced (Spann *et al.*, 1967; Parmely *et al.*, 1968).

The Role of Mitochondria in Myocardial Failure

Changes in mitochondrial respiration also are encountered in myocardial failure. Mitochondrial respiration is depressed, particularly in the ADP/O ratios. Several investigations have shown this depression in heart failure, and we have demonstrated this in the myocardium of alcohol-exposed dogs (Schwarz *et al.,* 1973; Weishaar *et al.,* in press). This finding in alcohol-exposed animals is not surprising, because electron microscopic studies reveal severe mitochondrial structural alterations.

What do these techniques reveal concerning the causes and mechanisms of myocardial failure? I would like to refer once again to our studies on catheterization of the coronary sinus, which showed that in congestive heart failure the extraction of carbohydrate and noncarbohydrate material was normal. We prematurely drew the conclusion that nothing could be amiss with the energy production of the failing heart. Soon, however, we realized that we were looking at the stage door rather than on the stage. We have begun to realize that disturbances are involved in all these processes. The concept, stated in 1968, that myocardial failure is a spectrum of disturbances that depends on the type of failure and its production, is valid today.

MYOCARDIAL INFARCTION

In no other field has the study of myocardial metabolism progressed with such speed as in myocardial infarction, anoxia and hypoxia. Discussion in this chapter is limited to regional ischemia. Under clinical conditions, regional ischemia as it exists in myocardial infarction is accompanied by hypoxia and anoxia, although complete lack of oxygen is unlikely. The confusion in the literature has arisen because ischemia and hypoxia of the whole heart (global ischemia and global hypoxia) cannot be studied *in vivo* and rarely, if ever, are seen in clinical situations. Only under experimental preparations, such as those used by Neely or Kübler, can one differentiate among the effects of ischemia, hypoxia, and anoxia (Kübler and Spieckermann, 1970; Neely *et al.,* 1973). Because of adjustments of the coronary circulation, global ischemia and hypoxia are not encountered *in vivo.* In artificial perfusion systems, the oxygen tension of the perfusate and volume flux can be altered, and global ischemia and hypoxia can be induced. But the "real thing" encountered under clinical conditions (myocardial infarction) is regional ischemia.

A knowledge of the anaerobic glycolytic pathways is essential for the understanding of the biochemical events that take place in regional ischemia. When we consider the glycolytic pathway, special emphasis must be placed on the rate-limiting enzymes. These enzymes are phosphorylase, phosphofructokinase, glycerol-phosphate-dehydrogenase, and pyruvate kinase. Through the metabolic blocks induced by these rate-limiting enzymes, lactate accumulates, and, to a significant degree, fatty acid metabolism is changed either through changes in glycolytic flux or through inhibition of fatty acid oxidation. Other biochemical changes during regional ischemia have been described by Opie (1976).

In line with the metabolic block caused by inhibition of rate-limiting enzymes, intermediates of the glycolytic cycle show marked changes as illustrated in a rise of glucose-6-phosphate, fructose-6-phosphate, α-glycerolphosphate, and lactate.

It is easy to see that coronary flow is of overriding importance in determining the metabolic fate of the heart. One may falsely assume that in the center of the infarct the coronary blood flow is zero. In the dog, this is not the case (Opie, 1976; Weishaar et al., in press). When coronary flow is measured with radioactive spheres, it is seen that flow in the marginal areas of the infarct is not reduced markedly; even at the center of the infarct, one hour after occlusion of the anterior descending coronary artery, the reduction in flow is not absolute. We have heard a great deal of discussion about the importance of collateral circulation. Collaterals are certainly responsible for the fact that the flow in the center of the infarct remains relatively high. Therefore, although glycolytic flux may decrease as the rate-limiting enzymes initiate metabolic blocks, some oxidative functions remain.

When we study contractility in the infarcted and noninfarcted portions, we find that despite the persistence of adequate respiratory function of the mitochondria, and despite the persistent collateral flow in these regions, contractility is markedly diminished one hour after ligation of the coronary artery. All parameters are affected in the glycerinated heart muscle fiber including P_0 (the maximal isometric tension developed), t_0 (the zero time to peak time of contraction), and dP/dt_{max} (the maximal rate of tension developed). Marked alterations also occur in the force-velocity relationship. It is intriguing to compare these alterations with those in myocardial failure. The contractile state of the heart is diminished in both situations. But while alcohol affects only V_{max}, myocardial failure and ischemia reduce all parameters (P_0, t_0, dP/dt, and V_{max}).

It is uncertain whether the discoveries that have been made concerning the metabolic changes in heart muscle taking place during myocardial failure and myocardial infarction can be translated into clinical therapeutic realities. Unquestionably, in myocardial infarction the surgeon has a better answer than the internist, the latter basing his therapy on metabolic changes in heart muscle. The best way of reversing these metabolic changes is through reestablishment of blood flow or by shunting of blood to the ischemic area. A detailed discussion of the therapeutic approaches that have been recently attempted is beyond the scope of these introductory remarks. However, it is of great satisfaction to me, as one who has watched the science of cardiac metabolism develop, to see that myocardial failure and myocardial infarction can now be examined by a new approach that does not rely on clinical observation alone but stems from observations of fundamental processes taking place in heart muscle.

REFERENCES

BING, R. J., HAMMOND, M., HANDELSMAN, J. C., *et al.* 1949. The measurement of coronary blood flow, oxygen consumption and efficiency of the left ventricle in man. Am. Heart J. 38:1.

BING, R. J., VANDAM, L. D., GREGOIRE, F., *et al.* 1947. Catheterization of the coronary sinus and the middle cardiac vein in man. Proc. Soc. Exp. Biol. Med. 66:239.

BLAIN, J. M., SCHAFER, H., SIEGEL, A., and BING, R. J. 1956. Studies on myocardial metabolism. VI. Myocardial metabolism in congestive failure. Am. J. Med. 20:820.

HERRICK, J. B. 1942. A Short History of Cardiology. Charles C Thomas, Springfield, Ill.

HOPE, J. 1831. A Treatise on the Diseases of the Heart and Great Vessels. Lawrence W. Kidd, London.

HUXLEY, A. F. and SIMMONS, R. M. 1971. Proposed mechanism of force generation in striated muscle. Nature 233:533.

JULIAN, F. J. 1971. The effect of calcium on the force-velocity relation of briefly glycerinated frog muscle fibers. J. Physiol. 218:117.

KAKO, K., and BING, R. J. 1958. Contractility of actomyosin bands prepared from normal and failing human hearts. J. Clin. Invest. 37:465.

KÜBLER, W., and SPIECKERMANN, P. G. 1970. Regulation of glycolysis in the ischemic and the anoxic myocardium. J. Mol. Cell. Cardiol. 1:351.

LANDIS, H. R. M. 1912. Austin Flint, Bull. Johns Hopkins Hosp. 23:182.

MACKENZIE, J. 1910. Diseases of the Heart, 2nd Ed. Oxford Medical Publications, New York.

MARUYAMA, Y., SARMA, J. S. M., FISCHER, R., BERTUGLIA, S., and BING, R. J. Effect of alcohol on the contractile and elastic properties of glycerinated heart muscle from rats. *In* Currents in Alcoholism. Grune and Stratton, New York. In press.

NAYLER, W. G. 1967. Some factors involved in the maintenance and regulation of cardiac contractility. Circ. Res. (suppl. III)21:213.

NEELY, J. R., ROVETTO, M. J., WHITMER, J. T., and MORGAN, H. E. 1973. Effects of ischemia on ventricular function and metabolism in the isolated working rat heart. Am. J. Physiol. 225:651.

OPIE, L. H. 1976. II. Metabolic regulation in ischemia and hypoxia. Effects of regional ischemia on metabolism of glucose and fatty acids. Circ. Res. 38:52.

PARMELY, W. W., SPANN, J. F., TAYLOR, R. R., and SONNENBLICK, E. H. 1968. The series elasticity of cardiac muscle in hyperthyroidism, ventricular hypertrophy and heart failure. Proc. Soc. Exp. Biol. Med. 127:606.

PAUL, C. 1883. Diagnostic et Traitement des Maladies du Coeur. Asselin Cic., Paris.

SCHWARTZ, A., SORDAHL, L. A., ENTMAN, M. L., *et al.* 1973. Abnormal biochemistry in myocardial failure. Am. J. Cardiol. 32:407.

SPANN, J. F., BUCCINO, R. A., SONNENBLICK, E. H., and BRAUNWALD, E. 1967. Contractile state of cardiac muscle obtained from cats with experimentally produced ventricular hypertrophy and heart failure. Circ. Res. 21:341.

WEISHAAR, R., SARMA, J. S. M., MARUYAMA, Y., *et al.* Regional blood flow, contractility and metabolism in early myocardial infarction. Cardiology. In press.

WEISHAAR, R., SARMA, J. S. M., MARUYAMA, Y., *et al.* Reversibility of mitochondrial and contractile properties of heart muscle after prolonged alcohol administration. Am. J. Cardiol. In press.

Mailing address:
Richard J. Bing, M.D.,
100 Congress Street,
Pasadena, California 91105 (USA).

MYOCARDIAL PROTEIN
AND
NUCLEOPROTEIN METABOLISM

Recent Advances in Studies on
Cardiac Structure and Metabolism, Volume 12
Cardiac Adaptation
Edited by T. Kobayashi, Y. Ito, and G. Rona
Copyright 1978 University Park Press Baltimore

TISSUE SPECIFICITY OF MYOCARDIAL GLYCOPEPTIDES SYNTHESIZED DURING EARLY EMBRYONIC DEVELOPMENT

F. J. MANASEK and J. W. LACKTIS

Department of Anatomy, The University of Chicago,
Chicago, Illinois, USA

SUMMARY

[^{3}H]Glucosamine-labeled glycopeptides synthesized by hearts from stage 14–16 chick embryos were separated on DE-52 by ion-exchange chromatography and compared to those synthesized in other parts of the embryo at the same stage. Relatively few molecular species were present in all tissues, and they appeared closely homologous. There were no glycopeptides unique to any embryonic region examined, suggesting that tissue specificity may result from quantitative rather than qualitative differences in glycopeptides.

INTRODUCTION

During early embryonic cardiogenesis, developing muscle cells increase their areas of close apposition, differentiate to produce myofibrils, and undergo shape changes that probably result in primary morphogenesis (looping). We are attempting to understand these events more clearly to determine whether or not they are causally related (for review, see Manasek, 1976a).

As part of our studies of the factors that control myocyte apposition, migration, and shape, we have begun to examine the synthesis of embryonic cardiac glycoproteins (Manasek, 1975, 1976b). In this chapter the synthesis of glucosamine containing glycopeptides by the embryonic heart is demonstrated, and evidence is presented suggesting that the parent glycoproteins may be tissue specific.

MATERIALS AND METHODS

Fertile, white, Leghorn eggs were incubated at 38°C to yield embryos of stage 14–16. Eggs were opened and embryos placed in Tyrode's medium to facilitate precise staging. Hearts, heads, and trunks were dissected free and transferred to

This work was supported by Grant HL 13831 from the U.S. Public Health Service.

Tyrode's medium containing 1 mCi/ml of [6-^{3}H] glucosamine. The large amount of radioactivity permitted the use of relatively few (10) hearts. Incubation was continued for 5 hr. All hearts continued beating normally for the duration of labeling. Following incubation, tissues were washed several times with Tyrode's medium to remove most of the unincorporated radioactivity. Tissues were sonicated and digested overnight with papain. Aliquots were placed on 0.9 X 10 cm DE-52 columns and eluted first with 30 ml of 0.002 M Tris-HCl, pH 7.2, then with a linear 200 ml 0–0.15 M LiCl gradient in 0.002 M Tris buffer, pH 7.2 (Brown, 1972). Three-milliliter fractions were collected, and radioactivity was determined using a Searle MK-III liquid scintillation counter.

RESULTS

Stage 14–16 Embryo Hearts

Relatively few anionic glucosamine-labeled glycopeptides were recovered from DE-52 (Figure 1). The first peak, eluting with 0.002 M Tris-HCl, represented residual unincorporated label, as well as *possible* neutral or possibly cationic glycopeptides. This material also could be eluted from DE-52 by water. The

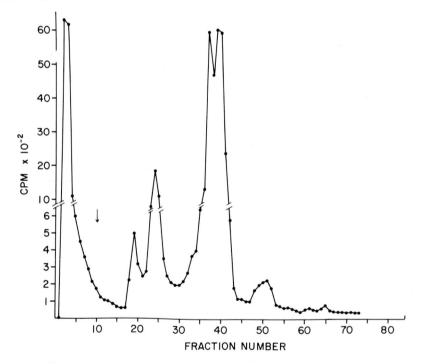

Figure 1. Elution of papain-released stage 14–16 cardiac glycopeptides from DE-52. Gradient begun at fraction 10 after buffer elution and terminated at fraction 73. Glycopeptides 1, 2, 3, and 4 elute at 0.021 M, 0.032 M, 0.07 M, and 0.10 M LiCl, respectively.

subsequent peaks eluted at different LiCl concentrations, and the individual ionic strengths at which they eluted were quite specific and repeatable.

Heads

Glycopeptides obtained from head regions of the same embryos eluted similarly to those from hearts (Figure 2). However, the relative heights of the individual glycopeptide peaks were markedly different. For example, the ratio between peaks 3 and 2 was 9.2, whereas this ratio in the heart was 5.7.

Trunks

Trunk glycopeptides were fewer in number (Figure 3), but the two major species were recognizable in both head and heart on the basis of the elution positions.

DISCUSSION

This study demonstrates the synthesis of glucosamine-containing embryonic cardiac glycopeptides that have some homologies with those from other regions.

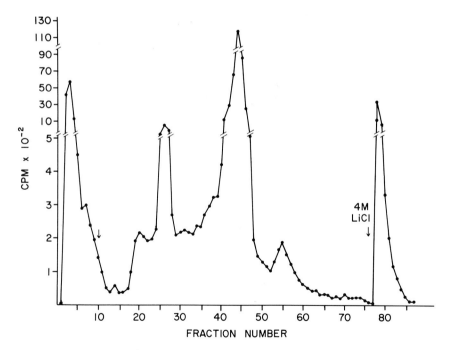

Figure 2. Glycopeptides from stage 14–16 head. Glycopeptides are qualitatively similar to those of heart but are present in relatively different amounts. This gradient was slightly different from that used for Figure 1, which accounts for the different fractions in which peaks appear, but their elution occurs at precisely the same ionic strength. 4 M LiCl removes all the more highly charged glycosaminoglycans.

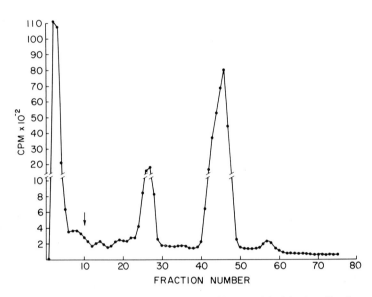

Figure 3. Glycopeptides from stage 14–16 trunk. Glycopeptide 1 is virtually absent but 2 and 3 (the dominant ones) and 4 are present.

At stage 14–16 the myocardium is still a homogeneous layer of developing muscle cells. Earlier radioautographic studies of only slightly younger hearts have shown that the myocardium is the principal site of [³H]glucosamine incorporation. Thus, we can be relatively certain that most of the glycopeptides recovered from stage 14–16 hearts represent molecules synthesized by myocytes. All of the cells in the myocardium have differentiated by stage 14–16 and are functional cardiac muscle. Preliminary studies have suggested homology between papain- and trypsin-released glycopeptides, indicating that we are indeed examining surface and matrix molecules.

At the level of resolution afforded by this study, the initial comparisons of cardiac glycopeptides to those synthesized by other tissues suggest that several of the embryonic glycopeptides may be ubiquitous. The entire array of glycopeptides differs quantitatively between tissues. We must emphasize the fact that this procedure separates molecules on the basis of their charge, and that we do not yet know how heterogeneous, by other criteria, each peak is. Preliminary studies in this laboratory suggest that use of an extended gradient can further separate some peaks, suggesting some additional degree of charge heterogeneity. If the glycopeptide elution profiles are considered both qualitatively (peak position) and quantitatively (relative peak heights), then it appears that each tissue has a unique set of glycopeptides, even though some glycopeptides are common.

Despite the rather small number of glycopeptides recovered from each tissue, they could represent a vast number of different parent glycoproteins. If the parent glycoproteins are involved in conveying surface specificity to different cell types, then it is suggested that this specificity may be determined by only a small number of independently sorted components. The words of the code would thus contain relatively few letters (on the order of five). A similarly small number of glycopeptides has been described earlier for different cell types (Brown, 1972).

Continued characterization of myocyte surface glycoproteins may enable us to understand further the regulation of cell-cell interactions within the myocardium and may permit us to place some events of myocardial ontogenesis in a molecular framework. For example, it has recently been noted that administration of the cardiac teratogen, trypan blue, results in rapid changes in cardiac glycoproteins (Satow and Manasek, 1977). It is consistent with current ideas about the role of these molecules in normal development (Moscona, 1974) to propose that their alterations may be reflected in abnormal myocardial form and function.

REFERENCES

BROWN, J. C. 1972. Cell surface glycoproteins I. Accumulations of a glycoprotein on the outer surface of mouse LS cells during mitosis. J. Supramol. Struct. 1:1–7.

MANASEK, F. J. 1975. The extracellular matrix of the early embryonic heart. *In* M. Lieberman and T. Sano (eds.), Developmental and Physiological Correlates of Cardiac Muscle, pp. 1–20. Raven Press, New York.

MANASEK, F. J. 1976a. Heart development: Interactions involved in cardiac development. *In* G. Poste and G. L. Nicolson (eds.), The Cell Surface in Aminal Embryogenesis and Development. North Holland, Amsterdam.

MANASEK, F. J. 1976b. Glycoprotein synthesis and tissue interactions during establishment of the functional embryonic chick heart. J. Mol. Cell. Cardiol. In press.

MOSCONA, A. A. 1974. Surface specification of embryonic cells: Lectin receptors, cell recognition and specific cell ligands. *In* A. A. Moscona (ed.), The Cell Surface in Development, pp. 67–94. John Wiley & Sons, New York.

SATOW, Y., and MANASEK, F. J. 1977. Direct effects of trypan blue on cardiac extracellular macromolecule synthesis. Lab. Invest. 36:100–105.

Mailing address:
F. J. Manasek, D.M.D.,
Department of Anatomy, The University of Chicago,
1025 East 57th Street, Chicago, Illinois 60637 (USA).

Recent Advances in Studies on
Cardiac Structure and Metabolism, Volume 12
Cardiac Adaptation
Edited by T. Kobayashi, Y. Ito, and G. Rona
Copyright 1978 University Park Press Baltimore

THE PATHWAYS OF PROTEIN SYNTHESIS AND DEGRADATION IN NORMAL HEART AND DURING DEVELOPMENT AND REGRESSION OF CARDIAC HYPERTROPHY

J. M. SIMS, B. PATZER, M. KUMUDAVALLI-REDDY,
A. F. MARTIN, M. RABINOWITZ, and R. ZAK

Cardiology Section of the Department of Medicine and the Department
of Biochemistry, The University of Chicago, and the Franklin
McLean Memorial Research Institute,[1] Chicago, Illinois, USA

SUMMARY

The half-life of cardiac myosin heavy chains (HC) was determined, with leucyl-tRNA as precursor, to be 5.4 days. Myosin HC are labeled more rapidly than actin; myosin light chains (LC_1 and LC_2) are labeled more slowly than HC. The observed differences are attributable to heterogeneity in the half-lives, e.g., actin, and to the effect of dilution by the existing macromolecular precursor pool (LC_1 and LC_2).

Cardiac and skeletal muscle contain a population of filaments that can be released from myofibrils by ATP-relaxing solution. The easily released filaments (ERF) are devoid of α-actinin and M-protein. Labeling of ERF is more rapid than that of residual myofibrils. Cardiac and skeletal muscle contains calcium-activated neutral protease, which selectively removes α-actinin when incubated with isolated myofibrils.

During development of pressure-induced cardiac hypertrophy, the labeling of LC_2 is increased. In regressing cardiac hypertrophy the activities of free and total cathepsin D and of acidic RNase are unaltered.

INTRODUCTION

The problems of myofibrillar assembly and degradation are outlined in Figure 1. It is well documented (Sarkar and Cooke, 1970) that the individual myofibrillar proteins are synthesized by distinct classes of polysomes. What happens after termination of polypeptide synthesis, however, is less clear. It is conceivable that the nascent protein or its subunits are added directly to existing myofibrils.

This work was supported in part by U.S. Public Health Service Grants HL-09172, HL-04442, HL-16637, and 1-P17-HL-17648 (Specialized Center of Research in Ischemic Heart Disease) from the National Heart and Lung Institute, grants from the Muscular Dystrophy Association of America, the Chicago and Illinois Heart Association, and the Louis Block Fund of The University of Chicago.

[1] Operated by The University of Chicago for the U.S. Energy Research and Development Administration under Contract E(11-1)-69.

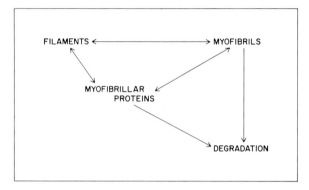

Figure 1. Possible pathways of myofibrillar assembly and degradation. For explanation, see text.

Alternatively, it is possible that the filaments are assembled in the cytoplasm before their association with myofibrils. The myofibrils are not static cellular components but are in a state of flux, being constantly degraded and resynthetized; therefore, the outlined processes have to be reversible. Several pathways for myofibrillar degradation can by postulated. The whole myofibrils (or rather parts of the myofibrillar mass) could be engulfed by limiting membranes of autophagic vacuoles and digested by cathepsins. Another possibility is that the proteins constituting the myofibrils are released into the cytoplasm, either separately or as filaments. Specific enzymes can participate in this process. Once released, the proteins can be digested by lysosomal hydrolases.

RESULTS AND DISCUSSION

Turnover of Myofibrillar Proteins in the Steady State

The extent to which myofibrils turn over is documented in Figure 2. Myosin, which constitutes nearly half of the content of myofibrillar proteins, has a half-life of 5.4 days, as determined with leucyl-tRNA used as precursor. This value corresponds to about 10% of the cardiac myosin being replaced per day.

Comparison of the half-life of myosin with that of other myofibrillar proteins is potentially a very important tool for delineation of pathways of myofibrillar assembly and degradation. If the turnover is the same for all myofibrillar proteins, a model of digestion is suggested that involves the degradation of myofibrils as a unit. On the other hand, if the turnover is heterogeneous, it is likely that the individual proteins leave the myofibrils before being digested. Several laboratories have attempted comparisons of the turnover of myofibrillar proteins in both skeletal and cardiac muscle (see Table 1). It can be seen that there is no agreement among the data obtained. One of the reasons for the discrepancies may be that it was generally unrecognized that no good precursor

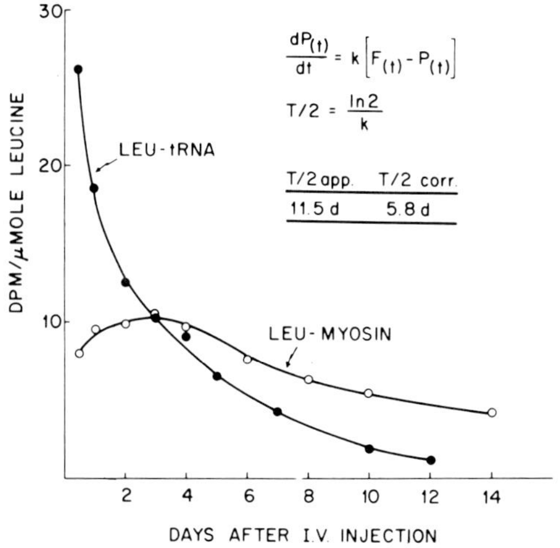

Figure 2. Apparent and corrected half-life of rat cardiac myosin. Female rats (200 g) were injected with 100 μC of [^{3}H]leucine. The first order rate constant of myosin degradation (k) was obtained by solving the equation given on the graph, in which $F_{(t)}$ and $P_{(t)}$ represent specific radioactivities of precursor and myosin leucine, respectively, as a function of time. The T/2app. was obtained from the semilogarithmic plot of myosin radioactivity. Leucine-specific radioactivity was determined as described by Martin, Prior, and Zak, 1976.

for labeling of myofibrillar proteins is available. Injected amino acids do not follow pulse-label kinetics; on the contrary, their concentration remains high in the circulation for an extended period of time, being constantly replenished by degradation of radioactive proteins. The complications arising from amino acid reutilization are demonstrated in Figure 3. It is self-evident that the labeling of a given protein will continue only to the point at which its radioactivity equals

Table 1. Relative half-lives of myofibrillar proteins

Myosin					Actin	Muscle type	Authors
HC	1		LC	1	1	H	Zak *et al.*, 1971
		1			1	Sk	Funabiki and Cassens, 1972
HC	1		LC_1	1.4		Sk	Morkin *et al.*, 1973
			LC_2	0.9			
			LC_3	0.6			
HC	1		LC	2		H	Wikman-Coffelt *et al.*, 1973
HC	1		LC	0.5		Sk	Low and Goldberg, 1973
	1		LC	0.8	2.5	Sk	Koizumi, 1974

The data given by authors were expressed as ratios to myosin heavy chains (HC); LC = myosin light chains; H = heart; Sk = skeletal muscle.

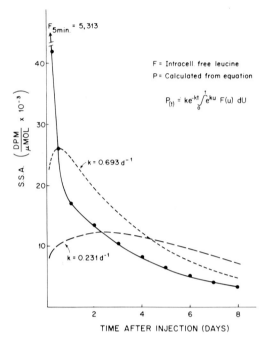

Figure 3. Specific radioactivity of precursor F and product P as a function of time. These are computer projected curves based on experimentally obtained values of intracellular free leucine (F). The projected values of P (protein standard specific radioactivity, S.S.A.) were obtained by substituting k (shown for the two examples) into the equation given at the top.

that of its precursor (crossover point). The radioactivity incorporated in proteins with a slower turnover rate will continue to rise for a longer time, but at the lower rate (see lower curve). It is thus possible that two proteins, when compared, will have a relative radioactivity larger than, smaller than, or equal to unity, depending entirely on the time interval chosen by the investigator.

Comparison of the turnover of several intracellular proteins can be facilitated by the double-isotope method (Glass and Doyle, 1972). In this procedure, the injection schedule is such that one radioisomer of an amino acid is left in the experimental animal long enough so that its radioactivity starts to decay. The second radioisomer, on the other hand, is injected shortly before sacrifice of the animal. If the ratio of radioactivities of the two isomers is calculated for several proteins, the difference in their turnover will become evident because decay and labeling are measured simultaneously. This procedure was analyzed in detail by Poole (1971), who demonstrated that the approach has severe limitations, especially when applied to studies of proteins with long half-lives. The problem is demonstrated by our data, as shown in Figure 4. By using the specific radioactivity of the precursor leucyl-tRNA, we projected what the double-iso-

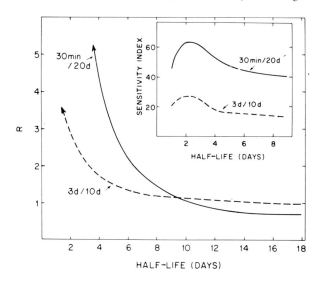

Figure 4. Sensitivity of the double-isotope technique. R corresponds to the double-isotope ratio obtained for two injection schedules. In the first schedule (3d/10d), the first radio-isomere of leucine was administered 10 days and the second 3 days before sacrifice. In the second schedule (30 min/20d), the labeling intervals were 20 days and 30 minutes, respectively. Sensitivity index is defined in the text.

tope ratio would be for proteins with different half-lives. To evaluate the sensitivity of the method, we determined the percentage difference in the isotope ratio for two proteins that differ in half-life by 50% (sensitivity ratio). From the data obtained (insert of Figure 4), several important facts are apparent: 1) the sensitivity of the method depends on the injection schedule; 2) the sensitivity is higher for proteins with a faster turnover; 3) there is no linear relationship between the protein half-life and the double-isotope ratio, i.e., a 50% difference in the isotope ratio does not mean a 50% difference in half-life.

Despite these limitations a suitable injection schedule nevertheless can be selected that allows a meaningful comparison of several myofibrillar proteins. The results are shown in Table 2. Differences in protein half-life become apparent only in experiment 3, during which the injection schedule was such that [^{3}H] leucine labeling lasted for 20 days and [^{14}C] leucine labeling for 30 minutes. Myosin heavy chains (HC) turn over faster than actin, and myosin light chains (LC) turn over more slowly than heavy chains.

A similar comparison can be made when the incorporation of labeled amino acids into proteins is measured, provided that enough time points are collected to ensure that the measurements are done before the crossover point is reached. A comparison of HC and LC and of actin is shown in Table 3. Although the trend is similar to that in Table 2, there are important quantitative differences,

Table 2. Comparison of the turnover of myofibrillar proteins by the double-isotope technique

Protein	$^{14}C/^{3}H$ ratio		
	Experiment 1	Experiment 2	Experiment 3
Myosin	0.51	0.52	
Myosin HC	–	0.51	2.25
Myosin LC$_1$	–	0.44	1.27
Myosin LC$_2$	–		1.14
Actin	0.48		1.53
Injection schedule ^3H	10 days	10 days	20 days
^{14}C	3 days	3 days	30 min

Two radioisomers of leucine were injected consecutively and animals were sacrificed at the intervals given, as per injection schedule. For determination of radioactivity the proteins were isolated from purified myofibrils (Experiments 1 and 2) or were separated electrophoretically and the radioactivity was determined directly on polyacrilamide gels (Experiment 3).

especially in the case of LC. At the 10-min labeling interval the radioactivity of LC was 62% less than that of HC; four days later the difference was only 32%. A similar convergence of LC and HC radioactivity with time has been reported by Yazaki (Yazaki and Raben, 1977). Such kinetic behavior is consistent with the existence of a macromolecular precursor that dilutes the radioactivity of newly formed LC.

The complexity of myofibrillar assembly is indicated by our recent observation (Etlinger *et al.,* 1975) that, in addition to a soluble pool of myosin LC,

Table 3. Incorporation of [^{3}H]leucine into myofibrillar proteins

Protein	Labeling time:	Leucine-specific radioactivity (dpm/nmol)	
		10 min	4 days
Myosin HC		6.2 ± 0.5	15 ± 1.1
Myosin LC$_1$		2.7 ± 0.3	10 ± 0.8
Myosin LC$_2$		2.4 ± 0.3	11.7 ± 0.9
Actin		4.7 ± 1.0	9.6 ± 0.3

Leucine-specific radioactivity was determined as described by Martin, Prior, and Zak, 1976. Rats received a single intravenous injection of [^{3}H]leucine (2 μCi per 200 g rat for the 10-min period and 1 μCi for the 4-day period). The results are given as the average of five determinations $\pm$ S.D.

Table 4. Labeling kinetics of myosin heavy chains in easily released filaments and in core myofibrils

Time	Specific radioactivity (dpm/nmol)		
	Leucyl-tRNA	ERF	CF
10 min	5,600	19	6.2
20 min	2,200	20	9.6
60 min	250	24	11.9
3 hr	140	19	13.0
24 hr	26	17	17.2

ERF = easily released filaments; CF = core myofibrils. Purified myofibrils were treated by ATP-relaxing low-ionic-strength solution, as described by Etlinger *et al.,* 1975, to obtain ERF and CF. Leucine-specific radioactivity in heavy chains was determined in electrophoretically separated protein bands. Rats received intravenously 500 μCi of [^{3}H] leucine per 100 g of body weight.

there is a population of myofilaments that is distinct from that of the remaining myofibrils. When isolated myofibrils are treated with low-ionic-strength relaxing solution, filaments are released that have a length similar to that seen in intact myofibrils. The quantity of protein released in the form of filaments is finite, amounting to about 10% of the total myofibrillar mass. The protein composition of easily released filaments (ERF) differs from the composition of core filaments (CF) in that the ERF are devoid of α-actinin and M-protein (Etlinger *et al.,* 1976). The incorporation of [^{3}H] leucine into myosin HC of ERF is also distinct from that of core filaments; 10 minutes after the administration of label, the specific radioactivity of ERF is about three times higher than in CF. Although more data need to be collected for a better understanding of the participation of ERF in myofibrillar assembly, at present, we favor a model in which the pool of ERF receives both the nascent myosin molecules and the filaments from existing myofibrils. This model explains why the radioactivity of ERF declines before it becomes equal to that of leucyl-tRNA (see Table 4). If ERF were an obligatory intermediate of myofibrillar assembly (not receiving existing filaments from myofibrils), this would not occur; instead, the radioactivity of ERF would continue to increase until the crossover point with leucyl-tRNA was reached.

Protein Synthesis and Degradation in Non-Steady-State Myocardium

We have studied several aspects of synthesis and degradation of myofibrillar proteins during development and regression of cardiac hypertrophy. Our model consists of constriction of the ascending aorta in adult female rats to about 40%

Table 5. Relative labeling of myosin heavy and light chains in developing cardiac hypertrophy

	Control	Sham operation	Banding
LC$_1$/HC	0.62 ± 0.04	0.65 ± 0.03	0.72 ± 0.07
LC$_2$/HC	0.59 ± 0.03	0.63 ± 0.04	1.09 ± 0.06
Number of animals	3	12	5

Ascending aorta was constricted for four days; the average heart enlargement was 40%. Rats received intravenously 250 μCi of [^{3}H]leucine per 100 g of body weight and were sacrificed 30 min later. Leucine-specific radioactivity was determined in electrophoretically separated proteins by the method of Martin, Prior, and Zak, 1976.

of its original lumen; thus, a pressure gradient of 70 mm Hg is produced. The overloaded myocardium enlarges rapidly, so that the heart weight is increased by about 40% on the third post-operative day. During the period of rapid cardiac growth, the labeling pattern of myosin heavy chains (HC) and light chain 2 (LC$_2$) differs from that in control or sham-operated rats. The specific radioactivity of LC$_2$ equals that of HC at 30 minutes after administration of [^{3}H]leucine. In control hearts, on the other hand, the LC$_1$ and LC$_2$ radioactivity amounts to about 70% of that of HC (see Table 5). Thus, it seems that the rate of synthesis of LC$_2$ is increased during the development of hypertrophy. It is also possible, however, that the pool of soluble light chains that is responsible for the dilution of radioactivity of nascent LC molecules is smaller in the hypertrophic heart. More data are needed so that these two possibilities can be differentiated.

When the constricting band on the ascending aorta is removed, the pressure gradient disappears and the size of the myocardium rapidly regresses to normal values (Cutilletta *et al.*, 1975). The level of RNA generally follows that of the cardiac mass (see Figure 5). It was of interest to examine whether or not the activities of cathepsin D and of acidic RNase are increased under these vasting conditions. The data shown in Figure 5 indicate that this is not so. Neither free nor total activities of both lysosomal enzymes show statistically significant differences from the activity in the sham-operated, hypertrophic, and regressing myocardium.

It is therefore conceivable that some other enzymes are involved in myofibrillar degradation. Two lines of evidence indicate that this might be so. First, as described in this volume by Dr. Ferrans (Ferrans *et al.*, 1977), Z-line abnormalities commonly accompany cardiac overload. Indeed, any disease of both skeletal and cardiac muscle leads to some alterations of Z-line structure. Second, a factor was isolated from a post-mitochondrial supernatant of muscle that removes Z lines when incubated with isolated myofibrils (Busch *et al.*, 1972). We have shown that this factor is a neutral, calcium-activated protease (CaAP) that selectively removes α-actinin from myofibrils (Kumudavalli-Reddy

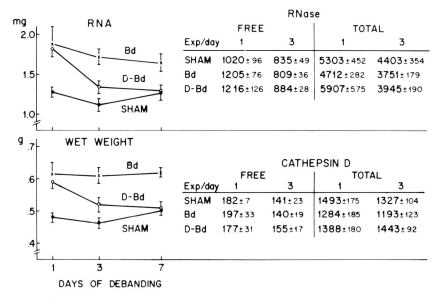

Figure 5. Activity of lysosomal enzymes during regression of cardiac hypertrophy. Bd = banded; D-Bd = debanded. Constriction of ascending aorta was performed 10 days before the experiment. "Total" and "Free" refer to presence or absence of Triton X-100 (0.2% final concentration). Cathepsin D was assayed in the left ventricular homogenate by the splitting of [³H]acetyl-hemoglobin at pH 5. Ribonuclease was assayed in the same homogenate by the splitting of yeast [³H]RNA at pH 6. Reprinted with permission from Cutilletta *et al.,* 1975.

et al., 1975). The involvement of CaAP in myofibrillar degradation, however, is still speculative. It remains to be determined whether myofibrils devoid of Z lines are indeed less stable structures or whether their proteins are more susceptible to degradative processes.

REFERENCES

BUSCH, W. A., STROMER, M. H., GOLL, D. E., and SUZUKI, A. 1972. Calcium activated specific removal of Z lines from rabbit skeletal muscle. J. Cell Biol. 52:367–381.

CUTILLETTA, A. F., DOWELL, R. T., RUDNIK, M., ARCILLA, R. A., and ZAK, R. 1975. Regression of myocardial hypertrophy. I. Experimental model, changes in heart weight, nucleic acids and collagen. J. Mol. Cell. Cardiol. 7:767–781.

ETLINGER, J. D., ZAK, R., FISCHMAN, D. A., and RABINOWITZ, M. 1975. Isolation of newly synthesized myosin filaments from skeletal muscle homogenates and myofibrils. Nature 255:259–261.

ETLINGER, J. D., ZAK, R., and FISCHMAN, D. A. 1976. Compositional studies of myofibrils from rabbit striated muscle. J. Cell Biol. 68:123–141.

FERRANS, V. J., MARON, B. J., JONES, M., and THIEDEMANN, K.-U. 1978. Ultrastructural aspects of contractile proteins in cardiac hypertrophy and failure. *In* G. Rona (ed.),

Recent Advances in Studies on Cardiac Structure and Metabolism. Vol. 12: Cardiac Adaptation, pp. 129–140. University Park Press, Baltimore.

FUNABIKI, R., and CASSENS, R. G. 1972. Heterogeneous turnover of myofibrillar proteins. Nature (New Biol.) 236:249.

GLASS, R. D., and DOYLE, D. 1972. On the measurement of protein turnover in animal cells. J. Biol. Chem. 247:5234–5242.

KOIZUMI, T. 1974. Turnover rates of structural proteins of rabbit skeletal muscle. J. Biochem. (Tokyo) 76:431–439.

KUMUDAVALLI-REDDY, M., ETLINGER, J. D., FISCHMAN, D. A., RABINOWITZ, M., and ZAK, R. 1975. Removal of Z lines and *a*-actinin from isolated myofibrils by a calcium-activated neutral protease. J. Biol. Chem. 250:4278–4289.

LOW, R. B., and GOLDBERG, A. L. 1973. Nonuniform rates of turnover of myofibrillar proteins in rat diaphragm. J. Cell Biol. 56:590–595.

MARTIN, A. F., PRIOR, G., and ZAK, R. 1976. Determination of specific radioactivity of amino acids in proteins directly on polyacrylamide gels: An application to *l*-leucine. Anal. Biochem. 72:577–585.

MORKIN, E., YAZAKI, Y., KATAGIRI, T., and LaRAIA, P. L. 1973. Comparison of the synthesis of the light and heavy chains of adult skeletal myosin. Biochim. Biophys. Acta 324:420–429.

POOLE, R. 1971. The kinetics of disappearance of labeled leucine from the free leucine pool of rat liver and its effect on the apparent turnover of catalase and other hepatic protein. J. Biol. Chem. 246:6587–6591.

SARKAR, S., and COOKE, P. H. 1970. *In vitro* synthesis of light and heavy polypeptide chains of myosin. Biochim. Biophys. Acta 41:918–925.

WIKMAN-COFFELT, J., ZELIS, R., FENNER, C., and MASON, D. T. 1973. Studies on the synthesis and degradation of light and heavy chains of cardiac myosin. J. Biol. Chem. 248:5206–5207.

YAZAKI, Y., and RABEN, M. S. 1978. Comparison of the synthesis of the light and heavy chains of cardiac myosin. *In* G. Rona (ed.), Recent Advances in Studies on Cardiac Structure and Metabolism. Vol. 12: Cardiac Adaptation, pp. 39–45. University Park Press, Baltimore.

ZAK, R., RAKITZIS, E., and RABINOWITZ, M. 1971. Evidence for simultaneous turnover of four cardiac myofibrillar proteins. Fed. Proc. 30 (abst.):1147.

Mailing address:
Dr. R. Zak, Assoc. Prof.,
Cardiology Section of the Department of Medicine,
The University of Chicago, Chicago, Illinois 60637 (USA).

Recent Advances in Studies on
Cardiac Structure and Metabolism, Volume 12
Cardiac Adaptation
Edited by T. Kobayashi, Y. Ito, and G. Rona
Copyright 1978 University Park Press Baltimore

TURNOVER RATES OF MUSCLE PROTEINS IN CARDIAC, SKELETAL, AND SMOOTH MUSCLE: TURNOVER RATE RELATED TO MUSCLE FUNCTION

M. P. SPARROW, C. A. EARL, G. L. LAURENT, and A. W. EVERETT

Department of Pharmacology, University of Western Australia,
Nedlands, Western Australia

SUMMARY

The turnover rate of muscle proteins was related to the physiological function of the muscle in dogs, fowl, rats, and mice. The turnover rates of mixed muscle proteins were most rapid in cardiac muscle, intermediate in red tonic and mixed fiber-type muscles, and slowest in white twitch skeletal muscle. This same progression in turnover rates also was shown in the subcellular fractions of muscle—sarcoplasmic and myofibrillar proteins—as well as in purified proteins, myosin, and tropomyosin. The RNA concentration of muscle was highly correlated with the protein turnover rate, and the RNA activity, i.e., the translational efficiency of the RNA, was similar in the different muscle types.

INTRODUCTION

There is now substantial evidence to show that muscle proteins turn over at different rates in different muscle tissues. Goldberg (1967) reported a greater incorporation of [14C]leucine into proteins in red tonic muscles than in white twitch muscles. Swick and Song (1974) have determined a half-life of 4–6 days for myosin from ventricle and of 25–45 days for white skeletal myosin in rats. The present study compares the turnover rates of proteins in muscles performing different physiological functions in different species.

MATERIALS AND METHODS

Turnover rates of mixed muscle proteins were measured in adult animals, maintained in a steady state, by determining either the rate of synthesis or the rate of degradation. In dogs the synthesis rate was measured directly by giving a continuous infusion of 50 μCi of [14C]tyrosine intravenously for 6 hr, and the specific activities of the free intracellular tyrosine and the protein-bound tyrosine were determined, from which a protein synthesis rate constant was calculated as described by Garlick, Millward, and James (1973).

Table 1. Average protein synthesis rates of mixed muscle proteins from canine muscle expressed as half-life ($t_{1/2}$) in days

	$t_{1/2}$ (days)	S.E.M.
Ventricle	8.4	± 0.3 (19)
Diaphragm	12.2	± 1.1 (11)
Vastus lateralis	18.1	± 0.8 (16)
Jejunum (circular smooth)	6.5	± 0.5 (8)

Number of dogs shown in parentheses. Each value is the mean ± S.E.M.

RESULTS AND DISCUSSION

The turnover rate of mixed muscle proteins was most rapid in canine ventricle (Table 1), intermediate in diaphragm, a predominantly red tonic fiber-type muscle, and slowest in the vastus lateralis, a predominantly white twitch fiber-type muscle. The circular layer of smooth muscle separated from the jejunum turned over as rapidly as cardiac muscle. Animals were in a steady state, and

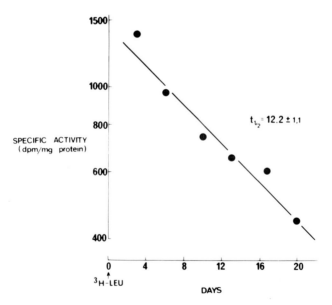

Figure 1. Turnover of mixed muscle proteins of mouse ventricle. The specific activity of the [³H]leucine incorporated into protein is shown as the mean of at least five animals at each time point. From the slope of the regression line, a $t_{1/2}$ = 12.1 ± 1.1 (S.D.) days was calculated.

therefore the rate of protein synthesis was equal to the rate of protein degradation. These differences in turnover rates also were seen in muscles of mice, rats, and fowl for which the rate of protein degradation was measured by pulse-labeling. An intravenous injection of [^{3}H]leucine was given, and the rate of loss of protein-bound radioactivity followed with respect to time (Figure 1). No evidence was obtained to suggest that this $t_{1/2}$ of 12.2 days was significantly influenced by intracellular recycling of leucine. Dietary manipulation with a high protein diet plus additional leucine intraperitoneally (125 mg/kg body weight) did not affect the turnover rate. Using [^{3}H]aspartate, a similar result of 12.0 days was obtained, irrespective of whether the radioactivity was counted in the total protein or in the aspartate fraction following protein hydrolysis. Figure 2 shows that mixed proteins from ventricle turned over more rapidly than those of the anterior latissimus dorsi, a red tonic muscle (Page, 1969), and turned over most slowly in the posterior latissimus dorsi, a white twitch muscle. The mixed

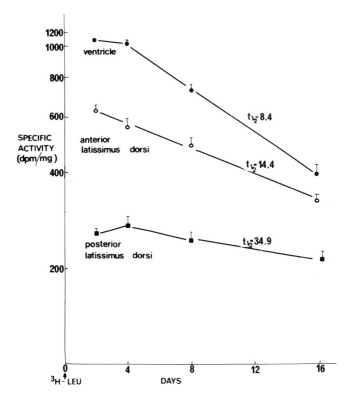

Figure 3. The relationship between protein turnover rate and RNA concentration in muscles of fowl. Turnover rate is expressed as a rate constant (days^{-1}). ALD = anterior latissimus dorsi; PLD = posterior latissimus dorsi.

Table 2. Average turnover rates of mixed muscle proteins from cardiac, skeletal, and smooth muscle

		$t_{1/2}$ (days)	S.E.M.
Cardiac			
Ventricle:	dog	8.4	± 0.3
	fowl	8.4	± 0.6
	rat	10.8	± 1.1
	mouse	12.1	± 1.1
Skeletal—red tonic			
Soleus:	mouse	10.9	± 1.0
Diaphragm:	dog	12.2	± 1.1
	mouse	13.0	± 1.2
	rat	13.6	± 1.2
Anterior latissimus dorsi:	fowl	14.4	± 0.2
Skeletal—mixed			
Levator ani:	dog	16.1	± 2.0
Vastus:	dog	18.1	± 0.8
	mouse	21.1	± 2.8
Gastrocnemius:	fowl	23.9	± 4.4
Skeletal—white twitch			
Posterior latissimus dorsi:	fowl	35	± 9
Pectoralis:	fowl	41	± 11
Smooth—gastrointestinal			
Jejunum circular:	dog	6.5	± 0.5
Gizzard circular:	fowl	7.7	± 1.7

In rats, fowl, and mice the rate of degradation was determined by pulse-labeling with [^{3}H] leucine using 20 or more animals and the $t_{1/2}$ ± S.E.M. of the gradient measured from the curve relating loss of radioactivity with time. In dogs the protein synthesis rates were determined directly for each dog using [^{14}C] tryosine. The $t_{1/2}$ is shown as the mean ± S.E.M. of not less than eight dogs.

proteins of the ventricle were the most highly labeled, and the loss of label occurred most rapidly, whereas those in the posterior latissimus dorsi were labeled least and declined the slowest. Table 2 lists these turnover rates in muscles from dogs, fowl, rats, and mice.

The reliability of an average turnover rate, when used to compare one tissue with another, could be influenced by small differences in protein compositions combined with heterogeneity of turnover rates. However, no evidence of gross heterogeneity of turnover rates of muscle components was observed. Table 3

Table 3. Protein synthesis rates of sarcoplasmic and myofibrillar protein fractions compared with the mixed muscle proteins from canine and fowl ventricle

	Dog $t_{1/2}$ (days) $\pm$ S.E.M.	Fowl $t_{1/2}$ (days) $\pm$ S.E.M.
Sarcoplasmic	7.6 ± 0.3(16)	7.6 ± 0.6
Myofibrillar	11.6 ± 0.5(16)	8.0 ± 0.5
Mixed	8.4 ± 0.3 (16)	8.4 ± 0.6

shows that the turnover rate of canine sarcoplasmic protein fraction was a little faster ($p < 0.001$) than that of the myofibrillar fraction, but the $t_{1/2}$ of the mixed proteins was intermediate. In fowl, the difference between myofibrillar and sarcoplasmic protein fractions was not statistically significant. However, the turnover rates of these subcellular fractions showed the same pattern as observed with the mixed muscle proteins (Table 3) when compared in different muscles. Purified myofibrillar proteins also showed this progression in turnover rates. Tropomyosin from rat heart turned over at least five times more quickly than tropomyosin from the vastus muscle. Myosin from canine ventricle turned over twice as fast as myosin from canine vastus lateralis; this observation supports the results of Swick and Song (1974), who used myosin from rat tissues. Furthermore, protein turnover rates reflected the RNA concentrations of the muscles. Figure 3 shows that the muscles in fowl with a more rapid turnover had a higher RNA concentration. A similar relationship was found in canine muscles; that is, the higher the rate of protein turnover, the more protein synthesizing machinery present. The RNA activities (Millward *et al.,* 1973) of each tissue were consistent, ranging from 9.6 ± 0.5 in the ventricle to 8.3 ± 0.9 g of protein/g of RNA/day in the levator ani in dogs, indicating that the translational efficiency of the RNA is similar.

These different turnover rates in different muscles in which the protein molecules are very similar in their physical properties indicate that the lifespan of a protein is a function of its intracellular proteolytic environment. Is the nature of the macromolecule that the more it is used, i.e., the more it interacts with other macromolecules, the greater is the chance of its denaturation and subsequently its degradation? Heart muscle performs continuous mechanical work and is replaced faster than the less frequently used white skeletal twitch muscle. To replace each tissue once a week with all new amino acids requires significant energy expenditure, and calculations indicate that the turnover of total body protein could account for almost all of the basal metabolic energy (Millward *et al.,* 1976). What evolutionary significance this apparent extravagant degradation of tissue components has is open to speculation. Perhaps a dynamic

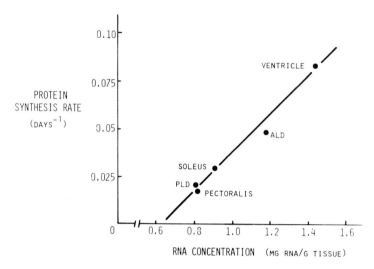

Figure 2. Turnover of mixed muscle proteins of muscles of the fowl after pulse-labeling with [³H]leucine intravenously. Each point is a mean of five animals.

state of destruction and reconstruction has evolved as a means by which a tissue rapidly adapts to stress. The mechanism that copes with the large amount of degradation is still largely not understood. It will be interesting to see whether or not the proteolytic environment of the tissues described here correlates with their degradation rates.

REFERENCES

GARLICK, P. J., MILLWARD, D. J., and JAMES, W. P. T. 1973. The diurnal response of muscle and liver protein synthesis *in vivo* in meal-fed rats. Biochem. J. 136:935–945.

GOLDBERG, A. L. 1967. Protein synthesis in tonic and phasic skeletal muscles. Nature 216:1219–1220.

MILLWARD, D. J., GARLICK, P. J., JAMES, W. P. T., NNANYELUG, D. C., and RYATT, J. W. 1973. Relationship between protein synthesis and RNA content in skeletal muscle. Nature 241:204–205.

MILLWARD, D. J., GARLICK, P. J., JAMES, W. P. T., SENDER, P., and WATERLOW, J. C. 1976. Protein turnover. *In* D. J. A. Cole, K. N. Boorman, P. J. Buttery, D. Lewis, R. J. Neale, and H. Swan (eds.), Protein Metabolism and Nutrition, pp. 49–69. Butterworths, London and Boston.

PAGE, S. G. 1969. Structure and some contractile properties of fast and slow muscles of chicken. J. Physiol. 205:131–145.

SWICK, R. W., and SONG, H. 1974. Turnover rates of various muscle proteins. J. Anim. Sci. 38:1150–1157.

Mailing address:
M. P. Sparrow, Ph.D.,
Department of Pharmacology, University of Western Australia,
Nedlands, Western Australia, 6009 (Australia).

Recent Advances in Studies on
Cardiac Structure and Metabolism, Volume 12
Cardiac Adaptation
Edited by T. Kobayashi, Y. Ito, and G. Rona
Copyright 1978 University Park Press Baltimore

INCREASED PROTEIN SYNTHESIS DURING RIGHT VENTRICULAR HYPERTROPHY FOLLOWING PULMONARY STENOSIS IN THE DOG

A. W. EVERETT, R. R. TAYLOR, and M. P. SPARROW

Departments of Pharmacology and Medicine, University of
Western Australia, Nedlands, Western Australia

SUMMARY

The synthesis rates of mixed protein in the left and right ventricles were the same in normal dogs, averaging 7.8% per day. After five days, pulmonary stenosis protein synthesis rate in the right ventricle increased rapidly to 13.6% per day and subsequently decreased to near normal by 12 days, during which time the right ventricle protein mass increased by 48% after five days and by 73% after 12 days. Similarly the synthesis rate of the myofibrillar and sarcoplasmic proteins was almost doubled after five days of stenosis. The protein synthesis rate in the left ventricle did not change significantly during the 24 days of pulmonary stenosis.

INTRODUCTION

Proteins comprising the myocardium are in a dynamic state, being continuously synthesized from amino acids and then degraded. Swick and Song (1974) and Martin *et al.* (1974) report a half-life of myosin from rat heart of 4–6 days. A half-life of 6–8 days for myosin from rabbit heart also has been reported (Morkin and Kimata, 1974).

The object of this study was, first, to measure protein synthesis and degradation rates in the myocardium of mongrel dogs, and, second, to measure changes in these parameters during right ventricular hypertrophy following stenosis of the pulmonary artery.

MATERIALS AND METHODS

Measurement of protein synthesis involved intravenously infusing the conscious dog with 50 μCi of [^{14}C] tyrosine for 6 hr. By 30 min the specific activity of plasma tyrosine had reached a plateau level and remained at that level thereafter. At the completion of the infusion, the dog was sacrificed; the right ventricular wall was dissected from the septum and from the left ventricle, weighed, and homogenized in 5% trichloroacetic acid, and the specific activity of the free and protein-bound tyrosine was determined. From the ratio of these specific activities, a protein synthetic rate constant was determined according to the method of Garlick, Millward, and James (1973).

Right ventricular hypertrophy was induced in dogs by tightening a polyethylene tube around the pulmonary artery until there was a visible right ventricular distension but just short of the point at which marked arrhythmia occurred. The right ventricular pressure increased from 40 ± 5 mm Hg (mean ± S.E.M., n = 5) before stenosis to 76 ± 6 mm Hg (n = 8) after stenosis.

RESULTS AND DISCUSSION

The synthesis rate of mixed proteins in the left and right ventricle of normal dogs was 7.6 ± 0.5% and 8.0 ± 0.6% per day (mean ± S.E.M., n = 8),respectively. There was no significant difference in the synthesis rate of both ventricles, and, because these animals were in a steady-state condition, protein degradation also had to equal approximately 8% per day, which corresponds to a $t_{1/2}$ of 8.7 days.

Five days after pulmonary stenosis (Figure 1), the wet weight of the right ventricle had increased by 48% after which the rate of increase slowed until, by 24 days, it was 83% above normal. In the five-day, sham-operated animals, the right ventricular mass was not significantly different from normal. Furthermore, there was no change in the left ventricular mass of stenotic animals throughout

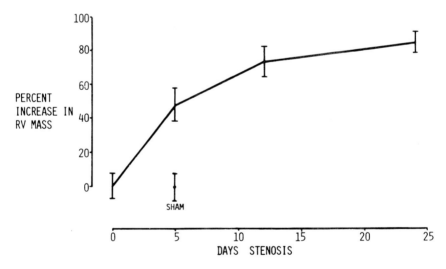

Figure 1. Increase in right ventricular mass above normal after pulmonary stenosis in dogs. Each point is the mean ± S.E.M. of at least four dogs. RV = right ventricle.

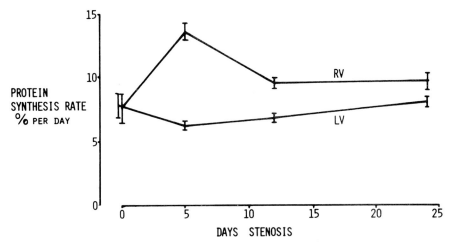

Figure 2. Synthesis rates of mixed proteins in the left and right ventricles after pulmonary stenosis. Each point is the mean ± S.E.M. of at least four dogs.

the 24 days of stenosis. The protein synthesis rates in the left and right ventricles during the 24 days of hypertrophy are shown in Figure 2.

After five days of stenosis, the synthesis in the right ventricle was almost double that of the normal, having increased from an average of 7.8% to 13.6% per day, an increase which was highly significant ($p < 0.001$). By day 12 the synthesis rate had decreased to a level that was still elevated but not significantly different from the normal. In five-day, sham-operated animals, protein synthesis was not significantly different from normal nor was there any significant change in protein synthesis of the left ventricle throughout the 24 days of stenosis.

The synthesis rates of myofibrillar and sarcoplasmic protein of five-day stenotic animals are shown in Figure 3. The synthesis of myofibrillar protein doubled in the right ventricle relative to the control left ventricle, while that of the sarcoplasmic protein was almost doubled. The synthesis rate in the right ventricle of both these fractions had decreased, returning to normal, by day 12.

These experiments show that right ventricular hypertrophy following pulmonary stenosis is accompanied by a rapid and marked increase in protein synthesis which then returns to near normal after compensation. Some indication of the changes in degradation during hypertrophy can be qualitatively seen by comparing the change in mass and the protein synthesis rate at each time period. Between days 5 and 12 the average synthetic rate is elevated and mass is increasing slightly, although not significantly, so degradation is not decreased and is possibly elevated.

Additional measurements of protein synthesis during the early phase of ventricular growth are needed to obtain more precise protein degradation rates.

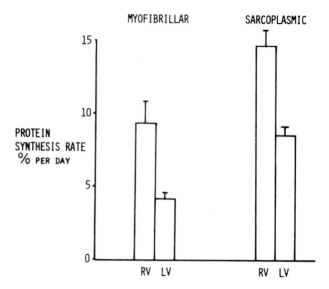

Figure 3. Protein synthesis rates of myofibrillar and sarcoplasmic protein in the left and right ventricles of five-day stenotic dogs. Shown is the mean ± S.E.M. of four observations. RV = right ventricle; LV = left ventricle.

REFERENCES

GARLICK, P. J., MILLWARD, D. J., and JAMES, W. P. T. 1973. The diurnal response of muscle and liver protein synthesis *in vivo* in meal-fed rats. Biochem. J. 136:935–945.

MARTIN, A. F., REDDY, M. K., RADOVAN, Z., DOWELL, R. T., and RABINOWITZ, M. 1974. Protein metabolism in hypertrophied heart muscle. Circ. Res. 34 and 35 (Suppl. III)32–40.

MORKIN, E., and KIMATA, S. 1974. Replacement of myosin during development of cardiac hypertrophy. Circ. Res. 34 and 35 (Suppl. III)50–56.

SWICK, R. W., and SONG, H. 1974. Turnover rates of various muscle proteins. J. Anim. Sci. 38:1150–1157.

Mailing address:
A. W. Everett, B. Pharm.,
Departments of Pharmacology and Medicine,
University of Western Australia, Nedlands, Western Australia 6009 (Australia).

Recent Advances in Studies on
Cardiac Structure and Metabolism, Volume 12
Cardiac Adaptation
Edited by T. Kobayashi, Y. Ito, and G. Rona
Copyright 1978 University Park Press Baltimore

COMPARISON OF THE SYNTHESIS OF LIGHT AND HEAVY CHAINS OF CARDIAC MYOSIN

Y. YAZAKI[1] and M. S. RABEN[2]

[1] The Third Department of Internal Medicine, Faculty of Medicine,
University of Tokyo, Tokyo, Japan
[2] New England Medical Center Hospital and Department of Medicine,
Tufts University, School of Medicine, Boston, Massachusetts, USA

SUMMARY

The synthesis of the light and heavy chains of cardiac myosin has been compared in rats injected with 0.1 mCi/200 g of [^{3}H]lysine. The two species of light chains with molecular weights of 27,000 (light chain I) and 20,000 (light chain II) were fractionated by preparative gel electrophoresis. The specific activity of myosin chains increased rapidly until about three days after injection of the label and then decreased gradually. Analysis of the protein isotope decay curves indicates that myosin chain degradation can be approximated using first-order kinetics, with the rate constants for degradation of the heavy chain, light chain I, and light chain II being 0.121, 0.099, and 0.101, respectively. These results indicate that the heavy chain is synthesized at a somewhat faster rate than the two light chains, which are synthesized at approximately the same rate. On the other hand, unequal chain labeling occurred in very brief labeling periods. The ratio of specific activity of each of the light chains to the heavy chain was the lowest at 10 min after isotope injection, and it increased following longer labeling times, particularly in the case of light chain II. These results demonstrate the evidence of pools of uncombined light chains, especially light chain II, in the cardiac muscle cell, because proteins with larger pools would be expected to become labeled more slowly.

INTRODUCTION

It is well known that the cardiac myosin molecule is composed of two large polypeptide chains (heavy chains) and two classes of low molecular weight polypeptide chains (light chains) (Sarkar, Sreter, and Gergely, 1971; Weeds and Pope, 1971). It is also generally accepted that cardiac myosin has a rapid turnover rate and can increase markedly in response to work overload. These characteristics of cardiac myosin raise interesting questions regarding the degree to which synthesis of the individual subunits of cardiac myosin is distinctive. Recently, we have found that preparative gel electrophoresis achieves the most complete separation of individual cardiac light chains and permits their isolation

This work was supported by Grants AM01567 and HL06924 from the National Institutes of Health, USPHS, and by a grant from the Japan Heart Foundation, 1975.

from small amounts of starting material (Yazaki, Mochinaga, and Raben, 1973). By using this method, we compared the rate of isotope incorporation into polypeptide chains of cardiac myosin and also compared the rate of isotope disappearance from polypeptide chains of cardiac myosin.

MATERIALS AND METHODS

Normal male rats (180–210 g) were fasted overnight and then injected intravenously via the tail vein with 0.1 mCi/200 g of L-[4,5-^{3}H]lysine. After different intervals of time, groups of rats were killed and ventricular muscle from 10 rat hearts was used for the extraction of each cardiac myosin preparation. Myosin was prepared by the dilution technique described previously (Yazaki and Raben, 1974). Cardiac myosin was dissociated into light and heavy chain fractions by guanidine denaturation. The two species of light chains with molecular weights of 27,000 (light chain I) and 20,000 (light chain II) were fractionated by preparative gel electrophoresis as previously reported (Yazaki, Mochinaga, and Raben, 1973). Polyacrylamide gel electrophoresis was run in the presence of sodium dodecyl sulfate (SDS).

Lysine was isolated from hydrolysates of the proteins by high-voltage electrophoresis, and its content and radioactivity were measured by quantitative ninhydrin assay and liquid scintilation counting (Kimata and Morkin, 1971). Free lysine also was isolated from homogenates of cardiac muscle by using ion exchange chromatography (Morgan et al., 1971).

RESULTS

Specific Activity of Free Lysine in Tissue

The free lysine concentration of heart muscle was 25.2 ± 2.1 μmol/100 g wet weight. The disappearance of free radioactive lysine from the tissue after injection is shown in Figure 1. The semi-logarithmic plot shows a rapid initial disappearance phase lasting the first day, followed by a slower decrease in radioactivity thereafter. The decay of free radioactive lysine from 3–25 days (Af) has a very gradual slope and may be approximated as an exponential with rate constant R and coefficient C (Henriques, Henriques, and Neuberger, 1954).

$$Af = Ce^{-R(t-3)}$$

Equating t to time in days, least-squares fitting of the date for the disappearance of free radioactive lysine gives the following expression:

$$Af = 0.642 \times 10^4 \, e^{-\cdot 107(t-3)}$$

The calculated disappearance curve for free [^{3}H]lysine using this expression is shown in Figure 1. This decay curve can be explained by the fact that free

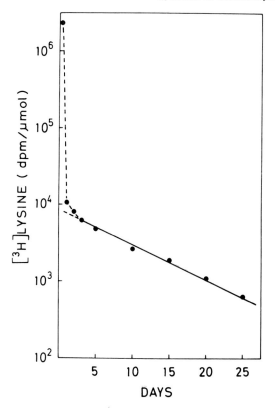

Figure 1. Specific radioactivity of free lysine in the ventricular muscle plotted against time. The rats were injected with [³H] lysine of 100 µCi/200 g at time 0. Least-squares fitting of experimental data is shown as a solid line.

radioactive lysine arising from protein breakdown is reutilized for protein synthesis.

Specific Activity of Lysine Contained in Cardiac Myosin Chains

Cardiac myosin is known to be synthesized rapidly in comparison to skeletal myosin (Kimata and Morkin, 1971). As would be anticipated, labeling of cardiac myosin polypeptide chains proceeded rapidly; their peak activities were attained at 48 hr and then decreased relatively rapidly (Figure 2). The disappearance rate of radioactivity from the heavy chain is slightly faster than radioactivity disappearance from the two light chains in which radioactivity decreased at about the same rate. A half-life for the peptide chain cannot be accurately determined directly from the isotope decay curve because of reutilization of the labeling compound. However, the degradation rate can be calculated from the decay curve, provided information is available concerning the specific activity of the

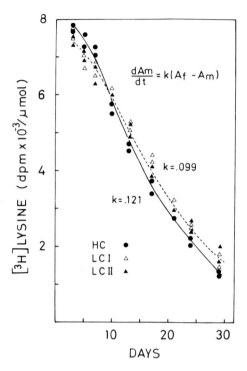

$$\frac{dAm}{dt} = k(A_f - A_m)$$

k = .099

k = .121

HC ●
LC I △
LC II ▲

[³H]LYSINE (dpm × 10⁻³/μmol)

DAYS

Figure 2. Specific radioactivity of [³H]lysine in the polypeptide chains of cardiac myosin 1–28 days after injection of [³H]lysine. ● = heavy chain; △ = light chain I; ▲ = light chain II. Curves represent computer fitting of experimental points using data on disappearance of free [³H]lysine and the equation (see text). —— = heavy chain; --- = two light chains.

precursor amino acid. Assuming the myosin content to be essentially constant throughout the period of the experiment, one can write:

$$dAm/dt = K \ (Af{-}Am)$$

where, Af and Am = specific radioactivities of free lysine and lysine contained in myosin chains respectively, dpm/μmol
K = rate constant for myosin chain degradation, day⁻¹

Using the date shown in Figure 1 for the variations in free [³H]lysine with time, we formulated the equation by a numerical technique using a digital computer (Figure 2). The degradation constant for cardiac myosin chain, K, which gave the best fit to the experimental date for the heavy chain, was 0.121 day⁻¹. This represents a half-life of 5.8 days (t₁/₂ = 0.693/K). The degradation constants for the two species of light chains (light chains I and II) were 0.099 and

Table 1. Incorporation of [³H]lysine into myosin light and heavy chains

Time	Specific activity dpm X 10^{-3}/μmol			Light chain/heavy chain ratios	
	Light chain I	Light chain II	Heavy chain	Light chain I/ Heavy chain	Light chain II/ Heavy chain
10 min	0.50	0.22	0.89	0.56	0.25
	0.70	0.41	1.31	0.53	0.31
	0.61	0.31	1.07	0.57	0.29
				Average: 0.55	0.28
30 min	2.16	1.29	3.05	0.71	0.42
	2.12	1.02	2.77	0.77	0.37
	2.49	1.37	3.35	0.74	0.41
				Average: 0.74	0.40
60 min	4.50	4.06	5.73	0.79	0.71
	4.88	4.32	5.94	0.82	0.73
	3.91	3.76	5.01	0.78	0.75
				Average: 0.80	0.73
2 hr	5.82	5.34	6.92	0.84	0.77
4 hr	6.74	6.56	7.81	0.86	0.84
	6.43	6.10	7.56	0.85	0.81

0.101 day^{-1}, which would give approximately the same half-life of 6.9 days. The exact values of degradation constants obtained are less certain; however, these results suggest that the heavy chain is synthesized at a slightly faster rate than the two light chains, which are synthesized at about the same rate. These calculations also illustrate that the isotope decay curves of cardiac myosin chains can be approximated using first-order kinetics.

The incorporation of radioactive lysine into myosin heavy and light chains in brief periods after injection is shown in Table 1. According to the values of their degradation constants obtained from the decay curves of the isotope, it would be expected that these polypeptide chains would tend to gain radioactivity at about the same rate. However, as shown in Table 1, the increase in the specific activities of these polypeptide chains, at 10 and 30 min after injection, revealed that unequal labeling occurred in very brief labeling periods. At a given time, the specific activities of these proteins varied such that heavy chain > light chain I > light chain II. Presence of pools of individual uncombined myosin chains could account for this unequal labeling. Polypeptide chains with larger pools would be expected to increase in specific activity more slowly until the pools equilibrate with newly synthesized radioactive chains. To test this possibility, the ratio of specific activity of each of the light chains to the heavy chains was compared, because the ratio of a chain with a larger pool to one with a smaller pool will be less after brief labeling periods than after longer periods. As shown in Table 1, the ratios were the lowest at 10 min after labeling—the values were 0.55 for light chain I and 0.28 for light chain II—and the ratios increased following longer labeling times, particularly in the case of the smaller light chain, light chain II. These results suggest the presence of pools of light chains, especially light chain II, in the cardiac muscle cell.

DISCUSSION

These results indicate that there is relative coordination between the rates of synthesis of myosin chains in cardiac muscle. Furthermore, the increase in ratios of light to heavy chain specific activities during the first 60 min after labeling suggests that there is a pool of light chains within the muscle cell.

Our previous studies have shown that the synthesis of skeletal myosin chains demonstrates no one-to-one coordination in the rabbit (Morkin et al., 1973); one light chain species (MW 12,000) is synthesized approximately as fast as one of the other species (MW 23,000). However, we found that the two cardiac light chains are synthesized at about the same rate. The rapid turnover rate of cardiac myosin chains could be reflected in this relative coordination of their syntheses, as compared to that of skeletal myosin chains. Recently, Wikman-Coffelt et al. (1973) reported that the heavy chains of cardiac myosin have a turnover rate twice that of the light chains. However, because they studied the relative rate of degradation of cardiac chains by the double-isotope technique, it is difficult to compare the synthesis rate of the proteins accurately. We found that the heavy chains are synthesized about 20% faster than the two light chains.

The increase in ratios of light to heavy chain specific activities in brief labeling periods suggests that there is a pool of uncombined cardiac light chains in the tissue, because polypeptide chains with larger pools would be expected to become labeled more slowly. However, it seems likely that the pool of the light chains is small because only one hour, at most, is required to achieve constant ratios of light to heavy chain specific activities, and myosin chain degradation then can be approximated by first-order kinetics. Whether or not the heavy chains have a pool is not elucidated by this study because the heavy chain fraction obtained by the dilution technique contained both uncombined and combined heavy chains.

REFERENCES

HENRIQUES, O. B., HENRIQUES, S. B., and NEUBERGER, A. 1954. Quantitative aspects of glycine metabolism in the rabbit. Biochem. J. 60:409–424.
KIMATA, S., and MORKIN, E. 1971. Comparison of myosin synthesis in heart and red and white skeletal muscles. Am. J. Physiol. 221:1706–1713.
MORGAN, H. E., EARL, D. C. N., BROADUS, A., WOLPERT, E. G., GIGER, K. E., and JEFFERSON, L. S. 1971. Regulation of protein synthesis in heart muscle. J. Biol. Chem. 246:2152–2162.

MORKIN, E., YAZAKI, Y., KATAGIRI, T., and LARAIA, P. J. 1973. Comparison of the synthesis of the light and heavy chains of adult skeletal myosin. Biochim. Biophys. Acta 324:420–429.

SARKAR, S., SRETER, F. A., and GERGELY, J. 1971. Light chains of myosins from white, red and cardiac muscle. Proc. Natl. Acad. Sci. USA 68:946–950.

WEEDS, A. G., and POPE, B. 1971. Chemical studies on light chains from cardiac and skeletal muscle myosin. Nature 234:85–88.

WIKMAN-COFFELT, Y., ZELIS, R., FENNER, C., and MASON, D. T. 1973. Studies on the synthesis and degradation of light and heavy chains of cardiac myosin. J. Biol. Chem. 248:5206–5207.

YAZAKI, Y., MOCHINAGA, S. and RABEN, M. S. 1973. Fractionation of the light chains from rat and rabbit cardiac myosin. Biochim. Biophys. Acta 328:464–469.

YAZAKI, Y., and RABEN, M. S. 1974. Effect of the thyroid state on the enzymatic characteristics of cardiac myosin. Circ. Res. 36:208–215.

Mailing address:
Y. Yazaki, M.D.,
Third Department of Internal Medicine,
Faculty of Medicine, University of Tokyo,
7-3-1 Hongo, Bunkyo, Tokyo (Japan).

Recent Advances in Studies on
Cardiac Structure and Metabolism, Volume 12
Cardiac Adaptation
Edited by T. Kobayashi, Y. Ito, and G. Rona
Copyright 1978 University Park Press Baltimore

MACROMOLECULAR METABOLISM OF NAD+
IN HEART NUCLEI

E. KUN and A. M. FERRO

Cardiovascular Research Institute, Departments of Pharmacology,
Biochemistry, and Biophysics, University of California, San Francisco,
California, USA

INTRODUCTION

The only macromolecular metabolite which until now has been isolated from
liver, thymus, and tumor cells is the nucleic acid type polymer: poly (adenosine-
diphosphoribose). Following the identification and isolation of an ADP-ribo-
sylated protein from mitochondria (Kun *et al.*, 1975), we have attempted to
clarify the following questions:

1. Is poly (ADP-R) formed in heart nuclei?
2. Is this macromolecule the only macromolecular derivative of NAD+ in cardiac
tissue?

RESULTS AND DISCUSSION

Phosphoribosyl-AMP and AMP were identified as the only degradation products,
and an average chain length of 16 was calculated for the poly (ADP-R) polymer
in heart. Based on DNA, poly (ADP-R) was formed more than twice as fast in
heart nuclei as in liver nuclei (108 nmol in liver, 250 nmol in heart per mg of
DNA). K_m for NAD+ for the polymerase was 330 μM. Macromolecular derivatives of ADP-ribose were formed directly, without the participation of NAD+, as
shown by incubation of labeled ADP-R with chromatin. Enzymatic degradation
of the macromolecular product revealed AMP as the single product, which
identified the macromolecular products of ADP-R as ADP-R proteins, in contrast to poly (ADP-R) (Ferro and Kun, 1976). Subsequent work showed that
histone f_1 and various proteins containing ϵ-NH$_2$ groups react directly with
ADP-ribose and with ribose-5-phosphate to form covalently modified products.
These were isolated and identified as Schiff bases as proved by selective tritiation

This work was supported by the USPHS Program Project and NIH Grant HL-06285.

with NaB^3H_4. The reaction of aldehydic metabolites of NAD^+ with nucleophylic NH_2 groups constitutes the molecular basis of regulation of nuclear and mitochondrial macromolecular metabolism, representing a signal system between metabolic and epigenetic cellular processes (Kun *et al.,* 1976).

REFERENCES

FERRO, A. M., and KUN, E. 1976. Biochem. Biophys. Res. Commun. 71:150–154.
KUN, E., CHANG, A. C. Y., SHARMA, M. L., FERRO, A. M., and NITECKI, D. 1976. Proc. Natl. Acad. Sci. USA 73:3131–3135.
KUN, E., ZIMBER, H. P., CHANG, A. C. Y., PUSCHENDORF, B., and GRUNICKE, H. 1975. Proc. Natl. Acad. Sci. USA 72:1436–1440.

Mailing address:
Ernest Kun,
Cardiovascular Research Institute, Departments of Pharmacology, Biochemistry, and Biophysics, University of California, San Francisco, California 94143 (USA).

Recent Advances in Studies on
Cardiac Structure and Metabolism, Volume 12
Cardiac Adaptation
Edited by George Rona and Yoshio Ito
Copyright 1978   University Park Press   Baltimore

INVESTIGATION INTO THE CAUSES OF INCREASED PROTEIN SYNTHESIS IN ACUTE HEMODYNAMIC OVERLOAD

S. S. SCHREIBER, M. A. ROTHSCHILD, and M. ORATZ

Department of Nuclear Medicine,
New York Veterans Administration Hospital,
New York, New York
Department of Medicine,
New York University School of Medicine,
New York, New York
Department of Biochemistry,
New York University College of Dentistry,
New York, New York, USA

SUMMARY

Prolonged increase in cardiac contractile effort results in increased protein synthesis. The effects of various stresses on ventricular protein synthesis in the left or right guinea pig heart were investigated in an *in vitro* guinea pig cardiac model in which the left ventricle was stressed with increased preload or afterload and also in a second model in which the right ventricle was stressed in the face of constant coronary flow. Assays of ventricular protein synthesis were made by perfusion with constant specific activities of labeled amino acids over periods of 1–3 hr utilizing the specific activity of the labeled amino acid in the intracellular space as the precursor label. After 3 hr of afterload pressure stress, protein synthesis in the stressed ventricle increased. Of the three specific proteins tested, myosin synthesis increased in this period while myoglobin and collagen synthesis were not changed with this acute stress. Microsomes isolated from the stressed ventricles showed increased peptide elongation after 1 hr, nuclear RNA polymerase activity was increased after 20 min of stress, and adenylcyclase activity increased after 10 min of stress. In contrast to the augmented protein synthesis in the acute stress, protein degradation was not increased with afterload. When contractility was increased by hypercalcemia, acetaldehyde perfusion, or fluid loading (preloading), protein synthesis was not increased after 3 hr. At the same time, when hearts were arrested with high K^+ but aerobically perfused, protein synthesis did not decrease. Hence, the model used demonstrated that there is a baseline of cardiac protein synthesis that does not depend on contractility per se, but that is significantly increased with work against increased pressure.

This work was supported in part by the U.S. Public Health Service Grants AA 00959 and HL 09562 and by the Bear Foundation.

INTRODUCTION

It is now well known that prolonged increases in cardiac contractile action result in increased protein synthesis leading to hypertrophy (Meerson, 1962; Gudbjarnason, Telerman, and Bing, 1964; Grimm, Kuboto, and Whitehorn, 1966; Schreiber et al., 1966; Hatt, Berjal, and Swynghedauw, 1970). This chapter presents data obtained from a perfused left or right ventricular perfusion model (Schreiber, Oratz, and Rothschild, 1972; Schreiber et al., 1975) in which various stresses such as increased pressure, fluid volume loading, inotropic actions of increased calcium or of acetaldehyde, and cardiac arrest were studied with respect to protein synthesis.

MATERIALS AND METHODS

Hearts from young male guinea pigs (250–300 g) were used in all *in vitro* studies. Preparation of the perfusion models has been described previously (Schreiber *et al.*, 1966, 1975; Schreiber, Oratz, and Rothschild, 1972). The perfusate was a modified Krebs-Henseleit solution containing added amino acids. Protein synthesis was determined from the incorporation of ^{14}C-amino acids, e.g., lysine or phenylalanine, into protein, utilizing the specific activity of the labeled amino acid in the intracellular precursor pool (Schreiber *et al.*, 1966, 1973, 1975; Schreiber, Oratz, and Rothschild, 1972). In the left ventricular model, perfusate was presented to the left ventricle, and the latter was studied with reference to increases in aortic pressure (Schreiber *et al.*, 1966). In the right ventricular model, coronary flow was maintained at a constant rate by a separate perfusion system, and the right ventricle received a combined load of the coronary perfusion and any desired additional fluid via the inferior vena cava. Right ventricular stress was obtained by raising the pulmonary artery pressure or by increasing the volume to the right heart via the vena cava (Schreiber *et al.*, 1975). Assays of radioactivity, chemical analysis, microsome isolation, and incubation methods have been described previously (Schreiber *et al.*, 1973, 1975, 1977; Hearse, Stewart, and Braimbridge, 1975).

RESULTS

Our initial direction of study investigated the response of the myocardium to pressure stress or increased afterload. After 3 hr of such stress *in vitro,* mixed cardiac protein synthesis was approximately 80% greater than that in the control (Figure 1) (Schreiber *et al.,* 1966, but all of the fractions isolated did not respond similarly, with most protein synthesis seen in the soluble supernatant (cell sap) fraction or myofibrillar fraction (Schreiber, Oratz, and Rothschild, 1971).

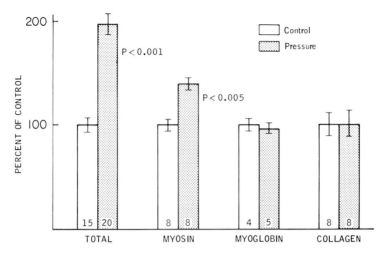

Figure 1. Incorporation of [14 C]-amino acids into specific proteins after 3-hr pressure loading. Incorporation of [14 C] lysine into mixed cardiac protein, myosin, and myoglobin in acute pressure stress *in vitro* is expressed as a percentage of controls. Collagen synthesis was determined from the conversion of [14 C] proline to [14 C] hydroxyproline (Schreiber *et al.,* 1966, 1970, 1973, 1975; Schreiber, Oratz, and Rothschild, 1971, 1972, 1976).

Analysis of three specific ventricular proteins also showed dissimilar response to afterload stress, with lysine incorporation into purified myosin increased and lysine incorporation into myoglobin unchanged (Figure 1) (Schreiber *et al.,* 1970. Similarly, the synthesis of connective tissues was not altered after 3 hr of afterload stress; the concentration of hydroxyproline remained the same as in the controls, and the conversion of [14 C] proline to [14 C] hyroxyproline also was the same as in the controls (Figure 1) (Schreiber *et al.,* 1970). Thus, of the three specific proteins studied, only myosin synthesis appeared increased after 3 hr of afterload stress (Schreiber *et al.,* 1970). The data did not preclude an increase in collagen synthesis after prolonged stress (Meerson *et al.,* 1968; Buccino *et al.,* 1969).

A study of the mechanisms by which protein synthesis was increased in acute afterload stress was begun with microsomes isolated from stressed ventricles. These microsomes demonstrated an increased capacity to incorporate labeled amino acids into microsomal protein (Moroz, 1967; Schreiber, Oratz, and Rothschild, 1967), which was not a function of the cell sap but of the microsomes themselves (Schreiber et al., 1967, 1968), and which could be demonstrated after only one hour of pressure stress. The addition of actinomycin (an inhibitor of synthesis of mRNA) to the perfusate of controls had no apparent effect on subsequent microsomal protein synthetic capacity. In contrast, actinomycin prevented the increased incorporation of amino acids into microsomal protein

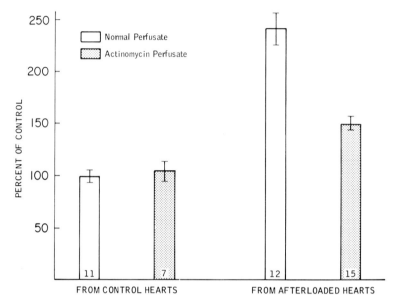

Figure 2. ^{14}C-Amino acids incorporation into protein by isolated microsomes. Microsomes, obtained from perfused control and afterload stressed left ventricles after perfusion with actinomycin, were incubated in cell free systems and the incorporation of labeled amino acids into microsomal protein was measured (Schreiber, Oratz, and Rothschild, 1967; Schreiber *et al.*, 1968).

by microsomes obtained from pressure-stressed ventricles (Figure 2). These studies strongly suggested that one of the early responses of the left ventricle to increased afterload was the increased synthesis of messenger RNA.

Further evidence supporting the above was obtained from nuclear polymerase studies. Although there was apparently no significant difference in total RNA labeling with uridine after 3 hr of increased afterload (Figure 3) (Schreiber *et al.*, 1968), polysome analysis with sucrose gradients showed that heavier aggregates had higher [3H]uridine activity, which was abolished by simultaneous actinomycin perfusion (Schreiber *et al.*, 1968). Finally, the stimulation of nuclear RNA polymerase activity in Mn^{2+} media after 20 minutes of increased afterload added support to the thesis that an early response to this stress was augmented mRNA (Figure 3) (Schreiber *et al.*, 1968). A later increase in Mg^{2+}-stimulated RNA polymerase activity supported subsequent increases in ribosomal RNA, as described by Nair *et al.* in *in vivo* studies (1967, 1968).

An apparent sequence of events following acute increases in afterload seemed to be increases in adenylcyclase activity (Figure 3) (Schreiber *et al.*, 1971), followed rapidly by polyamine synthesis (Russell *et al.*, 1971; Calderera *et al.*, 1975), mRNA synthesis (Schreiber *et al.*, 1968), and increased polysome formation of peptides, in turn leading to increased synthesis of proteins, particularly myosin, in this model.

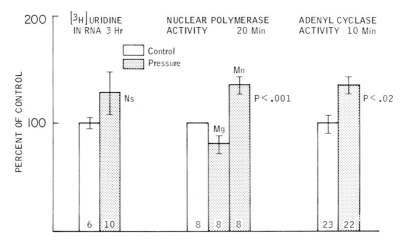

Figure 3. Although incorporation of [^{3}H] uridine into total RNA was not increased after three hours of afterload stress *in vitro*, nuclear RNA polymerase activity (Mn^{2+}-stimulated) was increased after 20 min and adenylcyclase activity was also increased after 10 min of this stress (Schreiber, Oratz, and Rothschild, 1969; Schreiber *et al.,* 1971).

A major problem in evaluating the effects of increased afterload on protein was the determination of protein degradation. This has been approximated from measurements of loss of radioactivity from the hearts prelabeled with amino acids *in vivo.* Earlier studies suggested that protein degradation was indeed slowed during afterload stress (Goldberg, 1969; Zak, Aschenbrenner, and Rabinowitz, 1971). However, these studies did not take into consideration the amino acids released by intracellular protein degradation being reutilized for the synthesis of new proteins (Millward, 1970; Righetti, Little, and Wolf, 1971; Schreiber *et al.,* 1973). [^{14}C] Lysine presented a particular problem: the intracellular precursor pool did not equilibrate rapidly with the extracellular amino acid because the intracellular pool was diluted with lysine of lower specific activity that was being released by protein degradation (Gan and Jeffay, 1967; Schreiber *et al.,* 1973), and it was evident that measurement of degradation by measuring the loss of radioactivity would give a false picture of the rate of degradation unless synthesis could be arrested (Figure 4). When protein synthesis was halted with puromycin, the rate of loss of [^{14}C] lysine from prelabeled perfused hearts increased from 0.6%/hr to 1.3%/hr, indicating that a very large degree of lysine, released by degradation, was reutilized in making new protein. With these methods, it was found that protein degradation was not slowed in cases of increased afterload but indeed remained unchanged (Figure 4) (Schreiber *et al.,* 1973). Similar results were obtained utilizing labeled phenylalanine (Schreiber *et al.,* 1973).

Although elevated left ventricular pressure rapidly increased protein synthesis, such rapid alterations were not consistently seen in volume loading. The

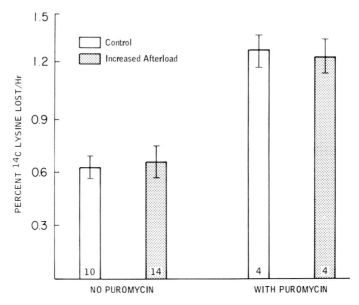

Figure 4. Degradation of protein in perfused hearts labeled with [¹⁴C]lysine. Hearts were prelabeled *in vivo* with [¹⁴C]lysine and were removed and perfused five days later under control and afterload stress conditions with and without puromycin in perfusate. The loss of radioactivity with synthesis arrested by puromycin showed that degradation was not altered in acute afterload stress (Schreiber *et al.,* 1973).

difference in response was difficult to clarify because it was not possible to alter left ventricular pressure or perfusion load without profoundly affecting coronary perfusion. With a right ventricle stress model in which coronary flow was controlled and fixed, increased pulmonary artery pressure was associated with increased protein synthesis, while excess fluid loading did not change synthesis (Figure 5) (Schreiber *et al.,* 1975).

Other causes of increased ventricular contractility have been studied with varied effects on cardiac protein synthesis. Thus, although the substance acetaldehyde, a metabolite of ethanol, has a profound inotropic and chronotropic effect, protein synthesis is not increased and, in fact, is actually significantly impaired (Schreiber, Oratz, and Rothschild, 1972). This inhibition apparently works directly at the microsome level (Figure 6) (Schreiber *et al.,* 1974; Schreiber, 1975). It is of interest that this inhibition was totally unlike the inhibition of ethanol, per se, on the liver, in which ethanol disaggregates polysomes. In the heart, polysome aggregation was untouched by acetaldehyde, and polysomes free of sarcoplasmic reticulum showed no inhibition of peptide elongation with acetaldehyde (Figure 6). At this time the data suggest that

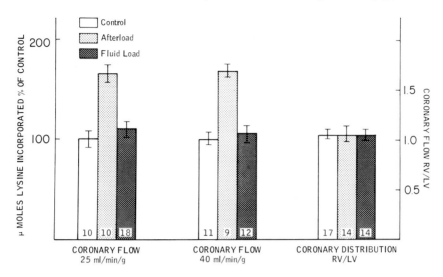

Figure 5. Incorporation of [^{14}C]lysine into protein of perfused hearts. At two levels of coronary flow, right ventricular protein synthesis was increased with afterload stress but not with increased fluid loading. Coronary distribution was not altered in these stresses (Schreiber *et al.*, 1975).

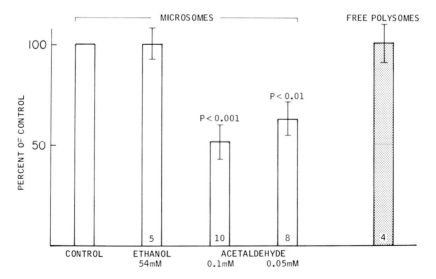

Figure 6. Incorporation of ^{14}C-amino acids into protein by microsomes and polysomes. Effect of acetaldehyde and alcohol in isolated cardiac microsomes is shown (Schreiber, Oratz, and Rothschild, 1972; Schreiber *et al.*, 1974).

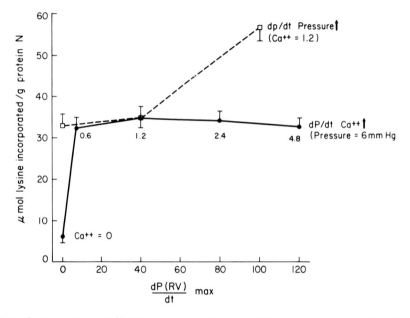

Figure 7. Comparison of [^{14}C]lysine incorporation into right ventricular protein after three hours of perfusion with increases in dP/dt (right ventricle) caused by elevation in pulmonary artery pressure or by increases in perfusate calcium (from 0.6 to 4.8 mM CaCl$_2$). Although protein synthesis increased with elevations of dP/dt caused by pressure stress, there was no change in synthesis when dP/dt was increased by calcium in the face of control pressures.

acetaldehyde inhibition of protein synthesis takes place only in the presence of sarcoplasmic reticulum.

Another type of inotropic action that has been investigated has been the ventricular response to increases in perfusate calcium. With the pulmonary artery pressure kept constant, as the calcium concentration increases from 0.6 to 4.8 mM CaCl$_2$, there is a progressive increase in contractility as indicated by increased amplitude of contraction (difference between systolic and diastolic pressure) and dP/dt$_{max}$ (right ventricle). Although similar increases in these parameters caused by pressure stress or afterload effect augmented protein synthesis, such increase in synthesis was not seen with the inotropic effects of calcium (Figure 7).

Because the increased contractility attributable to afterload augmented protein synthesis, it was of interest to see if arresting contraction would do the opposite, i.e., decrease synthesis. In the right ventricular model, in which aerobic perfusion was maintained through controlled coronary flow in high K$^+$ arrest (KCl = 16 mM), protein synthesis was not decreased (Figure 8). In contrast, in anoxic perfusion with normal K$^+$ (KCl = 4 mM) protein synthesis was diminished

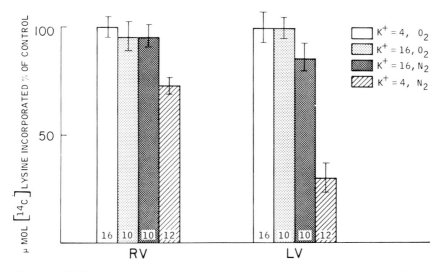

Figure 8. [^{14}C]lysine incorporation into proteins of perfused arrested hearts. Protein synthesis after three hours of cardiac arrest is compared to control beating hearts (Schreiber *et al.*, 1976). (See text.) The symbols $K^+ = 4$, O_2, etc., indicate the concentration of K^+ in the perfusate (mEq/liter) and the gas aerating the perfusate.

as expected. The drop in anoxia-induced arrest was minimized when the hearts were simultaneously arrested with high K^+ (Schreiber *et al.*, 1976) (Figure 8).

CONCLUSIONS

From the data obtained, it appears that, in acute experiments with an *in vitro* model, increases in afterload or pressure stress that increase contractile effort also augment protein synthesis. In contrast, fluid volume loading and increased contractility caused by increases in calcium concentration or by substances such as acetaldehyde do not increase protein synthesis. The maintenance of protein synthesis in viable high K^+-arrested hearts suggests that there is a baseline protein synthesis that is not dependent on contraction per se and that is not increased with low cardiac loads. Rather, it is the stress situation, particularly afterload, that is the most active initiator of protein synthesis in this model.

REFERENCES

BUCCINO, R. A., HARRIS, E., SPANN, J. F., JR., and SONNENBLICK, E. H. 1969. Response of myocardial connective tissue to development of experimental hypertrophy. Am. J. Physiol. 216:425–428.

CALDERERA, C. M., CASTI, A., GUARNIERI, C., and MORUZZI, G. 1975. Regulation of ribonucleic acid synthesis by polyamines. Biochem. J. 152:91–98.

GAN, J. C., and JEFFAY, H. 1967. Origins and metabolism of the intracellular amino acid pools in rat liver and muscle. Biochim. Biophys. Acta 148:448–459.

GOLDBERG, A. L. 1969. Protein catabolism during work induced hypertrophy and growth induced with growth hormone. J. Biol. Chem. 244:3217–3222.

GRIMM, A., KUBOTO, F., and WHITEHORN, W. V. 1966. Ventricular nucleic acids and protein levels with myocardial growth and hypertrophy. Circ. Res. 19:552–558.

GUDBJARNASON, S., TELERMAN, M., and BING, R. J. 1964. Protein metabolism in cardiac hypertrophy and heart failure. Am. J. Physiol. 206:294–298.

HATT, P., BERJAL, J., and SWYNGHEDAUW, B. 1970. Le myocarde ventriculaire dans l'insuffisance cardiaque experimentale par l'insuffisance aortique chez le lapin. Arch. Mal. Coeur 3:383–407.

HEARSE, D. J., STEWART, D. A., and BRAIMBRIDGE, M. V. 1975. Hypotheric and potassium arrest. Circ. Res. 36:481–489.

MEERSON, F. Z. 1962. Compensatory hyperfunction of the heart and cardiac insufficiency. Circ. Res. 10:250–258.

MEERSON, F. Z., ALEKHINA, G. M., ALEKSANDROV, P. N., and BAZARDJAN, A. E. 1968. Dynamics of nucleic acid and protein synthesis of the myocardium in compensatory hyperfunction and hypertrophy of the heart. Am. J. Cardiol. 22:337–348.

MILLWARD, D. J. 1970. Protein turnover in skeletal muscle. 1. The measurement of rates of synthesis and catabolism of skeletal muscle protein using ^{14}C-Na$_2$CO$_3$. Clin. Sci. 39:577–590.

MOROZ, L. A. 1967. Protein synthetic activity of heart microsomes and ribosomes during left ventricular hypertrophy in rabbits. Circ. Res. 21:449–459.

NAIR, K. G., RABINOWITZ, M., and CHEN TU, M. 1967. Characterization of ribonucleic acid synthesized in an isolated nuclear system from rat heart muscle. Biochemistry 6:1898–1902.

NAIR, K. G., CUTILETTA, A. F., ZAK, R., KOIDE, T., and RABINOWITZ, M. 1968. Biochemical correlates of cardiac hypertrophy. Circ. Res. 23:451–462.

RIGHETTI, P., LITTLE, E. P., and WOLF, G. 1971. Reutilization of amino acids in protein synthesis in Hela cells J. Biol. Chem. 246:5724–5732.

RUSSELL, D. H., SHIVERICK, K. T., HAMRELL, B. B., and ALPERT, N. R. 1971. Polyamine synthesis during initial phases of stress-induced cardiac hypertrophy. Am. J. Physiol. 221:1287–1291.

SCHREIBER, S. S. 1975. Stress and myocardial protein synthesis. The effect of alcohol and actaldehyde, In M. A. Rothschild, M. Oratz, and S. S. Schreiber (eds.), Alcohol and Protein Biosynthesis, pp. 273–291. Pergamon Press, New York.

SCHREIBER, S. S., BRIDEN, K., ORATZ, M., and ROTHSCHILD, M. A. 1966. Protein synthesis in the overloaded heart. Am. J. Physiol. 211:314–318.

SCHREIBER, S. S., HEARSE, D. J. ORATZ, M., and ROTHSCHILD, M. A. 1977. Protein synthesis in prolonged cardiac arrest. J. Mol. Cell. Cardiol. 9:87–100.

SCHREIBER, S. S., KLEIN, I., ORATZ, M., and ROTHSCHILD, M. A. 1971. Adenyl-cyclase activity and cyclic AMP in acute cardiac overload: A method for measuring cyclic AMP production based on ATP specific activity. J. Mol. Cell. Cardiol. 2:55–65.

SCHREIBER, S. S., ORATZ, M., EVANS, C. D., GUEYIKIAN, I., and ROTHSCHILD, M. A. 1970. Myosin, myoglobin and collagen synthesis in acute cardiac overload. Am. J. Physiol. 219:481–486.

SCHREIBER, S. S., ORATZ, M., EVANS, C., REFF, F., KLEIN, I., and ROTHSCHILD, M. A. 1973. Cardiac protein degradation in acute overload in vitro: Reutilization of amino acids. Am. J. Physiol. 224:338–345.

SCHREIBER, S. S., ORATZ, M., EVANS, C., SILVER, E., and ROTHSCHILD, M. A. 1968. Effect of acute overload on cardiac muscle mRNA. Am. J. Physiol. 449–459.

SCHREIBER, S. S., ORATZ, M., and ROTHSCHILD, M. A. 1967. Effect of acute overload on protein synthesis in cardiac muscle microsomes. Am. J. Physiol. 213:1552–1555.

SCHREIBER, S. S., ORATZ, M., and ROTHSCHILD, M. A. 1969. Nuclear polymerase activity in acute hemodynamic overload in the perfused heart. Am. J. Physiol. 217:1305–1309.

SCHREIBER, S. S., ORATZ, M. and ROTHSCHILD, M. A. 1971. Initiation of protein synthesis in the acutely overloaded perfused heart. In N. R. Alpert (ed.), Cardiac Hypertrophy, p. 215. 1st Ed. Academic Press, New York.

SCHREIBER, S. S., ORATZ, M., and ROTHSCHILD, M. A. 1972. Ethanol, acetaldehyde and myocardial protein synthesis. J. Clin. Invest. 51:2820–2826.

SCHREIBER, S. S., ORATZ, M., ROTHSCHILD, M. A., REFF, R., and EVANS, C. 1974. Alcoholic Cardiomyopathy. II. The Inhibition of cardiac microsomal protein synthesis by acetaldehyde. J. Mol. Cell. Cardiol. 6:207–213.

SCHREIBER, S. S., ROTHSCHILD, M. A., EVANS, C., REFF, F., and ORATZ, M. 1975. The effect of pressure vs flow stress on right ventricular protein synthesis in the face of constant and restricted coronary flow. J. Clin. Invest. 55:1–11.

ZAK, R. ASCHENBRENNER, V., and RABINOWITZ, M. 1971. Synthesis and degradation of myosin and cardiac hypertrophy. J. Clin. Invest. 50(abstr.):102a.

Mailing address:
Sidney S. Schreiber, M. S., M.D.,
Nuclear Medicine Service, Veterans Administration Hospital,
First Avenue at East 24th Street, New York, New York 10010 (USA).

Recent Advances in Studies on
Cardiac Structure and Metabolism, Volume 12
Cardiac Adaptation
Edited by T. Kobayashi, Y. Ito, and G. Rona
Copyright 1978 University Park Press Baltimore

THE EFFECT OF AEROBIC AND ANOXIC PERFUSION ON PROTEIN SYNTHESIS IN CARDIAC ARREST

S. S. SCHREIBER, D. J. HEARSE, M. ORATZ, and M. A. ROTHSCHILD

Radioisotope Service, New York Veterans Administration Hospital,
New York, New York; Department of Medicine, New York University School of Medicine;
Department of Biochemistry, New York University College of Dentistry,
New York, New York, USA; and Myocardial Metabolism Research Laboratories,
The Rayne Institute, St. Thomas' Hospital, London, S.E.1, United Kingdom

SUMMARY

When pressure stress is applied to the heart, there is an increase in protein synthesis leading ultimately to cardiac hypertrophy. However, the relationship between protein synthesis and contraction itself is not clear. To evaluate this contraction-protein synthesis relation, an *in vitro* preparation was used in which one could apply loads to the right ventricle used as the test ventricle and at the same time control the coronary flow through an independent perfusion system via the aorta. In contracting hearts and hearts arrested with K^+ (16 mEq/liter) and aerobically perfused, ATP, creatine phosphate, potassium, and glycogen levels were maintained and lactate produced was normal. Protein synthesis, measured from the incorporation of ^{14}C labeled lysine, was the same in contracting and in aerobically perfused high K^+-arrested hearts. Moreover, after 3 hr of such arrest, there was a 95% recovery of contractility when the K^+-arrested hearts were reperfused with normal perfusate (K^+ = 4 mEq/liter). In contrast, anoxic perfusion with normal K^+ (4 mEq/liter) induced arrest by 20–30 min, decreased incorporation of labeled lysine into protein and was associated with profound falls in ATP, creatine phosphate, glycogen, and potassium with sharp increases in lactate produced and no revival of contraction after 3 hr. The changes with anoxic perfusion were minimized when anoxic hearts were concomitantly perfused with high K^+ (16 mEq/liter), and there was also a recovery of 70% of contractility after 3 hr of such perfusion. The data suggested that cardiac arrest induced by K^+ (16 mEq/liter) with either aerobic or anoxic perfusion permits continuation of viability, recovery of contractility after 3 hr of such perfusion, as well as maintenance of near normal protein synthesis. The data also suggest that a baseline rate of protein synthesis occurs in cardiac tissue that is not dependent on contraction per se.

INTRODUCTION

In an *in vitro* cardiac perfusion model, in which the coronary artery perfusion could be kept constant in the face of right ventricular stress (Schreiber *et al.,*

This work was supported in part by grants from the U.S. Public Health Service, HL 09562 and AA 00959, the Veterans Administration, and the British Heart Foundation.

1975), it was found that right ventricular protein synthesis increased with afterload pressure stress. The data supported a relationship between pressure, contractile effort, and protein synthesis. Therefore, it was of interest to ascertain if cessation of all contraction would lead to the reverse effect, i.e., a decrease in protein synthesis.

MATERIALS AND METHODS

Young male guinea pigs, 260–300 g, were used in all perfusion studies. Preparation of the heart for perfusion has been described previously (Schreiber *et al.*, 1975). In essence, coronary perfusion in this model was controlled and fixed, and the right ventricle was presented with a load. The right atrium received a combined fluid load, which included coronary perfusion (4 ml/min/g ventricle) and a separate additional flow (2 ml/min) via the inferior vena cava, and emptied into the right ventricle which pumped the fluid out the cannulated pulmonary artery. Right ventricular pressures, heart rate, amplitude, and dP/dt_{max} were recorded. After operation, the heart was transferred to a perfusion chamber (Schreiber *et al.*, 1975) and was equilibrated with control perfusate for 15 min and then perfused for an additional 3 hr, as follows:

Group A (control):   4 mM KCl perfusate gassed with 95% O_2/5% CO_2
Group B: 16 mM KCl perfusate gassed with 95% O_2/5% CO_2
Group C: 16 mM KCl perfusate gassed with 95% N_2/5% CO_2
Group D: 4 mM KCl perfusate gassed with 95% N_2/5% CO_2

Chemical analyses for total cardiac ATP, creatine phosphate, glycogen, and potassium, and lactate production measurements were carried out in members of each group (Hearse, Stewart, and Chain, 1974; Hearse, Stewart, and Braimbridge, 1975; Schreiber *et al.*, 1975; Schreiber *et al.*, 1977).

The perfusate was modified Krebs-Henseleit solution with added amino acids (Schreiber *et al.*, 1977), 37–38°C, with a pH of 7.45 ± 0.05.

Protein synthesis was measured using [^{14}C]lysine in the perfusate and defined as µmol of lysine incorporated/g of protein N from the following:

$$\frac{\text{cpm } [^{14}\text{C}]\text{lysine/g of protein N}}{\begin{array}{c}\text{Intracellular } [^{14}\text{C}]\text{lysine specific activity}\\ (\text{cpm } [^{14}\text{C}]\text{lysine/µmol of lysine})\end{array}}$$

RESULTS

During the equilibration period, the cardiac rate averaged 170 beats/min, right ventricular systolic pressure 5–6 mm Hg, amplitude of contraction 4 mm Hg,

Table 1. Protein synthesis in both ventricles of beating and arrested hearts perfused for 3 hr with constant coronary perfusion[a] (coronary flow 4 ml/min and right ventricular pressure 5 mm Hg)

Group	Perfusate mM KCl	Perfusate Aeration	Coronary perfusion RV/LV	ATP levels at end of 3 hr (μmol/g of N) RV	ATP levels at end of 3 hr (μmol/g of N) LV	Incorporation of [^{14}C]lysine (μmol lysine/g of protein N) RV	Incorporation of [^{14}C]lysine (μmol lysine/g of protein N) LV	Intracellular free lysine pool ([^{14}C]lysine specific activity[b]) RV	Intracellular free lysine pool ([^{14}C]lysine specific activity[b]) LV
A	4	O_2	1.14 ± 0.06	122 ± 5	113 ± 4	29.7 ± 2.5	25.8 ± 1.0	0.70 ± 0.03	0.70 ± 0.03
B	16	O_2	1.49 ± 0.25	124 ± 14	113 ± 3	26.0 ± 1.4	25.0 ± 1.4	0.74 ± 0.06	0.72 ± 0.06
B v. A			$p < 0.001$	N.S.	N.S.	N.S.	N.S.	N.S.	N.S.
C	16	N_2	1.47 ± 0.20	125 ± 26	117 ± 20	25.2 ± 1.5	20.5 ± 1.2	0.75 ± 0.02	0.74 ± 0.03
C v. A			$p < 0.001$	N.S.	N.S.	N.S.	$p < 0.05$	N.S.	N.S.
D	4	N_2	2.32 ± 0.19	46 ± 12	10 ± 3	22.4 ± 1.3	9.4 ± 0.6	0.78 ± 0.06	0.86 ± 0.06
D v. A			$p < 0.001$	$p < 0.001$	$p < 0.001$	$p < 0.05$	$p < 0.001$	N.S.	$p < 0.02$

[a]Data taken from Schreiber et al., 1977.
[b][^{14}C]lysine specific activity in intracellular precursor pool is expressed as a fraction of that in the perfusate.
p represents significance of groups compared to control beating hearts in Group A (Student's t-test); O_2 = perfusate aerated with oxygen; N_2 = perfusate gassed with nitrogen; RV = right ventricle; LV = left ventricle. Values are mean ± S.E.M.

and dP/dt_{max} 40–50 mm Hg/sec. In the controls (Group A), these parameters of cardiac activity were maintained for 3 hr. Anoxic perfusion with 4 mM KCl in Group D resulted in slowly progressive failure with arrest by 30 min of perfusion. With high K^+ (16 mM KCl) (Groups B and C), there was immediate arrest. After 3 hr of perfusion, when experimental perfusate was replaced by aerobically gassed normal perfusate, there was a 90% recovery of amplitude and dP/dt_{max} (right ventricle) and of cardiac rate in the high K^+-arrested aerobically perfused hearts (Group B) and a 70% recovery in the high K^+-arrested anoxically perfused hearts (Group C).

There was no significant change of lysine incorporation into protein in either ventricle in high K^+-arrested aerobically perfusated hearts (Group B) after 3 hr of perfusion, and only a slight decrease in the left ventricle incorporation with high K^+ in nitrogen gassed perfusate (Group C) (Table 1). In contrast, in arrest induced by anoxia with normal K^+ (Group D) protein, synthesis decreased significantly in both ventricles with a more marked fall in the left.

In the control of this model, ATP was maintained at 60% of that seen in nonperfused hearts for 3 hr (Group A), and similar levels were seen in high K^+-arrested hearts with or without anoxia (Groups B and C). Similarly, creatine phosphate, glycogen and potassium contents, and lactate production in high K^+-arrested hearts, with or without anoxia, were similar to controls. In contrast, with anoxia-induced arrest in normal K^+ (Group D), there was a sharp rise in lactate production with a fall in ATP, creatine phosphate, and glycogen and potassium levels (Table 2). Coronary artery pressures were the same in all groups. In this model, the right ventricle received approximately 14% more flow per gram than the left (Schreiber *et al.*, 1975). With arrest, especially that induced by anoxia, there was an even more marked shift to the right ventricle (Table 1).

DISCUSSION

Studies conducted with various cardiac models concur that afterload stress initiates augmented protein synthesis (Meerson, 1962; Martin *et al.*, 1974; Schreiber *et al.*, 1975), but the fundamental pressure-protein synthesis relationship in the stressed ventricle has been difficult to separate from contraction per se. The question posed in work with the present model was, "If increased contractile effort, caused by afterload, augmented synthesis, did it follow that cessation of contraction effected a decrease in protein synthesis?" (Schreiber *et al.*, 1977).

The integrity of the high K^+-arrested aerobically perfused guinea pig heart was confirmed by the maintenance of ATP, creatine phosphate, glycogen, and potassium with low lactate production, as in the beating controls, and by the

Table 2. Cardiac ATP, creatine phosphate, and glycogen levels with lactate production during 3 hr of perfusion in beating and arrested hearts[a]

Experiment[b]	Perfusion time (min)	ATP (μmol/g dry wt)	Creatine phosphate (μmol/g dry wt)	Glycogen (μmol/g dry wt)	Lactate production (μmol/min/g wet wt)
A	0	17.5 ± 2.9	25.9 ± 2.9	70.6 ± 4.2	0.35 ± 0.12
	50	14.4 ± 2.0	20.6 ± 1.8	72.8 ± 13.6	0.29 ± 0.1
	150	14.4 ± 1.4	20.9 ± 2.2	55.0 ± 7.4	0.33 ± 0.1
B	0	17.5 ± 2.9	25.9 ± 2.9	70.6 ± 4.2	0.22 ± 0.02
	50	18.2 ± 0.7	31.9 ± 1.7	123.4 ± 12.4	0.32 ± 0.1
	150	15.5 ± 1.4	26.0 ± 4.4	114.9 ± 26.0	0.33 ± 0.2
C	0	17.5 ± 2.9	25.9 ± 2.9	70.6 ± 4.2	0.34 ± 0.07
	50	16.1 ± 1.3	22.0 ± 4.2	82.6 ± 8.7	0.35 ± 0.04
	150	15.6 ± 1.6	23.6 ± 3.3	82.5 ± 11.6	0.35 ± 0.05
D	0	17.5 ± 2.9	25.9 ± 2.9	70.6 ± 4.2	1.52 ± 0.14
	50	7.9 ± 1.5	6.5 ± 1.5	13.1 ± 2.9	0.84 ± 0.18
	150	3.2 ± 1.4	3.6 ± 0.8	6.5 ± 1.1	0.62 ± 0.07

[a]Data obtained from Schreiber et al., 1977.
[b]The groups A–D are identical to those in Table 1.

resumption of contraction with restoration of normal perfusate. In this type of arrest, $[^{14}C]$lysine incorporation into protein was unaltered in either ventricle.

In contrast, anoxia, with normal K^+, induced right ventricular failure and delayed cessation of contraction as in the anoxic left ventricle (Neely *et al.*, 1973) with a marked drop in ATP, creatine phosphate, glycogen, and potassium, and a sharp rise in lactate production (Scheuer, 1972; Neely *et al.*, 1973; Brachfeld, 1974; Hearse, Stewart, and Chain, 1974; and Hearse, Stewart, and Braimbridge, 1975) accompanied by decreased protein synthesis as seen in other models (Jefferson *et al.*, 1971; Peterson and Lesch, 1975). The decline in protein synthesis and ATP level was less in the right than in the nonworking left ventricle. This difference is puzzling because the increased tension on the right ventricle would be expected to increase demand for ATP in contraction during the early response to anoxia, with a more rapid depletion of the high-energy phosphates (Katz, 1971; Opie, Mansford, and Owen, 1971). One explanation may reside in the increased enzymatic activity found in the left ventricle (Cryer and Bartley, 1974).

The findings in anoxia were minimized in hearts simultaneously arrested with high K^+ (Group C), and they may be explained by the immediate cessation of contraction induced by high K^+ and decreased demand for ATP. Protein synthesis in this group was close to normal.

Thus, this study presents data indicating that a "normal" rate of protein synthesis is maintained in the high K^+-arrested, but viable, heart and suggests that a baseline rate of protein synthesis occurs in cardiac tissue that is not dependent on contraction per se. The rate of protein synthesis in this model is not increased when the heart is subjected to low workloads; but, under the stress of overwork, particularly pressure load, baseline synthesis is augmented (Schreiber *et al.*, 1975).

Acknowledgments The authors acknowledge with thanks the technical assistance of Carl Nadolney, Fran Reff, Carole Evans, and Deborah Smith, and the secretarial assistance of Jean Miller and Marie Hanley.

REFERENCES

BRACHFELD, N. 1974. Ischemic myocardial metabolism and cell necrosis. Bull. N.Y. Acad. Med. 50:261–293.

CRYER, A., and BARTLEY, W. 1974. Enzymatic makeup of left and right ventricles of the normal rat heart and the changes shown in exposure to exercise and hypoxic exercise. J. Mol. Cell. Cardiol. 6:61–71.

HEARSE, D. J., STEWART, D. A., and CHAIN, E. B. 1974. Recovery from cardiac bypass and elective cardiac arrest. Circ. Res. 35:448–457.

HEARSE, D. J., STEWART, D. A., and BRAIMBRIDGE, M. V. 1975. Hypothermic arrest and potassium arrest. Circ. Res. 36:481–489.

JEFFERSON, L. S., WOLPERT, E. B., GIGER, K. E., and MORGAN, H. E. 1971.

Regulation of protein synthesis in heart muscle. III. Effects of anoxia on protein synthesis. J. Biol. Chem. 246:2171–2178.

KATZ, A.M. 1971. Mechanical and biochemical correlates of cardiac contraction. Mod. Concepts Cardiovasc. Dis. 40:39–48.

MARTIN, A. F., REDDY, M. K., ZAK, R., DOWELL, R. T., and RABINOWITZ, M. 1974. Protein metabolism in hypertrophied heart muscle. Circ. Res. 111(suppl. 4):32–42.

MEERSON, F. Z. 1962. Compensatory hyperfunction of the heart and cardiac insufficiency. Circ. Res. 10:250–258.

NEELY, J. R., ROVETTO, M. J., WHITMER, T., and MORGAN, H. E. 1973. Effects of ischemia on function and metabolism of the isolated working rat heart. Am. J. Physiol. 225:651–658.

OPIE, L. H., MANSFORD, K. R. L., and OWEN, P. 1971. Effects of increased heart work on glycolysis and adenine nucleotides in the perfused hearts of normal and diabetic rats. Biochem. J. 124:475–490.

PETERSON, M. B., and LESCH, M. 1975. Studies on the reversibility of anoxic damage to the myocardial protein synthetic mechanism: Effects of glucose. J. Mol. Cell. Cardiol. 7:175–190.

SCHEUER, J. 1972. The effect of hypoxia on glycolytic ATP production. J. Mol. Cell. Cardiol. 4:689–692.

SCHREIBER, S. S. HEARSE, D. J., ORATZ, M., and ROTHSCHILD, M. A. 1977. Protein synthesis in prolonged cardiac arrest. J. Mol. Cell. Cardiol. 9:87–100.

SCHREIBER, S. S., ROTHSCHILD, M. A., EVANS, C., REFF, F., and ORATZ, M. 1975. The effect of pressure or flow stress on right ventricular protein synthesis in the face of constant and restricted coronary perfusion. J. Clin. Invest. 55:1–11.

Mailing address:
Sidney S. Schreiber, M.D.,
Nuclear Medicine Service, Veterans Administration Hospital,
First Avenue at East 24th Street, New York, New York 10010 (USA).

PACEMAKER
AND
CONDUCTION SYSTEM

Recent Advances in Studies on
Cardiac Structure and Metabolism, Volume 12
Cardiac Adaptation
Edited by T. Kobayashi, Y. Ito, and G. Rona
Copyright 1978 University Park Press Baltimore

MORPHOLOGICAL EVIDENCE FOR NEURAL CONTROL
OF THE ACTIVITY OF RAT HEART PACEMAKER

M. MORAVEC-MOCHET, J. MORAVEC, and P. Y. HATT

INSERM U.2, Unit of Cardiovascular Pathology Research,
Léon Bernard Hospital, 94450 Limeil-Brevannes, France

INTRODUCTION

The ultrastructure of the atrioventricular node of the rat heart was examined on serial thin sections. The hearts were fixed by an *in vivo* perfusion fixation as described in our previous paper (Mochet, Moravec, and Hatt, 1975). Special attention was paid to the neuromuscular interrelationships. The most significant data are discussed below.

RESULTS AND DISCUSSION

The density of neural elements was highest in the anterior part of the node, in accordance with previous findings of optical microscopy. In addition to the myelinated and unmyelinated axons, at least three different types of nerve terminals were present in the interstitial space:

1. "Freely located" neural endings, similar to those described previously by another researcher (Virágh and Porte, 1961), were observed (Figure 1).
2. "Efferent endings," some of which were tightly coupled to the muscle cell, were seen. In this case, the intermembrane space was about 75 μm, and there often was an agglomerate of synaptic vesicles localized in front of the neuro-muscular junction. The only element separating the two cells was the basement membrane of the myocytes. In certain cases, a rudimentary post-synaptic apparatus also was present under the sarcolemma of the nodal cell. Both, empty (ϕ 50 μm) and dense core vesicles (ϕ 120 μm) were observed in these endings (Figure 2).
3. "Afferent endings," containing only a few vesicles but numerous mitochondria and glycogen granules, also were recognized. In this case the intermembrane space was less than 30 μm, and the basement membrane of the two cells disappeared at the site of neuromuscular junction (Figure 3).

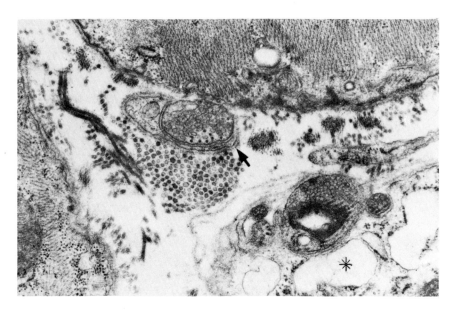

Figure 1. Two freely located neural endings containing the agglomerates of synaptic vesicles in contact with the thickening of the cell membrane can be noted (*). Another nerve terminal is much more tightly related to the nodal cell (↗). However, no pre- nor post-synaptic structure can be seen. × 24,000.

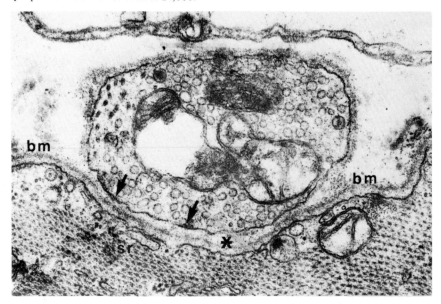

Figure 2. Synaptic neuromuscular junction: note the frequence of empty vesicles, thickening of the neurolemma (↗), enlargement of the intermembrane space containing the basement membrane (bm) of the muscle cell (*), as well as few tubules of the sarcoplasmic reticulum (sr) in front of the neural endings. × 53,000.

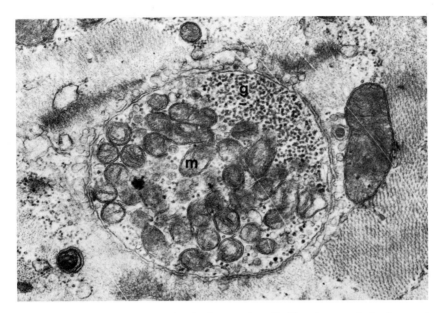

Figure 3. Sensory nerve terminal inside the muscle cell. The absence of the basement membrane (bm) should be noted in the latter. m = mitochondria; g = glycogen granules. × 24,500.

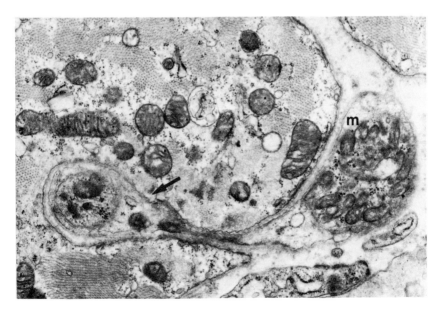

Figure 4. Sensory nerve terminal, with numerous mitochondria (m) and abundant glycogen stores, penetrates into a profound invagination of the sarcolemma of the nodal cell (↗). Only a few vesicles are visible. × 19,000.

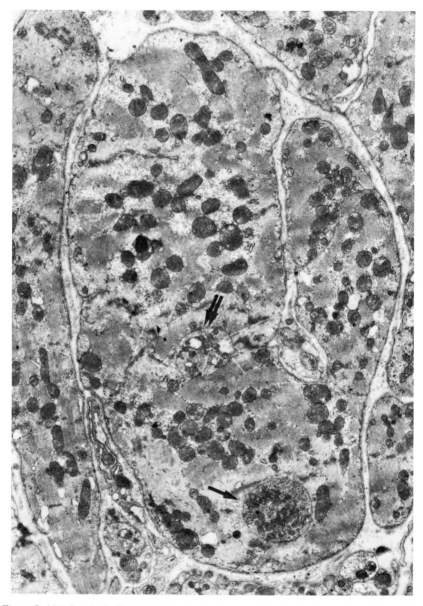

Figure 5. Muscle spindle-like structure: double innervation of a single muscle cell, i.e., both motor (⇒) and sensory nerve terminals (↗), supply the same nodal cell. A few free nerve terminals (*) also can be seen. × 8,900.

Some of these sensory terminals seemed to penetrate into the profound intracellular invaginations of the sarcolemma (Figure 4).

In a few cases, both motor and sensory innervation of one single nodal cell could be seen (Figure 5). This picture resembles the ultrastructural arrangement of skeletal muscle spindles, suggesting the possibility of neural feedbacks involved in the control of the pacemaker.

The analogy between nodal cells and muscle spindles is further suggested by the presence of leptomeric figures and centrioles in the perinuclear spaces and by close relationships between nodal cells and their connective environment, supplying a solid mechanical support (Mochet, Moravec, and Hatt, 1975). Furthermore, the existence of intracardiac ganglia in proximity to the pacemaker evokes the possibility that some of the "intrinsic" properties of the pacemaker may be of a neural nature.

REFERENCES

IRISAWA, A. 1977. Fine structure of the sinoatrial node of rabbit heart. This volume.

JAMES, T. N., and SHERF, L. 1971. Fine structure of the His bundle. Circulation 44:9–28.

MOCHET, M., MORAVEC, J., and HATT, P. Y. 1975. The ultrastructure of rat conductive tissue: An EM study of the atrioventricular node and bundle of His. J. Mol. Cell. Cardiol. 7:879–889.

THAEMERT, J. C. 1970. Atrioventricular node innervation in ultrastructural three dimensions. Am. J. Anat. 128:239–264.

THAEMERT, J. C. 1973. Fine structure of the atrioventricular node as viewed in serial sections. Am. J. Anat. 136:43–66.

VIRÁGH, S., and PORTE, A. 1961. Elements nerveux intracardiaques et innervation du myocarde. Etude au microscope électronique dans le coeur de rat. Z. Zellforsch. Mikrosk. Anat. 55:282–296.

Mailing address:
M. Moravec-Mochet, M.D.,
INSERM U.2, Unité de Recherches de Pathologie Cardio-vasculaire,
Hôpital Léon Bernard, 94450 Limeil-Brevannes (France).

Recent Advances in Studies on
Cardiac Structure and Metabolism, Volume 12
Cardiac Adaptation
Edited by T. Kobayashi, Y. Ito, and G. Rona
Copyright 1978 University Park Press Baltimore

FINE STRUCTURE OF THE SINOATRIAL NODE OF RABBIT HEART

H. IRISAWA

Department of Physiology, School of Medicine,
Hiroshima University, Hiroshima, Japan

SUMMARY

The structure of rabbit sinoatrial (SA) node cells has been studied with the electron microscope. There are three kinds of cells within the SA node region. Small nexus structures are found between nodal cells.

INTRODUCTION

Although a large number of studies have appeared on the structure and function of the sinoatrial (SA) node cells (Hayashi, 1962; Trautwein and Uchizono, 1963; James, 1967; Brooks and Lu, 1972), the description of the size and shape of SA node cells greatly varies from animal to animal. Even within the same animal species, there are some controversies over the description of the nodal tissue. Recently, the electrical coupling of SA node cells was observed with the space constant of 0.5 mm (Bonke, 1973) and 0.8 mm (Seyama, 1976). From these findings, the presence of nexus contacts is suggested between adjacent SA node cells. Nexus structures in the SA node, some of which were previously used in physiological experiments, were studied.

MATERIALS AND METHODS

Twelve rabbit hearts were used in this study. Specimens were obtained from a strip dissected perpendicular to the crista terminalis. Sections were cut parallel to the crita terminalis. Most specimens were fixed in 4% glutaraldehyde in 0.1 M cacodylate buffer (pH = 7.4) or in 0.1 M phosphate buffer (pH = 7.4), post-fixed in 1% OsO_4, and stained with 1% $KMnO_4$-acetone solution before embedding in Epon mixture. Thin sections were stained with uranyl acetate and lead hydroxide and examined by Hitachi HS-7 electron microscope. For light microscopy, sections less than 1 μm thick were prepared and stained with 1% toluidine blue.

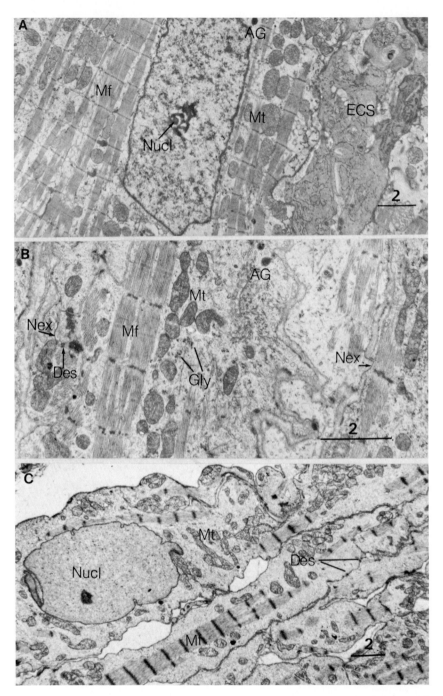

Figure 1. Electron micrograph of the three types of SA node cells. A: Type 1 cell: Myofibrils are separated by a row of mitochondria as commonly seen in atrial cardiocytes. ×
6,400. B: Type 2 cells: Fewer myofibrils, sparse mitochondria, pale sarcoplasm, two nexuses (arrows), and desmosomes are seen. × 10,000. C:Type 3 cells: A part of muscle network that appeared in the thinner portion of the node. Thin irregular cardiac muscle cells with intimate contacts, scattered small mitochondria, and sarcoplasmic reticulum are noted. ×
5,400. AG = atrial granules; CP = cell process; Des = desmosome; ECS = extracellular space; Gly = glycogen; Gol = Golgi complex; Mf = myofibril; Mt = mitochondria; Nex = nexus; Nucl = nucleus.

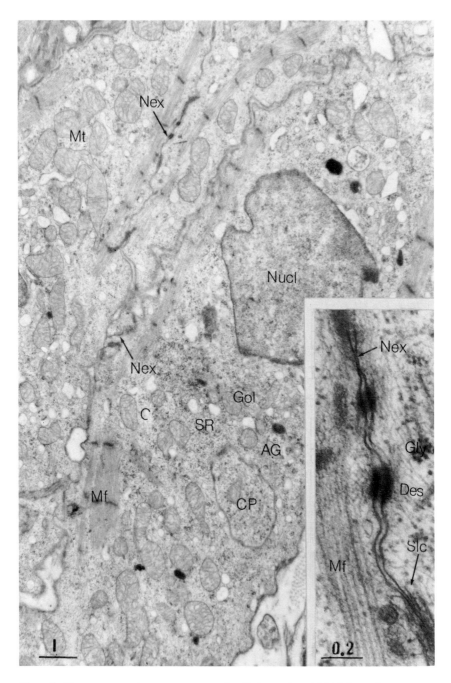

Figure 2. Nexus contacts between two type 3 cells (arrows). × 10,000. Inset shows a nexus contact in higher magnification. × 57,000. AG = atrial granules; CP = cell process; Des = desmosome; Gly = glycogen; Gol = Golgi complex; Mf = myofibril; Mt = mitochondria; Nex = nexus; Nucl = nucleus; Slc = ———; SR = sarcoplasmic reticulum.

RESULTS AND DISCUSSION

Three types of cells were observed within the SA node region. The first type of cells (type 1) have all the characteristics of the atrial cells (Figure 1A). The second type of cells (type 2) are slender and have fewer myofibrils and mitochondria than type 1 cells. The nexus contacts are observed between the adjoining cells, but they are shorter in length than those of the atrial myocardium. Short desmosomes are observed frequently (Figure 1B). The third type of cells (type 3) are small and are characterized by poorly developed myofibrils, large oval nuclei, sparse mitochondria, pale sarcoplasm, containing scattered filamentous structures, and glycogen granules (Figure 2, inset). The adjacent cells are in close contact with each other, with the gaps less than 200 Å; small desmosomal structures are observed frequently, but typical intercalated discs are not found. Nexus structures among type 3 cells are small in size and occur less frequently than within type 2 cells (Figure 1C and Figure 2).

These histological findings are in close agreement with electrophysiological findings (Noma and Irisawa, personal communication). Type 1 cells occur most frequently within the crista terminalis. As type 1 cells decrease in number, type 2 cells appear more frequently. Type 2 cells form thin strands that are separated by a broad band of collagenous connective tissue containing vascular and neural elements. In the thinnest part of the SA node region, type 3 cells are most abundant, and they form irregular networks surrounded by large interstitial spaces. In this region, type 2 cells also are found. Neuromuscular close apposition (less than 200 Å) is observed frequently in the type 3 cell area. Because the spontaneous activity and the electrical couplings are observed in the specimen containing mainly type 2 and 3 cells, the morphological identification of the "true" pacemaker cell remains to be elucidated.

REFERENCES

BONKE, F. I. M. 1973. Electrotonic spread in the sinoatrial node of the rabbit heart. Pfluegers Arch. 339:17–23.
BROOKS, C. M., and LU, H. 1972. The Sinoatrial Pacemaker of the Heart. Charles C Thomas, Springfield, Ill.
HAYASHI, K. 1962. An electronmicroscope study on the conduction system of cow heart. Jpn. Circ. J. 26:765–804.
JAMES, T. N. 1967. Anatomy of the cardiac conduction system in the rabbit. Circ. Res. 20:638–648.
SEYAMA, I. 1976. Characteristics of the rectifying properties of the sinoatrial node cell of the rabbit. J. Physiol. (Lond.) 255:379–397.
TRAUTWEIN, W., and UCHIZONO, K. 1963. Electronmicroscopic and electrophysiologic study of the pacemaker in the sinoatrial node of the rabbit heart. Z. Zellforsch. Mikrosk. Anat. 61:96–109.

Mailing address:
H. Irisawa,
Department of Physiology, School of Medicine,
Hiroshima University, Hiroshima (Japan).

Recent Advances in Studies on
Cardiac Structure and Metabolism, Volume 12
Cardiac Adaptation
Edited by T. Kobayashi, Y. Ito, and G. Rona
Copyright 1978 University Park Press Baltimore

FINE STRUCTURE OF THE CONDUCTION SYSTEM AND WORKING MYOCARDIUM IN THE LITTLE BROWN BAT, *MYOTIS LUCIFUGUS*

K. KAWAMURA, F. URTHALER, and T. N. JAMES

Cardiovascular Research and Training Center, University of Alabama
School of Medicine, Birmingham, Alabama, USA

SUMMARY

In the little brown bat, *Myotis lucifugus,* topography and ultrastructure of the sinus node and the atrioventricular (AV) node resemble those in larger mammalian hearts, except that the P cells in the sinus node are smaller than those in the bat AV node or those in the sinus node of slower hearts (e.g., dog, man). Despite rich innervation in the bat nodes, true neuromuscular synapses are rarely formed. Bat working cardiocytes have a well developed sarcoplasmic reticulum, but otherwise resemble working myocytes of larger mammals.

INTRODUCTION

Among all mammals, small bats appear to be unique in that they have a very rapid heart rate (over 1,000 beats/min) under some physiological conditions (Studier and Howell, 1969). Their resting heart rate of approximately 500 beats/min corresponds to that of the hummingbird (Figure 1). Furthermore, bat heart rates have been shown by telemetry to vary from one extreme to another in only a few seconds under normal physiological conditions (Studier and Howell, 1969). This high heart rate may be related to the small size of the heart, but the speed of variability also suggests that bats may have a specifically developed structure of the pacemaker and working myocardium for such prompt physiological responses. The purpose of this study was to investigate the fine structure of the sinus node, the atrioventricular (AV) node, and the working myocardium in the little brown bat, and to compare these observations to the heart in larger mammals (Kawamura, 1961; Hayashi, 1962; Torii, 1962; Traut-

This work was supported by the National Heart and Lung Institute, Program Project Grant HL 11310, and the Specialized Center for Research on Ischemic Heart Disease, No. 1 P17 HL 17667.

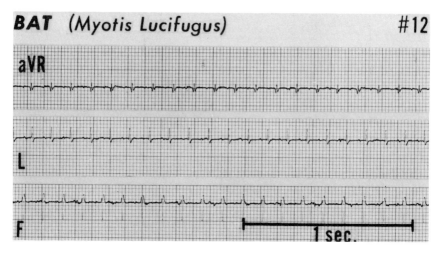

Figure 1. Electrocardiogram of a little brown bat under ether anesthesia. The heart rate is approximately 540 beats/min.

wein and Uchizono, 1963; James *et al.,* 1966; Maekawa *et al.,* 1967; Nilsson and Sporrong, 1970; James and Sherf, 1968, 1974; Cheng, Y.-P., 1971; Kawamura and James, 1971; Kim and Baba, 1971; Simpson, Rayns, and Ledingham, 1973; Thaemert, 1973; Virágh and Challice, 1973; McNutt and Fawcett, 1974; Mochet *et al.,* 1975; Tranum-Jensen, 1976).

MATERIALS AND METHODS

Thirteen little brown bats, *Myotis lucifugus,* 5.3 g in mean body weight, were captured in caves, during the period November through March, while they were hibernating. They were kept in a dark chamber at 10°C and sacrificed within three days. Following thoracotomy under ether anesthesia, the heart was removed and fixed *in toto* for 2–5 hr in either 2–6% glutaraldehyde in 0.1 M phosphate or cacodylate buffer, pH 7.2–7.5, or in a mixture of 4% paraformaldehyde and 3 or 5% glutaraldehyde in 0.1 M cacodylate buffer, pH 7.2–7.4. During fixation the heart was dissected under a stereomicroscope and the respective tissue blocks containing the sinus node, the AV node, and the working myocardium of atria, ventricular walls, and papillary muscles were obtained. The blocks were post-fixed in 1% osmium for 2 hr and embedded in epon or araldite. One micron section was stained with toluidine blue. Ultrathin sections were cut on a Porter-Blum MT-1 microtome. Electron microscopy was conducted in a Philips 300 electron microscope.

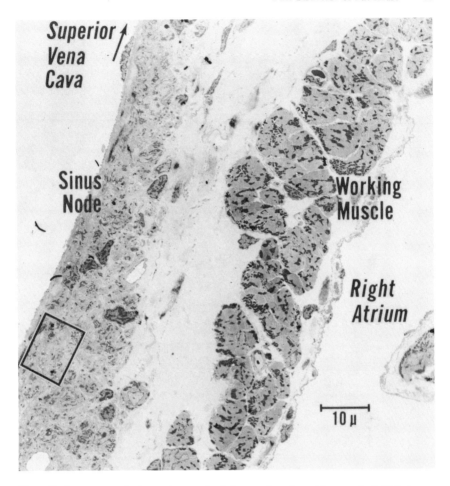

Figure 2. Low power electron micrograph of sinus node and working muscle in little brown bat. The sinus node appears pale, in contrast to the darker working myocardium. The area within the rectangle is magnified in Figure 3. × 1,300.

RESULTS

Sinus Node

The sinus node was a flattened and elongated structure with a transverse diameter of about 25 by 160 μm, located beneath the sulcus terminalis. The main nodal mass lay near the endocardium between the root of the right superior vena cava and the crista terminalis (Figure 2). The nodal artery had a single layer of smooth muscle cells in the tunica media. The sinus node con-

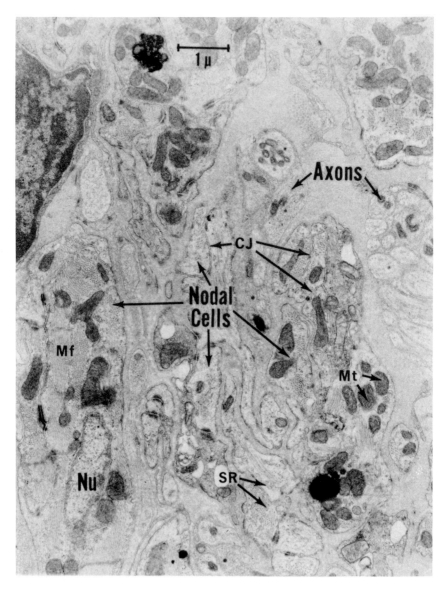

Figure 3. A typical profile of bat sinus node. CJ = cell junctions; Mf = myofibril; Mt = mitochondria; Nu = nucleus; SR = sarcoplasmic reticulum. (See text.) × 14,000.

tained numerous P cells and abundant nerve fibers. The P cells were pleo-morphic, containing sparse myofibrils, small mitochondria, poorly developed sarcoplasmic reticulum, and relatively large nuclei. There were no specific granules or T tubules in the P cells. The structural features of these P cells were basically the same as those of the P cells (probable pacemaker cells) designated in larger mammals (Trautwein and Uchizono, 1963; James et al., 1966; James and Sherf, 1968, 1974). In the bat, however, the P cells were much smaller, usually being less than 4 μm in transverse diameter, crossing through the nucleus. Many P cell profiles were less than 1 μm in diameter and thus comparable in size to the profiles of nerve axon varicosities (Figure 3). The P cells were organized into clusters in which the cell junctions contained only a few desmosomes, small fasciae adherentes, and very scarce rudimentary nexuses (Figure 3). In the periphery of the node the P cells were connected with the *transitional* cells, which in size, intracellular structure, and profiles of cell junctions were inter-mediate between the P cells and working cardiocytes in the atria. Transitional

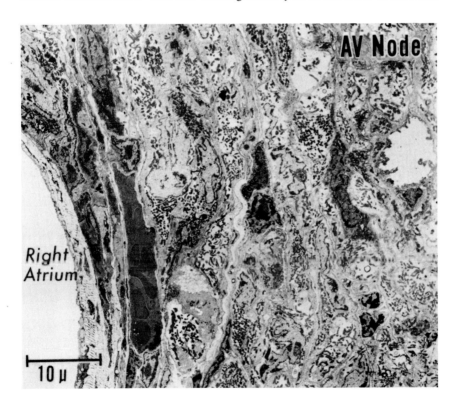

Figure 4. Low power electron micrograph of AV node in little brown bat. The AV nodal P cells are larger and more densely organized than the sinus nodal P cells (cf. Figure 2). × 2,050.

cells were then connected with other atrial cardiocytes. Nerve fibers appeared to be comparatively more numerous than those in sinus nodes of larger animals (Kawamura, 1961; James *et al.*, 1966; Maekawa *et al.*, 1967; James and Sherf, 1968). The axon varicosities usually contained numerous agranular or occasional granular vesicles. Although these axons were located near P cell surfaces, membrane-to-membrane synapses were rarely formed between them (Figure 3).

AV Node

The AV node lay subjacent to the attachment of the septal leaflet of the tricuspid valve. The main nodal mass occupied a relatively large space, having a transverse diameter of about 45 by 140 μm. In the main nodal tissue the myocytes resembled the P cells in the sinus node with regard to intracellular structure and intercellular junction. The AV nodal P cells were, however, usually

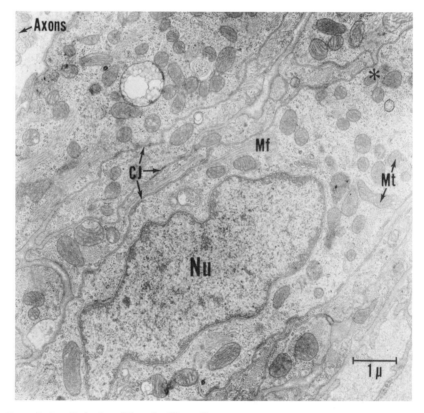

Figure 5. P cells in bat AV node. CJ = cell junction; Mf = myofibril; Mt = mitochondria; Nu = nucleus. Asterisk shows a point where three cell junctions come together at one point. (See text.) × 12,000.

larger (2–5 μm in transverse diameter, crossing through the nucleus) and more densely organized (Figure 4). Many cells were polyhedrally connected with one another so that three cell junctions frequently came together at one point in electron micrograph (Figure 5). Nerve axon varicosities were abundant but less dense in population than in the sinus node. The P cells were connected with *transitional* cells near the posterior portion of the AV node. In the anterior portion of the node, the P cells were connected with slender myocytes in the His bundle. Fine structure of the His bundle and its branches was not a subject of the present study.

Working Myocardium

In the left ventricular papillary muscle, the fibers varied between 8 and 14 μm in transverse diameter (Figure 6). Ultrastructural features of the contractile material, T system, lysosomes, glycogen granules, nuclei, and intercalated discs were essentially the same as those in larger mammalian hearts (Simpson, Rayns, and Ledingham, 1973; McNutt and Fawcett, 1974) (Figure 7). In bat working-cardiocytes, however, the sarcoplasmic reticulum was remarkably well developed. In transverse section of the muscle, numerous vesicular profiles of the sarcoplasmic reticulum were arranged in rows so that the myofibrils outlined by these vesicular rows were rather thin (Figure 7).

DISCUSSION

Within the bat sinus node the P cells resemble those of sinus nodes in larger mammalian hearts (Trautwein and Uchizono, 1963; James *et al.*, 1966; James and Sherf, 1968, 1974), except that P cells of bat sinus node are smaller (less than 4 μm) in transverse diameter than those (4–12 μm) in larger mammals (Trautwein and Uchizono, 1963; James *et al.*, 1966; Virágh and Challice, 1973). In bat sinus node, nerve axon varicosities are conspicuously abundant and more densely populated than in more slowly beating hearts (Kawamura, 1961; James *et al.*, 1966; Maekawa *et al.*, 1967; James and Sherf, 1968). This rich innervation, combined with the small size of the P cells, may help explain the speed of neurophysiological responses recorded in the bat heart. The AV nodal P cells in the bat are larger than the P cells of bat sinus node, being similar in size to the AV nodal P cells (ca. 5 μm) in larger mammals (Virágh and Challice, 1973; Mochet *et al.*, 1975). Working myocytes of bat ventricle (8–14 μm) are approximately the same size as ventricular myocytes in larger hearts, e.g., dog (5–16 μm) (Kawamura and James, unpublished observations) or man (10–15 μm) (Maron, Ferrans, and Roberts, 1975), despite the fact that the bat heart is much smaller in total myocardial mass. This indicates that the smaller size of the bat heart must be attributable to fewer, rather than smaller, cells, although it should be noted that the sinus node is an exception to this statement because its cells arc

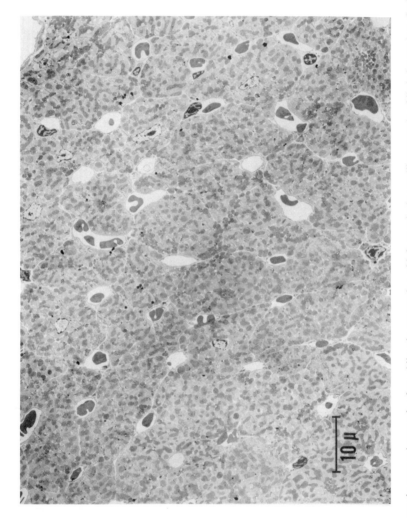

Figure 6. Low power electron micrograph of an obliquely cut section of left ventricular papillary muscle of little brown bat. Capillary to muscle fiber ratio is approximately one to one. × 1,500.

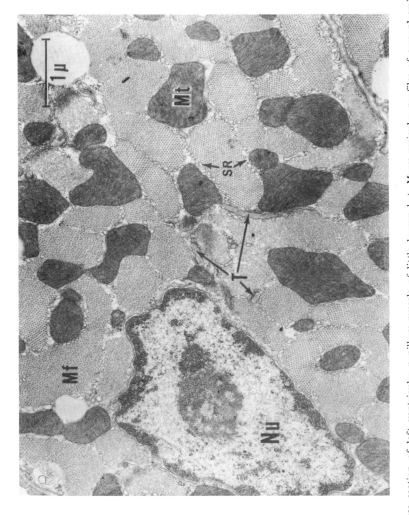

Figure 7. Transverse section of left ventricular papillary muscle of little brown bat. Many vesicular profiles of sarcoplasmic reticulum (SR) are arranged in rows so that the myofibrils (Mf) intervening between these vesicular rows and mitochondria (Mt) are slender. Nu = nucleus; T = T tubules. × 18,000.

genuinely smaller in size than its counterpart in larger hearts. Increased volume of well developed sarcoplasmic reticulum in bat working cardiocytes may provide the advantage of prompt release and sequestration of calcium, presumably required for the normally rapid bat heart.

REFERENCES

CHENG, Y.-P. 1971. The ultrastructure of the rat sino-atrial node. Acta Anat. Nippon. 46:339–358.

HAYASHI, K. 1962. An electron microscope study on the conduction system of the cow heart. Jpn. Circ. J. 16:765–842.

JAMES, T. N., SHERF, L., FINE, G., and MORALES, A. R. 1966. Comparative ultrastructure of the sinus node in man and dog. Circulation 34:139–162.

JAMES, T. N., and SHERF, L. 1968. Ultrastructure of the human atrioventricular node. Circulation 37:1049–1070.

JAMES, T. N., and SHERF, L. 1974. Ultrastructure of the myocardium. In J. W. Hurst, R. B. Logue, R. C. Schlant, and N. K. Wenger (eds.), The Heart, pp. 63–79. 3rd Ed. McGraw-Hill Book Co., New York.

KAWAMURA, K. 1961. Electron microscope studies on the cardiac conduction system of the dog. II. The sinoatrial and atrioventricular node. Jpn. Circ. J. 25:973–1013.

KAWAMURA, K., and JAMES, T. N. 1971. Comparative ultrastructure of cellular junctions in working myocardium and the conduction system under normal and pathologic conditions. J. Mol. Cell. Cardiol. 3:31–60.

KIM, S., and BABA, N. 1971. Atrioventricular node and Purkinje fibers of the guinea pig heart. Am. J. Anat. 132:337–354.

McNUTT, N. S., and FAWCETT, D. W. 1974. Myocardial ultrastructure. In G. A. Langer and A. J. Brady (eds.), Mammalian Myocardium, pp. 1–49. John Wiley & Sons, New York.

MAEKAWA, M., NOHARA, Y., KAWAMURA, K., and HAYASHI, K. 1967. Electron microscopy of the conduction system in mammalian hearts. In T. Sano, V. Mizuhira, and K. Matsuda (eds.), Electrophysiology and Ultrastructure of the Heart, pp. 41–54. Bunkodo, Tokyo.

MARON, B. J., FERRANS, V. J., and ROBERTS, W. C. 1975. Ultrastructural features of degenerated cardiac muscle cells in patients with cardiac hypertrophy. Am. J. Pathol. 79:387–434.

MOCHET, M., MORAVEC, J., GUILLEMOT, H., and HATT, P. Y. 1975. The ultrastructure of rat conductive tissue; an electron microscopic study of the atrioventricular node and the bundle of His. J. Mol. Cell. Cardiol. 7:879–889.

NILSSON, E., and SPORRONG, B. 1970. Electron microscopic investigation of adrenergic and non-adrenergic axons in the rabbit SA-node. Z. Zellforsch. 111:404–412.

SIMPSON, F. O., RAYNS, D. G., and LEDINGHAM, J. M. 1973. The ultrastructure of ventricular and atrial myocardium. In C. E. Challice and S. Virágh (eds.), Ultrastructure of the Mammalian Heart, pp. 1–41. Academic Press, New York.

STUDIER, E. H., and HOWELL, D. J. 1969. Heart rate of female big brown bats in flight. J. Mammal. 50:842–845.

THAEMERT, J. C. 1973. Fine structure of the atrioventricular node as viewed in serial sections. Am. J. Anat. 136:43–66.

TORII, H. 1962. Electron microscope observation of the S-A and A-V nodes and Purkinje fibers of the rabbit. Jpn. Circ. J. 26:39–77.

TRANUM-JENSEN, J. 1976. The fine structure of the atrial and atrioventricular (AV) junctional specialized tissues of the rabbit heart. In H. J. J. Wellens, K. I. Lie, and M. J. Janse (eds.), The Conduction System of the Heart, pp. 55–81. Lea and Febiger, Philadelphia.

TRAUTWEIN, W., and UCHIZONO, K. 1963. Electron microscopic and electrophysiologic study of the pacemaker in the sino-atrial node of the rabbit heart. Z. Zellforsch. 61:96–109.

VIRÁGH, S., and CHALLICE, C. E. 1973. The impulse generation and conduction system of the heart. *In* C. E. Challice and S. Virágh (eds.), Ultrastructure of the Mammalian Heart, pp. 43–89. Academic Press, New York.

Mailing address:
Dr. Thomas N. James,
Cardiovascular Research and Training Center, University of Alabama School of Medicine, University Station, Birmingham, Alabama 35294 (USA).

Recent Advances in Studies on
Cardiac Structure and Metabolism, Volume 12
Cardiac Adaptation
Edited by T. Kobayashi, Y. Ito, and G. Rona
Copyright 1978 University Park Press Baltimore

ELECTRON MICROSCOPIC CYTOCHEMISTRY
OF CYTOCHROME OXIDASE ACTIVITY
IN THE CONDUCTION SYSTEM OF THE CANINE HEART

K. KAWAMURA and T. N. JAMES

Cardiovascular Research and Training Center, University of Alabama
School of Medicine, Birmingham, Alabama, USA

SUMMARY

Histochemistry and electron microscopic cytochemistry of cytochrome oxidase in the conduction system were studied with the 3,3'-diaminobenzidine (DAB) method in adult canine hearts. This enzyme was distinctly less active in the entire conduction system than in the working myocardium. By electron microscopy, enzymatic activity per cristal membrane was apparently similar in both specialized and working cardiocytes. However, the volume fraction of cell occupied by mitochondria and the density of cristal membranes in mitochondria were smaller in the specialized cells in the sinus node, atrioventricular (AV) node, His bundle, and Purkinje fibers. These observations define the nature of decreased histochemical activity of cytochrome oxidase in cells of the conduction system, which is caused entirely by the decrease in activity per unit of mitochondrial volume and unit of cell volume in the specialized cardiac tissues.

INTRODUCTION

In most histochemical studies of cytochrome oxidase in the conduction system in various mammals (Schiebler, 1955, 1961, 1963; Schiebler and Doerr, 1963; Alcini, Lageron, and Wegmann, 1965; Morales and Fine, 1965; Wegmann and Suékané, 1966; Otsuka, Hara, and Okamoto, 1967), this enzyme has been reported to be much lower in activity in the conduction system than in the working myocardium. In these reports, the histochemical methods employed were invariably based upon the Nadi reaction. The osmiophilic properties of the indoanilines, an enzymatic product from the Nadi reaction, can be used to localize intracellular activity of cytochrome oxidase (Sabatini, Bensch, and Barrnett, 1963; Seligman et al., 1967). For example, in working myocardium, droplets of reaction product occur primarily in the mitochondria and occa-

This work was supported by the National Heart and Lung Institute, Program Project Grant HL 11310, and the Specialized Center for Research on Ischemic Heart Disease, No. 1 P17 HL 17667.

sionally in the sarcotubules. However, these droplets are so coarse that the method is of little value for precise localization of the enzymatic activity (Seligman *et al.*, 1968).

More recently, Seligman *et al.* (1968) published a report on a new method using 3,3'-diaminobenzidine (DAB) to demonstrate cytochrome oxidase activity. This method yields a nondroplet form of reaction product that is located on the outer surface of the inner membrane, in the intracristal spaces, and in the outer compartment between the inner and outer limiting membranes of mitochondria. This new method has significantly improved the accuracy of localization of cytochrome oxidase. The purpose of our study was to employ the Seligman method to determine the intracellular localization of cytochrome oxidase activity in the conduction system and to compare it with that in the working myocardium in canine hearts.

MATERIALS AND METHODS

Four adult mongrel dogs were anesthetized with sodium pentobarbital (30 mg/kg i.v.). After thoracotomy, both the sinus node and the atrioventricular (AV) node arteries were cannulated with small catheters (James and Nadeau, 1962; James *et al.*, 1970), and formaldehyde fixative described by Seligman *et al.* (1968) was perfused so that both nodes were selectively fixed. After removal of the heart, tissue blocks containing the sinus node, AV node, His bundle, false tendons, subendocardial Purkinje fibers, and papillary muscles were dissected and further fixed for up to 60 min, first as large pieces and then cut into smaller (about 1 mm) cubes. Some blocks were further cut into 50-μm sections on a vibratome. The specimens were incubated in the DAB medium and fixed with osmic vapor (Seligman *et al.*, 1968). Control study was conducted with KCN added to the incubation medium. The specimens were embedded in epon. Care was taken to assure that 5-μm sections for histochemistry and ultrathin sections for electron microscopic cytochemistry actually contained the specialized tissue and/or working myocardium lying within 20 μm of the section edge of tissue specimens. Examinations were made with a Philips 300 electron microscope. Quantitative analysis of the volume fraction of cell occupied by mitochondria was conducted with the point counting method described by McCallister and Page (1973).

RESULTS

Light Microscopic Histochemistry

In 5-μm sections, positive enzymatic reaction was shown as depositions of dark brownish pigments within cells in a whole section cut on a vibratome or in those which were cut within approximately 20 μm of the section edge of any tissue

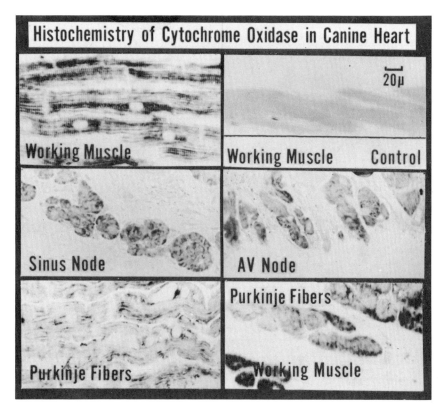

Figure 1. The right top shows control reaction. The others demonstrate enzymatic activity. In the left and right bottom, the Purkinje fibers in false tendon and left ventricular subendocardial space are shown, respectively. Magnifications are the same in all photomicrographs. (See text.) × 250.

block immersed in the DAB medium during incubation. No colored pigment was present in control specimens (Figure 1). Depositions of the reaction product appeared to be much less dense and more irregularly distributed in the specialized cardiocytes in the sinus node, AV node, His bundle, and Purkinje fibers than in the working myocardium (Figure 1).

Electron Microscopic Cytochemistry

Observations were limited to the sections cut on a vibratome or to those cells cut from within 20 μm of the section edge of tissue blocks. In both working and specialized cardiocytes, depositions of osmiophilic reaction produced from cytochrome oxidase activity were localized to the inner mitochondrial membranes, the intracristal spaces, and/or the outer compartment between the inner and

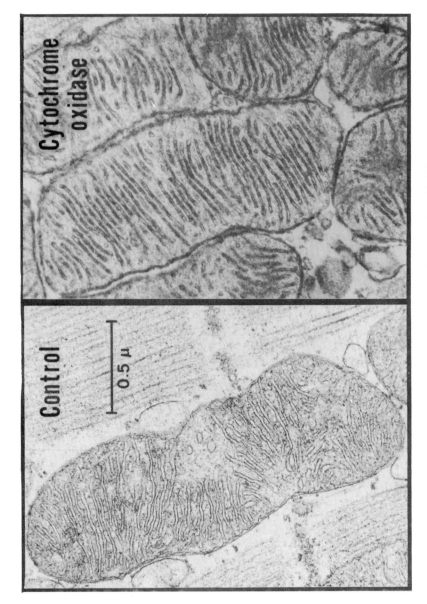

Figure 2. Mitochondria in working cardiocytes of left ventricular papillary muscle. × 50,000.

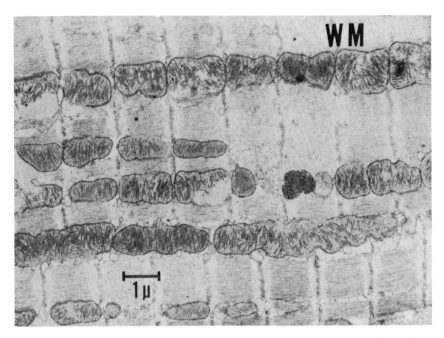

Figure 3. Cytochrome oxidase activity in working cardiocyte of left ventricular papillary muscle (WM). × 10,400.

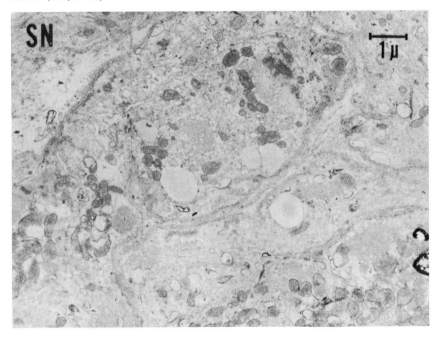

Figure 4. Cytochrome oxidase activity in P cells of sinus node (SN). × 10,400.

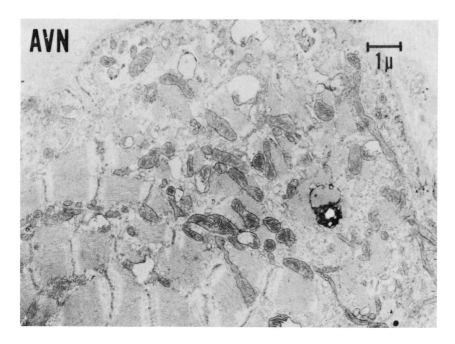

Figure 5. Cytochrome oxidase activity in P cells of AV node (AVN). × 10,400.

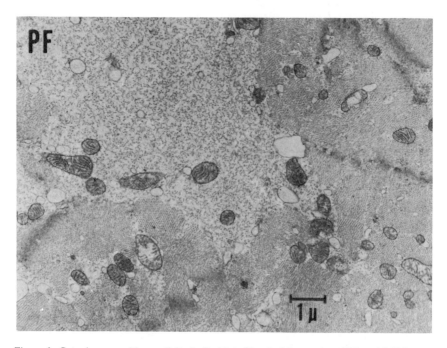

Figure 6. Cytochrome oxidase activity in Purkinje fiber in false tendon (PF). × 10,400.

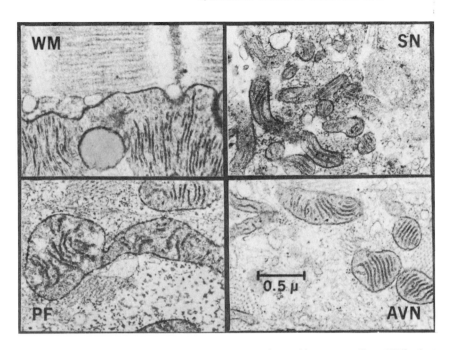

Figure 7. Cytochrome oxidase activity in cardiocyte in working myocardium (WM), sinus node (SN), AV node (AVN), and Purkinje fiber (PF). Compared with those in working myocytes (WM), the cristae mitochondriales are less dense in many mitochondria in the conduction system (SN, AVN, and PF). Magnifications are the same in all electron micrographs. × 26,000.

outer limiting membranes of mitochondria (Figures 2–7). Individual mitochondria were, however, smaller in size in the specialized cardiocytes in the sinus node, AV node, His bundle, and Purkinje fibers than in the working cardiocytes (Figures 3–6).

The volume fraction of cell occupied by mitochondria in the working myocytes of the left ventricular papillary muscle (26.4 ± 0.5% (mean ± S.E.M.)) was significantly greater than that in the Purkinje fibers in the false tendon (13.1 ± 0.6%) or than that in the specialized cardiocytes in the His bundle (16.0 ± 0.7%). In the sinus node and AV node, the mitochondrial population tended to be highly variable not only among the specialized cells but also in distribution within the same cell. The volume fraction of cell occupied by mitochondria was significantly smaller on the average in the sinus node (15.6 ± 0.4%) and the AV node (14.2 ± 0.5%) than in the working myocytes.

Densities of the cristal membranes also appeared to differ considerably when mitochondria were compared between the specialized and working myocytes. In the working myocytes the cristae were more numerous and tightly packed, whereas in the specialized cells the cristae were much less dense, particularly when the cristae were oriented along the long axis of a mitochondrion (Figure 7).

DISCUSSION

Cytochrome oxidase in individual cristal membranes appeared to be similarly active in both working and specialized cardiocytes. In all the specialized cardiocytes, however, the size of mitochondria, the volume fraction of cell occupied by mitochondria, and the density of mitochondrial cristae were smaller than those in the working cardiocytes. These observations suggest that there may be less cytochrome oxidase activity per unit of mitochondrial volume and unit of cell volume in the specialized cardiocytes compared to that in the working myocytes. If this is true, then energy metabolism in the specialized cells may either be quantitatively less or of a different type (e.g., less aerobic) in the conduction system than in working myocardium.

REFERENCES

ALCINI, E., LAGERON, A., and WEGMANN, R. 1965. Étude histoenzymologique du métabolisme glucidique du faisceau de Hiss (a différents niveaux) et du myocarde ventricularie, chez le rat. Ann. Histochem. 10:127–144.

JAMES, T. N., BEAR, E. S., FRINK, R. J., LANG, K. F., and TOMLINSON, J. C. 1970. Selective stimulation, suppression or blockade of the atrioventricular node and His bundle. J. Lab. Clin. Med. 76:240–256.

JAMES, T. N., and NADEAU, R. A. 1962. Direct perfusion of the sinus node: An experimental model for pharmacological and electrophysiologic studies of the heart. Henry Ford Hosp. Med. J. 10:21–25.

McCALLISTER, L. P., and PAGE, E. 1973. Effects of thyroxin on ultrastructure of rat myocardial cell, a stereological study. J. Ultrastruct. Res. 42:136–155.

MORALES, A. R., and FINE, G. 1965. Enzyme histochemistry of the sinus and atrioventricular nodes of the human heart. Lab. Invest. 14:321–329.

OTSUKA, N., HARA, T., and OKAMOTO, H. 1967. Histotopochemische Untersuchungen am Reizleitungssystem des Hundeherzens. Histochemie 10:66–73.

SABATINI, D. D., BENSCH, K., and BARRNETT, R. J. 1963. Cytochemistry and electron microscopy. The preservation of cellular ultrastructure and enzymatic activity by aldehyde fixation. J. Cell Biol. 17:19–58.

SCHIEBLER, Th. H. 1955. Herzstudie, II. Mitteilung: Histologische, histochemische und experimentelle Untersuchungen am Atrioventrikularsystem von Huf. und Nagetieren. Z. Zellforsch. 43:243–304.

SCHIEBLER, Th. H. 1961. Histochemische untersuchungen am Reizleitungssytem tierischer Herzen. Naturwissenschaften 48:502–503.

SCHIEBLER, Th. H. 1963. Über den histochemischen Nachweis von atmungsfermenten im Reizleitungssystem. Verh. Anat. Ges. 57:103–112.

SCHIEBLER, Th. H. 1963. Uber den histochemischen Nachweis von Atmungsfermenten in Bargmann and W. Doerr (eds.), Das Herz des Menschen Band I, pp. 165–227. Georg Thieme Verlag, Stuttgart.

SELIGMAN, A. M. KARNOVSKY, M. J., WASSERKRUG, H. L., and HANKER, J. S. 1968. Nondroplet ultrastructural demonstration of cytochrome oxidase activity with a polymerizing osmiophilic reagent, diaminobenzidine (DAB). J. Cell Biol. 38:1–14.

SELIGMAN, A. M., PLAPINGER, R. E., WASSERKRUG, H. L., DEB, C., and HANKER, J. S. 1967. Ultrastructural demonstration of cytochrome oxidase activity by the Nadi reaction with osmiophilic reagents. J. Cell Biol. 34:787–800.

WEGMANN, R., and SUÉKANÉ, K. 1966. Modifications histoenzymologiques comparées entre le noeud sino-atrial et le muscle auriculaire en anoxie, chez le lapin. Arch. Histol. Jpn. 27:139–152.

Mailing address:
Dr. Thomas N. James,
Cardiovascular Research and Training Center, University of Alabama School of Medicine, University Station, Birmingham, Alabama 35294 (USA).

HEART GROWTH
AND
ITS DISTURBANCES

Recent Advances in Studies on
Cardiac Structure and Metabolism, Volume 12
Cardiac Adaptation
Edited by T. Kobayashi, Y. Ito, and G. Rona
Copyright 1978 University Park Press Baltimore

FACTORS ACCOUNTING FOR GROWTH AND ATROPHY OF THE HEART

R. L. KAO, D. E. RANNELS,
V. WHITMAN, and H. E. MORGAN

Department of Physiology, The Milton S. Hershey
Medical Center, The Pennsylvania State
University, Hershey, Pennsylvania, USA

SUMMARY

Growth of the rat heart was induced by intrathoracic aortic banding, while atrophy followed hypophysectomy. During the early phase of hypertrophy, RNA concentration increased markedly. During the period of atrophy, RNA concentration was reduced. These changes in RNA concentration seemed to account for either the increased or the decreased rate of protein synthesis that was observed during hypertrophy or atrophy, respectively. Rates of protein degradation were unaffected during changes in heart size. These findings suggest that alterations in synthesis, processing, or degradation of RNA play a key role in modification of heart size.

INTRODUCTION

Variations in cardiac size depend upon changes in either the rates of protein synthesis or the rates of degradation. These rates are affected by the availability of hormones and substrates and by the rate of ventricular pressure development (for review, see Rannels, McKee, and Morgan, 1976). In heart and skeletal muscle, ribosome-catalyzed reactions, especially those involved in peptide-chain initiation, seem to limit synthesis of myocardial proteins (Earl and Korner, 1966; Schreiber *et al.*, 1968; Wool *et al.*, 1968; Morgan *et al.*, 1971b). The availability of amino acids (Morgan *et al.*, 1971a), insulin (Morgan *et al.*, 1971b), the supply of noncarbohydrate substrates (Rannels, Hjalmarson, and Morgan, 1974), and an increase in heart work (Hjalmarson and Isaksson, 1972) accelerate peptide-chain initiation in isolated hearts. In normal animals, plasma levels of amino acids, fatty acids, and insulin seem to be sufficient to maintain optimal rates of initiation. Under these circumstances, rates of protein synthesis are determined by the number of ribosomes and other components of the synthetic

This research was supported by Grant HL–11534 from the National Institutes of Health.

pathway. Similarly, protein degradation is regulated by the availability of insulin and by the supply of amino acids and other substrates (Rannels, Kao, and Morgan, 1975). In the perfused rat heart, insulin both inhibited protein degradation and increased latency of lysosomal enzymes (Rannels, Kao, and Morgan, 1975). Regression of cardiac hypertrophy, following cessation of thyroxine treatment of thyrotoxic rats, was accompanied by a 40% increase in activity of cathepsin D (Wildenthal and Mueller, 1974).

The present experiments were undertaken to assess the roles of protein synthesis and degradation in modifying heart size. Our approach has been to induce a rapid change in size either by aortic banding or by hypophysectomy and to estimate rates of synthesis and degradation during *in vitro* perfusion. This approach has the advantage of measuring these rates under controlled conditions, but the disadvantage that these measured rates may not reflect those rates occurring *in vivo*.

RESULTS AND DISCUSSION

Factors Accounting for Cardiac Atrophy in Hypophysectomized Rats

Removal of the pituitary results in cessation of body growth and a 25% decrease in the ratio of heart weight to body weight within the first week after operation

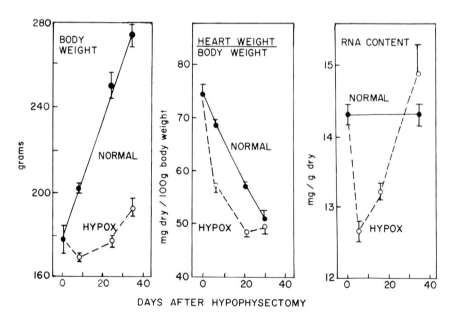

Figure 1. Effect of hypophysectomy on body weight, heart weight/body weight ratio, and RNA content. Values represent the mean ± S.E. of at least six determinations.

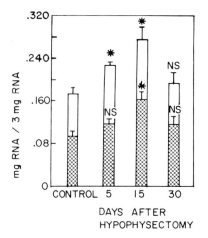

Figure 2. Effect of hypophysectomy on the proportion of RNA in ribosomal subunits in rat heart. Levels of 60S subunits are indicated by the full height of the bar, while levels of 40S subunits are indicated by the cross-hatched portion. As indicated by the asterisk, levels of 60S subunits were increased significantly ($p < 0.05$) five and 15 days after hypophysectomy, while levels of the 40S subunit rose at 15 days. The vertical lines indicate one S.E.M. (Adapted from Hjalmarson *et al.,* 1975.) N.S. = not significantly different ($p > 0.05$).

(Hjalmarson *et al.,* 1975). The number of ribosomes, as reflected by RNA concentration, fell during the period of atrophy but returned to normal as heart size stabilized (Figure 1). In addition to fewer ribosomes, a larger fraction of RNA was present as ribosomal subunits, suggesting that peptide-chain initiation was slow relative to rates of elongation and termination of chains (Figure 2). When hearts of normal and hypophysectomized rats were removed and perfused under conditions simulating those found *in vivo,* rates of protein synthesis were reduced approximately 20% in hearts of hypophysectomized rats when expressed per g of heart protein, but were unchanged when expressed per mg of RNA (Table 1). These findings suggest that a reduction in the number of ribosomes accounted for the slower rates of synthesis. The relationship between rates of protein synthesis and RNA concentration was explored further by perfusion of hearts from normal and hypophysectomized rats under conditions that resulted in maximal rates of synthesis (Figure 3). In addition, normal and hypophysectomized rats were treated with a combination of growth hormone and thyroxine to restore growth of the body and the heart. In normal, hypophysectomized, and hormone-treated animals, rates of protein synthesis were a linear function of RNA concentration, supporting the suggestion that rates of synthesis depended upon the numbers of ribosomes that were present.

The contributions of protein synthesis and degradation to changes in heart size also were assessed by measuring the net release of phenylalanine and the rate

Table 1. Effect of perfusion under simulated *in vivo* conditions on rates of protein synthesis in hearts of normal and hypophysectomized rats

	Protein synthesis	
Condition of animal	μmol of phenylalanine/g of protein · hr	μmol of phenylalanine/mg RNA · hr
Normal	1.14 ± 0.08	0.063 ± 0.004
Hypophysectomized	0.92 ± 0.03[a]	0.057 ± 0.002[b]

Hearts were perfused for one hour using Langendorff preparations with Krebs-Henseleit bicarbonate buffer containing 0.8 mM [^{14}C] phenylalanine and normal plasma levels of other amino acids. Other additions were made to the perfusate, and performance of the heart was adjusted to simulate conditions in normal and hypophysectomized rats. These additions were as follows: normal conditions–6.7 mM glucose, 0.5 mM palmitate, 4% albumin, 40 μU of insulin/ml, 120 mm Hg peak systolic pressure, 360 beats/min; hypophysectomized conditions–4.4 mM glucose, 0.3 mM palmitate, 4% albumin, 15 μU of insulin/ml, 100 mm Hg peak systolic pressure, 270 beats/min. Adapted from Hjalmarson *et al.*, 1975.
[a]$p < 0.05$.
[b]N.S. = not significantly different ($p > 0.05$).

of protein degradation. Because net release represents the difference between synthesis and degradation, protein synthesis could be calculated (Figure 4). Perfusion under conditions simulating those in normal and hypophysectomized rats revealed that the rate of protein degradation and net phenylalanine release were not changed significantly during the period of cardiac atrophy; however, protein synthesis was reduced in hormone-deficient hearts. Rates of protein degradation are underestimated by this method because a portion of the non-radioactive phenylalanine derived from proteolysis is reincorporated into protein before mixing with the pools of [^{14}C] phenylalanine. As a result, rates of protein synthesis also are underestimated, amounting to about 60% of those reported in Table 1.

In other experiments in which cycloheximide was added to block protein synthesis, protein degradation was found to be unaffected by perfusion *in vitro* under conditions simulating those in normal or hypophysectomized rats. These studies confirmed and extended those findings reported in Table 1 and Figure 3 in that they demonstrated that protein synthesis was inhibited during the period of cardiac atrophy but that protein degradation was unaffected. In other experiments, the total activity of cathepsin D, as assayed in the presence of Triton X-100, increased approximately 18% during the period of atrophy when expressed per g of heart. When expressed per total heart, no change in activity was found. These changes in cathepsin D activity could have resulted from a slower rate of degradation of this lysosomal enzyme than of whole heart protein.

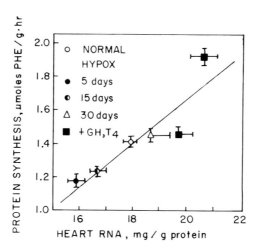

Figure 3. Effect of RNA content on rates of protein synthesis. Hearts were removed from normal and hypophysectomized rats and from rats treated for seven days with growth hormone (100 μg/day) and thyroxine (5 μg/day). Rates of synthesis were measured over a perfusion period of one hour using buffer containing five times the normal plasma levels of all amino acids, 1.5 mM palmitate, and 4% albumin. Hypophysectomized rats were used 5–30 days after operation. Vertical and horizontal lines around each data point indicated one S.E.M. (Adapted from Hjalmarson *et al.,* 1975.) PHE = phenylalanine.

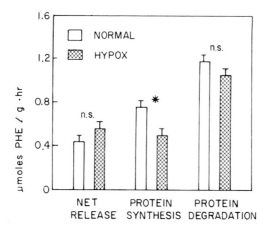

Figure 4. Effect of perfusion under simulated *in vivo* conditions on net release of phenylalanine, protein synthesis, and protein degradation in hearts of normal and hypophysectomized rats. Hearts were perfused for one hour as outlined in Table 1 except that the concentration of [^{14}C] phenylalanine was reduced to 0.01 mM. Net release of phenylalanine was estimated from the appearance of the amino acid in the heart and perfusion medium. Protein degradation was estimated from the rates of dilution of [^{14}C] phenylalanine specific activity. Protein synthesis was calculated by subtracting net release from protein degradation. (Adapted from Hjalmarson *et al.,* 1975.) * = $p < 0.05$; N.S. = not significantly different ($p > 0.05$).

Factors Accounting for Cardiac Hypertrophy Following Aortic Banding

Banding of the ascending aorta results in acute supravalvular aortic stenosis (Nair *et al.*, 1968), which is followed by a progressive increase in the heart weight/body weight ratio (Figure 5). RNA concentration, expressed per g of heart, increased markedly three days after aortic banding but returned to normal during the next month. After 30 days, RNA content, expressed per total heart, was 50% higher in rats subjected to aortic banding than in sham-operated animals. In other experiments, the proportion of RNA in ribosomal subunits was unchanged one and seven days after banding, indicating that rates of peptide-chain initiation and elongation remained in balance during the period of rapid cardiac growth.

When hearts were removed from sham-operated and aortic-banded rats and perfused under simulated *in vivo* conditions, rates of protein synthesis were increased approximately 30% when expressed per g of heart protein, but were unchanged when expressed per mg of RNA (Table 2). These findings complemented those reported for hypophysectomized rats in that they indicated that changes in the rate of protein synthesis were correlated with the concentration of RNA.

The contribution of protein degradation to hypertrophy of the heart was evaluated using the same methods applied to atrophy of the heart following

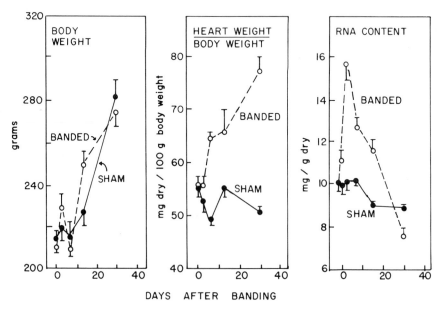

Figure 5. Effect of aortic banding on body weight, heart weight/body weight ratio, and RNA content. Control rats were subjected to sham-operations in which the chest was opened but a band was not applied. Banding was performed as described by Nair *et al.* (1968). Values represent the mean ± S.E. of at least six determinations.

Table 2. Effect of perfusion under simulated *in vivo* conditions on rates of protein synthesis in hearts of sham-operated and aortic-banded rats

	Protein synthesis	
Animal	μmol of phenylalanine/g of protein · hr	μmol of phenylalanine/mg of RNA · hr
Sham-operated	0.76 ± 0.05	0.048 ± 0.003
Aortic-banded	1.00 ± 0.09[a]	0.046 ± 0.004[b]

Hearts were removed from rats seven days after operation and perfused as described in Table 1. The perfusate contained 0.8 mM [¹⁴C]phenylalanine, normal plasma levels of other amino acids, ɩ mM glucose, 0.7 mM palmitate, 4% albumin, 1 mM lactate, and 100 μU of insulin/ml. Peak systolic pressure was 70 mm Hg and the rate was 240 beats/min.
[a]$p < 0.05$.
[b]N.S. = not significantly different ($p > 0.05$).

hypophysectomy (Figure 4). Perfusion of hearts from sham-operated and aortic-banded rats under simulated *in vivo* conditions revealed that net release of phenylalanine was reduced while protein degradation was unchanged in hearts from aortic-banded rats. Protein synthesis, as represented by the difference between the rate of degradation and net release, was increased in hypertrophying hearts. These results confirmed that protein synthesis was accelerated during growth of the heart, while degradation appeared to be unaffected. In other

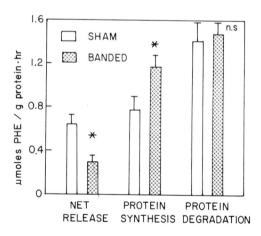

Figure 6. Effect of perfusion under simulated *in vivo* conditions on net release of phenylalanine, protein synthesis, and protein degradation in hearts of sham-operated and aortic-banded rats. Hearts were removed from rats three days after operation and perfused as outlined in Table 2 except that [¹⁴C]phenylalanine was reduced to 0.01 mM. Measurements were made as described in Figure 4. * = $p < 0.05$; N.S. = not significantly different ($p > 0.05$).

studies, activity of cathepsin D was measured in heart homogenates in the presence and in the absence of Triton. One or two days following banding, activity of cathepsin D, assayed in the absence of detergent and expressed per g of heart, was significantly reduced. Total activity, measured in the presence of detergent, was lower but the change was not statistically significant. These findings suggest that lysosomal fragility was reduced in the hypertrophying heart even though the rate of protein degradation was unchanged. Seven days after banding, activity of cathepsin D, measured in either the presence or absence of Triton, was the same as in sham-operated animals.

Common Factors Accounting for Growth or Atrophy of the Heart

These studies indicate that growth of the heart is associated with increased rates of protein synthesis, while atrophy is accompanied by a decrease in this rate. The major factor leading to a change in synthesis seems to be a change in RNA content. This suggestion is supported by the observation that the rate of synthesis was unaffected during atrophy or hypertrophy when expressed per mg of RNA. In the atrophying heart, a decrease in the rate of peptide-chain initiation, as compared to elongation and termination of chains, contributed to the impairment of synthesis. Protein degradation was unaffected during either atrophy or hypertrophy. In most instances, changes in the activity of cathepsin D, as expressed per g of heart, could be accounted for by a relatively long life for this enzyme as compared to the half-life of whole heart protein.

Earlier studies of protein turnover during hypertrophy have been carried out in intact rats (Morkin, Kimata, and Skillman, 1972; Albin *et al.*, 1973; Zak *et al.*, 1976). These experiments have the advantage that the rates of synthesis and degradation are observed *in vivo*, but the disadvantage that rates of synthesis and degradation are difficult to measure because of reutilization of radioactive amino acids and because of uncertainty as to the specific activity of the precursor pool serving protein synthesis. Studies from the Rabinowitz laboratory (Albin *et al.*, 1973; Zak *et al.*, 1976) have demonstrated that accumulation of cytochrome c following aortic banding results from both an increased rate of synthesis and a markedly decreased rate of degradation. In studies of the degradation of myofibrillar protein, Morkin, Kimata, and Skillman (1972) found that the rate of degradation was unchanged and that the increase in myofibrillar mass was attributable to increased rates of synthesis. The present experiments, based upon turnover of whole heart protein during *in vitro* perfusion, are in agreement with the conclusions of Morkin, Kimata, and Skillman (1972). The possibility that tissue levels of specific proteins, such as cytochrome c, change as a result of modifications in rates of both synthesis and degradation is not excluded.

REFERENCES

ALBIN, R., DOWELL, R. T., ZAK, R., and RABINOWITZ, M. 1973. Synthesis and degradation of mitochondrial components in hypertrophied rat heart. Biochem. J. 136:629–637.

EARL, D. C. N., and KORNER, A. 1966. Effect of rat hypophysectomy and growth hormone treatment on cardiac polysomes and ribonucleic acid. Arch. Biochem. Biophys. 115:445–449.

HJALMARSON, A. C., and ISAKSSON, O. 1972. *In vitro* work load and rat heart metabolism: III. Effect on ribosomal aggregation. Acta Physiol. Scand. 86:342–352.

HJALMARSON, A. C., RANNELS, D. E., KAO, R., and MORGAN, H. E. 1975. Effects of hypophysectomy, growth hormone and thyroxine on protein turnover in heart. J. Biol. Chem. 250:4556–4561.

MORGAN, H. E., EARL, D. C. N., BROADUS, A., WOLPERT, E. B., GIGER, K. E., and JEFFERSON, L. S. 1971a. Regulation of protein synthesis in heart muscle: I. Effect of amino acid levels on protein synthesis. J. Biol. Chem. 246:2152–2162.

MORGAN, H. E., JEFFERSON, L. S., WOLPERT, E. B., and RANNELS, D. E. 1971b. Regulation of protein synthesis in heart muscle: II. Effect of amino acid levels and insulin on ribosomal aggregation. J. Biol. Chem. 246:2163–2170.

MORKIN, E., KIMATA, S., and SKILLMAN, J. J. 1972. Myosin synthesis and degradation during development of cardiac hypertrophy in the rabbit. Circ. Res. 30:690–702.

NAIR, K. G., CUTILLETTA, A. F., ZAK, R., KOIDE, T., and RABINOWITZ, M. 1968. Biochemical correlates of cardiac hypertrophy. I. Experimental model; changes in heart weight, RNA content, and nuclear RNA polymerase activity. Circ. Res. 23:451–462.

RANNELS, D. E., HJALMARSON, A. C., and MORGAN, H. E. 1974. Effects of non-carbohydrate substrates on protein synthesis in muscle. Am. J. Physiol. 226:528–539.

RANNELS, D. E., KAO, R., and MORGAN, H. E. 1975. Effect of insulin on protein turnover in heart muscle. J. Biol. Chem. 250:1694–1701.

RANNELS, D. E., McKEE, E. E., and MORGAN, H. E. Regulation of protein synthesis and degradation in heart and skeletal muscle. *In* G. Litwack (ed.), Biochemical Actions of Hormones. Vol. 4. In press.

SCHREIBER, S. S., ORATZ, M., EVANS, C., SILVER E., and ROTHSCHILD, M. 1968. Effect of acute cardiac overload on cardiac muscle RNA. Am. J. Physiol. 215: 1250–1259.

WILDENTHAL, K., and MUELLER, E. A. 1974. Increased myocardial cathepsin D activity during regression of thyrotoxic cardiac hypertrophy. Nature 249:478–479.

WOOL, I. G., STIREWALT, W. S., KURIHARA, K., LOW, R. B., BAILEY, P., and OYER, D. 1968. Mode of action of insulin in the regulation of protein biosynthesis in muscle. Recent Prog. Horm. Res. 24:139–208.

ZAK, R., MARTIN, A. F., REDDY, M. K., and RABINOWITZ, M. 1976. Control of protein balance in hypertrophied cardiac muscle. Circ. Res. 38(suppl. I):145–150.

Mailing address:
Race L. Kao, Ph.D.,
Department of Surgery, The University of Texas Medical Branch,
Galveston, Texas 77550 (USA).

Recent Advances in Studies on
Cardiac Structure and Metabolism, Volume 12
Cardiac Adaptation
Edited by T. Kobayashi, Y. Ito, and G. Rona
Copyright 1978 University Park Press Baltimore

POLYPLOIDIZATION OF HEART MUSCLE NUCLEI AS A PREREQUISITE FOR HEART GROWTH AND NUMERICAL HYPERPLASIA IN HEART HYPERTROPHY

W. SANDRITTER and C. P. ADLER[1]

Institute of Pathology, University of Freiburg,
Freiburg, West Germany

SUMMARY

Although no regular mitotic figures appear in the heart muscle, heart weight increases from a birth weight of 20 g to 350 g in adult life. In hypertrophy, heart weights of more than 1,000 g can be reached. Cytophotometric DNA measurements (Feulgen-cytophotometry) have shown that, in normal adult hearts of 370 g, 44–60% of the muscle nuclei are tetraploid. In heart hypertrophy, a further polyploidization of the heart muscle nuclei takes place. In infant hearts, 85% of the muscle cells still are diploid and only 15% are tetraploid. At the age of 8 years, physiological polyploidization of the heart muscle cells occurs. It starts in the left ventricle (19% 2c-, 69.5% 4c-, and 6% 8c-nuclei), whereas the right ventricle still contains 80.7% diploid muscle cells. In the hearts of adolescents, beginning in the twelfth year of life, the polyploid DNA distribution pattern of the normal adult heart is reached. This physiological polyploidization of heart muscle nuclei is correlated with age and, at the same time, with increasing heart weight. In hearts with malformations, an earlier polyploidization occurs in the chronically overloaded chamber. This, however, can only happen after a certain age (at least three weeks) has been reached. Administration of cytostatics at the time of physiological polyploidization can hinder the synthesis of DNA.

In chronic hyperfunction of the heart, heart hypertrophy develops, and at the same time a pronounced polyploidization of the heart muscle nuclei occurs. This polyploidization is correlated with the weight of the heart and is independent of age. The highest degree of polyploidization is observed in hearts weighing 600–800 g, in which diploid cells are absent and 32-ploid cells are noted.

Polyploidization of heart muscle nuclei is irreversible, because we could not observe a decrease of the nuclear DNA content in atrophic hearts. In a 600-g heart from a patient with generalized splanchnomegaly, the DNA distribution pattern of a normal adult heart was present; this shows that the somatrotrophic hormone had no influence on the myocardial DNA content. A certain cause for polyploidization is obviously a chronic myocardial hyperfunction.

The size of the nuclei (area and volume) is correlated with the ploidy grade. With increasing areas of nuclei, a corresponding increase of the total areas of the nucleoli occurs. Polyploid cell nuclei have more nucleoli than diploid ones. This suggests an activated synthesis of ribosomal RNA and of contractile proteins within the heart muscle cells. It

---

[1] Supported by the Deutsche Forschungsgemeinschaft.

could be proved that in heart muscle cells, starting with a so-called "critical cell volume" of 20×10^3 μm^3, the DNA content has been doubled. The functional cell volume consequently represents the decisive factor of polyploidization. By means of the measurement data from the pure myocardial weight, the biochemically estimated amount of myocardial DNA, the ploidy grade of the heart muscle nuclei, and the ratio of heart muscle cells to connective tissue cells, the absolute cell number of the heart can be estimated. The number of connective tissue cells increases during physiological heart growth from 1×10^9 to 5×10^9 and can reach 10×10^9 in markedly hypertrophied hearts. In hypertrophied hearts, the number of heart muscle cells is increased to 4×10^9 (instead of the normal 2×10^9). This points to the fact that during normal heart growth and in cardiac hypertrophy a numerical hyperplasia of the heart cells takes place.

INTRODUCTION

The human myocardium is an irreversibly post-mitotic tissue, in which the number of cells is not augmented by regular mitoses. Mitotic cell division of heart muscle cells occurs only during intrauterine development and during early post-natal growth (Linzbach, 1955; Rumyantsey, 1963, 1964; Klinge, 1967). Nevertheless, the myocardium is capable of a considerable increase in size and weight by proliferation. During normal growth, the weight of the heart increases from 20 g immediately after birth to 350 g in adult life. In chronic hyperfunction (i.e., hypertension), the heart weight may increase to more than 1,000 g. Until now, whether the increase of the heart weight is caused by an enlargement

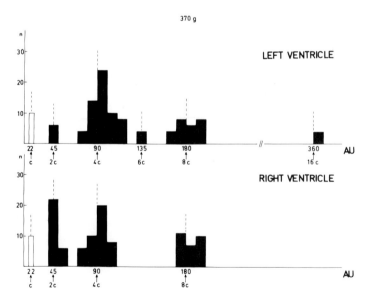

Figure 1. DNA distribution of muscle cell nuclei in the left and right ventricles of a normal heart weighing 370 g.

or by a numerical increase of the heart muscle cells was a questionable matter. A prerequisite for a numerical hyperplasia by nuclear division would be a synthesis of DNA in the heart muscle nuclei.

By the means of Feulgen-cytophotometric investigations on heart muscle nuclei, we were able to prove that a polyploidization of heart muscle nuclei occurs in human myocardium (Sandritter and Scomazzoni, 1964). In a normal adult heart (33-year-old male) with a weight of 370 g (Figure 1), 6% of the nuclei of the left ventricle are diploid. The tetraploid nuclei predominate by 60%. They contain a doubled amount of DNA. Moreover, we found 26% octoploid and 4% hexadecaploid nuclei in the same heart. The intermediate values (4% 6c-nuclei) represent *S*-phase cells. In the right ventricle, the polyploidization is less pronounced (Adler, 1971): we found 28% diploid, 44% tetraploid, and 28% octoploid nuclei.

In functional hypertrophy of the heart, a further augmentation of polyploidization of the heart muscle cells occurs that is correlated with the weight of the heart (Sandritter and Scomazzoni, 1964; Adler, 1971). In a 900-g heart of a 40-year-old male (Figure 2), diploid muscle nuclei are not observed at all. The tetraploid cells, too, are reduced to 26% in the left ventricle and to 36% in the right ventricle. The octoploid nuclei (*left:* 64% 8c-nuclei; *right:* 48% 8c-nuclei) and the hexadecaploid nuclei (*left:* 10% 16c-nuclei; *right:* 16% 16c-nuclei) predominate in both ventricles.

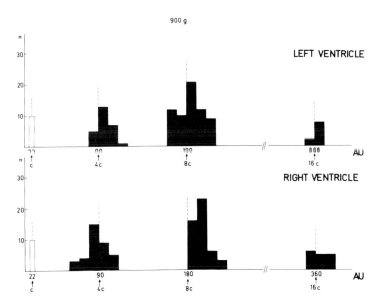

Figure 2. DNA distribution of muscle cell nuclei in the left and right ventricles of a hypertrophied human heart weighing 900 g.

MATERIALS AND METHODS

The aims of our present investigation were to analyze more exactly the process of polyploidization in human hearts by estimating the absolute cell number, and to try to determine if a numerical hyperplasia of heart muscle cells takes place. Our experiments were performed on 100 human hearts of various ages and weights. After preparation of the hearts, the pure myocardial weight was estimated. The total number of heart muscle nuclei was determined by biochemical and cytophotometric methods (Feulgen-cytophotometry) at eight selected sites in both ventricles. The quantitative relation between connective tissue nuclei and heart muscle nuclei was determined from histological slides.

RESULTS AND DISCUSSION

During our cytophotometric measurements on infantile hearts, we found that the heart muscle nuclei do not reveal a polyploid DNA amount in early infancy (Figure 3). The heart of a 3-year-old infant exhibits 85% diploid and only 15% tetraploid muscle cells.

In an 8-year-old child with a heart weight of 95 g (72 g pure myocardial weight), we found 80.7% diploid and only 17.3% tetraploid cell nuclei in the right chamber, while 19% diploid and 69.5% tetraploid cell nuclei were observed in the left ventricle. Six percent of the muscle cells were octoploid. Thus, at age 8, the right ventricle still reveals the DNA distribution pattern of infancy, while the left ventricle already presents an adult degree of polyploidization.

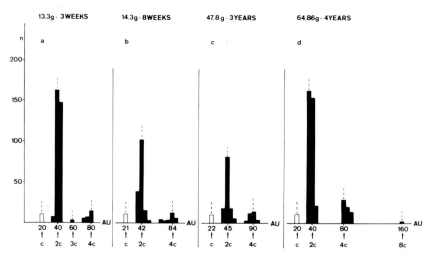

Figure 3. DNA distribution of muscle nuclei in hearts of infants of various ages and heart weights containing mainly diploid heart muscle cells.

In hearts of adolescents, the degree of polyploidization of normal adult hearts is already achieved. In a 285-g heart (pure myocardial weight: 253.1 g) of a 16-year-old, 77.75% of the heart muscle cells contain a tetraploid and 11% an octoploid DNA amount; 0.75% of the cell nuclei are hexadecaploid. Contrary to this, the portion of diploid cells is decreased to 10.25%.

From the diagram of the distribution of the ploidy classes (DNA modalities) expressed as percentages, a correlation of the DNA content of the heart muscle nuclei and the age of growing human hearts is evident. During normal growth of the heart in childhood, an increase in polyploidization of the heart muscle nuclei occurs that is correlated with the age and the increasing myocardial weight (Adler and Hueck, 1971; Adler, 1976). From birth to age 7, the diploid cells predominate by 83–93%. At age 7, corresponding to heart weights of about 100 g, the ratio of diploid nuclei is reduced to 56%, while that of the tetraploid nuclei increases to 42%. Hence, a decisive process of physiological polyploidization occurs between 8 and 12 years of age. First, the cardiac muscle cell nuclei of the left ventricle multiply their DNA content (at age 8); until age 12 most of the heart muscle cells also develop polyploidy. Beyond age 12 to adult life the predominance of tetraploid heart muscle nuclei persists.

In a cardiac malformation, a large number of high ploidy muscle cells with DNA values of up to 32c- and 48c-nuclei are noted in contrast to low diploid values. Thus, we are dealing with a heart that has developed a prominent premature polyploidization. In a heart with a Fallot-tetralogy, in harmony with the pronounced functional strain placed upon the right ventricle, an extra high degree of polyploidization was found with 39% tetraploid, 27% octoploid, and 75% hexadecaploid nuclei; even 32c- and 48c-nuclei occurred. The left ventricle also showed a marked polyploidization with 49.3% tetraploid, 11.3% octoploid, and 0.7% duodecaploid (12c-) nuclei. Only 36% of the nuclei were diploid. This observation demonstrates that an increased functional strain upon the heart muscle acts as a stimulus for polyploidization. In this connection, the duration of hyperfunction is important; in a malformed heart only 3 weeks old with a large atrial septal defect and patent ductus Botalli, a polyploidization of the heart muscle nuclei could not yet be demonstrated. In the right as well as in the left ventricle, 96% of the nuclei were found to be diploid, compared to 6.9% tetraploid nuclei (Staiger *et al.*, 1975).

Cytostatic drugs that inhibit DNA sythesis may also influence the DNA synthesis of heart muscle nuclei, if they are administered during the time of physiological polyploidization (Adler, 1972; Adler and Costabel, 1975). The heart of an 11-year-old child, who had been treated with Daunoblastin, weighed 141 g (pure myocardial weight). While the adult myocardium contains 27% diploid and 71% tetraploid nuclei, the heart of this child revealed only 56% diploid and 37% tetraploid nuclei in the right and 66% tetraploid nuclei in the left ventricle. This observation demonstrates that the physiological polyploidization of the right chamber was inhibited by Daunoblastin.

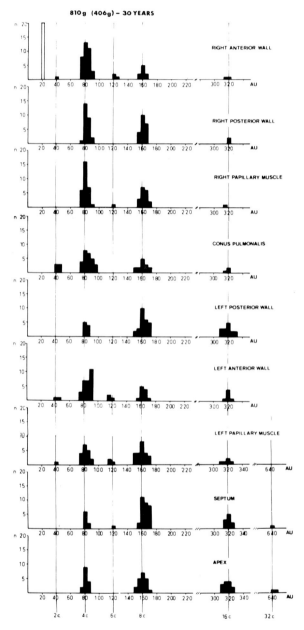

Figure 4. DNA distribution of muscle cell nuclei from different sites of a 30-year-old individual with extreme heart hypertrophy (heart weight: 810 g; pure myocardial weight: 406 g) and with a high grade of polyploidization.

From the diagram of the distribution of ploidy classes, expressed as a percentage of normal and hypertrophied human hearts, it is evident that the polyploidization increases proportionally with the degree of hypertrophy. While, in hearts weighing 300–400 g, tetraploid cell nuclei prevail and only 10–30% diploid nuclei exist, in hearts weighing over 450 g, 90% of the cell nuclei are tetra- and octoploid. Maximal polyploidization is found in hearts between 600 and 800 g, in which up to 28% hexadecaploid and even 6% 32-ploid cell nuclei occur. No diploid muscle cell nuclei are noted in these hypertrophied hearts. The degree of polyploidization in hearts of adults—contrary to hearts of children—is closely correlated with the weight of the myocardium and is independent of age (Adler, 1975).

Thus, we could demonstrate, in an 810-g heart of a 30-year-old (pure myocardial weight: 406 g), a pronounced polyploidization (Figure 4). In the right ventricle of this heart, only 3.5% diploid nuclei were found in contrast to 59.5% tetraploid, 31% octoploid, and 4% hexadecaploid nuclei. The left ventricle revealed a further polyploidization: here, 1.2% diploid and 31.2% tetraploid, 44% octoploid, 19.6% hexadecaploid, and 1.2% 32-ploid cell nuclei were measured.

In the heart of a 76-year-old man that weighed 720 g (Figure 5), the polyploidization of heart muscle cell nuclei also was pronounced: diploid muscle cells did not occur. In the left ventricle, 14% tetraploid, 42% octoploid, 36%

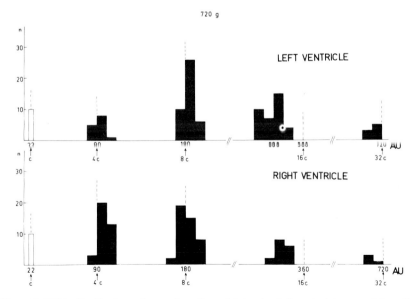

Figure 5. DNA distribution of muscle cell nuclei in the left and right ventricles of a 76-year-old man with heart hypertrophy and pronounced polyploidization.

hexadecaploid, and 8% 32-ploid nuclei were measured. A similar degree of polyploidization also was observed in the right ventricle (36% 4c-, 44% 8c-, 16% 16c-, and 4% 32c-nuclei) (Adler, 1975).

The polyploidization of heart muscle cells is an irreversible process as demonstrated by our investigations in atrophic hearts (Adler, 1975; Adler and Costabel, 1975). A heart weighing 125 g (pure myocardial weight: 85.3 g) from a 38-year-old female showed a normal DNA distribution pattern: in the left ventricle, 7.2% diploid, 86.4 tetraploid, and 5.2% octoploid cell nuclei were found; in the right ventricle, 26% 2c-, 71% 4c-, and 3% 8c-nuclei were found.

The results of these investigations raise many questions: What does polyploidization mean? Which mechanisms induce an augmentation of DNA content? Does a polyploid cell work more economically than a diploid cell? These questions are still unanswered. We have suggested the working hypothesis that an increased cytoplasmatic function leads to a doubling of the genome because certain sites of the genes—we think of ribosomal cistrons—probably can supply a certain amount of work per unit of time. Increased demand of ribosomal material in the cytoplasm may be the releasing factor for doubling of the whole genome. Hyperfunction of the heart muscle is, however, only one factor for polyploidization. For example, it offers no explanation for the physiological polyploidization in the hearts of 8- to 12-year-olds. Hormonal effects, primarily those of the somatotrophic hormone (Beznak, 1964; Morkin et al., 1968; Lipana and Fanburg, 1970) and the catecholamines (Barka, 1970), probably play a role.

In this connection, observations made of a heart obtained from a patient with splanchnomegaly are of interest. In this 600-g heart from a 61-year-old male (pure myocardial weight: 340 g), the DNA distribution pattern of heart muscle was normal, in spite of the cardiac enlargement: tetraploid cells predominated with 68.4% in the right ventricle. Only 20.8% (left ventricle) and 40% (right ventricle) of the cell nuclei were diploid; there were few octoploid nuclei (left ventricle, 8.4%, right ventricle, 2.5%). Thus, the degree of polyploidization was equivalent to a 300-g heart of an adult. In a hypertrophied 600-g heart of a 65-year-old individual with no splanchnomegaly, we found the usual increased polyploidization of heart muscle nuclei with 34% tetraploid, 46% octoploid, 12% hexadecaploid, and 8% 32-ploid heart muscle cells in the left ventricle (right ventricle: 58% 2c-, 36% 8c-, and 6% 16c-nuclei); diploid values were absent. Under the influence of the somatotrophic hormone, which induced the generalized splanchnomegaly, an enlargement of the heart muscle cells had taken place without a change of the DNA content of the heart muscle nuclei. Moreover, we could notice an increase of the number of heart muscle cells by 27.7%. Chronic hyperfunction, on the other hand, had effected a polyploidization of the heart muscle nuclei.

The polyploidization of the heart muscle cells goes along with an increase of the volume of the nuclei (Adler and Beckhove, 1971). The areas of the nuclei, measured on histological slides, show that nuclear areas have a distribution similar to the values of the DNA content (Fischer et al., 1970). Diploid cell nuclei have nuclear areas of about 65 μ^2. Accordingly, tetraploid nuclei have nuclear areas of about 130 μ^2, octoploid nuclei of about 260 μ^2, etc. With increasing DNA content, the size of the nuclei (nuclear area and volume) increases concomitantly.

In heart hypertrophy caused by hyperfunction, polyploidization of heart muscle nuclei takes place so that the synthesis of more contractile proteins can occur. Protein synthesis goes along proportionately with DNA synthesis (Adler et al., 1971; Adler, 1972; Pannen et al., 1973). There is a corresponding increase of ribosomal RNA synthesis, which is necessary for protein synthesis and the turnover of the myocardial structures. Using gallocyanine chromalumn staining, we were able to identify the nucleoli in heart muscle cell nuclei and determine their areas planimetrically. Comparing the areas of the nucleoli and the nuclei, we found an increase of the total area of the nucleoli in connection with the augmentation of the nuclear areas (Adler, 1975). In a heart of a 4-month-old child (heart weight: 35 g), containing only diploid nuclei with a nuclear area of 100−200 μ^2, 90% of the nucleoli showed areas of 4 μ^2. Eighty percent of the muscle nuclei of an atrophic heart (16 years of age, heart weight: 117 g) with a tetraploid DNA content had nucleolar areas of about 8 μ^2. In markedly hypertrophied heart (46 years of age, heart weight: 714 g), the nuclear areas amounted to more than 1,200 μ^2, with the concomitant nucleolar areas more than 40 μ^2. Therefore, we found the largest nucleolar areas in nuclei with the highest DNA content (16-ploid and 32-ploid values).

Polyploid cell nuclei reveal a higher number of nucleoli than diploid ones. In hearts of children, we found two nucleoli in 40% of the nuclei (five nucleoli in 2.9%, six nucleoli in 1.4%). In normal hearts from adults with mainly tetraploid cells, 30−50% of the nuclei had only one nucleolus, 22−26% of the nuclei contained two nucleoli, and 6−19% of the nuclei contained three nucleoli. More than 10 nucleoli per nucleus (in 3.3% of the nuclei) were found in an extremely hypertrophied heart weighing 890 g (pure myocardial weight: 577 g). The number and the size of the nucleoli allowed us to correlate the functional state of the heart muscle nuclei as well as the actual synthesis of ribosomal RNA and functional proteins within the cardiac muscle cells.

It is well known that the nucleus with its specific DNA content represents the navigation center of the cell. The cytoplasmic volume, supplied by a single nucleus, can be called "functional cell volume." It results from the ratio of myocardial volume to the number of nuclei. The volume of the myocardium is determined by the ratio of pure myocardial weight (in g) to specific myocardial weight (= 1.02 g/cm³; Karsner, Saphir, and Todd, 1925). In this calculation, 55% of the value must be substracted because of the nonmuscular structures of the myocardium (Ashley, 1945; Tadtkoro and Arai, 1972). Up to the pure myocardial weight of 400 g (concomitant to a total heart weight of 500 g), the cell volume increases proportionately to the myocardial weight. This means that up to the so-called "critical heart weight" of approximately 500 g (Linzbach, 1947), the growth of the heart muscle is accompanied by an enlargement of the muscle cells. Above this weight, only a small increase of the cell volume, which is insignificant, takes place.

Similar results can be demonstrated by estimations of the dry weight of heart muscle fibers (Sandritter, Grosser, and Schiemer, 1960; Sandritter *et al.*, 1971). Our cytophotometric investigations have shown that, in growing hearts of children, polyploidization of the cardiac muscle cell nuclei starts at the age of eight years, when the functional cell volume in the left ventricle is $20 \times 10^3 \mu^3$ (Figure 6). We call this value the "critical cell volume" at which a diploid cell nucleus is no longer able to supply the necessary amount of cytoplasm. The DNA content of the nucleus consequently must be doubled. The same process occurs with hypertrophied heart muscle cells, which have to double their DNA content when a certain cell size is reached. The functional cell volume consequently is the decisive factor in polyploidization of heart muscle cells.

Based upon cytophotometric DNA estimations of heart muscle cell nuclei, we succeeded in developing a new method for estimating the absolute number of cells (the respective number of nuclei) in different hearts (Adler and Sandritter, 1971; Sandritter and Adler, 1972). After autopsy, the heart is first freed from

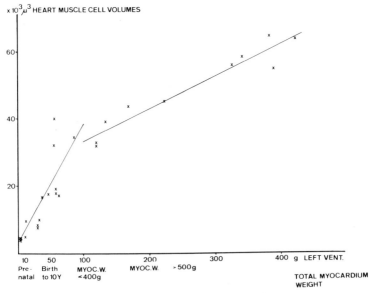

Figure 6. Increase of heart muscle cell volumes with increasing myocardial weight of the left ventricle.

fat and connective tissue, and then the pure ventricular myocardial weight (preparation weight) is determined. With different samples from both heart ventricles, the total DNA amount of the heart muscle is measured biochemically. Cytophotometric measurements (Feulgen-cytophotometry) give us the percentile distribution of the ploidy classes, and with that the DNA amount, which derives only from the heart muscle cell nuclei. Parenchymal and connective tissue cell nuclei are counted on histological slides to estimate the ratio of these two tissue elements. With these parameters, the total number of heart muscle and connective tissue cells in the hearts can be estimated.

The biochemically estimated total amount of DNA in the myocardium increases fivefold during normal growth of the heart, according to the increase of heart weight. In hypertrophied hearts weighing 900 g, the total amount of DNA is three times as high as in normal hearts of 300 g. In the same way, the amount of collagen increases concomitantly with the increasing heart weight. The number of connective tissue cells increases from 1×10^9 cells right after birth to 5×10^9 cells in adult life. In hypertrophied hearts of 700–900 g, we found 10×10^9 connective tissue cells. In the first hours after birth, the definite amount of 2×10^9 heart muscle cells is reached. In heart hypertrophy beginning at 450 g, the number of heart muscle cells increases and can be twice as high in high-degree hypertrophy (700–900 g) with 4×10^9 heart muscle cells. In atrophic hearts (100 g), on the other hand, a reduction of the cell number to 1.5×10^9 heart muscle cells is observed. This, the augmentation of the heart weight during heart hypertrophy, is a function of volume and weight increase of the muscle fibers and of an increase of the number of heart muscle cells.

REFERENCES

ADLER, C. P. 1971. Polyploidisierung und Zellzahl in menschlichen Herzen. Habilitationsschrift, Freiburg i. Br.

ADLER, C. P. 1972. Einfluss von Cytostatica auf den DNA-Gehalt und die Zellzahl in Herzen. Verh. Dtsch. Ges. Pathol. 56:656.

ADLER, C. P. 1972. Ultra-violet microspectrophotometric investigations on the cytoplasm in heart muscle cells. Folla Fac. Med. Univ. Comenianae Bratisl. 10.109–118.

ADLER, C. P. 1975. DNA-Gehalt und Zellzahl in alten Menschenherzen. Verh. Dtsch. Ges. Pathol. 59:328–335.

ADLER, C. P. 1975. Relationship between deoxyribonucleic acid content and nucleoli in human heart muscle cells and estimation of cell number during cardiac growth and hyperfunction. In P. E. Roy and P. Harris (eds.), Recent Advances in Studies on Cardiac Structure and Metabolism. Vol. 8: The Cardiac Sarcoplasm, pp. 373–386. University Park Press, Baltimore.

ADLER, C. P. 1976. DNS in Kinderherzen, biochemische und zytophotometrische Untersuchungen. Beitr. Pathol. 158:173–202.

ADLER, C. P., and BECKHOVE, P. 1971. Postmortale DNA-Veränderungen im Herzmuskel. Beitr. Pathol. 142:306–320.

ADLER, C. P., and COSTABEL, U. 1975. Cell number in human heart in atrophy, hypertrophy, and under the influence of cytostatics. In A. Fleckenstein and G. Rona (eds.), Recent Advances in Studies on Cardiac Structure and Metabolism. Vol. 6:

Pathophysiology and Morphology of Myocardial Cell Alteration, pp. 343–355. University Park Press, Baltimore.

ADLER, C. P., and HUECK, C. 1971. Der DNS-Gehalt in wachsenden Menschenherzen. Verh. Dtsch. Ges. Pathol. 55:464–470.

ADLER, C. P., and SANDRITTER, W. 1971. Numerische Hyperplasie der Herzmuskelzellen bei Herzhypertrophie. Dtsch. Med. Wochenschr. 96:1895–1897.

ADLER, C. P., SCHLUTER, G., and SANDRITTER, W. 1971. Ultraviolettmikrospektrophotometrische Untersuchungen am Cytoplasma von Herzmuskelzellen. Beitr. Pathol. 143:126–156.

ASHLEY, L. M. 1945. A determination of the diameters of ventricular myocardial fibers in man and others mammals. Am. J. Anat. 77:325.

BARKA, T. 1970. Further studies on the stimulation of deoxyribonucleic acid synthesis in the submandibular gland by isoproterenol. Lab. Invest. 22:73–80.

BEZNAK, M. 1964. Hormonal influences in the regulation of cardiac performance. Circ. Res. 15:141–152.

FISCHER, B., SCHLÜTER, G., ADLER, C. P., and SANDRITTER, W. 1970. Zytophotometrische DNS-, Histon- und Nicht-Histonprotein-Bestimmungen an Zellkernen von menschlichen Herzen. Beitr. Pathol. 141:238–260.

KARSNER, H. T., SAPHIR, O., and TODD, T. W. 1925. The state of the cardiac muscle in hypertrophy and atrophy. Am. J. Pathol. 1:351–371.

KLINGE, O. 1967. Die reaktiven Kernveränderungen beim experimentellen Herzinfarkt der Ratte. zugleich ein Beitrag zur Genese der Myocyten. Frankf. Z. Pathol. 77:185–206.

LINZBACH, A. J. 1947. Mikrometrische und histologische Analyse hypertropher menschlicher Herzen. Virchows Arch. Pathol. Anat. 314:534–594.

LINZBACH, A. J. 1955. Quantitative Biologie und Morphologie des Wachstums einschliechlich Hypertrophie und Riesenzellen. In F. Büchner, E. Letterer, and F. Roulet (eds.), Handbuch der allegemeiner Pathologie, VI/1:181–306. Springer, Berlin, Göttingen, Heidelberg.

LIPANA, J. G., and FANBURG, B. L. 1970. Heart growth in response to arotic constriction in the hypophysectomized rat. Am. J. Cardiol. 218:641–646.

MORKIN, E., GARRETT, J. C., and GISHMAN, A. P. 1968. Effects of actinomycin D and hypophysectomy on development of myocardial hypertrophy in the rat. Am. J. Physiol. 214.6–9.

PANNEN, F., ADLER, C. P., and SANDRITTER, W. 1973. Protein und Myoglobin in hypertrophierten und dilatierten Menschenherzen. Quantitative ultraviolett-zytophotometrische Untersuchungen. Beitr. Pathol. 149:70–83.

RUMYANTSEY, P. P. 1963. A morphological and autoradiographical study of the peculiarities of differentiation rate, DNA synthesis and nuclear division in the embryonal and postnatal histogenesis of cardiac muscles of white rats. Folia Histochem. Cytochem. 1:463–471.

RUMYANTSEY, P. P. 1964. An autoradiographic study of the problem of myocardial growth and regeneration using [^{3}H]Thymidine. Proc. II. Intl. Congr. Histo-Cytochemistry. Springer, Berlin, Göttingen, Heidelberg, New York.

SANDRITTER, W., and ADLER, C. P. 1972. A method for determining cell number of organs with polyploid cell nuclei. Beitr. Pathol. 146:99–103.

SANDRITTER, W., GROSSER, K. D., FRISCH, R., and BENEKE, G. 1971. Trockengewichtsbestimmungen on Herzmuskelfasern von atrophierten, normalen und hypertrophierten menschlichen Herzen (Röntgenhistographische Untersuchungen). Beitr. Pathol. 143:249–260.

SANDRITTER, W., GROSSER, K. D., RAST, D., SCHLÜTER, G., and BENEKE, G. 1971. Trockengewichtsbestimmung an Herzmuskelfasern bei experimenteller Herzhypertrophie (Röntgenhistographische Untersuchungen). Beitr. Pathol. 143:261–270.

SANDRITTER, W., GROSSER, K. D., and SCHIEMER, H. G. 1960. Trockengewichtsbestimmungen an normalen und pathologischen Herzmuskelfasern. 192–194.

SANDRITTER, W., and SCOMAZZONI, G. 1964. Deoxyribonucleic acid content (Feulgen photometry) and dry weight (interference microscopy) of normal and hypertrophic heart muscle fibers. Nature 202:100–101.

STAIGER, J., STOLZE, H., and ADLER, C. P. 1975. Nuclear deoxyribonucleic acid content in congenital cardiac malformations. *In* A. Fleckenstein and G. Rona (eds.), Recent Advances in Studies on Cardiac Structure and Metabolism. Vol. 6: Pathophysiology and Morphology of Myocardial Cell Alteration, pp. 357–363. University Park Press, Baltimore.

TADTKORO, M., and ARAI, S. 1972. Myocardial cell in right ventricular hypertrophy. Tohoku J. Exp. Med. 106:5–16.

Mailing address:
Professor C. P. Adler, M.D.,
Pathologisches Institut der Universität Freiburg,
Alberstr. 19, D 7800 Freiburg i. Br. (West Germany).

Recent Advances in Studies on
Cardiac Structure and Metabolism, Volume 12
Cardiac Adaptation
Edited by T. Kobayashi, Y. Ito, and G. Rona
Copyright 1978 University Park Press Baltimore

ULTRASTRUCTURAL ASPECTS OF CONTRACTILE PROTEINS IN CARDIAC HYPERTROPHY AND FAILURE

V. J. FERRANS, B. J. MARON, M. JONES, and K.-U. THIEDEMANN

Pathology Branch and Cardiology Branch,
National Heart, Lung, and Blood Institute, National Institutes of Health,
Bethesda, Maryland USA

SUMMARY

A review is presented in this chapter of morphological changes in contractile elements of cardiac muscle cells in hypertrophy and failure, with emphasis on alterations occurring in human hearts in the late stages of hypertrophy. The formation of new sarcomeres involves the synthesis of a variety of different proteins, their aggregation into filaments, and the organization of filaments into specific tridimensional arrays. Z-line material appears to play an organizer role in the formation of new sarcomeres. The ultrastructural appearance of contractile elements in hypertrophied muscle cells varies according to the cause and the stage of the hypertrophy. Myofibrillar lysis, with preferential loss of thick myofilaments, occurs in the late stages of hypertrophy in association with degenerative changes, including dissociation of intercellular junctions, proliferation of sarcoplasmic reticulum, cellular atrophy, and interstitial fibrosis.

Morphological changes in contractile elements of cardiac muscle cells in hypertrophy and failure, particularly as seen in human myocardium, are reviewed in this chapter. An analysis of changes related to formation of new sarcomeres is presented first, followed by reviews of alterations involving Z lines and other contractile elements of hypertrophied hearts.

CHANGES RELATED TO FORMATION OF NEW SARCOMERES

The formation of sarcomeres involves the synthesis of appropriate amounts of a variety of different proteins, their aggregation into filaments, and the organization of filaments into specific tridimensional arrays (sarcomeres). Most of our knowledge of these events in myocardium has been obtained from autoradiographic studies of incorporation of labeled amino acids and from studies of ultrastructural images that have been interpreted as representing various stages in the process of sarcomerogenesis. A continuous process of synthesis and breakdown of proteins goes on in fully developed sarcomeres of normal cardiac muscle, as evidenced by the fact that the half-life of cardiac myosin and actin is less than two weeks (Morkin, 1974). It is not clear whether different proteins in a sarcomere turn over simultaneously, or whether this turnover occurs evenly throughout different regions of myocardium. In any case, no ultrastructural evidence of turnover of contractile filaments is usually seen in normal myocardium of adult animals.

Autoradiographic studies of incorporation of labeled amino acids into myocardium have provided useful information concerning myofibrillogenesis, even though these investigations are limited by the large size of the developed silver grains with respect to the subcellular structures in question, by the relatively nonspecific nature of the labeling, and by the inability to distinguish between protein synthesis related to turnover in pre-existing myofilaments and that related to the addition of new ones. The localization of newly formed contractile proteins was studied by Morkin (1974) in normal rabbit right ventricular papillary muscle that had been labeled *in vitro* with [^{3}H]leucine and then glycerinated to extract soluble, noncontractile proteins. In these preparations, the developed grains were most frequently located a short distance from the margins of myofibrils and showed a distribution pattern similar to that expected to result from multiple point sources of radioactivity located on the surfaces of the myofibrils. Solubilization of contractile proteins removed most of the radioactivity, thereby providing support for the idea that the distribution of developed grains represents the location of newly synthesized contractile proteins.

Evidence also implicating peripheral regions of the myofibrils and Z lines as sites of rapid turnover of contractile proteins in hypertrophied myocardium was obtained by Anversa, Hagopian, and Loud (1973), who analyzed the distribution of radioactivity in cardiac muscle cells of rats given [^{3}H]leucine at 8, 13, and 40 days after aortic constriction and found that the periphery of the myofibrils and the Z lines had a consistently higher concentration of grains than would occur on a random basis. Anversa and his colleagues also found that developed grains in areas of accumulation of anomalous Z-line material were very few. This finding suggests that accumulations of Z-line material in hypertrophied hearts are not sites of selectively high incorporation of newly synthesized protein into contractile elements.

More direct information concerning mechanisms of sarcomere formation has been obtained from morphological studies of embryonic myocardium (for review, see Markwald, 1973). In very early stages of development of cardiac muscle cells, both the thick and thin myofilaments are free and located predominantly in subsarcolemmal regions. Organization of these filaments proceeds in association with dense, amorphous material that resembles that in Z lines. Such material forms either plaques along the inner aspect of the sarcolemma or isolated condensations that are free in the sarcoplasm. The association of filaments with organizing centers produces structures that consist of thin filaments which insert into one or both sides of a centrally located, widened Z line, and of thick filaments that are loosely associated with thin filaments. Primitive, branched myofibrillar bundles, characterized by widened Z lines and loosely aggregated filaments, are formed in later stages by the interconnection of these structures. Discrete A and I bands appear as these myofilaments come into closer contact and into closer registration with one another. I bands are seen only in those sarcomeres in which the Z lines have narrowed and the filaments have become more closely packaged. H bands and M lines do not appear until sarcomerogenesis is nearly complete. When myofibrils first develop in cardiac myoblasts, these cells are oval or stellate in shape. As more myofibrils develop, they fill the central regions of the cells and become oriented parallel to the longitudinal axis. Thus, the cells gradually become cylindrical in shape.

Role of Z-Line Material in Sarcomerogenesis

The possible role of Z-line material in the formation of new sarcomeres has received much attention in studies of cardiac hypertrophy. Considerable evidence supports the concept that accumulations of Z-line material are associated with the formation of new sarcomeres, and that these accumulations serve as templates upon which other sarcomeric components are brought into their proper three-dimensional relationships (Bishop and Cole, 1969; Legato, 1970). Nevertheless, accumulations of Z-line material also can occur as a result of disruption of myofibrils and reaggregation of their Z-line material, and in conditions unrelated to the formation of new sarcomeres. Thus, accumulations of Z-line material should not be regarded as necessarily indicative of a process of continuing synthesis of new sarcomeres.

Studies of Z lines and sarcomere formation in hypertrophying myocardium of newborn dogs (Bishop, 1973) are of special interest because they have a bearing on the question of whether or not the mechanisms of sarcomerogenesis differ in normal growth and in hypertrophy. In addition to incompletely organized myofilaments along the periphery of the cells (as in normal newborn dogs), myocardium from newborn dogs with aortic constriction showed increased folding and tortuosity of intercalated discs and various degrees of widening of the Z lines. The expansions of Z-line material appeared to displace adjacent sarcomeres in a longitudinal direction, resulting in a misalignment of these sarcomeres with respect to those of neighboring myofibrils. This type of change is shown in Figure 1. It should be pointed out that although these structures are referred to as expansions of Z-line material or widened Z lines, they consist of at least two morphologically distinct components, which are actin filaments and Z-line-like material (Figure 2). The lattice arrangement in these structures is complex and has not been fully elucidated. Although ac-

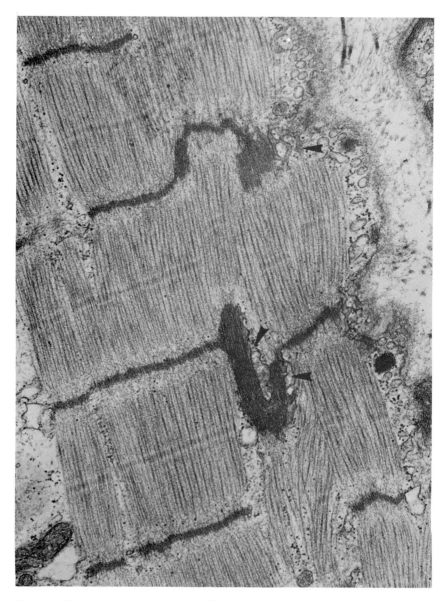

Figure 1. Electron-dense expansions of Z-line material that displace adjacent sarcomeres and are closely associated with tubules of sarcoplasmic reticulum (arrowheads), are present in left atrial myocardium from a 48-year-old woman who had mitral stenosis and atrial fibrillation and who underwent mitral commissurotomy. × 29,000.

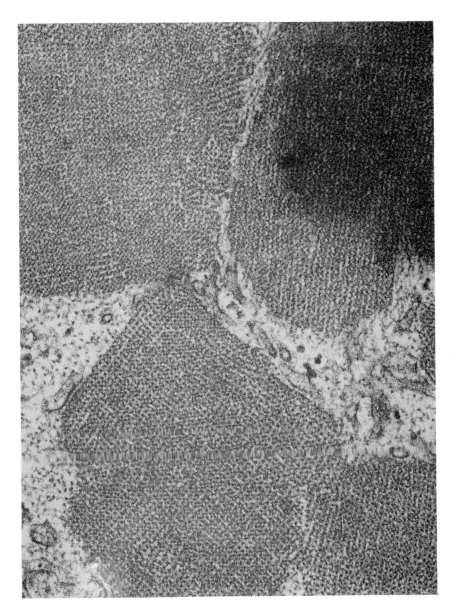

Figure 2. Cross-sectional view showing tetragonal lattice of large masses of Z-line material in muscle cell from crista supraventricularis of an 11-year-old boy with double outlet right ventricle and infundibular pulmonic stenosis. × 90,000.

cumulations of Z-line material were first regarded as being composed mainly of tropomyosin, more recent studies show that α-actinin is one of their major components (Schollmeyer *et al.,* 1973). Other components of these accumulations remain to be identified.

The anomalous expansions of Z-line material in hypertrophying myocardium of adult dogs with banding of the pulmonary artery (Bishop and Cole, 1969) and of newborn dogs with aortic constriction (Bishop, 1973) were especially prominent in animals with congestive heart failure, were less frequent in those with hypertrophy without failure, and were either very rare or absent in control animals. These correlations suggest that these Z-line expansions are related to cardiac failure. In a study of crista supraventricularis muscle from patients with congenital heart diseases associated with muscular obstruction to right ventricular outflow, we observed (Jones and Ferrans, 1977) frequent abnormalities of Z-line material in the eight patients who were at least 30 years old (most of whom had either cardiac failure or clinically significant arrhythmias), but not in any of the 11 patients who were less than six years old (all of whom were free of cardiac complications). We also found very extensive accumulations of Z-line material in severely degenerated muscle cells in large, dilated atria of patients who underwent operative treatment of mitral valvular disease. Other studies have shown, however, that anomalous Z-line material also occurs in circumstances which are unrelated to cardiac failure, and that it can assume several morphologically different forms.

The various alterations of material resembling that in Z lines of cardiac muscle can be classified as follows: 1) widening of Z lines, with or without periodicity, as described above; 2) extensions of Z-line material into adjacent regions of the sarcomeres; 3) accumulations of Z-line material, without periodic substructures, in areas adjacent to the sarcolemma and intercalated discs; 4) splitting of Z lines; 5) focal loss of Z-line material, and 6) clumping of Z-line material, in areas of myofibrillar damage or disorganization, into elongated masses that lack periodicity and are oriented parallel to the longitudinal axis of the cell. Of these six types of Z-line alterations (for review, see Maron, Ferrans, and Roberts, 1975a), the first three are known to occur in hypertrophying muscle cells in humans and experimental animals, in normal, specialized tissues of the atrioventricular conduction system of a variety of species, and in ventricular myocardium of old, but apparently healthy, cats and dogs. A relation has been found between the occurrence of these three types of changes and the degree of atrial hypertrophy in patients with rheumatic heart disease and, as mentioned previously, the presence of congestive heart failure in dogs. The fourth alteration, splitting of Z lines, represents the most direct evidence of actual replication of sarcomeres and has been observed consistently in hearts undergoing hypertrophy, but only very infrequently in normal hearts or in embryonic muscle. It is not certain that this change is related to normal sarcomerogenesis.

We believe that the basic changes in the first four types of Z-line alterations listed above are basically similar and related to an increased ability of actin filaments to associate with Z-line material. This increased association, which may be a response to excessive stretch, may lead to subsequent interactions with myosin and to eventual completion of formation of the sarcomeres. It is not certain, however, that masses of anomalous Z-line material do necessarily progress to actual completion of sarcomere formation. The presence of large amounts of Z-line material in some cells suggests that this material may be produced in quantities that are excessive, either from the absolute or relative standpoint, and that the cells fail to produce corresponding amounts of other sarcomeric components. Little is known of the mechanisms controlling the synthesis of different sarcomeric proteins. Studies of skeletal muscle have provided the most convincing evidence that accumulations of Z-line material are not necessarily related to normal sarcomerogenesis. Such accumulations are known to develop in many degenerative skeletal muscle diseases, myopathies, and experimentally produced types of damage (for review, see Maron, Ferrans, and Roberts, 1975a).

We regard the fifth and sixth alterations listed above as degenerative because we have found them frequently in degenerated left ventricular muscle cells from patients undergoing operation for treatment of aortic regurgitation, combined aortic stenosis and regurgitation, and hypertrophic obstructive cardiomyopathy, and from patients receiving anthracycline drugs for treatment of neoplasms.

Ultrastructure of Contractile Elements in Hypertrophied Hearts

The following generalizations can be drawn from ultrastructural studies of contractile elements in hypertrophied myocardium:

1. The hexagonal array of the myofilaments, the dimensions of the sarcomeres, and the diameters of the thick and thin myofilaments are similar in normal and in hypertrophied muscle cells (Richter and Kellner, 1963). Therefore, hypertrophy is not mediated by alterations in the size of the contractile elements.
2. The ultrastructural appearance of contractile elements in hypertrophied cardiac muscle cells varies according to the cause and stage of the hypertrophy.
3. The cardiac muscle in hypertrophic cardiomyopathy shows foci of disarray of cells and of their contractile elements. These alterations are present throughout the ventricles of symptomatic patients with the nonobstructive form of the disease, but are much more sharply restricted to the ventricular septum in patients with the obstructive form of hypertrophic cardiomyopathy (Maron *et al.*, 1974).
4. Electron microscopic study permits the recognition of a variety of myofibrillar degenerative changes that are not distinguishable by light microscopy.

In Meerson's first stage of hypertrophy, the cardiac muscle cells show evidence of increased synthesis of proteins. They also may show evidence of damage and destruction, involving mainly the myofibrils and mitochondria. The latter changes probably do not constitute a true manifestation of early hypertrophy; instead, they may occur as a consequence of the use of traumatic methods to induce hypertrophy.

In the second stage of hypertrophy (stage of stable hyperfunction), ultrastructural study of myocardium discloses cells that are larger than normal but show few or no qualitative abnormalities in their organelles. In several animal models of cardiac hypertrophy, morphometric study of electron micrographs has demonstrated that hypertrophied cells differ from normal-sized cells of normal animals in the volume fractions (i.e., percentages of the total cell volume) occupied by myofibrils, mitochondria, and other organelles (Page and McCallister, 1973). Such data are beyond the scope of this chapter.

In the third stage (Meerson's stage of cellular exhaustion), the morphological picture is dominated by degenerative changes in the muscle cells and by interstitial fibrosis. Although the exact relationship of these changes to myocardial failure has not been determined, it seems likely that they account for the irreversibility of cardiac failure in certain patients in whom operative correction of the hemodynamic lesion does not result in appreciable clinical improvement.

Based on study of myocardium from patients with congenital heart diseases (Jones *et al.,* 1975; Jones and Ferrans, 1977), aortic valvular disease (Maron, Ferrans, and Roberts, 1975b), hypertrophic cardiomyopathy (Maron, Ferrans, and Roberts, 1975a), mitral valvular disease (Thiedemann and Ferrans, 1976), and cardiotoxicity caused by antineoplastic agents (Buja and Ferrans, 1975; Buja, Ferrans, and Graw, 1976), we have classified cardiac muscle cells with evidence of degeneration as showing mild, moderate, or severe degeneration. This classification is based on the nature and extent of the morphological changes in such cells (Maron, Ferrans, and Roberts, 1975a, 1975b). Abnormalities of myofibrils in mildly degenerated cells consist of various alterations of Z-line material and of focal loss of myofilaments. The loss of myofilaments is unusual in that it affects the myosin filaments to a much greater extent than the actin filaments (Figures 3 and 4). This preferential loss of thick myofilaments results in the presence of disproportionately greater numbers of thin myofilaments in affected cells (Figure 3). Z-line changes in mildly or moderately degenerated cells consist of fragmentation of Z-line material, and spreading of Z-line material into adjacent regions of the sarcomeres, often in association with preferential loss of thick myofilaments. Mild, focal thickening of Z lines and subsarcolemmal accumulations of Z-line material are common in mildly or moderately degenerated cells.

The structure of myofibrils is markedly altered in cardiac muscle cells with severe degeneration. Myofibrils are almost completely absent in some of these cells and disrupted in others. Masses of Z-line-like material often are scattered randomly throughout these cells. These masses are traversed by thin myofilaments arranged either at random or in parallel, but thick filaments are rare or

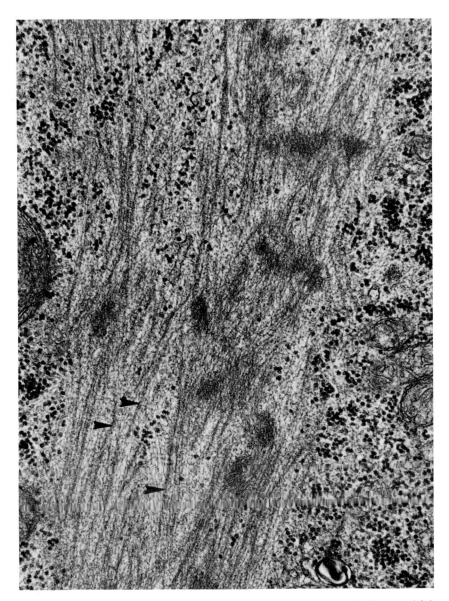

Figure 3. Area of myofibrillar lysis, with disorganization and clumping of Z-line material, is present in left ventricular muscle cell from a 43-year-old man with combined aortic stenosis and regurgitation. Note paucity of thick myofilaments (arrowheads). × 39,000.

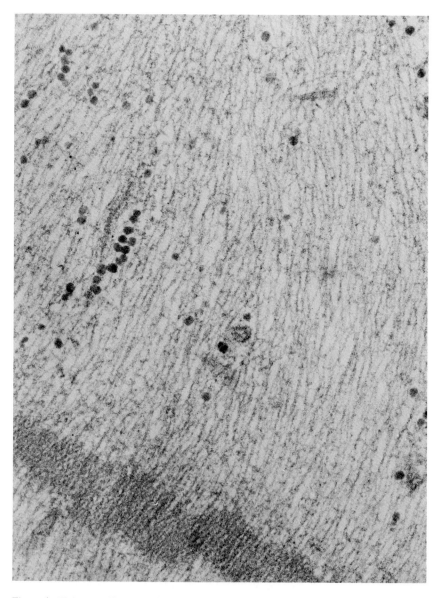

Figure 4. High magnification view of part of severely degenerated muscle cell from the same patient as in Figure 2. A widened Z line is the site of insertion of large numbers of thin myofilaments, but these filaments are not associated with thick (myosin) filaments. ×86,500.

absent in these areas (Figure 4). Cytoskeletal filaments measuring 100 Å in diameter frequently form tangled masses in these areas of myofibrillar disruption.

Myofibrillar loss in degenerated cardiac muscle cells may result from any of the following three types of alterations in contractile proteins: 1) abnormalities of synthesis; 2) acceleration of breakdown, and 3) disaggregation. The exact pathway and the relative importance of each of these mechanisms are uncertain. The loss of myofibrils that occurs in degeneration of hypertrophied cardiac muscle is associated with survival of other organelles, including the nuclei and mitochondria. These features distinguish this type of degeneration from a true phenomenon of necrosis. The degenerative alterations in hypertrophied cardiac muscle cells constitute part of the spectrum of changes described as myocytolysis by light microscopists. Both these degenerated cardiac muscle cells and other cells described as showing myocytolysis are characterized by loss of myofibrils. The alterations in hypertrophied, degenerated cardiac muscle cells differ from those in the usual type of myocytolysis, in which selective lysis of thick filaments does not occur and formation of contraction bands is a prominent phenomenon.

The ultrastructural features of moderately or severely degenerated cardiac muscle cells suggest that they are manifestations of the end stages of cellular hypertrophy. This concept is supported by the fact that cells with advanced degeneration often have few or no normal myofibrils or T tubules and have marked alterations in the sarcoplasmic reticulum. Furthermore, degenerated cells often lose their connections with adjacent cells and, therefore, do not have the capacity to directly transmit electrical activation to other muscle cells or to contribute to the contractile function of the heart. Our finding of cardiac muscle cells with similar degenerative features in dilated atria from patients with mitral valvular disease, in crista supraventricularis muscle from patients with congenital heart diseases associated with right ventricular outflow obstruction, and in ventricular myocardium from patients with hypertrophic cardiomyopathy, aortic valvular disease, or with neoplasms undergoing therapy with anthracycline drugs, suggests that these morphological alterations represent a final common pathway of cell injury in a variety of cardiac conditions.

REFERENCES

ANVERSA, P., HAGOPIAN, M., and LOUD, A. V. 1973. Quantitative radioautographic localization of protein synthesis in experimental cardiac hypertrophy. Lab. Invest. 29:282–292.

BISHOP, S. P. 1973. Effect of aortic stenosis on myocardial cell growth, hyperplasia, and ultrastructure in neonatal dogs. *In* N. S. Dhalla (ed.), Recent Advances in Studies on Cardiac Structure and Metabolism. Volume 3: Myocardial Metabolism, pp. 637–656. University Park Press, Baltimore.

BISHOP, S. P., and COLE, C.R. 1969. Ultrastructural changes in the canine myocardium with right ventricular hypertrophy and congestive heart failure. Lab. Invest. 20:219–229.

BUJA, L. M., and FERRANS, V. J. 1975. Myocardial injury produced by antineoplastic drugs. *In* A. Fleckenstein and G. Rona (eds.), Recent Advances in Studies on Cardiac Structure and Metabolism. Volume 6: Pathophysiology and Morphology of Myocardial Cell Alteration, pp. 487–497. University Park Press, Baltimore.

BUJA, L. M., FERRANS, V. J., and GRAW, R. G., JR. 1976. Cardiac pathologic findings in patients treated with bone marrow transplantation. Hum. Pathol. 7:17–45.

JONES, M., FERRANS, V. J., MORROW, A. G., and ROBERTS, W. C. 1975. Ultrastructure of crista supraventricularis muscle in patients with congenital heart diseases associated with right ventricular outflow tract obstruction. Circulation 51:39–67.

JONES, M., and Ferrans, V. J. 1977. Myocardial degeneration in congenital heart disease: A comparison of morphologic findings in young and old patients with congenital heart diseases associated with muscular obstruction to right ventricular outflow. Am. J. Cardiol. 39:1051–1063.

LEGATO, M. J. 1970. Sarcomerogenesis in human myocardium. J. Mol. Cell. Cardiol. 1:425–437.

MARKWALD, R. R. 1973. Distribution and relationship of precursor Z material to organizing myofibrillar bundles in embryonic rat and hamster ventricular myocytes. J. Mol. Cell. Cardiol. 5:341–350.

MARON, B. J., FERRANS, V. J., HENRY, W. L., CLARK, C. E., REDWOOD, D. R., ROBERTS, W. C., MORROW, A. G., and EPSTEIN, S. E. 1974. Differences in distribution of myocardial abnormalities in patients with obstructive and non-obstructive asymmetric septal hypertrophy (ASH): Light and electron microscopic findings. Circulation 50:436–446.

MARON, B. J., FERRANS, V. J., and ROBERTS, W. C. 1975a. Ultrastructural features of degenerated cardiac muscle cells in patients with cardiac hypertrophy. Am. J. Pathol. 79:387–434.

MARON, B. J., FERRANS, V. J., and ROBERTS, W. C. 1975b. Myocardial ultrastructure in patients with chronic aortic valve disease. Am. J. Cardiol. 35:725–739.

MORKIN, E. 1974. Activation of synthetic processes in cardiac hypertrophy. Circ. Res. 35(suppl. 2):37–48.

PAGE, E., and McCALLISTER, L. P. 1973. Quantitative electron microscopic description of heart muscle cells: Application to normal, hypertrophied, and thyroxin-stimulated hearts. Am. J. Cardiol. 31:172–181.

RICHTER, G. W., and KELLNER, A. 1963. Hypertrophy of the human heart at the level of fine structure. An analysis and two postulates. J. Cell Biol. 18:195–206.

SCHOLLMEYER, J. E., GOLL, D. E., ROBSON, R. M., and STROMER, M. H. 1973. Localization of α-actinin and tropomyosin in different muscles. J. Cell Biol. 59:306a.

THIEDEMANN, K.-U., and FERRANS, V. J. 1976. Ultrastructure of sarcoplasmic reticulum in atrial myocardium of patients with mitral valvular disease. Am. J. Pathol. 83:1–38.

Mailing address:
Victor J. Ferrans, M.D., Ph.D.,
Chief, Ultrastructure Section, Pathology Branch, National Heart, Lung, and Blood Institute,
National Institutes of Health,
Bethesda, Maryland 20014 (USA).

Recent Advances in Studies on
Cardiac Structure and Metabolism, Volume 12
Cardiac Adaptation
Edited by T. Kobayashi, Y. Ito, and G. Rona
Copyright 1978 University Park Press Baltimore

HISTOPATHOLOGICAL STUDY OF HYPERTROPHIED MYOCARDIUM OF KNOWN ETIOLOGIES WITH SPECIAL REFERENCE TO CORRELATION OF ECG CHANGES

R. OKADA and K. KITAMURA

Department of Internal Medicine, School of Medicine, Juntendo
University, Tokyo, Japan

SUMMARY

Sixty-two autopsied hearts, with left ventricular hypertrophy (LVH) caused by mitral regurgitation (MR), aortic failure (AR), combined valvular disease (CVD), hypertension (HHD), or ischemia (IHD), and 23 control hearts with normal left ventricles were studied morphologically for analysis of modes of hypertrophy and for ECG-pathology correlation. Basic disorders modify the mode of hypertrophy; that is, elongated AR-type LV makes muscle fiber orientation in the outer layer more vertical, and globular MR-type LV makes it more horizontal than normal. High-voltage QRS correlates with hypertrophy of the outer ayer which is often associated with that of the inner layer. ST depression and T changes correspond to relative deterioration of the inner and median layers, respectively.

INTRODUCTION

Only a few papers (Scott, 1960; Okada, 1976b) have been published concerning ECG-pathology correlation of myocardial hypertrophy. The aims of the present investigation were to study various modes of hypertrophy of the left ventricle to detect a common denominator or identify a difference among the modes, if present, and to compare the histological findings of the myocardium to ECG changes to facilitate clinical interpretation of ECG.

MATERIALS AND METHODS

Materials consisted of 85 autopsied hearts in which 62 had left ventricular hypertrophy caused by valvular failures, including 11 with mitral regurgitation (MR), 13 with aortic failure (AR), and 20 with combined valvular disease (CVD), or of a nonvalvular nature including 9 with hypertension (HHD) and 9 with ischemia (IHD). Twenty-three other hearts, 14 macroscopically normal with no clinical evidence of heart disease and 9 with mitral stenosis (MS) with almost normal left ventricles, were selected for control groups.

Heart weight and ventrical size were measured by using the base-apex distance (A) and the width of the ventricles at the median (B) after formalin fixation. Volume of the left ventricle was measured as injectable water volume into an ice bag that was inserted into the left ventricle. The wall thickness was determined as the thickness of the stratum compactum at the median portion of the anterior wall.

For microscopic examination, blocks, including vertical sections from base to apex, and horizontal sections were taken from the anterior wall; they were cut in 7-μm slices after paraffin embedding. Slices were stained with hematoxylin and eosin (H-E), Azan, and by Weigert van Gieson's methods.

Ante-mortem ECG records were checked carefully. At least two records of each case were utilized in which one was taken one month or more before death and another within one week of death. Criterion for high-voltage QRS, defined as $R_{V5\ or\ 6} + S_{V1}$, was more than 3.5 mV, and ST and T changes were estimated at the left precordial leads. Cases with bundle-branch blocks were excluded from this ST and T estimation.

RESULTS

Data from macroscopic examination are listed in Table 1. The shape of the left ventricle is quite different in each category. Globular enlargement in MR and CVD and elongated enlargement in AR are easily differentiated. Heart weight is increased markedly in AR and CVD, moderately in MR, and mildly in HHD and IHD. Wall thickness of the LV is most prominent in HHD and AR. The most marked increase of LV volume is seen in CVD and AR and the second largest increase in MR and HHD.

Results of microscopic study are summerized in Table 2. Categories, divided by ECG findings, are listed horizontally and vertical columns correspond to basic diseases. Each pathological finding, such as hypertrophy, degeneration, or fibrosis, is rated as 3 for +, 6 for ++, and 10 for +++ lesions, as well as 10 for normal state. The myocardial index is presented as a coefficient that is calculated by subtracting the degeneration and fibrosis count from the sum of the normal plus the hypertrophy count. A positive index indicates a good condition of the myocardium and a negative index means an altered state. The estimation is done separately for three layers, e.g., inner oblique, median circular, and outer oblique layers of the myocardium.

Even in the control groups, the condition of the outer layer shows the best score and that of the median and inner layers reflects some negative counts. The MR group shows rather uniform hypertrophy through the three layers, and degeneration and fibrosis predominate at the inner and median layers, as shown in Figure 1 d, e, and f. Muscle fiber orientation at the outer layer is more horizontal than in the normal group, and that at the inner layer is more vertical.

Table 1. Shape and size of the left ventricle

	Normal	MS	MR	AR	CVD	HHD	IHD
Shape	RV ⊌ LV	⊌	⊌	⊌	⊌	⊌	⊌
Heart weight (g)	272	438	501	620	618	469	451
A (Length) (cm)	10.4	11.3	12.2	13.0	12.7	11.3	11.5
B (Width) (cm)	8.4	8.4	11.0	10.8	10.3	9.8	9.8
LV wall (cm)	1.03	0.91	1.26	1.41	1.21	1.48	1.39
LV volume (ml)	27	27	38	59	71	35	34
Blood pressure	norm	norm	norm	syst high	norm	high	some high

MR = mitral regurgitation; AR = aortic failure; CVD = combined valvular disease; HHD = hypertension; IHD = ischemia; MS = mitral stenosis.

The AR group has hypertrophy at the outer layer and marked deterioration in the median and inner layers. Figure 1 g, h, and i indicate more vertical fiber orientation at the outer layer. The CVD group shows a similarity to MR but with more advanced myocardial lesions. The HHD group has hypertrophy with a count of 4:2:3 for the outer, median, and inner layers, respectively, as illustrated in Figure 1 a, b, and c. Degeneration and fibrosis are concentrated in the inner and median layers. Muscle fiber orientation at each layer is essentially normal in the HHD and IHD groups. The IHD group is characterized by deterioration of the median and inner layers.

From the viewpoint of ECG changes, ST depression corresponds to inner layer deterioration and T changes indicate median layer involvement. Some cases with ST and T change have normal QRS voltage in spite of the presence of histological hypertrophy. The explanation for this observation could be the cancellation of hypertrophy by myocardial fibrosis with a substantial loss of muscle fibers, as often seen in the IHD. High-voltage QRS correlates as a rule with hypertrophy at the outer layer which is often associated with that of the inner layer. The bundle-branch block group shows the most severe deterioration in the myocardium.

Table 2. Histology of left ventricular myocardium

ECG	Disease	N	MS	MR	AR	CVD	HHD	IHD	Total		N	H	D	F	Index (N+H)−(D+F)	Major lesions
Normal		8	5				1		14	i	4	1	1	1	+3	normal
										m	5	0	1	1	+3	
										o	6	0	1	1	+4	
ST↓		1			1	1			3	i	0	1	6	3	−8	i>m>o
										m	0	0	5	2	−6	
										o	0	0	3	1	−4	
T→		3	3	1		1	1		9	i	6	1	1	3	+3	median
										m	1	0	4	2	−5	
										o	6	1	1	2	+4	
T↓				2				3	5	i	0	2	5	5	−8	i<m>o
										m	0	1	6	6	−10	
										o	0	1	1	4	−4	
ST↓,T↓				1	1			3	5	i	0	4	5	7	−8	i=m>o H
										m	0	2	5	5	−8	
										o	0	4	3	4	−3	
HiV		1		1			1	1	4	i	0	3	3	3	−3	balanced, H
										m	3	3	3	3	0	
										o	0	3	3	2	−2	
HiV,ST↓		1		2	2	1			6	i	0	4	6	6	−6	i=m>o H
										m	0	3	4	5	−6	
										o	0	3	2	4	−3	
HiV,T→				1	1	3			5	i	0	4	5	5	−6	i<m H
										m	0	1	5	3	−7	
										o	0	4	1	3	0	

144

HiV, ST↓, T→	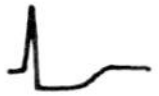			1	1	2	6	3		13	i 0 4 5 7 m 1 2 4 4 o 0 4 3 3	−8 −5 −2	i>m H
HiV, ST↓, T↓	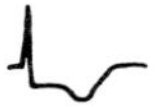				2	6	3	3	2	16	i 0 3 6 6 m 0 2 5 5 o 0 4 2 3	−9 −8 −1	i = m oH
cBBB	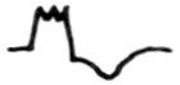						5			5	i 0 2 8 8 m 0 0 6 4 o 0 1 4 4	−14 −10 −7	i>m>o +++
Total			14	9	11	13	20	9	9	85			
Normal		i	5	2	1	0	0	0	0				
		m	3	3	3	0	0	1	0				
		o	5	6	2	0	0	1	0				
Hypertrophy		i	1	1	3	3	3	3	3				
		m	0	0	2	3	1	2	1				
		o	0	1	3	5	3	4	3				
Degeneration		i	2	2	5	7	5	4	5				
		m	3	2	4	5	4	4	6				
		o	1	1	3	2	2	2	2				
Fibrosis		i	0	3	7	7	6	5	7				
		m	0	2	5	4	4	3	5				
		o	0	2	4	3	3	2	4				
Index (N + H) − (D + F)		i	+4	−2	−8	−11	−8	−6	−9				
		m	0	−1	−4	−6	−7	−4	−10				
		o	+4	+4	−2	0	−2	+1	−3				

Index: + = 3; ++ = 6; +++ = 10; normal = 10

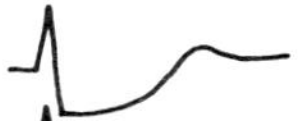
i>m>o

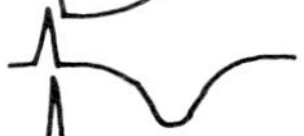
i<m>o

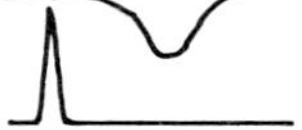
i>m<o oH

N = normal; H = hypertrophy; D = degeneration; F = fibrosis; i = inner layer; m = median layer; o = outer layer.
>indicates more involved.

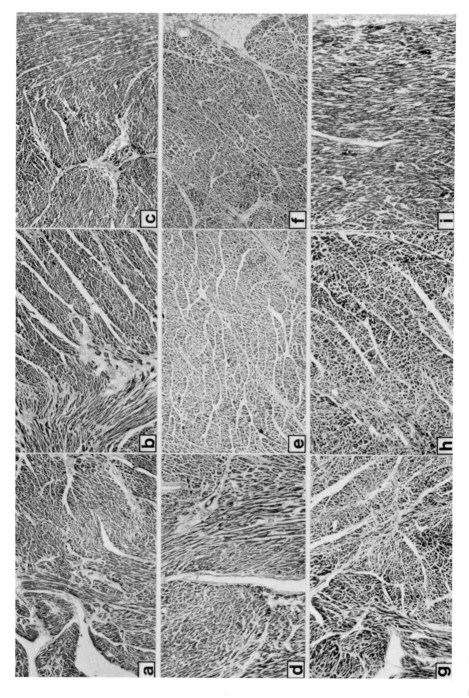

Figure 1. a, b, c = Vertical section of the left ventricular (LV) wall with hypertensive heart disease. d, e, f = mitral regurgitation. g, h, i = aortic regurgitation. 12 ×, Azan stain. a, d, g = inner oblique layer. b, e, h = median circular layer. c, f, i = outer oblique layer.

146

DISCUSSION

The layer-selective myocardial lesions seem to be closely related to the shape and size of the ventricle and to muscle fiber orientation. When ventricular size is increased, overstretching of the myocardium theoretically can cause median layer deterioration first (Okada, 1976a), because horizontally running muscle fibers cannot avoid the stretching overload by changing intercellular or inter-fascicular distance (Linzbach, 1960). When ventricular shape is changed, muscle fiber orientation should be altered for adaptation to new situation (Streeter *et al.*, 1969). The globular MR-type enlargement makes the outer oblique layer more horizontally oriented, and elongated AR-type enlargement makes this layer more vertically oriented than normal. The latter makes a sharp angulation between the hypertrophied outer layer and the fibrosing median layer, and it might augment a mechanical stress that accelerates median layer deterioration. The HHD and IHD groups usually show no particular alteration of fiber orientation because not as much dilation is expected.

The principle of ECG-pathology correlation presented here could be useful in the specification of the nature of hypertrophy and hypertrophy-related myocardial lesions.

REFERENCES

LINZBACH, A. J. 1960. Die pathologische Anatomie der Herzinsuffizienz. *In* G. Bergman, W. Frey, and H. Schwiegk (eds.), Handbuch der inn. Med. 4te Auflage, pp. 706–800. Springer-Verlag, Berlin.

OKADA, R. 1976a. Morphology of cardiac enlargement. Respir. Circ. 24:481–489.

OKADA, R. 1976b. Pathological approach to EKG reading. Sogo Rinsho 25:715–724.

SCOTT, R. C. 1960. The correlation between the electrocardiographic patterns of ventricular hypertrophy and the anatomic findings. Circulation 21:256–291.

STREETER, D. D., JR., SPOTNITZ, H. M., POTEL, D. P., ROSS, J., JR., and SONNENBLICK, E. H. 1969. Fiber orientation in the canine left ventricle during diastole and systole. Circ. Res. 24:339–347.

Mailing address:
Ryozo Okada, M.D.,
Department of Internal Medicine, School of Medicine, Juntendo University,
3-1-3 Hongo, Bunkyo-ku Tokyo 113 (Japan).

Recent Advances in Studies on
Cardiac Structure and Metabolism, Volume 12
Cardiac Adaptation
Edited by T. Kobayashi, Y. Ito, and G. Rona
Copyright 1978 University Park Press Baltimore

RIGHT VENTRICULAR HYPERTROPHY
IN TETRALOGY OF FALLOT

M. KATO, Y. KAWASHIMA, T. FUJITA, T. MORI, and H. MANABE

First Department of Surgery, Osaka University Medical School,
Fukushima-ku, Osaka, Japan

SUMMARY

Histopathological studies were carried out on right ventricular myocardium in 104 patients with tetralogy of Fallot (T/F). Detailed analysis of the correlation between morphological and clinical data was performed. Right ventricular hypertrophy in T/F was found to initiate immediately after birth, and the diameter of right ventricular muscle fiber (D) increased with age ($r = 0.74$). There was a correlation between D and the hemoglobin level. There was, however, no correlation between D, arterial oxygen saturation (SaO_2), and pulmonary trunk/aorta diameter (PA/Ao) ratio. Histopathological alterations were related directly to D and to the age of the patient, and were unrelated to hemoglobin, SaO_2, and PA/Ao ratio. Irreversible histopathological alterations were first observed when the D exceeded 15 μm, when most patients were four years old or more. From these findings, it is considered that the optimal age for corrective surgery to prevent irreversible alteration of the right ventricular muscle fibers in patients with T/F is less than three years.

INTRODUCTION

In tetralogy of Fallot (T/F), proliferation of stromal connective tissues, as well as degeneration of myocardial cells, often is associated with progressive right ventricular hypertrophy (Kato *et al.,* 1973). The time and the mechanisms of these alterations are unknown. Studies were carried out in 104 patients with T/F in an attempt to elucidate the mechanisms involved.

MATERIALS AND METHODS

Detailed analysis of the correlation between morphological and clinical data such as age, hemoglobin, arterial oxygen saturation (SaO_2), and pulmonary trunk/ aorta diameter ratio (PA/Ao) was carried out. Samples were taken from the crista supraventricularis for histopathological examination; the mean diameter of a series of 100 myocardial fibers was measured morphometrically according to the methods of Chalkley, Confield, and Park (1949) and Arai, Machida, and Nakamura (1968). Using a magnification of $\times$ 1,000, only fibers visible in an exact nucleated cross-section were measured.

RESULTS

There was a close correlation between the mean diameter of right ventricular myocardial fibers and the age of the patient. An identical relationship in 145 normal subjects of different ages can be seen in the lower part of Figure 1. Each value indicates a mean diameter of right ventricular fiber, obtained from two to nine normal hearts.

In normal subjects, the diameter of cardiac muscle fibers gradually increased approximately 6% in the first year after birth. In patients with T/F, the

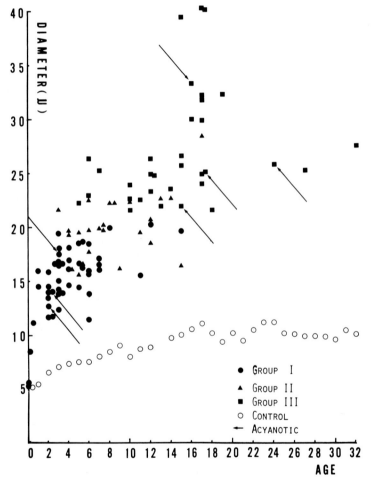

Figure 1. There was a close correlation between the mean diameter of right ventricular fibers and the age of the patient with tetralogy of Fallot (T/F) ($r = 0.74$, $p < 0.01$, Y = 0.76X + 13.764).

diameter at the time of birth was not significantly different from that of normal subjects. However, there was a rapid increase in the diameter of right ventricular fiber in the first year after birth, from 5.5 μm (at birth), to 8.6 μm (at 3 months), to 11.2 μm (at 6 months), to 15.3 μm (at 12 months), i.e., an increase of about 180% in the first year of life. Thereafter, the diameter of the right ventricular fiber in T/F continued to increase progressively with age, to as much as 40 μm or more (Figure 1).

The alteration of properties of blood, such as increased hemoglobin and decreased arterial oxygen saturation (SaO_2, also was considered. There was a positive correlation between the diameter of right ventricular muscle fiber and the hemoglobin level as shown in Figure 2. There was no correlation between SaO_2 and the PA/Ao diameter ratio nor between SaO_2 and the diameter of right ventricular muscle fibers. The histopathological alterations in the right ventricular myocardium in newborns with T/F (Figure 3) revealed hypertrophy of muscle fibers (Group I). The interstitial spaces between muscle bundles narrowed with progression of muscular hypertrophy, and connective tissues became dense. Ultimately, a prominent connective tissue septa developed around individual cardiac muscle fibers.

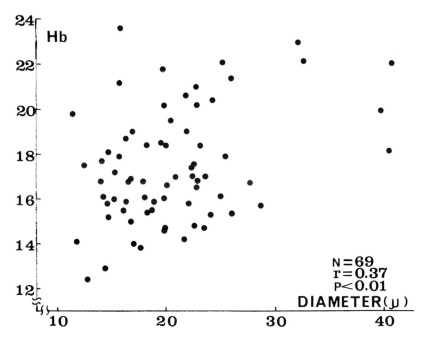

Figure 2. There was a positive correlation between the mean diameter of right ventricular muscle fiber and hemoglobin level ($r = 0.37, p < 0.01$, Y = 0.15X + 14.328).

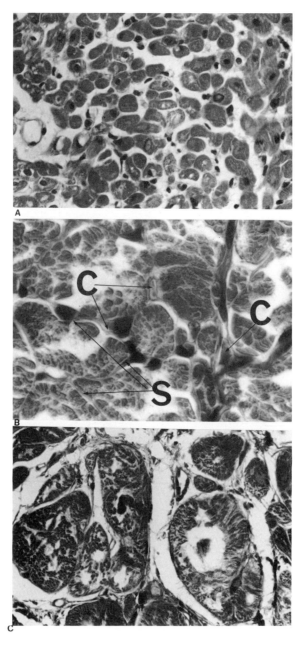

Figure 3. Typical photomicrographs. A: Group I (× 101), B: Group II (× 340), C: Group III (× 160). C = capillaries, which were encased by connective tissue septa (S).

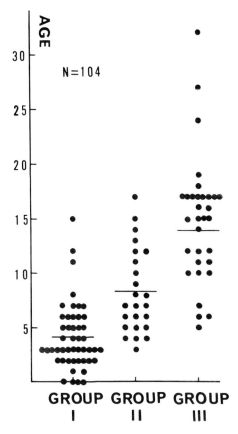

Figure 4. Relationship between age and histological grade of right ventricular muscle. Average age in the three groups increased from Group I → II → III ($p < 0.001$).

This histological picture was graded as Group II. The connective tissue continued to proliferate progressively with the hypertrophy of myocardial fibers; subsequently, degenerative changes occurred, such as the fragmentation of muscle fibers and the disappearance of cross-striation. This histological alteration was graded as Group III. As shown in Figure 4, average ages in these three groups increased with a statistical significance ($p < 0.001$). Histological alterations in patients classified as Group III were first seen at five years of age. Histological criteria of the three groups are summarized in Table 1.

With regard to the relationship between myocardial fiber diameter and the severity of the morphological alteration, all myocardial specimens showed histopathological alteration with a fiber diameter of 23 μm or more (Group III),

Table 1. Histological criteria

Histology group	Connective tissue septum formation	Myocardial degeneration
Group I	−	−
Group II	+	−
Group III	+	+

except for one patient. Average diameter increased in the order of Group I → II → III, respectively, with a statistical significance ($p < 0.001$). The severity of the morphological alteration correlated with age of the patients (Figure 1).

The degree of myocardial alteration seen in cyanotic T/F patients did not differ from that seen in acyanotic patients. From our data, hypoxia does not appear to influence myocardial alterations in T/F. There was no relationship between PA/Ao ratio, which is generally employed to express the morphological degree of pulmonary stenosis and the severity of myocardial alteration. The degree of pulmonary stenosis does not appear to influence the development of right ventricular muscular hypertrophy.

CONCLUSIONS

From the results of our investigations, the following was concluded: the development of right ventricular muscular hypertrophy and of associated myocardial alterations is attributable to the pressure overload exerted on the right ventricle, and closely parallels the age of the patients. However, this ventricular muscular hypertrophy is not influenced directly by changes in blood composition such as polycytemia and hypoxia.

From the findings obtained in the present study, it is concluded that corrective surgery for T/F should be performed at or before the age of three years to prevent irreversible alteration of the right ventricular muscle fibers.

Acknowledgment   Our gratitude is expressed to M. Ohara for her assistance in preparing the manuscript.

REFERENCES

ARAI, S., MACHIDA, A., and NAKAMURA, T. 1968. Myocardial structure and vascularization of hypertrophied hearts. Tohoku J. Exp. Med. 95:35.
CHALKLEY, H. W., CONFIELD, J., and PARK, H. 1949. A method of estimating volume-surface ratios. Science 110:295.
KATO, M., KAWASHIMA, Y., FUJITA, T., MIYAMOTO, T., HORIGUCHI, Y., OKA-MOTO, S., HASHIMOTO, S., FUDEMOTO, Y., SANDA, N., MATSUDA, H., and

MANABE, H. 1973. Infundibular stenosis in tetralogy of Fallot. J. Jpn. Assoc. Thorac. Surg. 21:104.

Mailing address:
Masaaki Kato, M.D.,
First Department of Surgery, Osaka University Medical School,
1-50, 1 Chyoume Fukushima, Fukushima-ku, Osaka (Japan).

Recent Advances in Studies on
Cardiac Structure and Metabolism, Volume 12
Cardiac Adaptation
Edited by T. Kobayashi, Y. Ito, and G. Rona
Copyright 1978 University Park Press Baltimore

EFFECTS OF LOW PROTEIN DIET ON CARDIAC FUNCTION AND ULTRASTRUCTURE OF SPONTANEOUSLY HYPERTENSIVE RATS LOADED WITH SODIUM CHLORIDE

Y. YOKOTA, K. OTA, M. AGETA, S. ISHIDA,
H. TOSHIMA, and N. KIMURA

Third Department of Internal Medicine, Kurume University,
School of Medicine, 67 Asahi-Machi, Kurume, Japan

SUMMARY

The effects of low protein diet on cardiac metabolic and structural changes subsequent to an extremely high pressure load were investigated. Spontaneously hypertensive rats(SHR) were divided into four groups, and fed the following diets for four weeks: 1) Group A: regular diet (23% protein) and water, 2) Group B: regular diet and 1% saline, 3) Group C: low protein diet (10% protein) and water, and 4) Group D: low protein diet and 1% saline.

Two weeks after the start of feeding, there was no significant difference in the left ventricular ultrastructures between the corresponding regular and low protein diet groups. Four weeks after, degenerative findings such as streaming of Z lines, dilatations of smooth endoplasmic reticulum, and disarrangements of myofilaments appeared in Group D, while in Group B electron microscopic findings indicated hypertrophy. Incorporation of $[^{14}C]$leucine into the myocardial myosin B in Group D was significantly low, with a resulting fall of the $LVdP/dt_{max}$ per integrated isometric pressure (IIP) and a rise of the left ventricular end-diastolic pressure (LVEDP), as compared to that in Group C at four weeks after the start of feeding. These observations suggest that, in the heart with an extremely high pressure load, low protein diet hinders the development of hypertrophy to the load with resulting heart failure.

INTRODUCTION

A series of metabolic alterations follows an abnormally high pressure load imposed on the ventricle, characterized by increases in energy production and myocardial protein synthesis (Meerson, 1962; Norman, 1962). Under such circumstances, the relatively low supply of dietary protein may interfere with renewal of the energy-producing and contractile structures of the myocardium, leading to heart failure (Zühlke *et al.,* 1966). This study was undertaken to determine the effects of low protein diet on cardiac metabolic and structural changes subsequent to an extremely high pressure load.

MATERIALS AND METHODS

Experiments were performed on 44 male, spontaneously hypertensive rats (SHR) with an average weight of 234 g. The animals were divided into four groups in such a way that the mean systolic pressure was approximately the same. Thereafter they were fed the following diets for four weeks:

1. Group A: regular diet (23% protein) and water
2. Group B: regular diet and 1% saline
3. Group C: low protein diet (10% protein) and water
4. Group D: low protein diet and 1% saline

Three parameters were investigated: 1) electron microscopic examinations at two and four weeks after the start of feeding; 2) measurements of cardiac function at zero, two, and four weeks after, and 3) incorporation of amino acid into myocardial myosin B at the end of the experiment. Fixed with 2% paraformaldehyde and 2.5% glutaraldehyde by using the vascular perfusion technique, samples for electron microscopic examination were taken from left ventricular (LV) anterior free wall, post-fixed with 2% OsO_4, and stained with uranyl acetate and lead citrate.

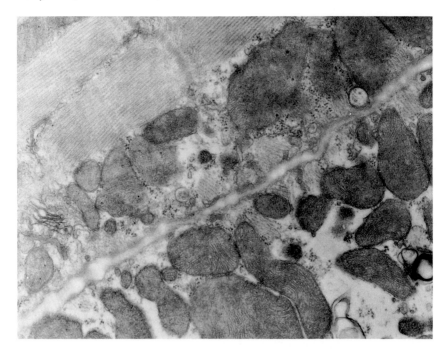

Figure 1. The ultrastructure of the myocardium from Group B four weeks after the start of feeding is shown. In the subsarcolemma, poorly organized myofilaments, indicating a renewal of myofibrils, can be seen. × 22,000.

Hemodynamic examination was carried out in rats anesthetized with ether; LVP and LVdP/dt measurements were taken by means of direct puncture of the LV through the chest wall. For studies on the incorporation of amino acid into myosin B, $[U-^{14}C]$ leucine was injected intravenously one hour before death; extraction of myosin B was carried out by the method of Straub-Feuer, modi-field by Ohsawa and Asakura (Matsumiya and Asakura, 1962).

RESULTS

Electron Microscopic Examination

Two weeks after the start of feeding, the left ventricular myocardium from Groups A and C presented normal ultrastructure, while those obtained from Groups B and D showed changes indicating hypertrophy. Four weeks after, clear differences were observed in the myocardial ultrastructure between Groups B and D, while there were no significant differences between the changes in Groups A and C.

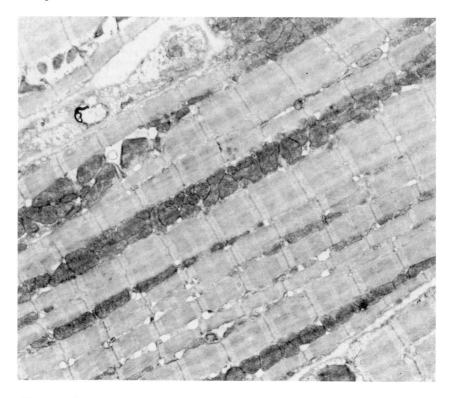

Figure 2. The ultrastructure of the myocardium from Group D four weeks after the start of feeding is shown. Mitochondria and myofilaments appear normal, but there is dilation of smooth endoplasmic reticulum. × 6,600.

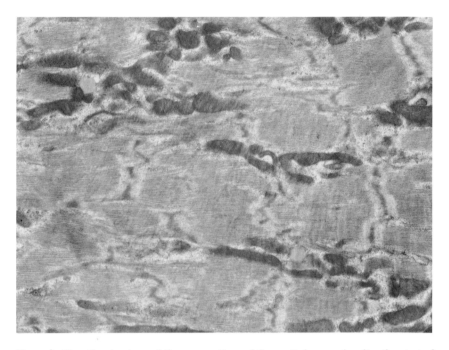

Figure 3. The ultrastructure of the myocardium of Group D four weeks after the start of feeding. Mitochondria appear smaller in size and abnormal in shape in comparison to those seen in Group B. Streaming of Z lines and disarrangements of myofilaments also are observed. × 12,000.

Figure 1 shows the ultrastructure of the myocardium from Group B after four weeks of feeding. Poorly organized myofilaments indicating renewal of myofibrils at subsarcolemma and an increase of ribosomes were observed. These findings, which were noted in most of the electron micrographs, suggested hypertrophy.

Figures 2 and 3 show the ultrastructures of the myocardium from Group D after four weeks. In Figure 2, mitochondria and myofilaments appear normal but the tubules of smooth endoplasmic reticulum are dilated. In Figure 3, mitochondria appear smaller in size and abnormal in shape in comparison to those from Group B. Streaming of Z lines and disarrangements of myofilaments also are evident, suggesting degenerative processes.

Hemodynamic Studies

In Group A, dP/dt_{max} per 11P and LVEDP did not change at two and four weeks after the start of feeding, while in Group B these parameters did not change at two weeks after, but showed a decrease in dP/dt_{max} per 11P and an

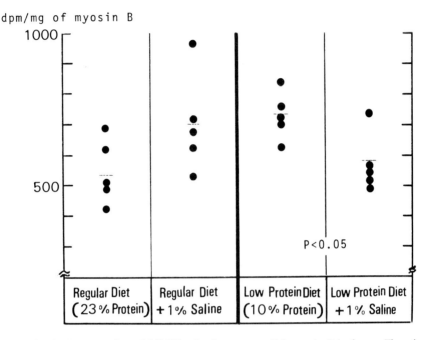

dpm/mg of myosin B

Figure 4. The incorporation of [^{14}C]leucine into myocardial myosin B is shown. There is no significant difference between Groups A and B. However, the values for Group D are significantly low in comparison to those for Group C.

increase in LVEDP by four weeks. On the other hand, in Groups C and D, a fall of dP/dt_{max} per 11P and a rise of LVEDP were found by two weeks feeding.

Incorporation of Amino Acid into Myocardial Myosin B

Figure 4 shows incorporation of [^{14}C]leucine into myocardial myosin B. Mean values and standard deviations for Groups A and B were 539 ± 103 and 707 ± 169 dpm/mg of myosin B, respectively. There was no significant difference between these two groups. On the other hand, the values for Group D were significantly low in comparison to those in Group C ($p < 0.05$)—730 ± 77 and 582 ± 103 dpm/mg of myosin B, respectively. This suggests a decrease in the rate of the cardiac myosin B synthesis.

DISCUSSION

The most significant findings of this study were that, in the heart with an extremely high pressure load, low protein diet caused a decrease in the rate of cardiac myosin B synthesis and caused degenerative ultrastructural changes, with resulting deterioration of the LV function. The mechanism of these changes is not clear at the present time. Wannemacher and McCoy (1969) reported that an increase in the rate of amino acid transport and in the concentration of amino acids has been associated with increased protein synthesis in cardiomegaly produced by treatment of unilaterally nephrectomized rats with desoxycortico-sterone (DOCA) and 1% saline. In view of the possibility that amino acids have a role in the stimulation of nucleic acid synthesis and subsequent cell growth (Nierlich, 1968), low concentrations of amino acids in myocardium, caused by low protein diet, may hinder the growth of heart muscle cells through the impairment of nucleic acid synthesis.

REFERENCES

MATSUMIYA, K., and ASAKURA, S. 1962. Kinniku tanpakushitsu no torikata (Extraction of muscle protein). Protein Nucleic Acid, Enzyme (Tokyo) 2:455–463.
MEERSON, F. Z. 1962. Compensatory hyperfunction of the hearts and cardiac insufficiency. Circ. Res. 10:250–258.
NIERLICH, D. P. 1968. Amino acid control over RNA synthesis. Proc. Nat. Acad. Sci. USA 60:1345–1352.
NORMAN, T. D. 1962. The pathogenesis of cardiac hypertrophy. Prog. Cardiovasc. Dis. 4:439–463.
WANNEMACHER, X., and McCOY, X. 1969. Regulation of protein synthesis in the ventricular myocardium of hypertrophic hearts. Am. J. Physiol. 216:781–787.
ZÜHLKE, V., ROCHEMONT, W. N., GUDBJARNASON, S., and BING, R. J. 1966. Inhibition of protein synthesis in cardiac hypertrophy and its relation to myocardial failure. Circ. Res. 18:558–572.

Mailing address:
Yasushi Yokota, M.D., Instructor,
Third Department of Internal Medicine, Kurume University, School of Medicine,
67 Asahi-machi, Kurume 830 (Japan).

ALTERED
MYOCARDIAL METABOLISM

Chemical Models

Recent Advances in Studies on
Cardiac Structure and Metabolism, Volume 12
Cardiac Adaptation
Edited by T. Kobayashi, Y. Ito, and G. Rona
Copyright 1978 University Park Press Baltimore

ISCHEMIC-LIKE CHANGE PRODUCED
IN CANINE HEART BY ATRACTYLOSIDE:
A CHEMICAL MODEL

N. BITTAR,[1] A. L. SHUG,[2] J. D. FOLTS,[1]
and J. R. KOKE[1]

[1] Department of Medicine, and [2] Department of Nutritional Science
and the Veterans Administration Hospital, Metabolic Research Laboratory,
University of Wisconsin, Madison, Wisconsin, USA

SUMMARY

Experiments were conducted in two canine models. Intracoronary infusion of atractyloside resulted in physiological, biochemical, and ultrastructural changes similar to those seen with ischemia. The fact that atractyloside, a specific inhibitor of adenine nucleotide translocase produces this change *in vivo* suggests that this inhibition is the key disturbance that initiates the metabolic derangements seen with ischemia. This chemical model seems to provide unique opportunities to study the possible factors that may reverse adenine nucleotide translocase inhibition and thus possibly prevent cell injury.

INTRODUCTION

It has been known from *in vitro* experimentation that atractyloside, the glycoside extracted from the plant *Atractylis gummifera* (Riccio, Scherer, and Klingenberg, 1973), when applied to isolated mitochondria, causes inhibition of the ADP-ATP carrier (Klingenberg, Grebe, and Scherer, 1975). Furthermore, we showed (Shug, Koke, Folts, and Bittar, 1975) that this carrier was inhibited during myocardial ischemia and that the likely cause for this inhibition was the accumulation of long chain, fatty acid, acyl-CoA esters. Beacuse ischemia and the application of atractyloside had the inhibition of the ADP-ATP carrier, otherwise known as adenine nucleotide translocase, in common, we reasoned that the infusion of atractyloside into the coronary circulation of the intact canine heart would produce cellular injury similar to that seen in ischemia, in spite of adequate blood flow and oxygen supply. The experiments described in this chapter show that atractyloside does produce cellular injury that is identical to that produced by interruption of coronary blood flow.

This research was supported in part by grants from the USPHS, NHLI-17736, NHLI-HL 17759, and NHLI-15681, and from the Wisconsin Heart Association.

MATERIALS AND METHODS

Experiments were conducted in two different canine models. The first has been described previously (Shug *et al.*, 1975). Briefly, 10 open-chest, anesthetized, artificially ventilated dogs were instrumented so that epicardial electrograms, coronary blood flow, and blood pressure were monitored, and catheters were placed in vessels to allow collection of arterial and great cardiac vein blood samples. Atractyloside was infused into the anterior descending branch of the left coronary artery at a rate of 75 μmol/ml/min through a 23-gauge catheter, introduced into the vessel using the method of Khouri, Gregg, and McGranahan (1971). Blood oxygen content was measured using a Lex O_2 Con oxygen analyzer, and M VO_2 was calculated from the arteriovenous difference. Tissue lactate (Hohorst, 1965), adenine nucleotide translocase activity (Shug, Koke, Folts, and Bittar, 1975), and ATP and creatine phosphate levels (Stanley and Williams, 1969) were measured in samples of myocardium obtained by transmural drill biopsy before, during, and after atractyloside infusion.

The second model was the isolated segment preparation described by Lajos *et al.* (1974), which has been shown to eliminate collateral flow and thus provide a segment of heart muscle in which all cells appear to be similarly affected, rather than the nonhomogeneous preparations commonly used for study of myocardial ischemia (Maroko and Braunwald, 1973). An area of left ventricle was incised and sutured (Figure 1) until an isolated segment was created with its own blood supply that could be entirely controlled. After recovery from surgery (usually two weeks), eight dogs were once again anesthetized, the chest opened, and the artery to the segment cannulated and connected to the femoral artery, thereby maintaining tissue perfusion. A Biotronex flow transducer was applied to the coronary artery and a Statham P23 db pressure transducer connected to the femoral artery. Four epicardial electrodes were attached to the myocardial surface, three to the isolated segment and the fourth to an adjacent area that served as a control. Data were recorded on a Sanborn Polyviso Recorder.

Atractyloside was infused as a 0.15 μM solution in 0.05 M Tris-HCl at pH 7.4, using a Harvard pump, directly into the coronary cannula at a rate sufficient to maintain a flow rate of 0.25–0.5 ml per min. The delivery rate averaged 6.0 mg/ml flow/min for 10 min.

Immediately following the infusion of atractyloside, a cold (4°C) fixative consisting of 4% formaldehyde, 2% glutaraldehyde, 0.5 mM $CaCl_2$ in 0.1 M Na cacodylate, pH 7.2, was infused via the same cannula at a rate of 5–15 ml/min, depending upon the segmental blood flow rate. Simultaneously with initiation of fixative perfusion, the femoral blood flow into the cannula was stopped. The isolated segment became cool and firm within 30–60 sec after initiation of fixative perfusion, and ventricular arrest usually occurred within 1–2 min.

After infusion of 150–300 ml of fixative, the segments were removed from the heart and cut into five equal-sized portions. Each portion was cut into

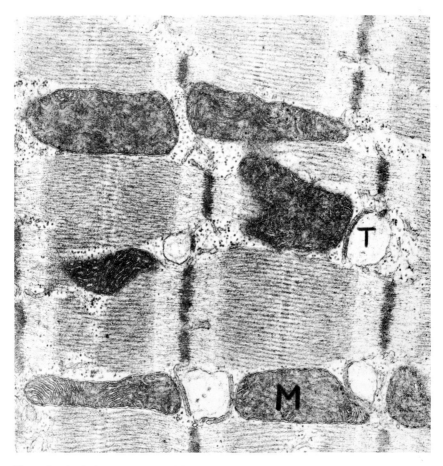

Figure 1. The isolated segment of left ventricle constructed by incision and suture around a diagonal branch of the left anterior descending artery.

epicardial, middle, and endocardial sections, and the epicardial and endocardial sections were discarded. The remaining portion was cut into pieces suitable for electron microscopy, and pieces from each of the five original portions were kept separate during processing. After trimming, the samples were washed in buffer, post-fixed in 2% osmium tetroxide, dehydrated in ethanol, and embedded in Spurr's low viscosity epoxy resin. Tissue blocks were oriented to allow selection of the sectioning plane. Sections were then cut with glass knives on a Porter-Blum MT-2 ultramicrotome, contrasted with methanolic uranyl acetate and lead citrate, and examined with a Hitachi HU-11B electron microscope. Thick (1.0 μm) sections also were cut and examined with a light microscope.

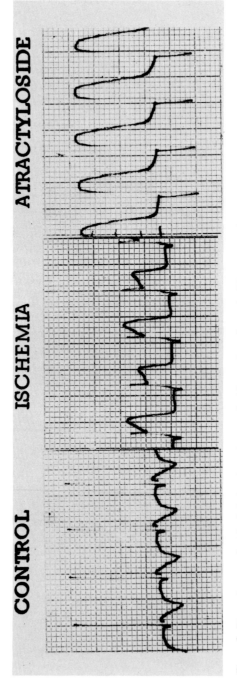

Figure 2. It can be seen that both ischemia and atractyloside produce dramatic ST-segment elevation in the isolated left ventricular segment electrogram recording.

Morphometric analysis was performed as described by Page, McCallister, and Power (1971). Volume-fraction and surface:volume determinations were performed on micrographs obtained at three different levels of magnification, calibrated by use of diffraction-grating replicas (obtained from Ernest Fullam Co.). Determinations were made at a magnification of X 4,500 with light microscopy, and at low magnification, X 14,750, and medium magnification, X 40,000, with electron microscopy, using a counting grid of 1-cm squares as described by Page, McCallister, and Power (1971).

RESULTS

The typical injury potential produced by infusion of atractyloside is shown in Figure 2. It can be seen that there is marked elevation of the ST segment, which is known to return to normal after cessation of atractyloside infusion. The identical result is obtained when a coronary artery is ligated, and this also returns to baseline once flow is restored.

The cumulative physiological derangements following atractyloside infusion and those produced by ischemia are shown in Table 1. It can be seen that the only difference involves the change in coronary blood flow; otherwise, both interventions produce electrogram injury without wide changes in blood pressure or heart rate.

The metabolic changes also are similar, as shown in Table 2. Infusion of atractyloside produced, as does ischemia, a rapid decline in cellular adenine nucleotide translocase activity, a decline in ATP and creatine phosphate levels, and a rise in muscle lactate.

The morphometric measurements carried out on atractyloside-injured cells are shown in Tables 3 and 4. It can be seen that a variety of changes take place in myocardial cells but that interstitial swelling and mitochondrial changes appear to be most significant.

Table 1. Physiological changes induced by atractyloside (ATR)

	Aortic pressure (mm Hg)	Coronary flow (cc/min)	Heart rate (beats/min)	ST elevation (mm)
Control	106 ± 13	40 ± 8	144 ± 18	0
ATR	96 ± 15[a]	52 ± 12[a]	151 ± 20	5.5 ± 2[b]
Ischemia	97 ± 14	10.7 ± 7[b]	149 ± 18	4.8 ± 2.7[b]

The similarity of the physiological changes is shown. Of course, in the atractyloside experiments, coronary flow is unrestricted and therefore registers a rise.
[a]$p < 0.01$.
[b]$p < 0.001$.

Table 2. Metabolic consequences of atractyloside (ATR) infusion

	ANT dpm/mg/g	ATP μm/g	CP μm/g	M VO$_2$[a] cc/min	A-V Lactate μg/100 cc
Control	31,387 ± 3,421	5.87 ± 0.15	8.21 ± 1.2	4.2 ± 1.2	1.42 ± 0.8
ATR	22,978 ± 1,897	4.66 ± 0.09	3.82 ± 0.71	4.9 ± 1.9	−11.4 ± 5.0
p Value	<0.05	<0.05	<0.05	<0.05	<0.05
Ischemia	21,373 ± 1,791	3.4 ± 0.14	2.94 ± 0.62	1.32	− 8.2 ± 4.1

The similarity of metabolic change produced by atractyloside infusion into the coronary circulation for two minutes, and the changes brought about by a five-minute interval of ischemia, are shown.
[a]LAD bed.

The mitochondrial changes consisted of compartmental volume changes with an increase in intracristal volume and a decrease in matrix volume. These changes are similar to those described by Stoner and Sirak (1973) in isolated beef heart mitochondria. Figure 3 shows an example of the fine structural change caused by atractyloside. It can be seen that there is intracellular swelling and a change in mitochondrial morphology.

DISCUSSION

These studies indicate the great similarities between cellular injury resulting from the application of atractyloside and that resulting from the interruption of the blood supply to myocardial cells. The fact that both types of injury have an inhibition of adenine nucleotide translocase in common suggests that this is the key lesion that triggers the commonly recognized cellular disturbances known to

Table 3. Morphometric analysis after atractyloside (light microscopy)

Cell component	Control	After atractyloside	Percent of control
Myocytes	79.6 ± 6.9	64.9 ± 8.8	81.5[a]
Interstitial space	0.5 ± 0.4	27.8 ± 7.2	5560.0[a]
Capillary lumen	14.8 ± 4.8	4.8 ± 1.3	32.4[a]
Capillary endothelium	4.3 ± 0.9	2.5 ± 0.4	58.1[a]
Ratio capillary lumen/ Capillary endothelium	3.39 ± 0.5	1.88 ± 0.4	55.5[a]

Morphometric measurements, carried out on cardiac muscle cells exposed to atractyloside for a period of 10 minutes, are shown. Striking changes in the intracellular space, T tubules, interstitial space, and capillary lumen have taken place, indicating a marked degree of swelling.
[a]*p* < 0.05.

Table 4. Morphometric analysis after atractyloside (electron microscopy)

Cell component	Control	After atractyloside	Percent of control
Mitochondria	24.8 ± 3.0	20.1 ± 1.8	81.0[a]
Myofilaments	63.0 ± 2.0	58.1 ± 2.9	922.0[a]
Ratio mito/myofilaments	0.39 ± 0.05	0.35 ± 0.03	89.7
T tubules	0.80 ± 0.20	2.42 ± 0.58	302.5[a]
Cytoplasm with glycogen	10.4 ± 1.0	9.12 ± 1.8	87.7
Intracell space	0.1 ± 0.1	9.60 ± 3.6	9600.0[a]
Sarcoplasmic reticulum	4.5 ± 0.7	3.28 ± 0.66	72.8[a]

Morphometric measurements, carried out on cardiac muscle cells exposed to atractyloside for a period of 10 minutes, are shown. Striking changes in the intracellular space, T tubules, interstitial space, and capillary lumen have taken place, indicating a marked degree of swelling.
[a]$p < 0.05$.

follow a brief period of ischemia. In these studies we have shown that adenine nucleotide translocase is inhibited within seconds after infusion of atractyloside, and this coincides with the development of ST-segment elevation in the epicardial electrogram. That the inhibition of adenine nucleotide translocase may cause cell membrane changes, most likely caused by the cessation of ATP efflux from the mitochondria, is suggested by the work of Bittar and Tallitsch (1976);

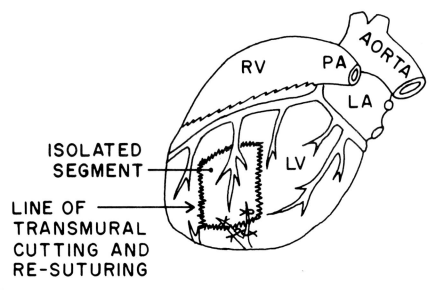

Figure 3. The fine structural change induced by infusion of atractyloside for 10 min. × 28,800. Slight intracellular swelling is apparent between the sarcomeres and around the mitochondria. Glycogen particles are diminished. Mitochondria (M) have dense appearing matrices and transparent intracristal space. The transverse tubules (T) are dilated.

they showed that the introduction of atractyloside into a single barnacle cell caused a decline in Na efflux and that this could be restored by the microinjection of ATP into the cell.

It is therefore suggested that these studies with atractyloside have brought forth what may be considered to be a chemical model of ischemic-like cell injury. This should allow wider opportunities at cellular component manipulation and drug analog studies in an effort to gain a better understanding of the pathogenesis of cellular injury.

Acknowledgments The authors wish to thank Cheryll Crosby, Judith Koke, Mary Schmidt, Susan Mitchell, and Denis Dahmen for technical assistance, and Mrs. Margaret Jorgensen for typing the manuscript.

REFERENCES

BITTAR, E. E., and TALLITSCH, R. B. 1976. Mode of the stimulation by aldosterone of the sodium efflux in barnacle muscle fibres: Effects of ouabain, ethacrynic acid, disphenyl-hydantoin, $(ATPMg)^{2-}$, adenine translocase inhibitors, pyruvate and oxythiamine. J. Physiol. 255:29–56.

HOHORST, H. J. 1965. Determination with lactic dehydrogenase and DPN. *In* Hans Ulrich Bergmeyer, Methods of Enzymatic Analysis. 1st Ed. Edited by Weinheim/Bergstrom, Verlag Chemie. Academic Press, New York.

KHOURI, E. M., GREGG, D. E., and McGRANAHAN, G. M. 1971. Regression and reappearance of coronary collaterals. Am. J. Physiol. 220:655–661.

KLINGENBERG, M., GREBE, K., and SCHERER, B. 1975. The binding of atractylate and carboxy-atractylate to mitochondria. Eur. J. Biochem. 52:351–363.

LAJOS, T. Z., CERRA, F. B., MONTES, M., and SIEGEL, J. H. 1974. A permanent experimental model for reversible myocardial anoxia. Ann. Thorac. Surg. 17:20–35.

MAROKO, P. R., and BRAUNWALD, E. 1973. Modification of myocardial infarct size after coronary occlusion. Ann. Intern. Med. 79:720–733.

PAGE, E., McCALLISTER, L. P., and POWER, B. 1971. Stereological measurements of cardiac ultrastructures implicated in excitation-contraction coupling. Proc. Natl. Acad. Sci. USA 68:1465–1466.

RICCIO, P., SCHERER, B., and KLINGENBERG, M. 1973. Isolation of a new atractyloside type compound. FEBS Lett. 31:11–14.

SHUG, A. L., KOKE, J. R., FOLTS, J. D., and BITTAR, N. 1975. Role of adenine nucleotide translocase in metabolic change caused by ischemia. *In* P. E. Roy and G. Rona (eds.), Recent Advances in Studies on Cardiac Structure and Metabolism. Volume 10: The Metabolism of Contraction, p. 365. University Park Press, Baltimore.

STANLEY, P. E., and WILLIAMS, S. G. 1969. Firefly method for ATP. Anal. Biochem. 29:381–392.

STONER, C. D., and SIRAK, H. D. 1973. Adenine nucleotide-induced contraction of the inner mitochondrial membrane. I. General characterization. J. Cell Biol. 56:51–64.

Mailing address:
Neville Bittar, M.D.,
Cardiovascular Section, Room 523,
420 N. Charter St., Madison, Wisconsin 53706 (USA).

Recent Advances in Studies on
Cardiac Structure and Metabolism, Volume 12
Cardiac Adaptation
Edited by T. Kobayashi, Y. Ito, and G. Rona
Copyright 1978 University Park Press Baltimore

EFFECTS OF L-LACTATE ON
GLYCERALDEHYDE-3-P DEHYDROGENASE
IN HEART MUSCLE

S. MOCHIZUKI,[1] K. KOBAYASHI, and J. R. NEELY

Department of Physiology, The Milton S. Hershey Medical Center,
The Pennsylvania State University, Hershey, Pennsylvania, USA

INTRODUCTION

The rate of glycolysis in hearts perfused with oxygenated perfusate is accelerated with moderate reductions in coronary flow, but becomes inhibited when
coronary flow is severely restricted (Neely, Whitmer, and Rovetto, 1975).
Inhibition of glycolysis in ischemic hearts is related to several changes in the
intracellular environment. In addition to a decrease in oxygen supply, tissue
levels of lactate, hydrogen ion, and NADH increase as coronary flow is reduced
(Rovetto, Whitmer, and Neely, 1973; Neely, Whitmer, and Rovetto, 1975;
Rovetto, Lamberton, and Neely, 1975). Restriction of glycolysis in the ischemic
hearts appeared to develop at the level of glyceraldehyde-3-phosphate dehydrogenase (GAPdh) (Rovetto, Lamberton, and Neely, 1975). Glycolytic inhibition can be produced in aerobic or anoxic hearts when coronary flow is
maintained at normal rates, either by lowering the extracellular pH or by adding
lactate to the perfusate.

The purpose of the present study was to investigate the mechanism of
glycolytic inhibition in ischemic hearts and to determine control of GAPdh
isolated from heart muscle.

MATERIALS AND METHODS

Heart Perfusion

Hearts were removed from 200–250-g male Sprague-Dawley rats and perfused by
the working heart technique as described previously (Neely *et al.*, 1967). The

This work was supported by NHLI Grant 5 RO1 HL 18206-02.
[1] Dr. Mochizuki was a Postdoctoral Fellow of The Pennsylvania Heart Association.

perfusate was gassed with 95% O_2/5% CO_2, and ischemia was induced by use of a one-way valve in the aortic outflow tract which prevented retrograde perfusion of the coronary arteries during diastole (Neely *et al.,* 1973). The perfusate consisted of Krebs-Henseleit bicarbonate buffer containing 11 mM glucose as substrate and other additions as indicated in the figures.

Analytical Procedures

Rates of glycolysis were determined by measuring the rate of production of ^3H_2O from [5-^{3}H]glucose as described earlier (Neely *et al.,* 1972). Tissue levels of glycolytic intermediates were determined on hearts that were quick frozen by clamping with a Wollenberg clamp cooled to the temperature of liquid nitrogen. The frozen heart was powdered and extracted in 6% perchloric acid, and the neutralized perchloric acid extract was used to measure levels of glycolytic intermediates and lactate by standard enzymatic procedures, as described by Bergmeyer (1963).

GAPdh was isolated from beef heart by the methods of Cori *et al.* (1948) or of Amelunxen and Carr (1967). The activity of GAPdh was assayed spectrophotometrically in a buffer containing 0.6 mM NAD, 3 mM cysteine, 1.3 mM arsenate, and 1.3 M TES buffer at pH 6.5 (Oguchi, Meriwether, and Park, 1973; Oguchi *et al.,* 1973). GAP was purchased from the Sigma Chemical Company, and the concentration in the assay mixture was varied as indicated in the figures. Neutralized solutions of sodium lactate and sodium pyruvate were added at the concentrations indicated in the text.

RESULTS

The rate of glycolysis in ischemic or anoxic hearts was inversely related to tissue levels of lactate, and maximum glycolytic inhibition occurred when the intracellular concentration of lactate was approximately 25 mM (Rovetto, Lamberton, and Neely, 1975). When the rate of coronary flow in aerobic hearts was reduced from the control level of 15 ml/min to 5 ml/min, glycolysis was accelerated (Neely, Whitmer, and Rovetto, 1975). This effect of reducing coronary flow is illustrated in Figure 1 by the solid line. During 20 min of ischemic perfusion the rate of glycolysis increased from about 4 μ mol/g of dry tissue per min to about 10 μmol/g/min. Addition of 20 mM L-lactate or 10 mM pyruvate to the perfusate prevented this effect of moderate ischemia on glycolysis. Therefore, lactate and pyruvate, both products of glycolysis, inhibit the rate of glucose utilization. However, pyruvate does not accumulate in ischemic hearts (Rovetto, Lamberton, and Neely, 1975; Figure 3), and it is unlikely that this compound could account for the inhibition of glycolysis that develops during severe ischemia. The effect of lactate is specific for the L-isomer. As indicated in Figure 1, D-lactate, at the same concentration as L-lactate, did not inhibit

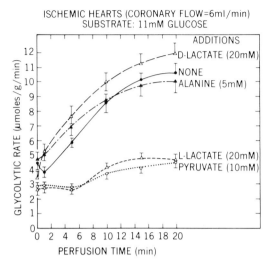

Figure 1. Effects of D- and L-lactate, pyruvate, and alanine on glycolytic rate in mildly ischemic hearts. The rate of coronary flow was decreased at zero time from 15–6 ml/min and perfusion was continued for 20 min with buffer containing 11 mM glucose and the additions as shown in the figure. The pH of all buffers was adjusted to 7.4.

glycolytic rate. This indicates that the effect of lactate is stereospecific and is probably not related to changes in cellular pH. Other three-carbon products of glucose metabolism, such as alanine, do accumulate during ischemia, but alanine was ineffective in reducing the glycolytic rate when added to the perfusate in 5-mM amounts (Figure 1). This amount of extracellular alanine resulted in the accumulation of intracellular alanine to concentrations above those found in severely ischemic hearts. Therefore, inhibition of glycolysis in ischemic hearts seems to be specifically related to the accumulation of lactate.

The relationship between glucose utilization and tissue lactate is illustrated in Figure 2. In this experiment, the rate of coronary flow was reduced to 5 ml/min and maintained at this level for 20 minutes. Tissue lactate was increased by adding various concentrations of L-lactate to the perfusate. The glycolytic rate was high in the ischemic hearts that were perfused without lactate in the perfusate, and these hearts had about 10 mM intracellular lactate. As intracellular lactate was increased by the addition of lactate to the perfusate, glycolysis became progressively inhibited. Maximum inhibition occurred when the intracellular lactate concentration was about 25–30 mM. This concentration of lactate is comparable to that found in ischemic hearts at lower rates of coronary flow when no lactate is added to the perfusate (Rovetto, Whitmer, and Neely, 1973). Thus, increased concentrations of intracellular lactate are associated with inhibition of glycolysis, whether the lactate is produced by the

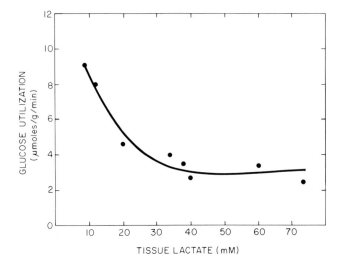

Figure 2. Relationship between glucose utilization and tissue lactate in mildly ischemic hearts. The rate of coronary flow was reduced to 6 ml/min and maintained at this level for 20 min of perfusion in each case. Those hearts perfused with glucose as the only substrate accumulated approximately 10 mM lactate in the tissue. Addition of L-lactate to the perfusate at concentrations ranging from 5–50 mM raised the tissue levels of lactate to as much as 70 mM. Glycolytic rate was measured between 18 and 20 min of perfusion and the hearts were frozen at 20 min for lactate determination.

tissue and accumulates because of the restriction of coronary flow or whether coronary flow is maintained and tissue lactate is increased by the addition of sodium lactate to the perfusate.

As indicated previously, the inhibition of glycolysis in ischemic hearts perfused with glucose as substrate seems to develop at the level of GAPdh (Rovetto, Lamberton, and Neely, 1975). This effect of ischemia is illustrated in Figure 3. In this experiment, the rate of coronary flow was reduced from a control rate of 15 ml/min to either 8 or 1 ml/min in ischemic hearts. These rates of flow were maintained for 20 min of perfusion with glucose as substrate and with no lactate added to the perfusate. At the end of a 20-min perfusion period, intracellular levels of glycolytic intermediates were determined. Restriction of coronary flow to either 8 or 1 ml/min caused an accumulation of glucose-6-phosphate (G-6-P), fructose-1,6-diphosphate (F,1-6,P), and triosphosphates. The level of these glycolytic intermediates was greater at 1 than at 8 ml/min coronary flow. These data indicate that GAPdh became the rate-limiting step for glycolysis in ischemic tissue. Accumulation of substrates for this enzyme associated with either a reduction or no change in the products of the enzyme indicates that inhibition of GAPdh occurred in the ischemic tissue. This inhibition was associated with accumulation of lactate and alanine but not of pyruvate.

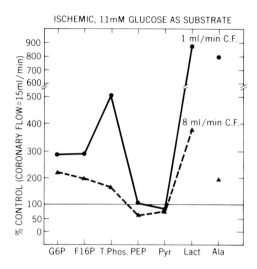

Figure 3. Crossover analysis of glycolytic intermediates in ischemic hearts. Coronary flows averaged 15 ml/min in control hearts and were reduced to 8 or 1 ml/min in ischemic hearts. The perfusate contained glucose (11 mM) as substrate. Levels of glycolytic intermediates were determined after 20 min of perfusion. Data for ischemic hearts are expressed as percentages of the control levels which are shown as 100%. G6P = glucose-6-phosphate; F16P-fructose-1,6-diphosphate; T. Phos = sum of glyceraldehyde-3-phosphate and dehydroxyacetone phosphate; PEP = phosphoenolpyruvate; Pyr = pyruvate; Lact = lactate; Ala = alanine. Each value represents the mean of data from 6–10 hearts.

Addition of L-lactate to the perfusate of mildly ischemic hearts (8 ml/min coronary flow) had a similar effect on glycolytic intermediates as did reducing flow to 1 ml/min (Figure 4). In this experiment, coronary flow was reduced to 8 ml/min and maintained at this rate for 20 min. The addition of 20 mM lactate caused an accumulation of glycolytic intermediates before the GAPdh step and reduced the level of phosphoenolpyruvate. This indicates that addition of lactate to the perfusate in mildly ischemic hearts causes an inhibition of glycolysis at the same step (GAPdh) as does severe ischemia. The inhibition of glycolysis that results from addition of pyruvate to the perfusate caused a somewhat different pattern of change in glycolytic intermediates. In this case, inhibition of glycolysis appears to develop at the level of phosphofructokinase. This is indicated by the increase in G-6-P associated with a decrease in the product, F,1-6,P, and with a reduction in the rate of glycolysis. Inhibition of glycolysis under this condition was associated with accumulation of high levels of citrate. Citrate increased from 0.5 μmol/g dry in ischemic hearts with glucose alone as substrate to 7 μmol/g dry in those hearts receiving glucose plus 10 mM pyruvate. Pyruvate levels were high, and the tissue levels of phosphoenolpyruvate and triosphosphate increased. These data indicate that lactate has a specific effect on GAPdh, whereas

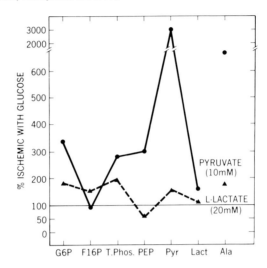

Figure 4. Effects of L-lactate and pyruvate on tissue levels of glycolytic intermediates in mildly ischemic hearts. Hearts were perfused for 20 min as described for Figure 1 with coronary flows of 6 ml/min. The data from hearts receiving lactate and pyruvate are expressed as percentages of the levels in hearts receiving only glucose. Intermediates are the same as those defined in Figure 3. Each value represents the mean of data from 6–10 hearts.

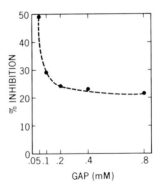

Figure 5. Inhibition of glyceraldehyde-3-phosphate dehydrogenase (GAPdh) by L-lactate at various concentrations of glyceraldehyde-3-phosphate. The reaction mixture contained NAD, 0.6 mM; cysteine, 3.0 mM; arsenate, 1.3 mM; TES buffer, 0.13 M; pH 6.5 and beef heart enzyme, 3.3 μg of protein. The reaction was run at 25°C. The reaction was started by the addition of glyceraldehyde-3-phosphate.

pyruvate may affect glycolysis indirectly at the level of phosphofructokinase by increasing the levels of citrate.

GAPdh isolated from beef heart was inhibited by L-lactate as illustrated in Figure 5. At substrate concentrations of 0.05 mM, 40 mM lactate caused a 50% inhibition of GAPdh activity. These concentrations of glyceraldehyde phosphate and lactate are approximately the same as those found in severely ischemic hearts. Therefore, inhibition of GAPdh in the ischemic hearts may be accounted for by a direct effect of lactate on the activity of this enzyme.

DISCUSSION

Accumulation of metabolic products in ischemic tissue seems to have effects on function and metabolism of the heart that are not directly related to a decrease in oxygen supply. The mechanisms of these effects of sluggish coronary flow are not well understood, but they are related to the accumulation of hydrogen ion, lactate, NADH, CO_2, and other products. In the present study, the inhibition of glycolysis that results from a reduction in coronary flow was shown to be associated with the accumulation of lactate in the tissue. Addition of lactate to the perfusate in hearts in which coronary flow is maintained at mildly ischemic levels also inhibited glycolysis. This inhibition developed at the level of GAPdh in either case. The effects of lactate did not appear to be related to changes in cellular pH and may have resulted from a direct effect of lactate on the activity of GAPdh. This conclusion is based on the observation that L-lactate inhibited the activity of GAPdh isolated from heart muscle.

REFERENCES

AMELUNXEN, R. E., and CARR, D. O. 1967. The crystallization and properties of glyceraldehyde-3-phosphate dehydrogenase isolated from rabbit muscle by a simplified procedure. Biochim. Biophys. Acta 132:256–259.

BERGMEYER, H. U. 1963. Methods of Enzymatic Analysis. Academic Press, New York.

CORI, G. T., SLEIN, M. W., and CORI, C. F. 1948. Crystalline D-glyceralde-hyde-3-phosphate dehydrogenase from rabbit muscle. J. Biol. Chem. 173.605 018.

NEELY, J. R., DENTON, R. M., ENGLAND, P. J., and RANDLE, P. J. 1972. Effects of increased heart work on the tricarboxylate cycle and its interactions with glycolysis in perfused rat heart. Biochem. J. 128:147–159.

NEELY, J. R., LIEBERMEISTER, H., BATTERSBY, E. J., and MORGAN, H. E. 1967. Effect of pressure development on oxyten consumption by isolated rat heart. Am. J. Physiol. 212:804–814.

NEELY, J. R., ROVETTO, M. J., WHITMER, J. T., and MORGAN, H. E. 1973. Effects of ischemia on ventricular function and metabolism in the isolated working rat heart. Am. J. Physiol. 225:651–658.

NEELY, J. R., WHITMER, J. T., and ROVETTO, M. J. 1975. Effect of coronary flow on glycolytic flux and intracellular pH in isolated rat hearts. Circ. Res. 37:733–741.

OGUCHI, M., GERTH, E., FITZGERALD, B., and PARK, J. H. 1973. Regulation of glyceraldehyde-3-phosphate dehydrogenase by phosphocreatine and adenosine triphosphate. IV. Factors affecting *in vivo* control of enzymatic activity. J. Biol. Chem. 248: 5571–5576.

OGUCHI, M., MERIWETHER, B. P., and PARK, J. H. 1973. Interaction between adenosine triphosphate and glyceraldehyde-3-phosphate dehydrogenase. IV. Mechanism of action and metabolic control of the enzyme under simulated *in vivo* conditions. J. Biol. Chem. 248:5562–5569.

ROVETTO, M. J., LAMBERTON, W. F., and NEELY, J. R. 1975. Mechanisms of glycolytic inhibition in ischemic rat hearts. Circ. Res. 37:742–751.

ROVETTO, M. J., WHITMER, J. T., and NEELY, J. R. 1973. Comparison of the effects of anoxia and whole heart ischemia on carbohydrate utilization in isolated, working rat heart. Circ. Res. 32:699–711.

Mailing address:
Dr. Seibu Mochizuki,
Department of Physiology, The Milton S. Hershey Medical Center,
The Pennsylvania State University, Hershey, Pennsylvania 17033 (USA).

Recent Advances in Studies on
Cardiac Structure and Metabolism, Volume 12
Cardiac Adaptation
Edited by George Rona and Yoshio Ito
Copyright 1978 University Park Press Baltimore

EFFECTS OF ACETATE ON MYOCARDIAL CONTRACTILITY AND EPICARDIAL ECG OF ISOLATED AND PERFUSED FELINE HEARTS

S. H. SONG[1]

Department of Biophysics, Faculty of Medicine,
University of Western Ontario, London, Ontario, Canada

SUMMARY

In isolated, perfused hearts, the effects of acetate on epicardial ECG and ventricular pressure were observed during various times of perfusion. Anions—Cl^- and acetate—caused changes of ECG configuration, especially in the ST segments. These were different in Phase I (fast compartment) and Phase II (slow compartment).

INTRODUCTION

Chronic or acute alcohol intake is known to be harmful to the heart, as well as to the overall cardiovascular system. In addition, it is well known that the concentration of acetate in the blood increases as a result of alcohol metabolism (Lindeneg *et al.,* 1964) and that the mammalian heart is a potential site of acetate utilization and production (Knowles *et al.,* 1974). Therefore, we attempted to investigate the indirect manifestations of alcohol consumption and the direct effects of acetate on the mammalian isolated heart. Using the modified Langendorff heart preparation for studies of washout kinetics, we have proposed a three-compartmental model for red blood cells (Song, 1975) and a two-compartmental model for plasma (Ng and Song, in preparation). In this study, we tried to determine if acetate could be used to demonstrate functional differences between compartments in the coronary microcirculation.

MATERIALS AND METHODS

After sodium pentobarbital anesthesia, the heart was exposed by thoracotomy, and major vessels surrounding the heart and aortic branches were tied off and

This investigation was supported by the Ontario Heart Foundation.
[1] The author is a Senior Research Fellow of the Ontario Heart Foundation.

Table 1. Concentrations of electrolytes in the perfusate

	Normal (g/liter)	Acetate ringer (g/liter)
[Cl]	145 mEq/liter	10 mEq/liter
$CaCl_2 \cdot 2H_2O$	0.32	0.32
KCl	0.42	0.42
NaCl	8.1	
$NaHCO_3$	0.019	0.019
$NaH_2PO_4 \cdot H_2O$	0.164	0.164
glucose	1.00	1.00
$NaC_2H_3O_2$		12.696
	310 mOsm/liter	310 mOsm/liter

cut. Inflow and outflow catheters were inserted into the sinus of valsalva and into the right auricle through the vena cava, respectively. Other details of the perfusion system have been described fully in a previous paper (Song, 1975). Two pressure transducers were connected to the inflow catheter and to the right ventricular chamber catheter, and two metal electrodes were fastened on the epicardium to record the epicardial ECG. Table 1 shows how the acetate concentrations were altered in the perfusate without changing the osmolality and cationic compositions. Both perfusates were adjusted to 310 mOsm/liter and 7.4 pH units. Before perfusion the solutions were freed by small particles by filtering three times through millipore filters (GSWP, 0.22 μM).

Three separate recordings of epicardial ECG, perfusion pressure (PP), and ventricular pressure (VP) were traced with a Beckman type RM Dynograph. The control recordings were obtained when the normal Ringer solution (Table 1) was used for at least 10 min at a flow rate of 5 ml/min or 10 ml/min. Effects of normal and acetate perfusion were compared in the same heart preparation with the same flow rate, although two rates were used.

RESULTS AND DISCUSSION

Figure 1 shows the alteration of epicardial ECG and VP when the perfusate was switched from the normal to the acetate solution. Usually the ST segment was the first part to change drastically with the acetate infusion. Then the T wave changed, with either inversion or upright peaking. Although it is not apparent in Figure 1, the amplitude of the whole ECG always was increased by the acetate perfusion. This increase in amplitude with acetate could be caused by synchronization of the myocardial cells or by inward Ca^{2+} currents enhancing the degree of depolarization at the membrane level. However, in this study it was

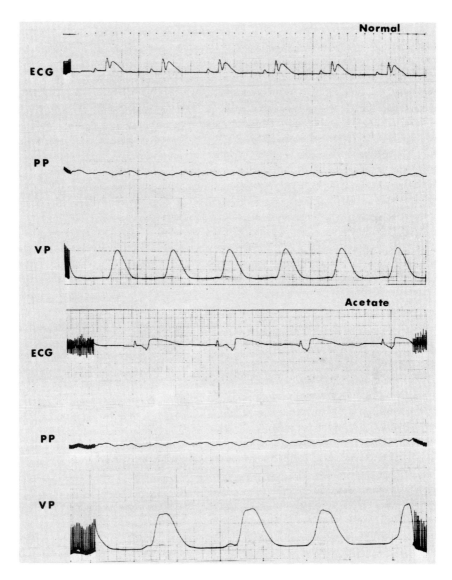

Figure 1. Tracings of epicardial ECG, perfusion pressure (PP), and ventricular pressure (VP) during perfusion with normal and acetate solutions. VP with acetate was recorded when the strain gauge coupler preamplifier was set at twice the normal sensitivity.

not possible to conclude that the involvement of Ca^{2+} is the exclusive factor of the acetate effects.

Because the concentration of acetate in the coronary microcirculation should have the same kinetics as the red cell washout (Song, 1975) or the plasma washout (Ng and Song, unpublished observations), the effective time may arbitrarily be divided into two phases: Phase I comprises a period of both fast and intermediate compartments and Phase II is a period of slow compartment washout. In Figures 2 and 3, successive recordings are shown from the control, Phase I of acetate, Phase II of acetate, and the control again. The amplitude of electrical activity was increased by the acetate perfusion, while the ventricular pressures were reduced by more than half.

The ST segment of the control in Figure 2 has downward sloping depression with T-wave inversion. With acetate the ST segment was elevated further during Phase II (Figure 3). The normal recovery in Figure 3 shows an ECG pattern similar to that of Phase I, while the mechanical contractility was restored completely to, or to even better than, the control level. This recovery of mechanical power of the myocardial cells eliminates the possibility that the effects of hypoxia or ischemia, caused by acetate perfusion, might act on the electromechanical properties of heart muscle cells.

To illustrate the mechanism by which the acetate can affect the myocardial cells, infusions of high K^+ or high Ca^{2+} were carried out in another series of experiments (Song and Aniol, unpublished observations). The ECG patterns obtained from the epicardium when a solution with 10 mEq/liter of Ca^{2+} was perfused were very similar to the changes obtained when the acetate was perfused in the same heart. The results showed conclusively that there was an association between the effects of acetate and Ca^{2+} on the epicardial ECG. This relationship also was demonstrated in the frog ventricular muscle by Anderson and Foulks (1974). They stated that substitution of acetate for external Cl^- induces an increase in the resting membrane potential, a prolongation of the action potential, and a possible increase in Ca influx. However, the reduction of mechanical contractility because of acetate probably is not one of the Ca^{2+} effects unless there is a distinction between the action potential and the muscular contraction caused by the Ca^{2+} involvement during the acetate perfusion.

The difference in ECG between Phases I and II also may occur from the different rates of molecular movement of Cl^- and acetate ions through the cell membrane; but, obviously, Phase I occurs during the fast compartment, while Phase II is limited to the slow compartment. This phase difference may result either from uneven distribution of coronary flow in the microcirculation (Kirk and Honig, 1964) or from different permeabilities of Cl^- and acetate. Realizing that the effects of alcohol intake may act on different parts of the heart, we plan to assess the full effect of the slow compartment by prolonged perfusion.

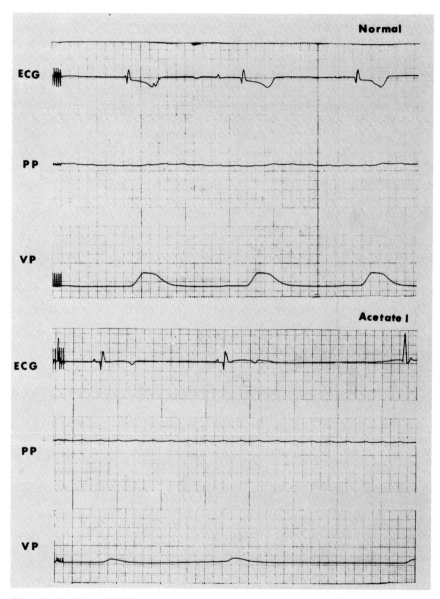

Figure 2. Tracings of ECG, PP, and VP from another heart during the perfusion with normal and within 10 min of acetate perfusion (Phase I, Acetate I).

188   Song

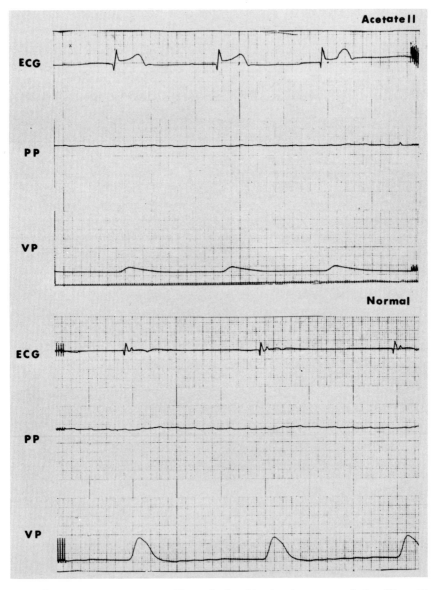

Figure 3. The same tracings as in Figure 2 after 30 min of acetate perfusion (Phase II, Acetate II) and the control perfusion (normal) again.

Acknowledgment   The author is grateful to Professor Margot R. Roach for her valuable comments.

REFERENCES

ANDERSON, E. R., and FOULKS, J. G. 1974. Mechanism of the effect of acetate on frog ventricular muscle. Can. J. Physiol. Pharmacol. 52:404–423.

KIRK, E. S., and HONIG, C. R. 1964. Nonuniform distribution of blood flow and gradients of oxygen tension within the heart. Am. J. Physiol. 207:661–668.

KNOWLES, S. E., JARRETT, I. G., FILSELL, O. H., and BALLARD, F. J. 1974. Production and utilization of acetate in mammals. Biochem. J. 142:401–411.

LINDENEG, O., MELLEMGAARD, K., FABRICIUS, J., and LUNDQUIST, F. 1964. Myocardial utilization of acetate, lactate, and free fatty acids after ingestion of ethanol. Clin. Sci. 27:427–435.

NG, C. E., and SONG, S. H. Compartmental analysis of ^{125}I labeled albumin washout from the coronary vessels of isolated, perfused hearts. In preparation.

SONG, S. H. 1975. Kinetics of the red cell washout from coronary vessels of isolated feline hearts. Can. J. Physiol. Pharmacol. 53:755–762.

SONG, S. H., and ANIOL, V. 1974. Effects of K and Ca on the red cell clearance from coronary vessels of isolated, feline hearts. Presented at the 58th FASEB meeting, Atlantic City, New Jersey.

Mailing address:
S. H. Song, Ph.D.,
Department of Biophysics, Faculty of Medicine,
University of Western Ontario, London, Ontario N6A 5Cl (Canada).

Recent Advances in Studies on
Cardiac Structure and Metabolism, Volume 12
Cardiac Adaptation
Edited by T. Kobayashi, Y. Ito, and G. Rona
Copyright 1978 University Park Press Baltimore

ALTERATION IN CALCIUM METABOLISM IN CARDIAC HYPERTROPHY AND FAILURE CAUSED BY BACTERIAL INFECTION

C. W. TOMLINSON and N. S. DHALLA

Pathophysiology Laboratory, Department of Physiology,
Faculty of Medicine, University of Manitoba, Winnipeg, Canada

SUMMARY

Left ventricular hypertrophy was seen in catheterized, uninfected rabbits, whereas contractile failure superimposed upon hypertrophy was observed in catheterized animals after injection with *Streptococcus viridans* within six days. The infected animals showed marked changes in the ultrastructure of the left heart in comparison to the uninfected rabbits. The levels of calcium and potassium were decreased, whereas sodium was increased in both infected and uninfected hearts; however, magnesium levels did not change in uninfected hearts but were decreased at three days and increased at six days of infection. The microsomal calcium uptake was decreased in six-day uninfected as well as three- and six-day infected hearts. On the other hand, the mitochondrial calcium uptake was increased in six-day uninfected and three-day infected hearts but decreased in six-day infected hearts. The sarcolemmal calcium binding and (Na^+,K^+)ATPase activities were decreased in six-day uninfected as well as three- and six-day infected hearts. These results suggest dramatic changes in intracellular calcium metabolism in myocardial hypertrophy and failure caused by bacterial infection.

INTRODUCTION

In view of a crucial role played by calcium in different processes regulating myocardial function and metabolism, most of the changes in the contractile properties, ultrastructure, and metabolism in different types of failing hearts have been explained on the basis of either intracellular calcium deficiency or intracellular calcium overload (Dhalla, 1976). Recently, we have suggested that changes in the intracellular calcium metabolism may be involved in the pathogenesis of myocardial failure and ultrastructural damage caused by bacterial infection (Tomlinson and Dhalla, 1975, 1976). It should be mentioned that congestive heart failure superimposed upon myocardial hypertrophy has

This work was supported by the Manitoba Heart Foundation. Dr. Tomlinson was the recipient of a Medical Scientist Award from the Canadian Heart Foundation.

been shown to occur in 100% of the cases of catheterized rabbits upon injecting *Streptococcus viridans,* whereas myocardial hypertrophy occurs in uninfected animals in which a catheter is inserted through the carotid artery and placed in the left ventricle for six days. Therefore, in the study discussed in this chapter, we wished to gain some information concerning the calcium-accumulating abilities of the hypertrophied and failing heart sarcoplasmic reticulum, mitochondria, and sarcolemma because these membrane systems are considered to be intimately involved in the regulation of intracellular calcium. Furthermore, myocardial calcium contents and other electrolytes were measured, and the activity of the sarcolemmal $(Na^+,K^+)ATPase$, which controls the movements of sodium and potassium in the cell (McNamara *et al.,* 1974), was determined in hypertrophied and failing hearts.

MATERIALS AND METHODS

Polyethylene catheters were inserted into the left ventricles through the right carotid artery of albino rabbits weighing about 2 kg each. Twenty-four hours after recovery, one group of these animals received a saline injection while the other was given a dose of *Streptococcus viridans* (10^7 organisms/kg) through the ear vein. These uninfected and infected animals were sacrificed three and six days after the injection. Sham-operated animals served as controls. These methods for inducing myocardial hypertrophy in the uninfected rabbits and both hypertrophy and failure in the infected animals have been described elsewhere (Tomlinson and Dhalla, 1975, 1976).

Small pieces of the left ventricle were fixed in 1% glutaraldehyde for 12–16 hr for electron microscopic investigation. The tissue specimens were washed overnight in 0.1 M phosphate buffer, fixed for 1 hr with 1% osmium tetroxide, dehydrated in a graded ethanol series, and embedded in Epon 812. The sections were stained with uranyl acetate and lead citrate and examined with a Zeiss electron microscope (EM9S).

For the determination of myocardial electrolytes, the hearts were removed and quickly perfused with 20 ml of ice-cold, Dowex-treated, sucrose-histidine buffer (0.32 M sucrose, 5 mM histidine, pH 7.4) via an aortic cannula. This method was found to eliminate most of the extracellular fluid because no red blood cells were detectable upon histological examination. Portions of the left ventricle from sham-operated, uninfected, and infected rabbits were homogenized in sucrose-histidine buffer, and ions were extracted by boiling in the presence of 2 N HCl. The total ion contents in the clear supernatant after centrifugation at 5,000 × *g* were determined by employing a Zeiss atomic absorption spectrophotometer. Lanthanum chloride (1%) and strontium chloride (0.25%) were used in the determination of calcium and magnesium, respectively, to prevent interference by other ions. Similarly, cesium chloride (0.1%) was added to the supernatant samples when potassium and sodium were determined.

Both mitochondrial and sarcoplasmic reticular (heavy microsomal) fractions were isolated and purified by methods described earlier (Sulakhe and Dhalla, 1971), whereas the sarcolemmal fraction was isolated by the hypotonic shock-LiBr treatment method (McNamara *et al.*, 1974) and purified by extracting with 0.6 mM KCl for 15 min. For calcium uptake studies, microsomes (about 0.05 mg of protein/ml) were incubated in a medium containing 100 mM KCl, 10 mM $MgCl_2$, 20 mM Tris-HCl (pH 6.8), 4mM ATP, and 5 mM potassium oxalate. Mitochondrial (about 0.2 mg of protein/ml) calcium uptake also was carried out in the above medium, except 4 mM succinate and 4 mM phosphate were present instead of potassium oxalate. The medium for the sarcolemmal (0.5 mg of protein/ml) calcium binding contained 100 mM KCl and 20 mM Tris-HCl, pH 6.8. The reactions were started by the addition of 0.1 mM $^{45}CaCl_2$ and were stopped by Millipore filtration after one minute of incubation at $37°C$. The method for determining (Na^+, K^+)-ATPase activity was the same as described earlier (McNamara *et al.*, 1974).

RESULTS

Assessment of the cardiovascular system according to the method of Mason, Spann, and Zelis (1970) revealed that the contractile state of the intact myocardium was depressed by 40 and 75% of the control values in rabbits three and six days after infection, respectively, whereas no appreciable changes were seen in the uninfected catheterized animals. The left ventricle weight increased by 21 and 42% in three- and six-day uninfected rabbits, whereas it increased by 40 and 70% in three- and six-day infected rabbits, respectively. No ultrastructural changes in three-day uninfected left ventricles were seen, whereas areas with myofibrillar contracture, sarcotubular swelling, and occasional mitochondrial damage were observed in six-day uninfected hearts. Marked alterations in the ultrastructure of myofibrils, the sarcotubular system, and mitochondria were noted in animals six days after infection, but these changes were of less magnitude in three-day infected animals. Typical electron micrographs from six-day uninfected and infected hearts are shown in Figure 1.

Electrolyte contents of the left ventricular muscle from control, uninfected catheterized, and infected hearts are shown in Table 1. The levels of calcium and potassium were decreased ($p < 0.05$), whereas the sodium level was increased ($p < 0.05$) six days after saline injection in catheterized animals without any significant ($p > 0.05$) changes in the magnesium level ($p > 0.05$). Three and six days after bacterial injection, myocardial potassium and calcium were decreased ($p < 0.05$) and sodium was increased ($p < 0.05$) in comparison to controls.

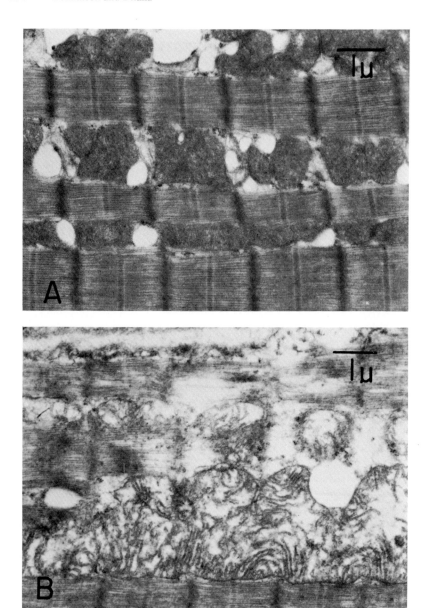

Figure 1. A: Electron micrograph of the left ventricle from the heart of an uninfected catheterized rabbit six days after injection of saline. B: Electron micrograph of the left ventricle from the heart of a rabbit six days after injection of *Streptococcus viridans* showing swelling and disruption of mitochondria and dissolution of myofilaments. X 16,500.

Table 1. Myocardial electrolytes in control, uninfected, and infected rabbits

	Myocardial electrolytes (μmol/g heart dry weight)			
	Calcium	Magnesium	Sodium	Potassium
Control	7.41 ± 0.28	31.75 ± 0.97	130.7 ± 9.6	342.7 ± 10.5
Uninfected (6 days)	5.69 ± 0.36[a]	33.66 ± 1.16	213.9 ± 14.5[a]	267.4 ± 14.8[a]
Infected (3 days)	3.87 ± 0.41[a]	28.45 ± 0.58[a]	171.3 ± 13.2[a]	278.5 ± 8.9[a]
Infected (6 days)	6.01 ± 0.29[a]	35.10 ± 0.72[a]	258.2 ± 11.9[b]	257.7 ± 12.3[a]

[a]Significantly different from control ($p < 0.05$).
[b]Significantly different from control and uninfected hearts ($p < 0.05$).
Each value represents the mean ± S.E.M. of four experiments.

Myocardial magnesium was decreased ($p < 0.05$) after three days and increased ($p < 0.05$) after six days of infection. On the other hand, calcium, magnesium, and potassium levels in six-day infected hearts were not significantly ($p > 0.05$) different from those of uninfected hearts; however, the level of sodium was significantly ($p < 0.05$) higher in infected hearts than in uninfected hearts.

The data shown in Figure 2 reveal that calcium uptake by the microsomal fraction was depressed in six-day uninfected as well as in three- and six-day infected hearts. On the other hand, mitochondrial calcium uptake was increased in six-day uninfected and three-day infected hearts but was decreased in six-day infected hearts. Calcium binding and (Na^+,K^+)-ATPase activities of the sarcolemmal fractions from the six-day uninfected as well as from three- and six-day infected hearts were decreased (Figure 3).

DISCUSSION

In this study, we have noted that the levels of sodium were increased and those of potassium were decreased in six-day uninfected as well as in three- and six-day infected hearts. These changes can be explained on the basis of a defect in the Na^+K^+ pump mechanism at the cell membrane because the sarcolemmal (Na^+, K^+)-ATPase activity in these hearts was significantly depressed. The leakiness of sarcolemma in these hypertrophied and failing hearts is further apparent from the observed changes in the myocardial calcium and magnesium contents, as well as from the elevated serum levels of different intracellular enzymes (Tomlinson and Dhalla, 1976). Furthermore, sarcolemmal calcium-binding activity was decreased in these hypertrophied and failing hearts. It is possible that aortic regurgitation, caused by the presence of a catheter in the left ventricle of these animals, and valvular stenosis, caused by vegetations in the case of infected animals, may be responsible for inducing these shifts in the electrolyte composition of the myocardium by producing certain defects in the sarcolemmal

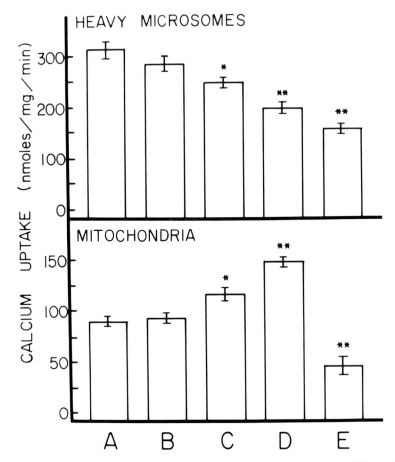

Figure 2. Calcium uptake activities of the heavy microsomal and mitochondrial fractions from the hearts of control, uninfected catheterized, and infected rabbits. A represents the control group; B and C denote uninfected catheterized animals after three and six days of saline injection, respectively; D and E refer to infected animals after three and six days of injection of *Streptococcus viridans.* Each value is the mean ± S.E.M. of four experiments. * = significantly different from control ($p < 0.05$); ** = significantly different from control and uninfected hearts ($p < 0.05$).

membrane. Thus, the failure and myocardial damage as seen in these situations are not surprising.

Decreased myocardial calcium contents in the hypertrophied and failing hearts may be taken to reflect an intracellular calcium deficiency, which has been shown to produce marked changes in heart function and ultrastructure (Tomlinson, Yates, and Dhalla, 1974; Yates and Dhalla, 1975). Depression in the abilities of heart sarcolemmal and microsomal fractions to accumulate calcium

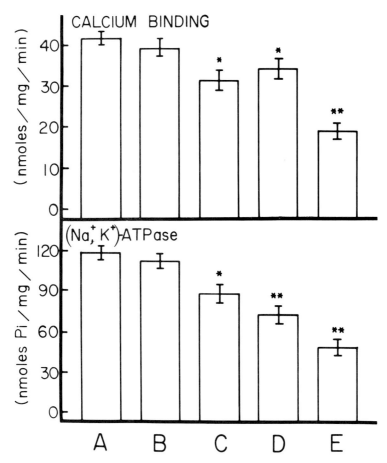

Figure 3. Calcium-binding and (Na^+,K^+)-ATPase activities of the sarcolemmal fractions from the hearts of control (A), uninfected catheterized (B and C) and infected (D and E) rabbits. Abbreviations and symbols as in Figure 2. Each value is a mean ± S. E. of four experiments.

can be assumed to result in a decrease of calcium stores that are available for release upon excitation. This would explain the contractile failure in the infected hearts where these changes are of greater magnitude than those in the uninfected hearts. Our inability to observe depression in the contractile state of the intact heart in the uninfected animals may be attributable to the compensatory effect of the myocardial hypertrophy. It also should be noted that the abilities of mitochondria to accumulate calcium in the six-day uninfected and three-day infected hearts were greater than the control values but were markedly depressed in the six-day infected hearts. It is likely that mitochondria in the hypertropied and early-infected hearts may be playing a compensatory role in conserving intracellular calcium, but this may eventually become a problem and result in deterioration of the structure and function of these organelles. Such a result is exactly what was seen in the late stages of bacterial infection.

Impaired abilities of sarcolemmal and microsomal fractions to accumulate calcium represent changes in the intracellular calcium regulatory mechanisms in the early and late stages of myocardial hypertrophy and failure caused by bacterial infection. This situation is further complicated by the observed increase and decrease in the abilities of mitochondria to accumulate calcium in early and late stages of infection. Alterations in mitochondrial and microsomal functions also have been reported in cardiac hypertrophy and failure caused by genetic cardiomyopathy (Sulakhe and Dhalla, 1971) and aortic stenosis (Sordahl *et al.,* 1973). However, the exact manner in which these defects in calcium regulatory mechanisms are related to myocardial hypertrophy and failure remains to be established.

REFERENCES

DHALLA, N. S. 1976. Involvement of membrane systems in heart failure due to intracellular calcium overload and deficiency. J. Mol. Cell. Cardiol. 8:661–667.

McNAMARA, D. B., SULAKHE, P. V., SINGH, J. N., and DHALLA, N. S. 1974. Properties of heart sarcolemmal Na^+–K^+ ATPase. J. Biochem. 75:795–803.

MASON, D. T., SPANN, J. F., JR., and ZELIS, R. 1970. Quantification of the contractile state of the intact human heart: Maximal velocity of contractile element shortening determined by the instantaneous relation between the rate of pressure rise and pressure in the left ventricle during isovolumic systole. Am. J. Cardiol. 26:248–257.

SORDAHL, L. A., McCOLLUM, W. B., WOOD, W. G., and SCHWARTZ, A. 1973. Mitochondria and sarcoplasmic reticulum function in cardiac hypertrophy and failure. Am. J. Physiol. 224:497–502.

SULAKHE, P. V., and DHALLA, N. S. 1971. Excitation-contraction coupling in heart. VII. Calcium accumulation in subcellular particles in congestive heart failure. J. Clin. Invest. 50:1019–1027.

TOMLINSON, C. W., and DHALLA, N. S. 1975. Myocardial cell damage during experimental infective endocarditis. Lab. Invest. 33:316–323.

TOMLINSON, C. W., and DHALLA, N. S. 1976. Alterations in myocardial function during bacterial infective cardiomyopathy. Am. J. Cardiol. 37:373–381.

TOMLINSON, C. W., YATES, J. C., and DHALLA, N. S. 1974. Relationship among changes in intracellular calcium stores, ultrastructure, and contractility of myocardium. *In* N. S. Dhalla and G. Rona (eds.), Recent Advances in Studies on Cardiac Structure and Metabolism. Vol. 4: Myocardial Biology, pp. 331–345. University Park Press, Baltimore.

YATES, J. C., and DHALLA, N. S. 1975. Structural and functional changes associated with failure and recovery of hearts after perfusion with Ca^{++}-free medium. J. Mol. Cell. Cardiol. 7:91–103.

Mailing address:
Naranjan S. Dhalla, Ph.D.,
Professor of Physiology, University of Manitoba,
Winnipeg, Manitoba, R3E OW3 (Canada).

Recent Advances in Studies on
Cardiac Structure and Metabolism, Volume 12
Cardiac Adaptation
Edited by T. Kobayashi, Y. Ito, and G. Rona
Copyright 1978 University Park Press Baltimore

SPECIES DIFFERENCE OF MITOCHONDRIAL RESPIRATION IN EXPERIMENTALLY INDUCED HEART FAILURE

H. SAITO, Y. MONMA, and T. TANABE

Department of Pharmacology, Hokkaido University,
School of Medicine, Sapporo, Japan

SUMMARY

In guinea pigs with acute heart failure, a decrease in oxygen consumption (QO_2) at state 3 and an increase in QO_2 at state 4 were seen and the respiratory control index (RCI) was markedly lowered; ADP/O ratio was not affected. In rabbits with acute heart failure, both RCI and ADP/O ratio showed a statistically significant decrease. In dogs with acute and chronic heart failure, no impairment of respiratory function of mitochondria was seen. These conflicting results may be attributed to the difference in experimental conditions, namely, the species difference and the difference in methods to produce experimental heart failure. With special regard to species difference, it was confirmed that the RCI of myocardial mitochondria of healthy dogs was much lower than that of healthy guinea pigs. It is suggested that the difficulty of obtaining intact mitochondria may be responsible for the species difference in experimentally induced heart failure.

INTRODUCTION

In studies of the experimentally induced failing heart of animals, emphasis has been laid on changes in respiratory function of the myocardial mitochondria by previous workers. Several investigators (Schwartz and Lee, 1962; Wollenberger, Kleitke, and Raabe, 1963; Argus *et al.*, 1964; Sordahl *et al.*, 1973) reported that mitochondria obtained from the failing heart showed an impairment of respiratory function. Other workers (Plant and Gertler, 1959; Olson, 1964; Sobel, Spann, and Pool, 1967; Yamamura, 1968) demonstrated that oxidative phosphorylation of heart mitochondria was normal in experimentally induced heart failure and in the failing heart of a patient with valvular rheumatic disease (Chidsey *et al.*, 1966).

These conflicting results may be attributed to experimental conditions, namely, the species difference and the difference in methods to produce experimental heart failure. The present investigation discussed in this chapter was designed based upon the hypothesis that the species difference in mitochondrial respiration of heart failure might be relevant to the conflicting data reported by previous workers.

MATERIALS AND METHODS

Heart Failure in Animals

The procedure for inducing heart failure was essentially similar to that used by Gertler (1959). Animals used included guinea pigs, rabbits, and dogs. The operative technique involved intrathoracic incision and restriction of aortic blood flow by ligature surrounding the aorta. The basic principle of this operation is to reduce the size of the aorta by one-third by means of a ligature. In animals with acute heart failure, the heart was removed eight to 12 days after aortic constriction. In dogs with chronic heart failure, the heart was removed 60 to 90 days after aortic constriction.

Restriction of blood flow through the aorta caused ECG and pathological changes. Pathological changes showed chronic passive venous congestion in liver, kidney, and spleen and cardiac hypertrophy.

Method for Determination of Mitochondrial Respiration

Ventricular muscle was homogenated in a cool system with a loose homogenizer to obtain myocardial mitochondria (Chance and Hagihara, 1961). Glutamic acid was added as the substrate to the medium described by Chance and Hagihara (1961), and ADP was added as the phosphate acceptor. The oxygen consumption of mitochondria was measured polarographically with a rotating electrode, after the method of Hagihara (1961). The temperature of the reaction mixture was $25°C$ and the pH was adjusted to 7.2 with Tris-HCl and K-phosphate buffers. As the criteria for the respiratory function of mitochondria, oxygen consumption (QO_2) at states 3 and 4, RCI, and ADP/O ratio were calculated.

RESULTS

Changes in Mitochondrial Respiration of
Heart with Experimentally Induced Failure in Several Species of Animals

In guinea pigs with acute heart failure, a decrease in QO_2 at state 3 $(p < 0.01)$ and an increase in QO_2 at state 4 were seen $(p < 0.01)$. The RCI was markedly lowered when compared with the control $(p < 0.01)$. No influence was seen in ADP/O ratio. In rabbits with acute heart failure, oxygen consumption at state 3 and ADP/O ratio were lowered as compared to control $(p < 0.05)$.

In dogs with acute heart failure and chronic heart failure, the oxygen consumption at state 3 and at state 4 was not affected. Accordingly, the value of RCI was not affected.

Effect of Hypoxia on Respiratory Function of
Mitochondria of Isolated Guinea Pig Heart in Physiological Saline Solution

The relation of the oxygen deficit to the onset of impairment of mitochondrial respiration was studied. Nontreated, healthy guinea pigs were sacrificed, and the heart was immediately isolated and placed in physiological saline at 20°C to produce hypoxic damage of heart mitochondria. The heart, placed in saline for 10 min, showed a marked decrease in RCI resulting from the increase in QO_2 of state 4. In the isolated heart exposed to oxygen deficit for 30 min, QO_2 decreased in state 3 ($p < 0.05$) and increased in state 4 ($p < 0.01$). Accordingly, the RCI was markedly decreased ($p < 0.01$). RCI showed a rapid decrease during the first 30 min, followed by a gradual decrease ($p < 0.01$). The decrease in ADP/O ratio was relatively slight and was of the same degree during the period from 10 to 60 min ($p < 0.01$).

DISCUSSION

Of interest in this experiment is the observation that the results from different species were not always coincidental. Both guinea pigs and rabbits showed an impairment of respiratory function of mitochondria obtained during heart failure. In dogs, however, such a finding was never noted. Concerning the species difference of respiratory function of mitochondria, we clearly found that RCI obtained from healthy dogs was much lower than that from healthy guinea pigs. An explanation for this observation would be relevant to the difficulty of obtaining intact mitochondria from canine heart, because of the interrelated adhesiveness of myofibrils and mitochondria at the cellular level. Hence, the assumption was made that it is difficult to find a difference in the respiratory function of myocardial mitochondria between dogs with or without heart failure. Therefore, it is concluded that the experiment using canine mitochondria cannot provide an appropriate model for investigating the biochemical function of heart failure under present experimental conditions.

With regard to experimentally induced heart failure in guinea pigs, no conclusions have been reached by earlier investigators (Plant and Gertler, 1959; Schwartz and Lee, 1962; Sobel, Spann, and Pool, 1967). The question of why these conflicting results of heart failure have come only from this species was posed, and attempts were made to understand the factors that are involved in the pathological mechanisms underlying experimental heart failure.

Finally, it is noted that hypoxia induced a remarkable change in the respiratory function of guinea pig heart mitochondria. Therefore, if the impairment of myocardial mitochondria observed in failing heart of guinea pigs is associated with the continuing hypoxia, the extent of mitochondrial damage induced by such hypoxia seems to be responsible for the divergent results as aforementioned (Plant and Gertler, 1959; Schwartz and Lee, 1962; Sobel, Spann, and Pool, 1967).

REFERENCES

ARGUS, M. F., ARCOS, J. C., SARDESAI, V. M., and OVERBY, J. L. 1964. Oxidative rates and phosphorylation in sarcosomes from experimentally induced failing rat heart. Proc. Soc. Exp. Biol. Med. 117:380–383.

CHANCE, B., and HAGIHARA, B. 1961. Direct spectroscopic measurements of interaction of components of the respiratory chain with ATP, ADP, phosphate, and uncoupling agents. Proc. 5th Intl. Cong. Biochem. (Moscow), Sump. 5:3–37.

CHIDSEY, C. A., WEINBACH, E. C., POOL, P. E., and MORROW, A. G. 1966. Biochemical studies of energy production in the failing human heart. J. Clin. Invest. 45:40–50.

GERTLER, M. M. 1959. Production of experimental congestive heart failure in the guinea pig. Proc. Soc. Exp. Biol. Med. 102:396–397.

HAGIHARA, B. 1961. Techniques for the application of polarography to mitochondrial respiration. Biochem. Biophys. Acta 46:134–142.

OLSON, R. E. 1964. Abnormalities of myocardial metabolism. Circ. Res. 14(suppl. 2): 109–119.

PLANT, G. W. E., and GERTLER, M. M. 1959. Oxidative phosphorylation studies in normal and experimentally produced congestive heart failure in guinea pigs: A comparison. Ann. N.Y. Acad. Sci. 72:515–517.

SCHWARTZ, A., and LEE, K. S. 1962. Study of heart mitochondria and glycolytic metabolism in experimentally induced cardiac failure. Circ. Res. 10:321–332.

SOBEL, B. E., SPANN, J. F., Jr., and POOL, P. E. 1967. Normal oxidative phosphorylation in mitochondria from the failing heart. Circ. Res. 21:355–363.

SORDAHL, L. A., McCOLLUM, W. B., WOOD, W. G., and SCHWARTZ, A. 1973. Mitochondria and sarcoplasmic reticulum function in cardiac hypertrophy and failure. Am. J. Physiol. 224:497–502.

WOLLENBERGER, A., KLEITKE, B., and RAABE, G. 1963. Some metabolic characteristics of mitochondria from chronically overloaded, hypertrophied hearts. Exp. Mol. Pathol. 2:251–260.

Mailing address:
H. Saito,
Department of Pharmacology, Hokkaido University,
School of Medicine, Sapporo (Japan).

Recent Advances in Studies on
Cardiac Structure and Metabolism, Volume 12
Cardiac Adaptation
Edited by T. Kobayashi, Y. Ito, and G. Rona
Copyright 1978 University Park Press Baltimore

EXPERIMENTAL STUDIES ON THE EFFECT
OF GLUCOCORTICOIDS ON CARDIAC MUSCLE

T. ITO,[1] K.-M. SU,[1] M. MURATA,[1] T. KOIZUMI,[1]
S. MATSUMOTO,[1] Y. ITO,[1] and A. KAMIYAMA[2]

[1] Fourth Department of Internal Medicine,
University of Tokyo, Tokyo, Japan
[2] Department of Physiology, Yokohama City
School of Medicine, Yokohama, Japan

SUMMARY

Abnormal electrocardiographic changes were found in some patients on long-term glucocorticoid treatment. In experimental animals, chronic glucocorticoid administration resulted in an increase of amplitude of the QRS complex and abnormal ST and T changes. Changes of action potential were somewhat different in the subendocardial and the subepicardial layers. Diffuse mitochondrial alterations were found, particularly in the subepicardial layer. In rabbits treated with glucocorticoids, no significant changes were found in either serum or myocardial potassium content. Slightly decreased V_{max} was the observed hemodynamic change.

INTRODUCTION

Steroid myopathy has been well documented in skeletal muscle, but the effects of steroids in cardiac muscle have not been well elucidated (Byers, Bergman, and Joseph, 1962; Tice and Engel, 1967; Peter, Varhaag, and Worsfold, 1970). In some patients, treated with glucocorticoids for long terms, abnormal electrocardiographic changes, such as reversible ST and T changes (Figure 1), have been observed, which prompted us to investigate the effect of glucocorticoids on cardiac muscle in animal experiments.

MATERIALS AND METHODS

Five dogs were given 2 mg/kg of predonisolone daily for 6–10 months and ECG of standard limb leads were recorded. Light and electron microscopic and histochemical studies were carried out. In rabbit experiments, 40 rabbits were injected with 0.5–3 mg/kg of triamcinolone acetonide daily for 3–6 weeks. Fifteen rabbits were placed on a low potassium diet for six weeks. The following studies were carried out: 1) ECG: standard limb leads were recorded during the

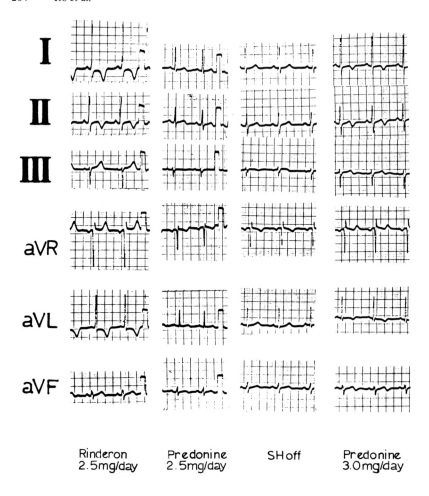

I

II

III

aVR

aVL

aVF

Rinderon   Predonine   SHoff   Predonine
2.5mg/day   2.5mg/day   3.0mg/day

Figure 1. Young female patient treated with steroid for nephrotic syndrome previously. From left to right: the first ECG revealed apparent tall R waves and ST and T changes during treatment with 2.5 mg of β-methasone; the second ECG has less tall R waves and no significant changes of ST and T; the third ECG, after discontinuation of steroid administration, seems almost normal; the fourth ECG, after readministration of glucocorticoid, again with abnormal changes.

course of the experiment; 2) electrophysiological studies: action potentials of cardiac muscle cells were recorded by using the routine microelectrode technique, perfusing at 37°C in a modified Tyrode solution that contained five times more glucose than the original solution; 3) electron microscopic studies: specimens from the left ventricle were fixed with 2.5% phosphate-buffered glutaraldehyde and stained with osmium and uranyl; 4) potassium values: potassium

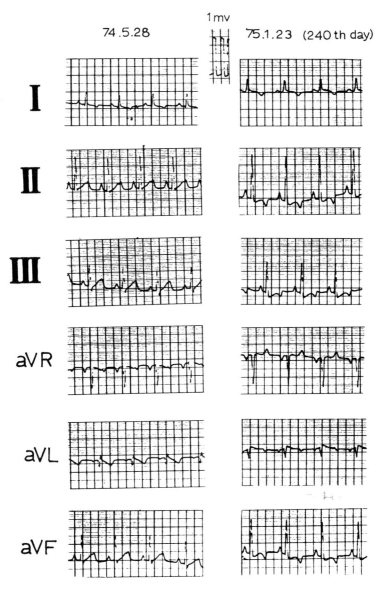

Figure 2. ECG of a dog treated with predonisolone for 240 days. ECG on the right after treatment: tall R waves, depression of ST segments, and inversion of T waves, as compared with ECG on the left taken before administration.

content was determined in serum and in left ventricular myocardium, dissolved in 1 N NaOH solution; 5) hemodynamic measurements: V_{max} was calculated by using a logarithmic amplifier with continuous on-line recording of dP/dt/kp (k = 28).

RESULTS

Electrocardiographic Findings

ECG of dogs, taken after treatment with predonisolone, showed tall R waves, depressed ST segments, and inversion of T waves (Figure 2). Rabbits, treated with triamcinolone, also showed similar ECG changes, but not as distinctly as in the dogs. Rabbits with low potassium diet only showed flattening of T waves.

Electrophysiological Studies

Figure 3 shows the effect of glucocorticoids on transmembrane action potentials of cardiac muscle cell. As shown in Figure 3, when 10^{-6} M dexamethasone was

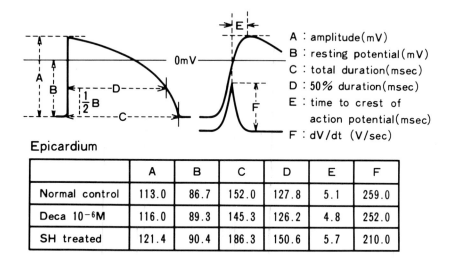

A : amplitude(mV)
B : resting potential(mV)
C : total duration(msec)
D : 50% duration(msec)
E : time to crest of action potential(msec)
F : dV/dt (V/sec)

Epicardium

	A	B	C	D	E	F
Normal control	113.0	86.7	152.0	127.8	5.1	259.0
Deca 10^{-6}M	116.0	89.3	145.3	126.2	4.8	252.0
SH treated	121.4	90.4	186.3	150.6	5.7	210.0

Endocardium

	A	B	C	D	E	F
Normal control	116.3	85.8	201.8	152.0	3.8	245.0
Deca 10^{-6}M	114.3	85.2	159.0	103.2	3.3	252.0
SH treated	131.8	100.8	216.7	180.5	3.8	273.0

Figure 3. Action potentials of rabbit myocardium. Deca = dexamethasone. SH treated = steroid hormone treated; i.e., treated with glucocorticoids.

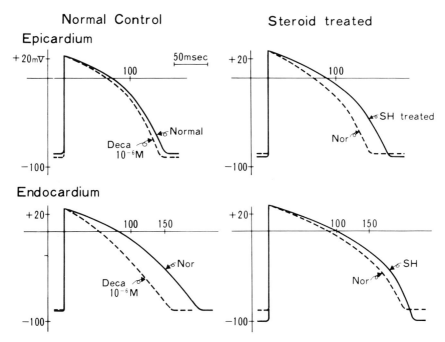

Figure 4. Scheme of action potentials of rabbit cardiac muscle. Deca = dexamethasone. Nor = normal control. SH = steroid hormone (treated with triamcinolone). Duration of action potential increased, particularly in the subepicardial layer, in the rabbits treated with glucocorticoids. On the other hand, duration in the subendocardial layer decreased when dexamethasone was added to perfusing solution *in vitro*.

added directly to the perfusing solution, total and half duration of action potentials decreased, particularly in the subendocardial layer, in comparison to control levels. Duration of action potentials of the rabbits chronically injected with triamcinolone increased, particularly in the subepicardial layer. Furthermore, a deeper subendocardial resting potential was observed in triamcinolone-injected rabbits. The differences of action potentials between control and steroid-treated rabbits are compared in Figure 4. These action potential discrepancies between the various myocardial layers may be the explanation for electrocardiographic changes during glucocorticoid treatment.

Morphological Studies

No significant light microscopic or histochemical changes were observed. However, electron microscopic studies disclosed cardiac muscle cell changes following glucocorticoid treatment. While the arrangement of myofilaments was preserved, mitochondrial changes were found diffusely and especially in the subepicardial layer; the mitochondrial cristae were irregular and swollen (Figure 5A). More

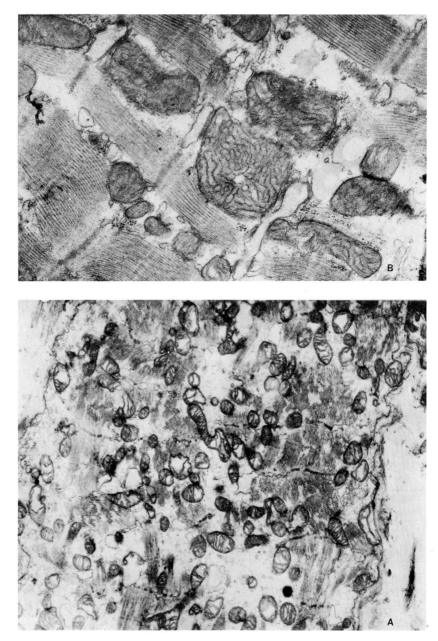

Figure 5. Electron micrograph taken from the left ventricle of rabbit treated with triamcinolone for four weeks. 5A: Cristae of mitochondria are irregular and swollen, while
arrangement of myofilaments appears normal. × 16,000. 5B: Massive cell damage with
vacuolization of mitochondria and destruction of myofilaments. × 9,000.

severe changes consisted of vacuolization of mitochondria and myofilament disarray (Figure 5B).

Other Findings

In rabbits, body weights increased during the first week of experimental study followed by a decline in weight; however, the treatment had no effect on heart weight. The serum potassium level was significantly lower in the low potassium diet group, but the potassium content of myocardium did not show any difference among the three groups. As for hemodynamic studies, there was no difference in left ventricular pressure and dP/dt, but V_{max} values decreased slightly in the steroid-treated group. (Refer to Table 1.)

DISCUSSION

Mineralocorticoid-induced changes of cardiac muscle have been well studied (D'Agostino, 1964; Engel, 1966; Kovács, Blascheck, and Gardell, 1969). However, there are only a few reports on glucocorticoid-induced changes of cardiac muscle (Ellis, 1956; Nickerson, Karr, and Dresel, 1961; Smith, 1964).

The pathogenesis of changes in electrophysiological parameters and mitochondria have not yet been elucidated. It is not likely that potassium imbalance plays a role, because no significant changes were found in serum or cardiac tissue potassium levels of the steroid-treated rabbits. Furthermore, the ECG changes were different from those observed in the low potassium diet group with significant hypopotassemia. While, according to previous reports, hypopotassemia induces some derangements of cardiac myofilaments in the early stage (Molnar, Larsen, and Spargo, 1962), in our steroid experiments the myofilaments were

Table 1. Mean body weight, heart weight, heart weight/body weight ratio, serum and cardiac muscle potassium content, and V_{max} of the left ventricle of rabbits

	Normal control $n = 6$	Steroid hormone treated $n = 6$	Low potassium diet $n = 7$
Body weight (g)	2,460	2,470	2,470
Heart weight (g)	5.4	6.2	5.2
Heart weight/Body weight (%)	0.22	0.25	0.21
Serum K^+ (mEq)	3.3	3.1	2.7[a]
K^+ content in cardiac muscle (mEq)	76.2	74.6	79.9
V_{max} (K = 28)	5.6	5.0[b]	5.4

[a] $p < 0.01$.
[b] $p < 0.05$.

intact. It is possible that adrenal insufficiency, induced by chronic glucocorticoid treatment, may contribute to the ECG and myofilament changes. In adrenalectomized animals, changes of mitochondria and intact myofilament were reported but the potassium transmembrane gradient of cardiac cell decreased (Kôrge, Masso, and Rooson, 1974). Moreover, electrophysiologically, in adrenalectomized rat, the duration of action potential decreased as compared to intact control (Rovetto, 1974). Steroid effect may be attributed to metabolic changes; glucocorticoids also may produce cell membrane changes responsible for the electrophysiological changes described (Baxter and Forsham, 1972). Electrophysiological, as well as morphological, alterations in the subepicardial layer of the myocardium caused by steroid treatment might serve as the basis for electrocardiographic and hemodynamic changes observed in man and experimental animals.

REFERENCES

BAXTER, J. D., and FORSHAM, P. H. 1972. Tissue effects of glucocorticoids. Am. J. Med. 53:573–589.

BYERS, R. K., BERGMAN, A. B., and JOSEPH, M. C. 1962. Steroid myopathy. Pediatrics 29:20–36.

D'AGOSTINO, A. N. 1964. An electron microscopic study of cardiac necrosis produced by 9-alpha-fluorocortisol and sodium phosphate. Am. J. Pathol. 45:633–644.

ELLIS, J. T. 1956. Necrosis and regeneration of skeletal muscle in cortisone treated rabbits. Am. J. Pathol. 32:993–1013.

ENGEL, A. G. 1966. Electron microscopic observations in thyroxim and corticosteroid induced myopathies. Mayo Clin. Proc. 41:785–796.

KORGE, P., MASSO, R., and ROOSON, S. 1974. Changes in myocardial water, electrolytes and ultrastructure after adrenalectomy. Acta Biol. Med. Ger. 32:363–374.

KOVÁCS, K., BLASCHECK, J. A., and GARDELL, G. 1969. Electron microscopic study of myocardial changes produced in rats by the concurrent administration of 9-alpha-fluorocortisol, Na$_2$HPO$_4$ and corn oil. Cardiology 54:16–29.

MOLNAR, Z., LARSEN, K., and SPARGO, B. 1962. Cardiac changes in the potassium-depleted rat. Arch. Pathol. 74:339–347.

NICKERSON, M., KARR, G. W., and DRESEL, P. E. 1961. Pathogenesis of "Electrolyte-Steroid-Cardiopathy." Circ. Res. 9:209–217.

PETER, J. B., VARHAAG, D. A., and WORSFOLD, M. 1970. Studies of steroid myopathy. Biochem. Pharmacol. 19:1627–1636.

ROVETTO, J. 1974. Myocardial cell function in adrenal insufficiency. *In* T. M. Glenn (ed.), Steroid and Shock, pp. 33–51. University Park Press, Baltimore.

SMITH, B. 1964. Histological and histochemical changes in the muscle of rabbits given the corticosteroid triamcinolone. Neurology (Minneap.) 14:854–863.

TICE, W., and ENGEL, A. G. 1967. The effects of glucocorticoid on red and white muscle in the rat. Am. J. Pathol. 50:311–333.

Mailing address:
Takashi Ito, M.D.,
Internal Medicine, Branch Hospital of Tokyo University
3-28-6 Mejirodai, Bunkyo-ku, Tokyo (Japan).

Myocardial Ischemia

Recent Advances in Studies on
Cardiac Structure and Metabolism, Volume 12
Cardiac Adaptation
Edited by T. Kobayashi, Y. Ito, and G. Rona
Copyright 1978 University Park Press Baltimore

EFFECT OF GRADED CORONARY STENOSIS
ON REGIONAL MYOCARDIAL BLOOD FLOW
AND LEFT VENTRICULAR FUNCTION

M. NAKAMURA, H. MATSUGUCHI, A. MITSUTAKE,
A. TAKESHITA, Y. KIKUCHI, M. MORI,
Y. KOIWAYA, Y. NOSE, and A. KUROIWA

Research Institute of Angiocardiology and Cardiovascular Clinic,
Kyushu University Medical School, Fukuoka, Japan

SUMMARY

Dogs with 70% stenosis of the left circumflex coronary artery showed a reduction of myocardial blood flow with a minimal impairment of left ventricular wall motion. Eighty to ninety percent stenosis produced a marked reduction of flow and wall motion, and ST elevation close to 100% occlusion, but delayed antegrade run-off was found. The effectiveness of collaterals to protect against left ventricular dysfunction was supported.

INTRODUCTION

To evaluate coronary arterial disease, selective coronary arteriography and left ventricular angiography have been used widely. However, interrelationships between wall motion in left ventricular angiography, regional myocardial blood flow, collateral flow, and a degree of stenosis in coronary cinearteriography have not been described previously. The present study was undertaken to determine critical stenosis by coronary cinearteriography in dogs, which causes regional ischemia and abnormalities of wall motion of the left ventricle at the resting state in the acute and chronic stages.

MATERIALS AND METHODS

Eighteen mongrel dogs were anesthetized, the left circumflex coronary artery (LCA) was isolated, and a constrictor was placed before arterial branching. The degree of stenosis of LCA was evaluated by selective coronary cinearteriography. Abnormalities of wall motion of the left ventricle (LV) and changes of regional myocardial blood flow and of collateral flow were measured by LV cineangiography and the tracer microsphere (TM) technique, respectively.

Changes of distribution of regional myocardial blood flow were measured by using 15-μm microspheres labeled with four different radioactive isotopes, [85]Sr, [46]Sc, [141]Ce, and [51]Cr. The first microsphere (TM_1) was injected 20 min after LCA stenosis to determine the effect of different degrees of stenosis on myocardial blood flow. A few minutes later, the second microsphere (TM_2) was injected with a temporary complete occlusion of LCA at the proximal site of the constriction in order to determine the area supplied by LCA and to measure collateral flow to the ischemic LCA area through the nonoccluded coronary arteries. The third and fourth microspheres (TM_3 and TM_4) were injected in a similar way three weeks after stenosis. The changes in distribution of myocardial flow were expressed as a flow-ratio of the LCA area to the left anterior descending coronary artery (LAD) area (LCA/LAD) and/or the posterior papillary muscle (PPM) to the LAD area (PPM/LAD). For example, the flow ratio of LCA/LAD of 0.3 indicates that flow in the LCA area was three-tenths of the flow in the LAD area. The ratio of subendocardial to subepicardial radioactivity was calculated as I/O ratio.

In order to evaluate changes of ejection fraction and wall motion of the LV after LCA constriction at the acute and chronic stages, the first, second, and third LV angiographies (Leighton, Wilt, and Lewis, 1974) were performed in the control period, 42 min, and 3 weeks after LCA constriction, respectively. Coronary cinearteriography was performed 15 min after the third LV angiography in the chronic stage.

The uptake of TM_2 or TM_4 that enters the ischemic LCA area from the nonoccluded coronary arteries during a complete LCA occlusion was used to calculate the collateral flow ratio.

RESULTS AND DISCUSSION

A significant reduction of mean blood pressure was found after more than 80% constriction of LCA, while stenosis of 50–70% did not alter it. In animals with 50–60% stenosis, the resting flow-ratio of the LCA area remained within normal range (Table 1). Seventy percent stenosis produced a mild reduction of the antegrade flow through the stenosed LCA, but wall motion of the postero-inferior wall showed a minimal impairment. A flow reduction of PPM was greater than that of LV free wall. In animals with 70% stenosis, flow through the stenosed LCA was found in a significant amount. This finding concerning flow corresponded well to the normal run-off in a coronary arteriogram. In animals with more than 80% stenosis, flow in the LCA area was decreased to 20% of LAD flow, which was almost the same extent of reduction as with 100% occlusion. In animals with more than 80% stenosis, a markedly delayed antegrade run-off in a coronary arteriogram was found, and the antegrade flow through the stenosed LCA was negligible.

Table 1. Changes of postero-inferior wall motion and flow distribution of left ventricle after stenosis (acute stage)

Degree of stenosis (%)	Number of dogs	Posterior-inferior wall motion (%)		Flow-ratio after stenosis			ST II, III (mV)	Antegrade run-off[a]
		Before	After stenosis	LCA/LAD	PPM/LAD	I/O		
50	3	44	36	1.1	1.3	1.1	0	++
60	2	29	33	1.0	1.1	1.2	0	++
70	5	33	30	0.8	0.6	0.9	0	++
80	2	38	1	0.2	0.2	0.5	+2.2	+
90	2	38	7	0.2	0.1	0.4	+0.8	±
100	4	42	1	0.1	0.1	0.4	+1.4	−

Values are the mean of each group.
[a] Appearance time of LCA distal to stenosis: ++ = same as LAD; + = delayed; ± = markedly delayed; − = not opacified.

In animals with more than 80% stenosis, a remarkable impairment of postero-inferior wall motion, as well as an ejection fraction of LV and a significant elevation of ST segment in ECG, limb II- and III-leads was found in the same extent as in the animals with complete occlusion of the LCA. There was a significant positive correlation between ejection fraction and the mean value of segmental wall motion ($r = 0.93$).

Collateral flow from the nonoccluded coronary arteries to the ischemic LCA area during an abrupt LCA complete occlusion was approximately 10–20% of LAD flow in the acute stage. In the LCA area the collateral flow was significantly smaller than the antegrade flow in animals with 70% or less stenosis, but not in animals with more than 80% stenosis.

These results may indicate that more than 80% abrupt stenosis produced a marked myocardial ischemia close to complete occlusion, although a delayed antegrade run-off was noted in coronary arteriograms.

Two dogs with 70% stenosis and one dog with 80% stenosis in the acute stage completed the entire experimental schedule up to three weeks. Three weeks after acute LCA stenosis, all these dogs showed 100% occlusion angiographically. In spite of progression of stenosis, an improvement of the flow, as well as wall motion of LV free wall, was markedly found three weeks after stenosis in all three dogs when compared with those at the acute stage. However, flow of the PPM in two out of three dogs did not show any increase. Thus, an increase of collateral flow and collaterals showed a wide individual variation. It seems that the papillary muscle is the region that rarely develops collaterals.

Increases of collateral flow, collateral vessels, and an improvement of wall motion were great in one dog, in which a good wall motion of LV and a mild decrease of flow were found in the acute stage even with the same 70% stenosis. Myocardial necrosis in this dog was negligible in contrast to others. This histological finding corresponded to good wall motion and well preserved myocardial flow through collaterals, and small and narrow Q waves in ECG of this animal. This preliminary result at the chronic stage may suggest that the degree to which collaterals are protective against LV dysfunction is determined by the congenital pattern of coronary distribution, as pointed out previously by Sheldon (1969). In the present study, I/O ratio of collateral flow was below unity at both the acute and chronic stages. Thus, the collateral flow distributed in subepicardium to a greater extent than in subendocardium.

REFERENCES

LEIGHTON, R. F., WILT, S. M., and LEWIS, R. P. 1974. Detection of hypokinesis by a quantitative analysis of left ventricular cineangiograms. Circulation 50:121–127.
SHELDON, W. C. 1969. On the significance of coronary collaterals. (Editorial). Am. J. Cardiol. 24:303–304.

Mailing address:
M. Nakamura, M.D.,
Research Institute of Angiocardiology and Cardiovascular Clinic,
Kyushu University Medical School, Fukuoka (Japan).

Recent Advances in Studies on
Cardiac Structure and Metabolism, Volume 12
Cardiac Adaptation
Edited by T. Kobayashi, Y. Ito, and G. Rona
Copyright 1978 University Park Press Baltimore

TRANSMURAL GRADIENTS IN MYOCARDIAL GAS TENSIONS IN REGIONALLY ISCHEMIC CANINE LEFT VENTRICLE

J. FLAHERTY,[1] J. O'RIORDAN, S. KHURI, and V. GOTT

Departments of Medicine and Surgery, The Johns Hopkins University
and Hospital, Baltimore, Maryland, USA

SUMMARY

Previous studies from this laboratory have demonstrated the usefulness of myocardial gas tensions as measured by mass spectrometry for the quantitative assessment of regional myocardial ischemia (Khuri *et al.*, 1975a). Progressive increases in myocardial carbon dioxide tensions were noted when progressive reduction in coronary blood flow was created by means of a variable constrictor. The present study was designed to determine if changes in myocardial oxygen and carbon dioxide tension were greater in deep, compared to more superficial, myocardial layers. In eight anesthetized dogs, progressive reduction in circumflex coronary flow was associated with a progressive reduction in myocardial oxygen tension and a progressive increase in myocardial carbon dioxide tension and intramyocardial ST-segment voltage. Evidence of a transmural gradient in the severity of ischemia was present at all degrees of flow reduction. These results confirm the findings of previous metabolic studies, which demonstrated gradients in lactate and high-energy phosphates. Myocardial carbon dioxide tension, which can be monitored continuously by mass spectrometry, would appear to provide a useful means of quantitatively assessing changes in regional myocardial metabolism.

INTRODUCTION

Our earlier work has demonstrated the usefulness of myocardial oxygen and carbon dioxide tensions as measured by mass spectrometry for the quantitative assessment of the severity of regional myocardial ischemia (Khuri *et al.*, 1975a). Progressive reduction in mean coronary blood flow resulted in a progressive increase in myocardial carbon dioxide tension and a parallel, progressive rise in unipolar intramyocardial ST-segment voltage as measured with multicontact plunge electrodes. Myocardial oxygen tension decreased 13 mm Hg and myocardial carbon dioxide tension increased 20 mm Hg following application of a

---

[1] J. Flaherty is supported by Research Career Development Award 5 KO4 HL 00019-02 from the National Heart and Lung Institute.

stenosis that abolished the hyperemic response to a transient total occlusion without significantly lowering mean flow ("critical stenosis"). Severe reduction in mean coronary flow to 14% of its control value resulted in only a 7-mm Hg further decrease in oxygen tension, in contrast to an 84-mm Hg further increase in carbon dioxide tension. Thus, myocardial carbon dioxide tension appeared to provide a more useful index of the severity of ischemia than did oxygen tension. Recent studies have demonstrated that myocardial carbon dioxide tension is also a useful index when regional ischemia is induced by atrial pacing in the presence of a flow-limiting coronary stenosis (O'Riordan *et al.*, 1977).

The present study was designed to test the hypothesis that regional ischemia is more severe in deep myocardial layers than in more superficial layers when ischemia is induced by a progressive reduction in regional coronary blood flow and that this gradient in ischemia can be demonstrated by the measurement of myocardial gas tensions.

MATERIALS AND METHODS

Eight adult mongrel dogs, weighing 20–25 kg, were anesthetized with chloralose (60 mg/kg I.V.), intubated, placed on a Harvard respirator, and ventilated with room air. Arterial pressure was monitored continuously via a catheter inserted into the femoral artery, utilizing a Statham P_{23} db transducer. A left thoracotomy extending across the sternum was performed, a pericardial cradle was created, and a 3-cm segment of the proximal left circumflex coronary artery (CCA) was dissected free. An electromagnetic flow probe (Biotronex Series 6000 with a Biotronex Model 610 Pulse logic flowmeter), a variable screw type constrictor, and a snare were placed around the exposed proximal CCA. Arterial gas tensions were monitored intermittently, and arterial oxygen tension was maintained in the 100–200-mm Hg range by varying the percentage of oxygen in the inspired air.

Mass spectrometer probes were inserted into the postero-lateral wall of the left ventricle, a region supplied by the constricted CCA. One probe was inserted in a deep position in the myocardial wall, and a second probe was placed more superficially. The probes consisted of 22-gauge stainless steel tubing slotted in the distal 2 cm and covered with heat-shrinkable teflon. A 19-mm segment near the distal tip was left in the expanded state. The probes were connected to a vacuum mass spectrometer (Med Spect Model MS-8) that sampled the mixture of dissolved gas in the interstitial fluid near the probe tip at a rate of 5×10^{-6} ml/sec. The probes were calibrated before each experiment in a glass tonometer at $37°C$ with two gas mixtures of known composition. Details of this method have been published previously (Khuri *et al.*, 1975b).

A multicontact plunge electrode also was placed in the postero-lateral wall adjacent to the mass spectrometer probes. The electrodes consisted of 10 teflon-coated silver wires, 0.0001 inches in diameter, inserted into the shaft of a 22-gauge needle that had side holes drilled at 1-mm spacings. Following insertion of the mass spectrometer probes and the plunge electrode, approximately one hour was allowed for stabilization of myocardial gas tensions and ST-segment voltages before applying the first of a series of 15-min periods of coronary constriction.

The proximal CCA then was progressively stenosed using the screw-type variable constrictor, and the degree of stenosis was assessed by recording mean circumflex coronary flow and the reactive hyperemic response following a 10-sec total occlusion. At the end of each experiment, the depth of each mass spectrometer probe, relative to the epicardial and endocardial surfaces, was recorded and the two plunge electrode contacts, which were located at comparable depths to the gas probes, were noted. All data are expressed as mean ± one S.E.M. and were analyzed using the paired Student's t test.

RESULTS

The mean position of the deeper mass spectrometer probe was 0.45 ± 0.03, expressed as a fraction of the endocardial to epicardial distance. The mean position of the more superficial probe was 0.72 ± 0.2. Before application of the first stenosis, control myocardial carbon dioxide tension was 44.8 ± 1.8 in the deeper layer and 41.1 ± 1.5 mm Hg in the more superficial layer. This difference in pCO_2 was significant at the 0.02 level. Control myocardial oxygen tension was 20.6 ± 1.6 mm Hg in the deeper layer and 21.9 ± 2.2 mm Hg in the superficial layer.

Reduction in mean flow in the circumflex coronary artery resulted in an increase in myocardial carbon dioxide tension, a decrease in myocardial oxygen tension, and a corresponding increase in intramyocardial ST-segment voltage. The mean myocardial carbon dioxide tension rose to 87.4 ± 9.6 mm Hg in the deep layers and to 72.0 ± 6.5 mm Hg in the superficial layers. This gradient in carbon dioxide tension was significant at the 0.01 level. Mean oxygen tension in the deeper layers fell to 11.2 ± 1.5, and the mean oxygen tension in the more superficial layers fell to 13.8 ± 1.6 mm Hg, but this difference did not reach statistical significance ($0.10 < p < 0.20$).

In the eight experimental animals, 29 different degrees of proximal coronary artery constriction were applied. The 29 stenoses were divided into six equal groups according to the percentage of reduction in mean circumflex coronary flow (Table 1; Figure 1). Progressive reduction in coronary flow resulted in a progressive rise in myocardial carbon dioxide tension that was greater in deep, compared to superficial, layers with all degrees of stenosis. Progressive reduction in coronary perfusion also resulted in a progressive decline in myocardial oxygen

Table 1. Changes in deep and superficial myocardial gas tensions and ST-segment voltages resulting from application of various stenoses

	Percentage reduction in mean circumflex coronary flow					
	0 $n = 4$	5.4 ± 3.3 $n = 5$	24.3 ± 1.8 $n = 6$	38.2 ± 1.5 $n = 5$	50.4 ± 1.9 $n = 5$	76.0 ± 5.2 $n = 4$
pCO_2 (mm Hg) Deep	40.8 ± 4.3	54.8 ± 6.3	65.0 ± 8.5	80.4 ± 7.8	130.2 ± 25.1	163.8 ± 21.2
Superficial	36.8 ± 3.5	52.4 ± 4.3	56.0 ± 6.3	72.9 ± 7.1	83.2 ± 3.9	140.5 ± 13.1
pO_2 (mm Hg) Deep	20.8 ± 3.3	14.9 ± 2.7	12.6 ± 3.1	8.6 ± 2.1	7.1 ± 3.4	4.2 ± 0.9
Superficial	24.0 ± 4.5	17.8 ± 3.3	13.1 ± 3.7	11.7 ± 3.2	10.8 ± 1.6	6.6 ± 2.2
ΔST (m V) Deep	−0.1 ± 0.1	0.9 ± 0.3	5.3 ± 3.3	11.1 ± 3.8	8.2 ± 1.3	21.8 ± 4.4
Superficial	−0.6 ± 0.6	1.0 ± 0.9	4.3 ± 3.3	7.8 ± 4.3	10.7 ± 1.8	21.8 ± 3.8

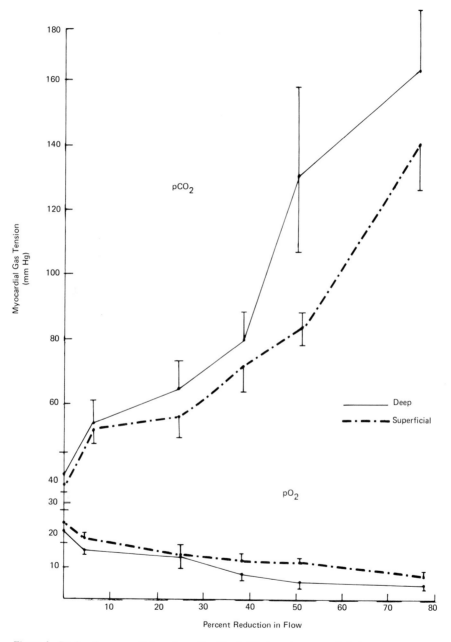

Figure 1. Regional myocardial carbon dioxide (pCO_2) and oxygen (pO_2) tensions associated with progressive degrees of reduction in mean circumflex coronary flow.

tension that, likewise, was greater in deep, compared to superficial, layers at all degrees of flow reduction.

Progressive reduction in mean circumflex coronary flow also produced changes in intramyocardial ST-segment voltages that paralleled the changes in myocardial carbon dioxide tension (Table 1). These ST-segment changes were of greater magnitude in deeper, compared to more superficial, layers with mild and moderate degrees of flow reduction. However, distal to more severe degrees of stenosis associated with 45–90% reduction in mean flow, superficial ST-segment changes were equal to, or exceeded, ST-segment changes in deep layers.

DISCUSSION

The changes in myocardial oxygen and carbon dioxide tension found in this study support our hypothesis that a transmural gradient in the severity of ischemia develops when coronary perfusion is reduced by proximal coronary artery stenosis. Progressive reduction in mean coronary artery flow resulted in a progressive increase in myocardial carbon dioxide tension and a progressive decrease in myocardial oxygen tension in the region of myocardium supplied by the stenosed artery.

Studies of regional myocardial metabolism have demonstrated uniform tissue levels of lactate and adenosine triphosphate (ATP) in the outer, middle, and inner myocardial layers when coronary perfusion is normal. In contrast, reduction in coronary perfusion pressure was shown to result in significant gradients in each of these substances as well as in a redistribution of regional myocardial blood flow with a lower flow to subendocardial than to subepicardial layers (Griggs and Nakamara, 1968; Griggs, Tchokoev, and Chen, 1972). Furthermore, wall stress and, thereby, energy demands of the contracting ventricle have been shown to be greater in subendocardial compared to subepicardial layers (Kirk and Honig, 1964a). Reduction in coronary blood flow therefore might be expected to result in a greater imbalance between oxygen supply and demand in the deeper subendocardial layers.

Measurement of oxygen tension by the polarographic technique has revealed gradients in deep, compared to superficial, myocardial layers under conditions of normal coronary perfusion (Kirk and Honig, 1964b). Gradients in oxygen tension under conditions of reduced coronary perfusion have not been reported.

The results of the present study confirm the presence of an endocardial to epicardial gradient in oxygen tension in both normally perfused and underperfused myocardium. However, the magnitude of this oxygen gradient was small and less consistent. More consistent, however, was an endocardial to epicardial gradient in carbon dioxide tension in both normally perfused and underperfused hearts. This gradient in myocardial carbon dioxide tension was 4 mm Hg, with normal coronary blood flow, and 47 mm Hg, with a 50% reduction in mean coronary flow. The greater consistency of this gradient with all degrees of coronary stenosis, coupled with the greater magnitude of changes in myocardial carbon dioxide tension with progressive reduction in coronary flow, seems to make myocardial carbon dioxide tension a more useful quantitative index of the severity of ischemia than myocardial oxygen tension.

Thus, these results confirm the findings of the previous metabolic studies that suggested increased vulnerability of the subendocardial layers to the development of ischemia. These studies demonstrated increased lactate and decreased ATP concentrations in deep, compared to superficial, layers. The gradient in myocardial carbon dioxide tension appears to parallel the previously reported gradient in lactate concentration in regionally ischemic myocardium. The increase in myocardial carbon dioxide tension under conditions of regional ischemia is probably related both to increased generation of CO_2 molecules caused by the buffering of the excess hydrogen ions generated by ATP hydrolysis by the bicarbonate buffer system, and to decreased washout of metabolic end products such as CO_2 caused by the local decrease in coronary flow.

Because myocardial carbon dioxide tension can be monitored continuously and lactate determinations must be intermittent, mass spectrometry seems to provide a more useful means of assessing changes in regional myocardial metabolism and should provide a valuable new tool for future studies of the pathophysiology of myocardial ischemia.

REFERENCES

GRIGGS, D. M., JR., and NAKAMARA, Y. 1968. Effect of coronary constriction on myocardial distribution of iodoantipyrine [131]-I. Am. J. Physiol. 215:1082–1088.

GRIGGS, D. M., JR., TCHOKOEV, V. V. and CHEN, C. C. 1972. Transmural differences in ventricular tissue substrate levels due to coronary constriction. Am. J. Physiol. 222: 705–709.

KHURI, S. F., FLAHERTY, J. T., O'RIORDAN, J. B., PITT, B., BRAWLEY, R. K., DONAHOO, J. S., and GOTT, V. L. 1975a. Intramyocardial ST segment voltage and gas tensions with regional myocardial ischemia in the dog. Circ. Res. 37:455–463.

KHURI, S. F., O'RIORDAN, J. B., FLAHERTY, J. T., BRAWLEY, R. K., DONAHOO, J. S., and GOTT, V. L. 1975b. Mass spectrometry for the measurement of intramyocardial gas tensions: Methodology and application to the study of myocardial ischemia. In T. E. Roy and G. Rona (eds.), Recent Advances in Studies on Cardiac Structure and Metabolism. Vol. 10: The Metabolism of Contraction, pp. 539–550. University Park Press, Baltimore.

KIRK, E. S., and HONIG, C. R. 1964a. An experiment and theoretical analysis of myocardial tissue pressure. Am. J. Physiol. 207:361–367.

KIRK, E. S., and HONIG, C. R. 1964b. Non-uniform distribution of blood flow and gradients of oxygen tension within the heart. Am. J. Physiol. 207:661–668.

O'RIORDAN, J. B., FLAHERTY, J. T., KHURI, S. F., BRAWLEY, R. K., PITT, B., and GOTT, V. L. 1977. Effects of atrial pacing on regional myocardial gas tensions with critical coronary stenosis. Am. J. Physiol. 232:H49–H53.

Mailing address:
John T. Flaherty, M.D.,
Cardiology Division, Johns Hopkins Hospital,
601 N. Broadway, Baltimore, Maryland 21205 (USA).

Recent Advances in Studies on
Cardiac Structure and Metabolism, Volume 12
Cardiac Adaptation
Edited by T. Kobayashi, Y. Ito, and G. Rona
Copyright 1978 University Park Press Baltimore

HEMODYNAMIC AND METABOLIC CHANGES CAUSED BY REGIONAL ISCHEMIA IN PORCINE HEART

P. D. VERDOUW, J. W. De JONG,[1] and W. J. REMME

Laboratories for Experimental Cardiology and Cardiochemistry,
Thoraxcenter and Department of Biochemistry I,
Erasmus University, Rotterdam, The Netherlands

SUMMARY

Myocardial ischemia was induced in the pig by reducing the left anterior descending coronary artery (LAD) flow to 26% of its control value. After one hour, the LAD was reperfused for 50 minutes. During ischemia and reperfusion, cardiac output correlated strongly with arterial levels of lactate and nucleosides (all $r < -0.85$). Myocardial inosine production seems to be a good marker of ischemia because it correlated very well with myocardial lactate production ($r = 0.99$).

INTRODUCTION

Most experimental studies dealing with hemodynamics and biochemistry during ischemia or during acute myocardial infarction have been carried out in the dog. However, the coronary vascular structure of the dog is quite different from that of man. Recent findings indicate that the pig may be a better animal for these studies (Bertho and Gagnon, 1964; Schaper, 1971; Brooks *et al.,* 1975). This study was undertaken to establish the relationship between hemodynamics and some biochemical parameters of myocardial metabolism (lactate and ATP breakdown products) in the porcine heart during acute regional ischemia.

MATERIALS AND METHODS

Experiments were performed on Yorkshire pigs (20–25 kg), fasted for 24 hr. The animals were anesthetized with 120 mg of azaperone, I.M., and 150 mg of metomidate, I.V. They were ventilated with a mixture of 33% O_2 and 67% N_2O. Arterial blood gases were measured intermittently to control the setting of the respirator. The temperature of the animals was kept between 36 and 37°C.

This study was supported in part by a grant from the Dutch Heart Foundation.
[1] Established Investigator of the Dutch Heart Foundation.

Three peripheral ECG leads were monitored continuously. An 8F Cournand catheter, positioned in the right atrium, was used for the administration of anesthetics. A catheter was positioned in the aorta for the withdrawal of arterial blood samples and for the measurement of mean aortic pressure. Left ventricular pressure was obtained from a micromanometer-tip catheter. Cardiac output (CO) was determined using the thermodilution technique.

The heart was exposed, and the left anterior descending coronary artery (LAD) was dissected from its origin to the first branch. This gave approximately 1.0 cm of free artery, a length sufficient to attach an electromagnetic flow probe and to place a J-shaped screw clamp around the vessel distal to the probe. The accompanying vein was cannulated and a polyethylene catheter was inserted. The blood was collected and returned directly to the animal via the vena cava inferior. Inosine and hypoxanthine determinations took place in neutralized samples (De Jong and Goldstein, 1974). For samples in which the inosine concentration was less than 5 μM, Olsson's method was used (Olsson, 1970). Lactate was assayed with an AutoAnalyzer II (Technicon, Tarrytown, N.Y.) according to Apstein et al. (1970). All determinations were carried out in duplicate.

After catheterization and surgery were completed, a stabilization period of 30 min was allowed before control values of the hemodynamic parameters were determined and before simultaneous arterial and coronary venous blood samples were drawn. Subsequently, the mean LAD blood flow was reduced and kept at about 25% of control by tightening the screw on the clamp. After 60 min, the clamp was released and the animal was studied for 50 more minutes.

RESULTS AND DISCUSSION

Coronary Blood Flow and Myocardial Oxygen Extraction

LAD blood flow during control was 26.5 ± 2.3 ml/min (mean ± S.E.M.). This was reduced to 7.0 ± 0.5 ml/min. After release of the clamp, there was considerable reactive hyperemia, with a peak after about 2 min (58.8 ± 8.7 ml/min, $p < 0.001$). There was only partial repayment of flow debt (Figure 1).

Cardiac Output (CO)

Cardiac output decreased sharply in the first 2 min of occlusion (from 2.0 ± 0.2 to 1.7 ± 0.2 liter/min, $p < 0.005$). Subsequently, it dropped more gradually until 1.34 ± 0.08 liter/min ($p < 0.005$) at the end of occlusion. There was no recovery after release.

Peak Left Ventricular Pressure (LVdP/dt)

Control values were 2,000 ± 200 mm Hg sec^{-1}. Immediately after the flow reduction, LVdP/dt started to drop, and, after 2 min, peak LVdP/dt was only

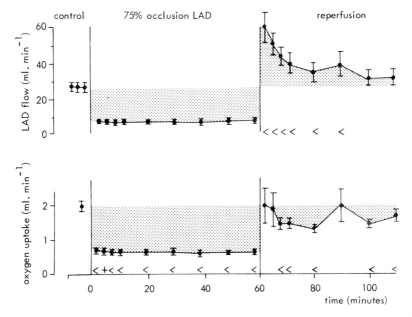

Figure 1. LAD blood flow (top) and myocardial oxygen uptake (bottom) during control, partial occlusion, and reperfusion. $<$ denotes $p < 0.05$.

1,430 ± 130 mm Hg sec^{-1} ($p < 0.005$). Gradually, peak LVdP/dt started to increase, and, after 40 min, no values significantly different from control were found. In the recovery period, there was an initial increase ($p < 0.05$) compared to the last ischemic values. In the following minutes, there was no significant change.

Arterial Levels of Lactate, Inosine, and Hypoxanthine

Arterial lactate was 3.84 ± 0.52 mM during control. This increased gradually to 6.29 ± 1.03 mM ($p < 0.05$) at the end of the experiment. Inosine levels during control were 17.9 ± 2.5 μM. This also increased by about 60% during the course of the experiment to 27.9 ± 5.1 μM ($p < 0.05$) at the end of the experiment (Figure 2). The same trend was found for hypoxanthine (from 38.0 ± 5.0 μM to 61.1 ± 10.5 μM, $p < 0.05$).

The increase in metabolic levels is reflected in the deterioration of CO (all $r < -0.85$), with hypoxanthine giving the best correlation ($r = -0.94$).

Myocardial Extraction of Lactate, Inosine, and Hypoxanthine

An extensive presentation of these data has been given elsewhere (De Jong *et al.*, 1976; De Jong *et al.*, 1977). Lactate extraction (20% during control) changed

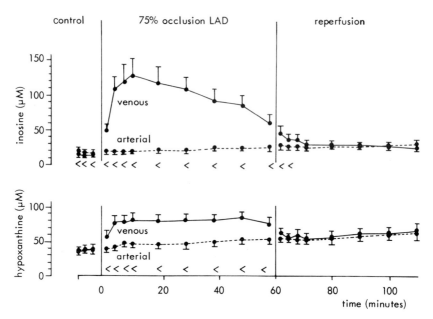

Figure 2. Arterial and coronary venous inosine (top) and hypoxanthine (bottom) during control, partial occlusion, and reperfusion. Note that coronary venous inosine returns gradually to arterial values, after 15 min of ischemia. < denotes $p < 0.05$.

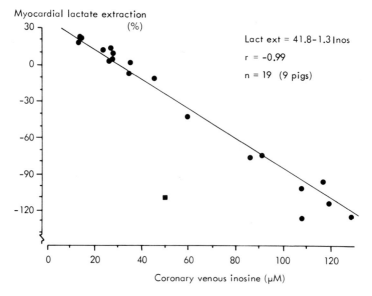

Figure 3. Relation between coronary venous inosine and lactate extraction. The value after 2 min of occlusion (■) was not taken into account for the determination of the correlation coefficient.

to production during ischemia. A peak was found after 10 min of occlusion (−125%), after which there was a decrease in production. In the release phase, there was a return to control levels. Inosine extraction, which was 24% during control, decreased to −67.2% in the first 10 min of ischemia (Figure 2). Subsequently, extraction started to decrease and returned to control values in the release period.

Throughout the experiment, there was an excellent correlation between coronary venous inosine and myocardial lactate extraction, with the exception of the values obtained after 2 min of ischemia (■ in Figure 3), at which time there was a much larger production than would be expected on the basis of the other data points. An explanation is that, in sudden ischemia, increased anaerobiosis precedes ATP breakdown. Furthermore, peak LVdP/dt correlated well with coronary venous metabolites—best with lactate extraction ($r = 0.76$).

REFERENCES

APSTEIN, C. S., PUCHNER, E., and BRACHFELD, N. 1970. Improved automated lactate determination. Anal. Biochem. 38:20–34.

BERTHO, E., and GAGNON, G. 1964. A comparative study in three dimensions of the blood supply of the normal interventricular septum in human, canine, bovine, porcine, and ovine hearts. Dis. Chest 46:251–262.

BROOKS, H. L., AL-SADIR, J. A., SCHWARTZ, J., RICH, B., HARPER, P., and RESNEKOV, L. 1975. Biventricular dynamics during quantitated anteroseptal infarction in the porcine heart. Am. J. Cardiol. 36:765–775.

De JONG, J. W., and GOLDSTEIN, S. 1974. Changes in coronary venous inosine concentration and myocardial wall thickening during regional ischemia in the pig. Circ. Res. 35:111–116.

De JONG, J. W., REMME, W. J., and VERDOUW, P. D. 1976. Myocardial arteriovenous difference in carbohydrates, purine nucleosides and electrolytes following occlusion and release of pig coronary artery. Am. J. Cardiol. 37(abstr.):130.

De JONG, J. W., VERDOUW, P. D., and REMME, W. J. 1977. Myocardial nucleoside and carbohydrate metabolism and hemodynamics during partial occlusion and reperfusion of pig coronary artery. J. Mol. Cell. Cardiol. 9:297–312.

OLSSON, R. A. 1970. Changes in content of purine nucleoside in canine myocardium during coronary occlusion. Circ. Res. 26:301–306.

SCHAPER, W. 1971. Comparative arteriography of the collateral circulation. In B. Dak ed.), The Collateral Circulation of the Heart, Chap. IV, pp. 39–49. North Holland Publishing, Amsterdam.

Mailing address:
P. D. Verdouw, Ph.D.,
Laboratory for Experimental Cardiology,
Eramus University, P.O. Box 1738, Rotterdam (The Netherlands).

Recent Advances in Studies on
Cardiac Structure and Metabolism, Volume 12
Cardiac Adaptation
Edited by T. Kobayashi, Y. Ito, and G. Rona
Copyright 1978 University Park Press Baltimore

CHANGES IN INTRAMYOCARDIAL OXYGEN TENSION AND LOCAL ELECTROGRAMS PRODUCED BY CORONARY OCCLUSION

M. M. WINBURY and B. B. HOWE

Department of Pharmacology, Warner-Lambert Research Institute,
Morris Plains, New Jersey, USA

SUMMARY

Coronary occlusion reduces oxygen tension of the subendocardium considerably more than of the subepicardium. Changes in surface electrograms do not reflect the changes in regional oxygen tension.

INTRODUCTION

In recent years, ST-segment elevation of surface or precordial electrograms (ECG) has been used in animals and man to estimate the degree of ischemia and/or infarction. The relevance of the surface ECG to measure the degree of tissue hypoxia and eventual damage has been questioned, particularly with regard to evaluation of drugs for treatment of myocardial infarction.

The subendocardium is highly susceptible to ischemia or infarction, but the relationship between subendocardial oxygen tension and the electrogram has not been demonstrated. Therefore, we undertook a study of the changes in the oxygen tension (pO_2) and in local ECGs in the subendocardium (endo), subepicardium (epi), and surface produced by varying degrees of coronary stenosis. This information is required before one is justified in using surface ECG to draw any conclusions regarding the effectiveness of a therapeutic intervention. The objectives of this study discussed here were: 1) to quantitate the relationship between changes in coronary blood flow (CBF) and regional pO_2; 2) to compare the vulnerability of endo and epi to coronary stenosis; 3) to determine the vasodilator reserve of endo and epi; 4) to compare changes in local ECG with local pO_2; and 5) to compare changes in surface ECG with changes in local pO_2.

MATERIALS AND METHODS

Intramyocardial pO_2 was determined polarographically with small platinum electrodes inserted to a depth of 3 mm (epi) and 9 mm (endo) below the surface of the left ventricle. Local unipolar ECGs were recorded simultaneously with pO_2 at the same depths and in the same area with similar electrodes; a flat electrode was sewn to the surface. An electromagnetic flowmeter probe was placed around the left anterior descending coronary artery (LAD), mid-way between the base and apex. Distal to the probe was a hydraulic occluder for graded stenosis and a snare for abrupt total occlusion. In several experiments, reactive hyperemia after release of total occlusion was determined at various degrees of stenosis to determine the autoregulatory reserve in both epi and endo. ECG and pO_2 were recorded in the central ischemic zone.

RESULTS

Gradual stenosis of the LAD was produced until resting coronary blood flow (CBF) began to decline. On further stenosis, endo pO_2 declined stepwise with

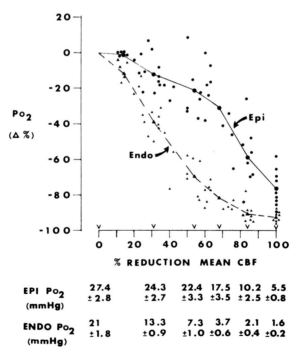

BLOOD FLOW vs REGIONAL Po_2

EPI Po_2 (mmHg)	27.4 ±2.8	24.3 ±2.7	22.4 ±3.3	17.5 ±3.5	10.2 ±2.5	5.5 ±0.8
ENDO Po_2 (mmHg)	21 ±1.8	13.3 ±0.9	7.3 ±1.0	3.7 ±0.6	2.1 ±0.4	1.6 ±0.2

Figure 1. Relationship of changes in coronary blood flow (CBF) produced by gradual stenosis to changes in oxygen tension (pO_2) of subepicardium (epi) and subendocardium (endo) of the canine left ventricle. Table at bottom shows pO_2 in torr.

each reduction of CBF. Epi pO_2 changed more slowly or declined transiently and recovered, suggesting compensatory autoregulation or the opening of superficial interarterial anastomosis.

The overall relationship of changes in regional pO_2 to changes in CBF is illustrated in Figure 1. The differences between animals were normalized by converting to percentage change. The rate of decline of endo pO_2 was considerably steeper than that of epi. When blood flow had diminished about 50%, endo pO_2 was reduced 70%, but epi pO_2 was reduced only 20%.

The reserve was estimated in endo and epi by determination of changes in resting flow, reactive hyperemia, and regional pO_2 during progressive stenosis. The reactive hyperemia response began to diminish before there was any change in resting flow or pO_2. Further stenosis affected resting flow, endo pO_2, and epi pO_2 in that order. Endo reserve was exhausted when resting flow was reduced by 10% and reactive hyperemia by more than 80%; a further decline in resting CBF caused a diminution in resting endo pO_2. Epi reserve was exhausted when resting flow was reduced approximately 50% and reactive hyperemia almost abolished; further reductions in CBF eliminated reactive hyperemia and caused reductions in pO_2 of both regions.

The sign of ischemia in the local or surface ECG is ST-segment elevation. In each region there was a good correlation between the changes in the local ECG

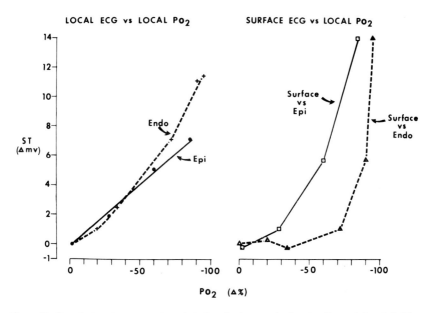

Figure 2. Correlation between stenosis-induced changes in local pO_2 and local (left) or surface (right) ST-segment elevation. Epi = ——; Endo = – – –.

and the changes in the local pO_2 (Figure 2—left). The first region to show ST-segment elevation was endo at a reduction of CBF of 30%; epi ECG changes occurred when CBF was reduced 70%. These changes are associated with a 40% decrease in pO_2 of each region. Surface ECG changes appeared at approximately the same point as epi changes. Comparison of changes in the surface ECG with the local pO_2 (Figure 2—right) shows some correlation with epi pO_2 but not with endo pO_2. These data indicate that the ST-segment changes in the surface ECG are not a good index of endocardial ischemia.

Partial release of the stenosis to permit blood flow to return to the control level caused an immediate return of surface ST segment to control; epi ST segment decreased toward control, but endo ST segment remained elevated. This correlates well with the oxygen tension because there was only a slight rise in the endo pO_2 but a marked increase in the epi. Total release led to reactive hyperemia after which the ST segments returned to control level in all regions.

DISCUSSION

The endo of the left ventricle is exceedingly vulnerable to any decrease in coronary blood flow. The reserve capacity of the endo to maintain oxygen tension in the face of decline in coronary blood flow is considerably lower than that of epi. This would explain why endo is the more frequent site of infarction.

Surface ECGs are not adequate indicators of regional ischemia based upon ST-segment elevation, even though local ECG in endo and epi may correlate with local changes in pO_2. The endo pO_2 is diminished by 90% before there is a significant change in the surface ECG. Therefore, the use of the surface ECG for the study of the severity and size of myocardial infarcts is questioned.

Mailing address:
Martin M. Winbury, Ph.D.,
Warner-Lambert Research Institute,
Morris Plains, New Jersey 07950 (USA).

Recent Advances in Studies on
Cardiac Structure and Metabolism, Volume 12
Cardiac Adaptation
Edited by T. Kobayashi, Y. Ito, and G. Rona
Copyright 1978 University Park Press Baltimore

LOCAL PULSATILE INTRAMYOCARDIAL PRESSURE (IMP) AS A VECTOR FORCE: SIMULTANEOUS MEASUREMENTS OF IMP AND TISSUE OXYGEN AVAILABILITY

T. KOYAMA, T. SASAJIMA, T. YAGI,
Y. KAKIUCHI, and T. ARAI

Laboratory of Physiology, Research Institute of Applied Electricity
Hokkaido University, Sapporo, Japan

SUMMARY

A directional nonuniformity of the intramyocardial pressure (IMP) was observed in anesthetized open-chest dogs using a piezoelectric pressure sensor implanted in the left ventricular myocardium. The nonuniformity seemed to be attributable to the variation in myocardial fiber orientation. The IMP, which developed in a direction parallel to the base-apex line, was measured in the deep portion of the myocardium, simultaneously with local O_2 availability. In some cases, IMP decreased quickly as soon as a decrement in O_2 availability had proceeded only slightly as a result of ligation of the anterior descending artery (LAD). In other cases, the once decreased IMP recovered gradually even when O_2 availability remained lowered by continuation of the ligation. These observations indicated that IMP had no direct dependency on O_2 availability in the case of acute LAD.

INTRODUCTION

The present study was initiated to investigate the effects of coronary occlusion on the local pulsatile intramyocardial pressure (IMP) in the deep portion of the left ventricular myocardium. To undertake this study successfully, it seemed necessary to first clarify the features of IMP as a vector force, because left ventricular myocardium consists of muscle layers running in various directions and probably develops its characteristic hoop tension by each contraction in a specified direction. Therefore, a small pressure sensor was constructed, using piezoelectric ceramics, that showed a clear anisotropic sensitivity. Such a pressure sensor seemed suitable for the determination of the orientation of local IMP. The sensor was applied to the measurements of the effects of ligation of the coronary anterior descending artery (LAD) on IMP in the deep portion of the ventricular myocardium.

MATERIALS AND METHODS

A thin rectangular bar (2.0 × 1.0 × 0.4 mm in length, width, and thickness, respectively) of piezoelectric ceramics with an electrical conductive coating on the upper and lower surfaces as electrodes for signal sampling was attached to a thin, flexible, polyvinyl tube and coated with resin for electrical insulation. This pressure sensor yielded a positive signal in response to a stress acting parallel to the direction of poling, which is preferable to the 3-axis (voltage output coefficient for this direction, $g_{33} = 3.81 \times 10^{-3}$ V·m/N). The lateral surfaces of this sensor, which are normal to 1-axis, yielded a negative signal in response to a stress acting on the 1-axis because of the negative coefficient ($g_{31} = -15.1 \times 10^{-3}$ V·m/N). If two kinds of stress, P_1 on the 3-axis and P_2 on the 1-axis, act on the sensor, the output signal is the summation of the positive and negative signals, respectively. The voltage amplitude V_1 of output signal is given by the following equation:

$$V_1 = (g_{33} \cdot P_1 + g_{31} \cdot P_2) \cdot d \tag{1}$$

where d is the thickness of the sensor.

When the sensor is rotated by 90 degrees, P_1 and P_2 act on the 1- and 3-axes, respectively. Then the voltage amplitude V_2 is given by the following equation:

$$V_2 = (g_{33} \cdot P_2 + g_{31} \cdot P_1) \cdot d \tag{2}$$

When V_1 and V_2 are measured, P_1 and P_2 can be obtained by simultaneously solving equations (1) and (2).

In the animal experiments using anesthetized dogs, the 3-axis of the sensor was alternately positioned approximately parallel to (but slightly deviated from) and nearly perpendicular to the base-apex line of the ventricle, as indicated by the arrows in the schematic illustration of the heart (Figure 1), so as to detect longitudinal and circumferential IMPs, respectively. The output signals obtained in these positions were denoted as V∥ and V⊥, respectively. Such a positioning was combined with the different depths of insertion of the sensor; the center of the sensitive surface was located 8 mm (V∥ deep and V⊥ deep) or 4 mm (V∥ middle and V⊥ middle) from the epicardial surface of the whole myocardial thickness of 10 mm. Thus, the signal for IMP calculation was obtained at four placements of the sensitive surfaces in each serial measurement for the study of the anisotropic aspects of IMP.

For the simultaneous measurements of IMP ∥ deep and local O_2 availability (abbreviated as O_2), an insulated Pt-wire 50 μm in diameter was attached to the pressure sensor. The tip of the Pt-wire protruded beyond the tip of the sensor by 0.5 mm. O_2 was expressed with O_2 current in the figures. V// deep was assumed to express IMP// deep.

RESULTS

A set of serial recordings obtained by a sensor placed in the myocardium is shown in Figure 1, in which the curves from top to bottom represent ECG, aortic blood pressure, and output signal Vs from the sensor. Each output signal shows a different amplitude and characteristic contour, specific for positioning of the sensor. IMPs were calculated using the peak amplitudes of Vs according to equations (1) and (2). On an average of seven serial measurements, IMP// deep was 121.0 ± 16.6 mm Hg, which was almost the same as the systolic aortic pressure and which highly exceeded IMP⊥ deep (6.4 ± 2.3 mm Hg). IMP⊥ middle and IMP// middle were 97.8 ± 13.9 and 72.6 ± 10.2 mm Hg, respectively.

Figure 2 shows recordings obtained in a dog whose ventricular wall was poor in collateral anastomoses from the coronary circumferential artery. IMP// deep decreased rapidly following LAD, although local O_2 was still high and remained suppressed during the continuation of LAD. Figure 3 shows another set of recordings obtained in canine ventricle in which collateral anastomoses were

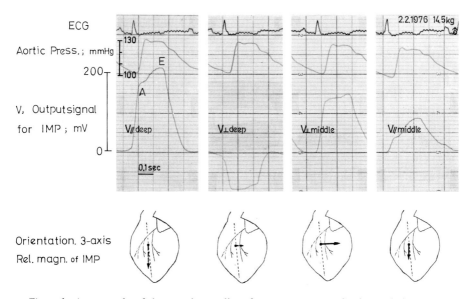

Figure 1. An example of the actual recordings for measurements of anisotropic intramyocardial pressure. The curves from top to bottom represent ECG, abdominal aortic pressure, and output signals, voltage amplitudes (V). Vs were recorded at four placements of the pressure sensor. The dotted and straight arrows in the schematically illustrated heart show directional positions of the 3-axis of the sensor.

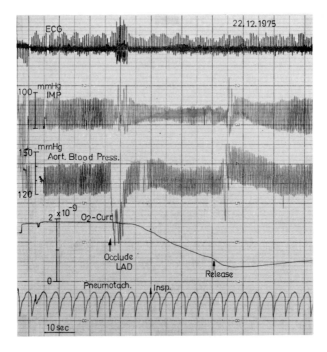

Figure 2. Simultaneous recordings of intramyocardial pressure (IMP) and local O$_2$ availability in the deep portion of myocardium after an acute ligation of the left anterior descending branch (LAD) of the coronary artery. Note the quick decline of IMP.

visible and local O$_2$ fell only partially. The arrows in Figure 3a indicate the location corresponding to each section in Figure 3b that was made by a low speed reproduction of the signals once stored in a data recorder. The IMP contour for one cardiac cycle, shown in Figure 3b, did not decrease uniformly after LAD, and the slow rise of the ejection phase of IMP was much affected; it disappeared quickly and was replaced by a transient fall, while the sharp rise to point A from the onset of systole remained less affected. Then IMP of the ejection phase recovered gradually, although the local O$_2$ remained lowered.

DISCUSSION

The present results indicate a directional nonuniformity of IMP, which is probably caused by the variation in myocardial fiber orientation. The ventricular shortening differs regionally according to myocardial fiber orientation (LeWinter *et al.*, 1975). The contractile forces observed using strain gauge arch are different when the directional position of the arch is altered (Sonnenblick and Kirk, 1971–72; Robie and Newman, 1974). The present results seem to coincide with

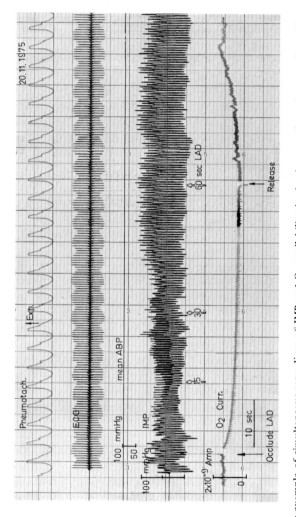

Figure 3a. Another example of simultaneous recordings of IMP and O_2 availability in the deep portion of myocardium. Note the recovery of IMP, while the O_2 level remained lowered. The open arrows indicate the location corresponding to each section of Figure 3b.

241

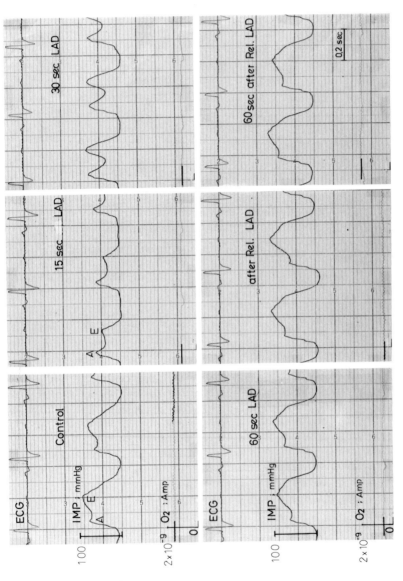

Figure 3b. Slow reproduction of the IMP curve of Figure 3a, showing the effects of ligation of the left anterior descending artery (LAD) on the IMP contour.

these investigations. Since IMP⊥ deep was small, it can be expected that the IMP deep developed mainly in the direction parallel to the base-apex line and that the signal V∥ deep directly represented IMP∥ deep.

The nonuniform changes in IMP contour seen in Figure 3b may indicate that the oxygen necessary for the initial rise of IMP can be recruited during diastole, but the amount of O_2 was insufficient for establishment of IMP of the ejection phase. The gradual recovery of IMP of the ejection phase, which occurred despite the lowered O_2 level, was probably made possible by the blood and O_2 supply through collateral anastomoses and by a new balance being introduced between IMP and the lowered O_2 level. But such a speculation seems unsatisfactory, because the rapid decline in IMP seen in Figure 2, which did not keep pace with changes in O_2, suggests that the IMP had no direct dependency on tissue O_2 in the case of acute LAD. Satisfactory explanation of IMP changes seen in Figures 2 and 3 remains for future study.

REFERENCES

LeWINTER, M. M., KENT, R. S., KROENER, J. M., CAREW, T. E., and COVELL, J. W. 1975. Regional differences in myocardial performance in the left ventricle of the dog. Circ. Res. 37:191–199.

ROBIE, N. W., and NEWMAN, W. H. 1974. Effects of altered ventricular load on the walton-brodie strain gauge arch. J. Appl. Physiol. 36:20–27.

SONNENBLICK, E. H., and KIRK, E. S. 1971–72. Effects of hypoxia and ischemia on myocardial contraction. Cardiology 56:302–313.

Mailing address:
Dr. T. Koyama,
Laboratory of Physiology, Research Institute of Applied Electricity,
Hokkaido University, Sapporo (Japan).

Recent Advances in Studies on
Cardiac Structure and Metabolism, Volume 12
Cardiac Adaptation
Edited by T. Kobayashi, Y. Ito, and G. Rona
Copyright 1978 University Park Press Baltimore

ABNORMAL MYOCARDIAL FLUID RETENTION
AS AN EARLY MANIFESTATION
OF ISCHEMIC INJURY

A. MUKHERJEE, L. M. BUJA, F. E. SCALES,
G. C. FINK, G. H. TEMPLETON, M. R. PLATT,
and J. T. WILLERSON

The Ischemic SCOR Research Unit, The University
of Texas, Southwestern Medical School, Dallas, Texas, USA

SUMMARY

Fifty-seven isolated, blood-perfused, continuously weighed canine hearts were utilized to study the development of abnormal myocardial fluid retention during early myocardial ischemic injury. Inflatable balloon catheters were positioned around the left anterior descending artery (LAD) or the proximal left circumflex coronary artery for coronary occlusion for periods of: 1) 10 min followed by 20 min of reflow, 2) 40 min followed by either no reflow or by 20 min of reflow, and 3) a fixed 60-min occlusion without reflow. Following 60 min of proximal LAD occlusion, histological and ultrastructural examination revealed mild swelling of many cardiac muscle cells in the absence of either interstitial edema or weight gain. After 40 min of coronary occlusion and 20 min of reflow, significant weight gain occurred, and interstitial edema, focal vascular congestion and hemorrhage, and swelling of cardiac muscle cells were noted in histological study. The development of abnormal myocardial fluid retention after 40 min of LAD occlusion occurred in association with a significant reduction in sodium-potassium ATPase activity in the ischemic region, but no significant alteration in either creatine phosphokinase on citrate synthase activity occurred. Thus, the data indicate that impaired cell volume regulation and interstitial fluid accumulation are early manifestations of ischemic injury with reflow, and that cell swelling without interstitial edema is an early manifestation of ischemic injury without reflow. The etiological importance of the reduction in sodium potassium ATPase activity with regard to its relationship to cell swelling remains to be determined.

INTRODUCTION

The temporal relationship among myocardial ischemia, alterations in myocardial sodium-potassium ATPase activity, and the development of abnormal myo-

This work was supported by NIH contract 72-2947, NIH grant HL-15522, NIH Ischemic Heart Disease Specialized Center of Research (SCOR) Grant HL-17669, and by the Harry S. Moss Heart Fund.

cardial fluid retention has not been elucidated. Accordingly, the present study was designed: 1) to explore the temporal relationship between the duration of acute myocardial ischemia and the development of abnormal myocardial fluid retention, and 2) to determine whether or not alterations in sodium potassium ATPase activity are present in isolated, blood-perfused canine hearts at the time that abnormal myocardial fluid retention develops.

MATERIALS AND METHODS

Two dogs were anesthetized simultaneously. One dog ("support animal") had cannulae inserted in both femoral veins and in one femoral artery. The heart from the other dog ("donor animal") was exposed, and the arterial catheter from the support dog was connected to the proximal aortic root of the donor; perfusion was begun as the sutures around the proximal pulmonary artery, superior, and inferior vena cavae were ligated and the remaining stump of the vessels severed. The isolated heart was removed to a cantilever beam that had been especially constructed so that the isolated hearts could be weighed continuously (Figure 1); this weighing device is capable of recognizing changes in weight of the isolated heart of 0.25 g. The perfusion pressure of the isolated heart was set at a constant value by using a Sarns roller pump (Model 6002) to pump to an overflow valve at a vertical height of 100 cm. Once the heart was positioned on the weighing stand, an inflatable balloon occlusive catheter was positioned around the proximal LAD or the circumflex coronary artery; when inflated, this device totally occluded the coronary artery. A "mitral button" was placed through the mitral valve orifice to prevent mitral regurgitation. A balloon filled with enough volume to provide a left ventricular end-diastolic pressure of 4–5 mm Hg was fastened to the mitral button. A drainage catheter was inserted into the apical dimple of the LV and allowed to drain any coronary blood flow that collected in the LV; this blood and that collected by catheter from the right ventricle (coronary venous drainage) were returned to the support dog. Thus, when all lines were appropriately connected, the isolated heart–support dog perfusion was a closed system.

Heart rate was kept constant by ventricular pacing. Total coronary blood flow was measured as the difference between blood pumped from the support dog and overflow from the vertical tubing (Figure 1).

Control hearts and hearts from various experimental groups either were processed for morphological examination or were used for various biochemical assays. In the hearts designated for morphological study, an intracoronary catheter was inserted for perfusion fixation with 1% glutaraldehyde in 0.1 M phosphate buffer. Following perfusion, the hearts were divided into multiple transverse slices, and large tissue blocks were obtained from the ischemic and nonischemic LV for histological and electron microscopic examination.

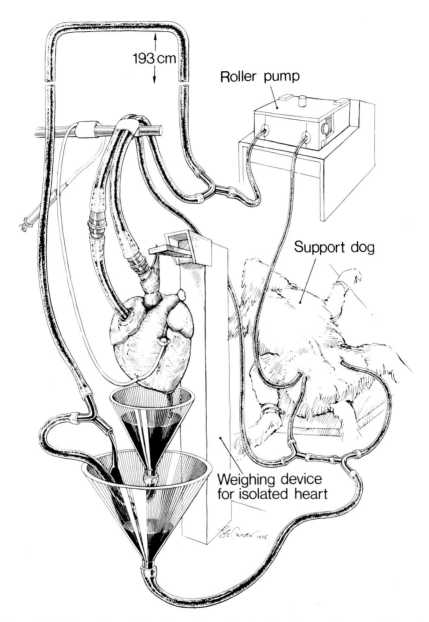

Figure 1. The figure demonstrates the cantilever beam utilized for continuous weighing of the isolated, blood-perfused, canine hearts and the isolated heart–support dog experimental model.

In 15 isolated hearts, in two hearts obtained from the support animals, and in three additional hearts obtained from normal, unoperated control dogs, myocardial sodium potassium ATPase activity was measured utilizing previously described methods (Matsui and Schwartz, 1968; Schwartz *et al.*, 1971). Both direct measurements of sodium potassium ATPase and, in six hearts, measurements of ouabain binding were obtained. Inorganic phosphate analysis was performed using the methods of Ames and Dubin (1960), and protein concentration was determined by the method of Lowry *et al.* (1951).

In six of these hearts, creatine kinase activity was measured, and in four hearts, citrate synthase activity also was measured (Srere, Brazil, and Gonen, 1963; Rosalki, 1967).

RESULTS

The paced heart rates for the isolated hearts were 85 ± 2.37 (S.E.) beats/min; the mean arterial perfusion pressure was 77 ± 1.07 mm Hg. Coronary blood flows were 95 ± 7.8 ml/min 100 g of LV precoronary occlusion, 51 ± 4.78 ml/min/ 100 g LV at the end of coronary occlusion, and 74 ± 6.35 ml/min/100 g LV after 20 min of reflow.

In the hearts with 10-min occlusions of the proximal LAD and reflow, there was no significant gain in weight.

Sixty-Minute, Permanent LAD Occlusion

There was no significant weight gain either during the initial 40-min period of occlusion or during the last 20 min of the occlusion.

Histological and ultrastructural study of nonischemic and ischemic myocardium demonstrated that 60 min of fixed LAD occlusion was associated with the development of cell swelling; in addition, a few cells contained mitochondria that also demonstrated electron dense inclusions indicative of advanced, irreversible injury. Swollen muscle cells had ultrastructurally intact plasma membranes. Interstitial edema was not noted in these hearts.

Forty-Minute LAD Occlusion with Reflow

There was no significant gain in weight during the 40-min occlusion. However, with reflow, significant weight gain occurred after 10 min ($7 \pm 2.6\%$, 1.25 ± 0.55 g, $p < 0.05$) and after 20 min ($14 \pm 0.9\%$, 2.6 ± 0.78 g, $p < 0.01$), as compared to weight noted after 1 min of reflow. Ten minutes of reflow resulted in coronary blood flow decreasing to $82 \pm 4\%$, $p < 0.01$; by 20 min of reflow, coronary blood flow had fallen to $73 \pm 7.0\%$. $p < 0.01$, of the value obtained after 1 min of reflow. The weight gained by the isolated hearts with reflow at a time when coronary blood flow was decreasing demonstrates that the weight

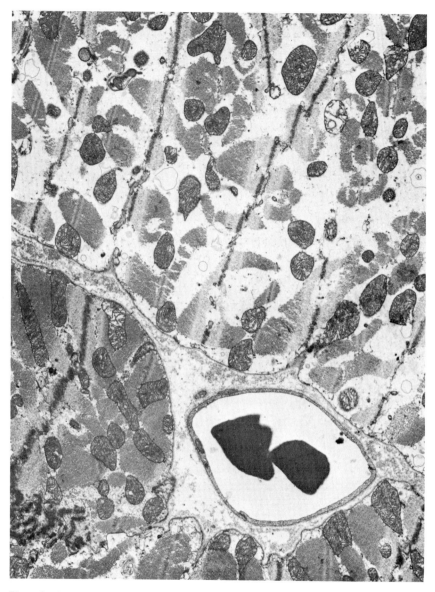

Figure 2. Area of moderate structural damage in ischemic left ventricular myocardium of isolated heart following 40-min temporary coronary occlusion and 20-min reflow. One muscle cell shows glycogen depletion and prominent edematous swelling, indicated by separation of organelles; some mitochondria are swollen, and myofibrils and plasma membrane are intact. The interstitial space is widened and contains percipitated edema fluid. The capillary is patent and exhibits normal endothelium. × 5,000.

gain was not simply the result of an increase in coronary blood volume as part of the hyperemic response.

Microscopic studies confirmed that the weight gain in these hearts did indeed represent abnormal myocardial fluid retention in the ischemic region. Histologically, ischemic myocardium from the hearts with 40-min LAD occlusion and reflow (and also from the three hearts with proximal circumflex occlusion and reflow) exhibited marked interstitial edema, focal vascular congestion and hemorrhage, and multiple foci of damaged muscle cells (Figure 2). The interstitial and intracellular alterations were more extensive in the subendocardial than in the subepicardial region. Some muscle cells showed prominent cell swelling and glycogen depletion but were otherwise structurally normal. Others exhibited edema, vacuolar dilatation of sarcoplasmic reticulum and T tubules, accumulation of lipid droplets, mitochondrial damage with swelling or stacking of cristae, and formation of subsarcolemmal blebs. Some muscle cells also had focal defects in the plasma membranes (Figure 3).

Measurement of sodium-potassium ATPase activity in ischemic and nonischemic regions of the LV in nine hearts demonstrated a value of 9.5 ± 0.52 in the subendocardial portion of the ischemic area as compared to 12.7 ± 0.35 μmol of Pi/hr/mg of protein at 37°C in the subendocardial portion of the nonischemic LV ($p < 0.01$). In ischemic epicardium, sodium-potassium ATPase activity was 10.3 ± 0.43 as compared to 12.5 ± 0.60 μmol of Pi/hr/mg of protein at 37°C in nonischemic epicardium ($p < 0.01$). In addition, in the six hearts that were tested, ouabain uptake also was decreased significantly in the subendocardial and subepicardial portions of the ischemic area of the LV. There was no significant depression of either creatine kinase or citrate synthase activity in the same areas in the six hearts. In the control hearts there was no significant difference in sodium-potassium ATPase activity in the anterior and posterior LV regions.

DISCUSSION

The data demonstrate that the potential for abnormal myocardial fluid retention occurs within 40 min after proximal LAD or left circumflex coronary occlusion and that abnormal myocardial fluid retention can be demonstrated by reflow and recognized as significant weight gain in the isolated heart. The morphological studies demonstrate that abnormal myocardial fluid retention following temporary coronary occlusion and reflow was caused by intracellular and interstitial edema and focal vascular congestion and hemorrhage. The fluid accumulation probably was mediated, at least in part, by functional abnormalities in vascular permeability unmasked by reperfusion. The mild swelling of muscle cells following 60 min of permanent LAD occlusion was not associated with interstitial edema and appeared to represent an abnormal redistribution of fluid

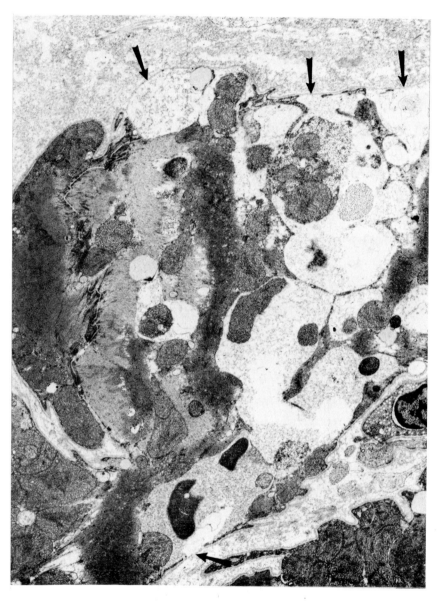

Figure 3. Area of severe structural damage in ischemic left ventricular myocardium of isolated heart following 40-min temporary coronary occlusion and 20-min reflow. The widened interstitial space contains abundant edema fluid. The muscle cells exhibit vacuolated and edematous cytoplasm, myofibrillar disruption with contraction bands, and extensive disruption of the plasma membrane (arrows). × 8,500.

in the absence of an overall cardiac weight gain. Only a minority of the muscle cells showed changes indicative of irreversible injury following either permanent or temporary coronary occlusion.

In our model the abnormal myocardium fluid retention occurred in association with a reduction in sodium-potassium ATPase activity in both the subendocardial and subepicardial regions of the ischemic area, thereby suggesting a potential functional defect in cell membrane integrity occurring within 40 min of proximal LAD occlusion. Whether this small reduction in sodium-potassium ATPase activity is a major reason for the development of cell swelling is presently uncertain; in fact, defects in plasma membrane integrity could be demonstrated in hearts subjected to 40 min of coronary occlusion and reflow, but similar structural alterations in cell membrane integrity were not apparent with 60-min fixed coronary occlusion. While the average reduction in ischemic region sodium-potassium ATPase activity appeared small, the significance of the abnormality would increase if future studies demonstrate that some ischemic region swollen cells have marked reductions while nonswollen cells retain almost normal sodium-potassium ATPase activity. Time and additional studies will be needed to further evaluate this possibility.

REFERENCES

AMES, B. N., and DUBIN, D. T. 1960. The role of polyamines in the neutralization of bacteriophage deoxyribonucleic acid. J. Biol. Chem. 225:769–775.

LOWRY, O. H., ROSENBROUGH, N. J., FARR, A. C., and RANDALL, R. J. 1951. Protein measurement with the Folin phenol reagents. J. Biol. Chem. 193:265–275.

MATSUI, H., and SCHWARTZ, A. 1968. Mechanism of cardiac glycoside inhibition of the [Na$^+$,K$^+$] dependent ATPase from cardiac tissue. Biochem. Biophys. Acta 151:655–663.

ROSALKI, S. B. 1967. Improved procedure for serum creatine phosphokinase determination. J. Lab. Clin. Med. 69:696–705.

SCHWARTZ, A., NAGANO, K., NAKAO, M., LINDENMAYER, C. E., and ALLEN, J. C. 1971. The sodium and potassium activated adenosine triphosphatase system. *In* Methods in Pharmacology. Appleton-Century-Crofts, Educational Division, Meredith Corp., New York. 1:361–388.

SRERE, P. A., BRAZIL, H., and GONEN, L. 1963. The citrate condensing enzyme of pigeon breast muscle and moth flight muscle. Acta Chem. Scand. 17(suppl.):129–134.

Mailing address:
Amal Mukherjee, Ph.D.,
Ischemic Heart Center, L5-134, The University of Texas Health Science Center at Dallas,
5323 Harry Hines Boulevard, Dallas, Texas 75235 (USA).

Recent Advances in Studies on
Cardiac Structure and Metabolism, Volume 12
Cardiac Adaptation
Edited by T. Kobayashi, Y. Ito, and G. Rona
Copyright 1978 University Park Press Baltimore

METABOLIC CONSEQUENCES OF
SEPHADEX-INDUCED REDUCTION OF CORONARY FLOW
IN ISOLATED RAT HEART

H. STAM, J. W. De JONG, and H. L. VAN DER WIEL

Department of Biochemistry I and Thoraxcenter,
Erasmus University, Rotterdam, The Netherlands

SUMMARY

With a polysaccharide microsphere suspension (Sephadex), coronary flow of isolated perfused rat hearts was reduced by approximately 70%. During this Sephadex-induced ischemia, the energy charge and creatine phosphate content of the myocardial tissue dropped significantly, while total nucleoside and lactate release from the heart increased. During hypoxia (30% O_2), changes in high-energy phosphate content and lactate and nucleoside release were similar to the changes induced by ischemia. During hypoxia, coronary flow rate was increased by 47%. Thus, Sephadex-induced reduction of coronary flow could be a useful model in studies of metabolic changes during ischemia.

INTRODUCTION

In the past, several methods were used to impair coronary flow in isolated heart preparations (Bester, Bajusz, and Lochner, 1972; Neely *et al.*, 1973; Hough and Gevers, 1975; Lai and Scheuer, 1975) and *in vivo* (Degenring, Rubio, and Berne, 1975) in order to create an ischemic state. Investigations were carried out concerning the metabolic and hemodynamic consequences of this ischemia.

The reduced coronary flow during ischemia impairs oxygen and energy substrate supply and prevents an adequate removal of catabolites. During hypoxia, as well as during ischemia, high-energy phosphates are depleted (Olson, Dhalla, and Sun, 1971/72), ATP catabolites (adenosine, inosine, and hypoxanthine) are released from the heart, and the enhanced anaerobic glycolytic flux is reflected in a higher lactate production and release (Rovetto, Whitmer, and Neely, 1973).

In the study presented here, whole heart ischemia in nonworking, retrogradely perfused rat hearts was induced by injecting Sephadex G-25 micro-

This work was supported by the Dutch Heart Foundation.

spheres into the coronary arteries. The alteration in tissue levels of high-energy phosphates and nucleoside and lactate release during Sephadex-induced ischemia were compared with results from hypoxic hearts.

METHODS AND MATERIALS

Rat hearts were perfused according to De Jong (1972) at a perfusion pressure of 100 cm H_2O. Hypoxia was induced by substituting O_2 (partially) with N_2. Ischemia was introduced by injecting 0.7-mg Sephadex G-25 microspheres (20–80 μm) into the cannula. Ischemia and hypoxia were introduced after a 30-min control perfusion. Effluent was collected, and at the end of the experiment the hearts were freeze-clamped. Creatine phosphate, ATP, ADP, and AMP were determined according to Lamprecht et al. (1970), lactate according to Apstein, Puchner, and Brachfeld (1970), and adenosine, inosine, and hypoxanthine according to Olsson (1970). Protein was determined by the biuret method. Results are given in mean values ± S.E.M. Significance was calculated with Student's t-test; $p > 0.05$ was considered to be not significant.

RESULTS AND DISCUSSION

As Figure 1 indicates, the effects of hypoxia (30% O_2) and ischemia on the coronary flow of isolated, perfused rat hearts are inverse. Injection of the microspheres into the coronary system caused a rapid reduction of the flow from 53.0 ± 2.8 to 17.0 ± 1.8 ml·min^{-1}·g of myocardial protein^{-1} ($p < 0.001, n = 8$), while during hypoxia the flow rate increased to 78.2 ± 7.9 ml·min^{-1}·g of myocardial protein^{-1} ($p < 0.001, n = 8$). The metabolic effects of the impaired coronary flow are drastic.

Because of the lower oxygen supply, the glycolytic flux is enhanced, resulting in a high rate of lactate production and release. As Figure 2 illustrates, lactate release increased from 1.82 ± 0.24 to 13.07 ± 0.91 μmol·min^{-1}·g of myocardial protein^{-1} ($p < 0.001, n = 8$) after the first 10-min period of ischemia. The lactate release after the same period of hypoxia (16.44 ± 1.30 μmol·min^{-1}·g of myocardial protein^{-1}) is significantly higher compared to the control ($p < 0.001, n = 6$) as well as to the ischemic values ($p < 0.05, n = 8$). This significant difference shows the improved catabolite removal under conditions of increased coronary flow occurring during hypoxia.

The impaired energy metabolism after 10 min of ischemia is responsible for the rapid decline of the creatine phosphate and ATP levels of the myocardial tissue, as is illustrated in Figure 3a. Creatine phosphate breakdown is faster than ATP breakdown, but they are in the same order of magnitude for hypoxia (30% O_2) and ischemia. The decrease in tissue levels of ATP is accompanied by a rise of ADP and AMP levels (Figure 3b). The low energetic state of ischemic and

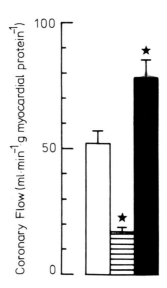

Figure 1. Coronary flow in isolated, perfused rat hearts during control (□), Sephadex-induced ischemia (⊟), and hypoxia (30% O) (■). (X + SEM, *n* = 8.) * = *p* 0.001 for comparison with control.

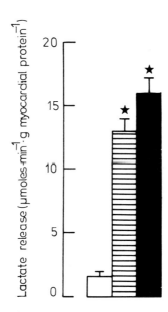

Figure 2. Lactate release during control (□), ischemia (⊟), and hypoxia (■). (*n* = 6–8, * = *p* < 0.001.)

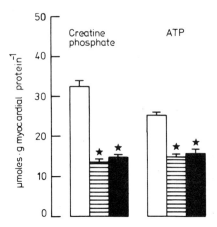

Figure 3a. Myocardial tissue levels of creatine phosphate and ATP during control (□), ischemia (⊟), and hypoxia (■). ($n = 4$, * = $p < 0.01$.)

hypoxic tissue is demonstrated by the drop of the energy charge ([ATP] + ½[ADP])/([ATP] + [ADP] + [AMP]). During ischemia, energy charge fell from 0.87 ± 0.01 to 0.77 ± 0.01 ($p < 0.005$, $n = 4$), and to 0.75 ± 0.02 ($p < 0.005$, $n = 4$) during hypoxia.

The ATP breakdown is not only reflected in the higher ADP and AMP tissue levels, but also in the release of AMP breakdown products, adenosine, inosine, and hypoxanthine from the heart (Berne and Rubio, 1974). In Figure 4 the release of these purine nucleosides during control and after 10 min of ischemia or hypoxia (30% O_2) is shown. As can be seen, no adenosine is released from the

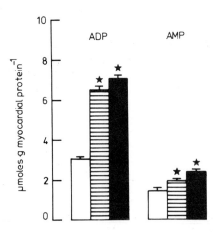

Figure 3b. Myocardial tissue levels of ADP and AMP during control (□), ischemia (⊟), and hypoxia (■). ($n = 4$, * = $p < 0.01$.)

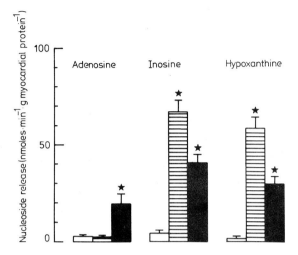

Figure 4. Nucleoside release from perfused rat hearts during control ($\square$), ischemia ($\boxminus$), and hypoxia ($\blacksquare$). ($n = 4$, * = $p < 0.001$.)

hearts after this period of ischemia, although high intramyocardial concentrations could be detected then (1.21 ± 0.23 μmol·g of myocardial protein). After 20 min of ischemia, however, large amounts of adenosine were released (35.26 ± 2.61 nmol·min^{-1}·g of myocardial protein^{-1}). The lack of adenosine release during the first period of ischemia is probably attributable to high adenosine deaminase activity in rat heart (De Jong, 1972) in combination with the severe reduction of flow. No adenosine deaminase activity was found in the effluents during ischemia. When adenosine production further increases, even the high rate of deamination is insufficient and adenosine appears in the effluent. An immediate release of purine nucleosides after the onset of hypoxia (30% O_2) could be seen, which approached a constant level after 20 min. The clear correlation between adenosine release and coronary flow rate ($r = 0.94, p < 0.001$) during different degrees of oxygenation (0, 30, 60, and 95% O_2) illustrates the vasoactive properties of this compound (Berne and Rubio, 1974). Nucleoside release is in the same order of magnitude during hypoxia and ischemia.

Comparing the consequences of hypoxia and Sephadex-induced ischemia in isolated, perfused rat hearts, it can be concluded that metabolic changes induced by hypoxia (30% O_2) and ischemia are in the same order of magnitude for creatine phosphate and adenine nucleotides, and for the release of lactate, inosine, and hypoxanthine. Hypoxia-induced release of adenosine is absent during the first period of ischemia.

The Sephadex-induced reduction of coronary flow is a new model for ischemia and may be used to create the combination of decreased oxygen supply and impaired coronary flow, as is observed in ischemic heart disease.

REFERENCES

APSTEIN, C. S., PUCHNER, E., and BRACHFELD, N., 1970. Improved automatic lactate determination, Anal. Biochem. 38:20–34.

BERNE, R. M., and RUBIO, R. 1974. Adenine nucleotide metabolism in the heart. Circ. Res. 34 and 35(suppl. 3):109–120.

BESTER, A. J., BAJUSZ, E., and LOCHNER, A. 1972. Effect of ischaemia and infarction on the metabolism and function of the isolated, perfused rat heart. Cardiovasc. Res. 6:284–294.

DEGENRING, F. H., RUBIO, R., and BERNE, R. M. 1975. Adenine nucleotide metabolism during cardiac hypertrophy and ischemia in rats. J. Mol. Cell. Cardiol. 7:105–113.

De JONG, J. W. 1972. Phosphorylation and deamination by the isolated, perfused rat heart. Biochim. Biophys. Acta 287:252–259.

HOUGH, F. S., and GEVERS, W. 1975. Catecholamine release as mediator of intracellular enzyme activation in ischaemic perfused rat hearts, S. Afr. Med. J. 49:538–543.

LAI, F., and SCHEUER, J. 1975. Early changes in myocardial hypoxia: Relation between mechanical function, pH and intracellular compartment metabolites. J. Mol. Cell. Cardiol. 7:289–303.

LAMPRECHT, W., STEIN, P., HEINZ, F., and WEISSER, H. 1970. In H. U. Bergmeyer (ed.), Methods of Enzymatic Analysis, Verlag Chemie, Weinheim.

NEELY, J. R. ROVETTO, M. J., WHITMER, J. T., and MORGAN, H. E. 1973. Effects of ischemia on function and metabolism of the isolated working rat heart. Am. J. Physiol. 225:651–658.

OLSON, R. E., DHALLA, N. S., and SUN, C. N. 1971/72. Changes in energy stores in the hypoxic heart. Cardiology 56:114–124.

OLSSON, M. D. 1970. Changes in content of purine nucleoside in canine myocardium during coronary occlusion. Circ. Res. 26:301–306.

ROVETTO, M. J., WHITMER, J. T., and NEELY, J. R. 1973. Comparison of the effects of anoxia and whole heart ischemia on carbohydrate utilization in isolated, working rat hearts. Circ. Res. 32:699–711.

Mailing address:
Dr. H. Stam,
Department of Cardiovascular Research, Erasmus University,
P. O. Box 1738, Rotterdam (The Netherlands).

Recent Advances in Studies on
Cardiac Structure and Metabolism, Volume 12
Cardiac Adaptation
Edited by T. Kobayashi, Y. Ito, and G. Rona
Copyright 1978 University Park Press Baltimore

CARDIAC MUSCLE TAURINE:
EFFECTS OF ACUTE LEFT VENTRICULAR ISCHEMIA IN
THE DOG AND ANOXIC PERFUSION OF THE RAT HEART

M. F. CRASS III, W. SONG, and J. B. LOMBARDINI

Departments of Physiology and Pharmacology,
Texas Tech University School of Medicine,
Lubbock, Texas, USA

SUMMARY

It has been proposed that taurine, or one of its metabolites, may exert anti-arrhythmic effects in cardiac muscle. The present studies examined the effects of acute left ventricular ischemia in the dog (*in vivo*) and whole heart anoxia in the perfused rat heart (*in vitro*) on the content and distribution of taurine. In control dogs an increasing outer-to-inner gradient in taurine content was observed in the left ventricle. Left circumflex artery ligation for four hours markedly decreased tissue taurine content, the greatest disappearance occurring in the inner zone. Anoxic perfusion resulted in a similar decrease in rat ventricular taurine levels. Recovery of taurine in the heart perfusates indicated that tissue disappearance, secondary to oxygen deficiency, involved leakage into the extracellular fluid rather than metabolic conversion.

INTRODUCTION

Taurine administration has been shown to modify electrocardiographic changes induced by various pharmacological interventions (Read and Welty, 1963; Chazov *et al.*, 1974) and to stabilize membrane potentials (Gruener *et al.*, 1975). It would seem, therefore, that taurine may be functionally involved in maintenance or modification of the cardiac conduction system.

The present studies were designed to examine the response of endogenous taurine levels to alterations in normal cardiac function, specifically, the responses to 1) acute coronary artery occlusion and 2) whole heart anoxia.

MATERIALS AND METHODS

Acute Left Ventricular Ischemia in Dogs

Mongrel dogs of both sexes weighing 15–35 kg were given free access to food and water. The animals were anesthetized with sodium pentobarbital, 30 mg/kg, and ventilated with room air with a positive pressure respirator. A left thorocot-omy was performed, and a length of the circumflex branch of the left coronary artery was dissected free of surrounding tissue. At zero time the vessel was ligated (ischemic) or left patent (control) for a period of 4 hr. Following this interval, transmural punch biopsies were obtained from the posterolateral wall of the left ventricle, and frozen and sectioned into zones representing subepi-cardium, midventricle, and subendocardium (Crass and Sterrett, 1975). The frozen tissue samples were analyzed for taurine content.

Anoxic Perfusion of Isolated Rat Hearts

Male albino Sprague-Dawley rats weighing 250–300 g were given free access to food and water. The hearts were excised and perfused as described previously (Crass and Pieper, 1975). One group of hearts was perfusion-washed in a nonrecirculated system with Krebs-Henseleit bicarbonate buffer containing 5.5 mM glucose for 5 min only. These hearts were freeze-clamped in liquid nitrogen and analyzed for "initial" taurine content. Other groups of hearts were perfused in recirculated fashion for an additional 30 min followed by freeze-clamping and taurine analysis ("residual"). In one group of experiments, the perfusion medium was equilibrated with 95% O_2/5% CO_2 (oxygenated controls). In another group, the perfusate was equilibrated with 95% N_2/5% CO_2 (anoxia). Perfusate samples were obtained at 10-, and 20-, and 30-min intervals during perfusion and analyzed for taurine content.

Estimation of Tissue and Perfusate Taurine

Taurine was determined by enzymatic, double-isotope assay (Lombardini, 1975) and on a Beckman 121 amino acid analyzer.

RESULTS AND DISCUSSION

Regional Taurine Content in Posterolateral Wall of Canine Left Ventricle

In control dogs, an increasing subepicardial to subendocardial gradient was observed (Table 1).

Four hours of left circumflex artery occlusion resulted in an overall 47% decline in taurine within the ischemic zone (Table 1). All regions of the wall lost substantial quantities of taurine. However, the losses were not quantitatively uniform. Disappearance of taurine after the ischemic interval was greatest in the subendocardial region, the loss amounting to approximately 32 μmol/g dry weight. The mode of loss or fate of the taurine that disappeared from the ischemic hearts was not immediately apparent in these studies. For example, was there loss of taurine per se to the extracellular fluid or did taurine undergo metabolic transformation? The latter possibility was unlikely in these acute

Table 1. Transmural distribution of taurine in normal and ischemic canine left ventricle[a]

| | Taurine (μmol/g dry weight)[b] | | |
	Subepicardium	Midventricle	Subendocardium
Control	44.97	53.73	68.00
	±3.76	±3.11	±2.05
Ischemic	25.26	27.74	35.57
	±2.60	±2.55	±4.37

[a]After 4 hr with (Ischemic) or without (Control) left circumflex artery ligation, punch biopsies were performed in the posterolateral wall of the left ventricle. Transmural sections were cut and taurine determined as described in Materials and Methods.
[b]Each value represents the mean of five hearts ± S.E.

studies because of the reportedly slow rate of metabolic conversion (Peck and Awapara, 1967; Huxtable and Bressler, 1972).

Effects of Anoxia in Isolated Perfused Rat Heart

Table 2 shows the effects of whole heart anoxia on rat heart taurine content. It can be seen that 30 min of perfusion under well oxygenated conditions was without effect on tissue taurine content. On the other hand, a similar duration of anoxic perfusion resulted in a significant decrease in the heart taurine level.

Perfusates of both well oxygenated and anoxic hearts were examined for a possible concomitant appearance of taurine (Table 3). A small quantity of

Table 2. Effects of anoxic perfusion on rat heart taurine content[a]

| | Taurine (μmol/g dry weight)[b] | |
	Initial	Residual
95% O_2/5% CO_2	154.4	159.6
	±2.6 (8)	±2.7 (11)
95% N_2/5% CO_2	146.4	132.2
	±3.7 (4)	±3.6 (9)

[a]Hearts were perfused with Krebs-Henseleit bicarbonate buffer containing 5.5 mM glucose for 5 min only (Initial) or for an additional 30 min (Residual) with the indicated gas mixture.
[b]Values are means of the number of hearts shown in parentheses ± S.E.

Table 3. Release of tissue taurine into medium during anoxic perfusion of the isolated rat heart[a]

	Time (min)	Taurine in medium (μmol/g dry weight)
95% O_2/5% CO_2	10	3.88 ± 0.22
	20	4.24 ± 0.32
	30	3.90 ± 0.25
95% N_2/5% CO_2	10	12.98 ± 1.60
	20	16.66 ± 2.95
	30	19.44 ± 2.57

[a]After a 5-min perfusion washout, hearts were perfused with Krebs-Henseleit bicarbonate buffer containing 5.5 mM glucose for an additional 30 min with the indicated gas mixture. Each value represents the mean of six hearts ± S.E.

taurine was detected in oxygenated control hearts after 10 min of perfusion. In this group the total amount of taurine released did not change further throughout the 30 min period. Recovery of taurine in control heart perfusates amounted to less than 3% of the initial tissue values, i.e., within methodological error. Release of taurine was increased three- to four-fold in anoxic hearts after 10 min and continued to increase through 30 min of perfusion. Perfusate taurine recovery in anoxic hearts after 30 min approximated 100% of the observed tissue taurine loss.

Perhaps the principal event in ischemia is a reduction of tissue oxygen tension in the affected myocardium. Release of taurine from the anoxic, but hyperemic, rat heart suggested that a similar mechanism of loss may occur in the acutely ischemic canine left ventricle. The possible functional significance of taurine loss in the oxygen-deficient heart and its potential correlation with ischemia-induced electrocardiographic changes are currently under investigation.

REFERENCES

CHAZOV, E. I., MALCHIKOVA, N. V., LIPINA, N. V., ASAFOV, G. B., and SMIRNOV, V. N. 1974. Taurine and electrical activity of the heart. Circ. Res. 34(suppl. III):11–21.

CRASS, M. F., III, and PIEPER, G. M. 1975. Lipid and glycogen metabolism in the hypoxic heart: Effects of epinephrine. Am. J. Physiol. 229:885–889.

CRASS, M. F., III, and STERRETT, P. R. 1975. Distribution of glycogen and lipids in the ischemic canine left ventricle: Biochemical and light and electron microscopic correlates. *In* P.-E. Roy and G. Rona (eds.), Recent Advances in Studies on Cardiac Structure and Metabolism. Vol. 10: The Metabolism of Contraction, pp. 251–263. University Park Press, Baltimore.

GRUENER, R., MARKOVITZ, D., HUXTABLE, R., and BRESSLER, R. 1975. Excitability modulation by taurine. Transmembrane measurements of neuromuscular transmission. J. Neurol. Sci. 24:351–360.

HUXTABLE, R., and BRESSLER, R. 1972. Taurine and isethionic acid: Distribution and interconversion in the rat. J. Nutr. 102:805–814.

LOMBARDINI, J. B. 1975. An enzymatic derivative double isotope assay for measuring tissue levels of taurine. J. Pharmacol. Exp. Ther. 193:301–308.

PECK, E. J., JR., and AWAPARA, J. 1967. Formation of taurine and isethionic acid in rat brain. Biochim. Biophys. Acta 141:499–506.

READ, W. O., and WELTY, J. D. 1963. Effect of taurine on epinephrine and digoxin induced irregularities of the dog heart. J. Pharmacol. Exp. Ther. 139:283–289.

Mailing address:
M. F. Crass, III, Ph.D.,
Department of Physiology, Texas Tech University School of Medicine,
Lubbock, Texas 79409 (USA).

Recent Advances in Studies on
Cardiac Structure and Metabolism, Volume 12
Cardiac Adaptation
Edited by George Rona and Yoshio Ito
Copyright 1978   University Park Press   Baltimore

CORONARY CIRCULATION, MYOCARDIAL METABOLISM, AND HEMODYNAMICS OF PACING-INDUCED ANGINA

K. TAMURA,[1] N. HIGUMA,[1] S. BANNAI,[1]
R. AOYAGI,[1] T. IZUMI,[1]
M. MATSUOKA,[1] and S. EGUCHI[2]

[1] First Department of Medicine, Niigata University, School of Medicine,
Niigata, Japan
[2] Second Department of Surgery, Niigata University, School of Medicine, 1-Asahimachi,
Niigata City, Niigata, Japan

SUMMARY

The following changes were noted during pacing-induced angina: The coronary sinus blood flow was less than it was during the control period and less than that in the myocardial ischemic group without induced angina. While myocardial oxygen consumption did not increase, myocardial metabolism became anaerobic. The possibility of myocardial dysfunction also was noted.

INTRODUCTION

The pathophysiology of the angina pectoris still is not entirely clear in spite of many contributions to this field. Therefore, the purpose of this study was to determine changes that occur in coronary circulation, myocardial metabolism, and systemic hemodynamics when anginal pain is induced by pacing-stress test in patients with coronary heart disease.

MATERIALS AND METHODS

Twenty-three patients, 18–75 years of age, were examined. Coronary antiography was performed according to the method of Judkins (1968). A coronary sinus thermodilution flow catheter with bipolar pacing electrodes was inserted into the coronary sinus. The coronary sinus pacing-stress test using an external pacemaker with these pacing electrodes was performed following the method proposed by Sowton *et al.* (1967). The coronary sinus blood flow was measured by the continuous local thermodilution method, as previously described (Ganz *et al.,* 1971). Both the arterial and coronary sinus blood samples were withdrawn before and during the stress test for analysis of myocardial oxygen consumption

265

by oxymetry and by the myocardial lactate extraction ratio established by enzymatic determination. The Swan-Ganz flow-directed thermodilution catheter was inserted into the pulmonary artery. By this catheter, the left ventricular filling pressure and the cardiac output were measured during the test. The patients who had at least one of the following criteria were classified as the myocardial ischemic group: 1) definitively abnormal electrocardiogram at rest, with either abnormal ST and T changes or abnormal Q wave, 2) positive response to the maximal exercise treadmill stress test, and 3) definite anatomic changes by the selective coronary angiography. The rest of the patients without the above mentioned criteria were classified as the control group.

RESULTS

Changes in the following groups were compared: 1) the control group (Group 1), 2) the ischemic heart disease group without induced anginal pain (Group IIA), and 3) the ischemic heart disease group with induced anginal pain (Group IIB). Comparisons of heart rate were made at the control period and at either the maximal pacing rate or at angina. Pacing-stress test increased the heart rate significantly in all groups ($p < 0.001$). However, the increase of the heart rate was less in Group IIB than in Group I ($p < 0.05$). The coronary sinus blood flow increased in all groups according to the increase of the heart rate by pacing. The increment of the coronary sinus blood flow by pacing-stress was examined in percentile changes compared to the control period. In the control group, the increment was $62.3 \pm 44.5\%$ (mean $\pm$ 1 S.D.) compared to the control period. In Group IIA, there was no difference in the increment of the flow from that in the control group. However, in Group IIB, the increment of the flow was $29.9 \pm 20.2\%$, and this was significantly lower than Group I ($p < 0.05$). Furthermore, as shown in Figure 1, there was a significant difference between the increase of the coronary sinus flow per increment of heart rate in the control subjects and in the two myocardial ischemic groups ($p < 0.01$). These data indicated that there was a significant increase of the coronary sinus blood flow by using the pacing-stress method in the face of a lower supply of blood to the myocardial ischemic area (Yoshida *et al.*, 1971).

The myocardial oxygen extraction ratio, as shown in Figure 2, calculated from the arteriovenous oxygen content difference divided by the arterial oxygen content, remained the same in each group. However, myocardial oxygen consumption, calculated from the arteriovenous oxygen content difference times the coronary sinus blood flow, increased in Groups I and IIA. In Group IIB, myocardial oxygen consumption remained the same as in controls. This indicated that the myocardial ischemic area consumed less oxygen than the rest of the myocardium.

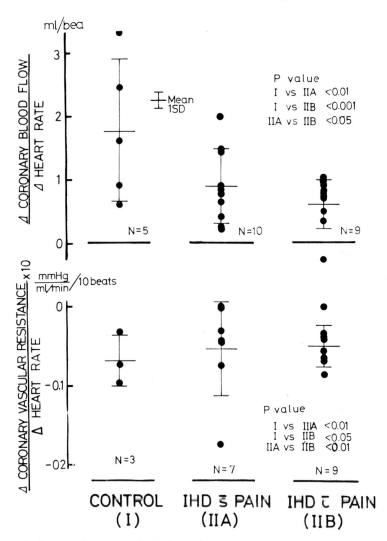

Figure 1. Coronary hemodynamics during pacing-stress.

The changes of myocardial lactate during pacing-stress are shown in Figure 3. The top panel shows that the arterial lactate content remained the same in the three groups. The coronary sinus content of lactate also remained the same in Groups I and IIA. However, in Group IIB, coronary sinus lactate increased significantly ($p < 0.05$). Therefore, the myocardial lactate extraction ratio, calculated from the arteriovenous content of the lactate divided by the arterial

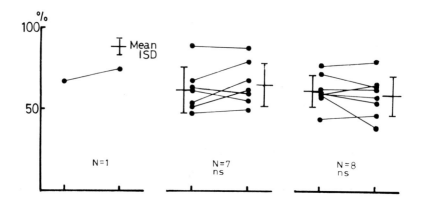

Myocardial Oxygen Consumption

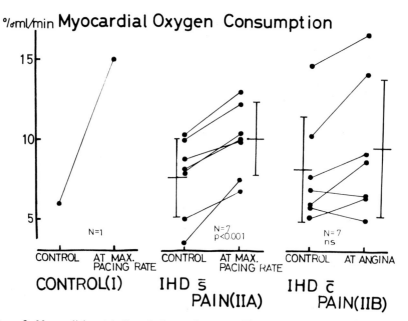

Figure 2. Myocardial metabolism during pacing-stress. The upper panel shows the myocardial oxygen extraction ratio and the lower panel shows myocardial oxygen consumption.

lactate content, decreased in Group IIB compared to Groups I and IIA ($p <$ 0.001), indicating that myocardial metabolism became anaerobic during the period of anginal pain. All patients in Group IIB were proved by coronary angiography to have significant coronary arterial involvement.

The cardiac index increased significantly during the pacing period at angina in Group IIB. The left ventricular filling pressure, however, increased only in one

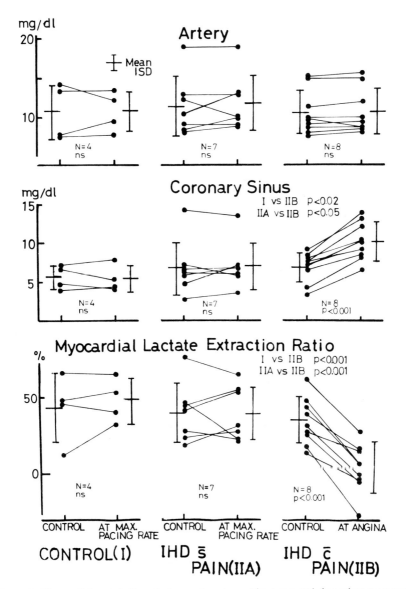

Figure 3. Myocardial metabolism during pacing-stress. The top panel shows lactate content in the arterial blood. The middle panel shows lactate content in coronary sinus, and the bottom panel shows the myocardial lactate extraction ratio.

of three cases. Therefore, this finding might explain the occurrence of the left ventricular dysfunction when anginal pain was induced by pacing-stress. The mean arterial pressure remained the same throughout the entire procedure.

REFERENCES

GANZ, W., TAMURA, K., MARCUS, H. S., DONOSO, R., YOSHIDA, S., and SWAN, H. J. C. 1971. Measurement of the coronary sinus blood flow by continuous local thermodilution in man. Circulation 44:181.
JUDKINS, M. P. 1968. Percutaneous transfemoral selective coronary arteriography. Radiol. Clin. North Am. 6:467.
SOWTON, G. E., BALCON, R., CROSS, D., and FRICK, M. H. 1967. Measurement of the anginal threshold using atrial pacing. Cardiovasc. Res. 1:301.
YOSHIDA, S., GANZ, W., DONOSO, R., MARCUS, H. S., and SWAN, H. J. C. 1971. Coronary hemodynamics during successive elevation of heart rate by pacing subjects with angina pectoris. Circulation 44:1062.

Mailing address:
K. Tamura, M.D.,
First Department of Medicine, Niigata University, School of Medicine,
1-Asahimachi, Niigata City, Niigata 951 (Japan).

Recent Advances in Studies on
Cardiac Structure and Metabolism, Volume 12
Cardiac Adaptation
Edited by T. Kobayashi, Y. Ito, and G. Rona
Copyright 1978 University Park Press Baltimore

ARRHYTHMOGENIC EFFECTS OF ACUTE FREE FATTY ACID MOBILIZATION ON ISCHEMIC HEART

N. YAMAZAKI,[1] Y. SUZUKI,[1] T. KAMIKAWA,[1] K. OGAWA,[2] K. MIZUTANI,[2] N. KAKIZAWA,[2] and M. YAMAMOTO[2]

[1] The Third Department of Internal Medicine, Hamamatsu Medical
University, Hamamatsu, Japan
[2] The Second Department of Internal Medicine, Nagoya University,
School of Medicine, Nagoya, Japan

SUMMARY

The mechanism of action of the acute abnormal rise of plasma free fatty acids (FFA) in the provocation of arrhythmia in ischemic heart was studied by means of electron spin resonance (ESR) spectrometer. A sudden and abnormal rise of plasma FFA caused a significant fall of the respiratory control index (RCI) of the amount of free radical myocardial mitochondria in state 4 respiration.

Based on these findings, a sudden and abnormal rise of plasma FFA seems to further facilitate the uncoupling of oxidative phosphorylation in the myocardial mitochondria of the ischemic portion of the heart. These observations indicate that it may play an important role in the provocation of arrhythmia by high plasma FFA on the ischemic heart.

Nicomol (2,2,6,6,-tetrakis (nicotinoyloxymethyl) cyclohexanol), an inhibitor for the rapid rise of plasma FFA, was effective in the treatment and prevention of arrhythmia in ischemic heart disease and diabetes mellitus.

INTRODUCTION

As a result of recent studies, a rapid and abnormal elevation of plasma free fatty acid (FFA) is considered to be an important provoking factor of arrhythmia in the ischemic heart (Kurien, Yates, and Oliver, 1969; Hoak, Warner, and Conner, 1972), but the mechanism of such provocation is still only poorly understood. In a previous paper (Suzuki, 1975), we reported that the free radical concentration of mitochondria in state 4 respiration is a good indicator to use in the evaluation of the function of the myocardial mitochondria. In the present study, to clarify the mechanism by which high plasma FFA provokes arrhythmia in relation to the function of myocardial mitochondria, the free radical concentration of myocardial mitochondria in state 4 respiration following a sudden rise of plasma FFA was studied by means of electron spin resonance (ESR) spectrometer.

Nicotinic acid is known to inhibit the release of FFA from adipose tissue (Carlson and Orö, 1962). Consequently, nicotinic acid or its analogs might be useful for the prevention or treatment of arrhythmia in ischemic heart disease. Therefore, we also clinically investigated the preventive effect of a nicotinic acid analog (2,2,6,6-tetrakis (nicotinoyloxymethyl) cyclohexanol) on the appearance of arrhythmia.

MATERIALS AND METHODS

Mongrel dogs, weighing 10–15 kg, were anesthetized with pentobarbital sodium (30 mg/kg, I.V.). Sixty minutes after intravenous administration of 50 ml of triglyceride suspension (Intralipid) and 2,000 U of heparin, the heart was removed. The myocardial mitochondria were separated by the method of Chance and Hagihara (1963). Mitochondrial respiration was measured polarographically with a Beckman oxygen analyzer. For the measurement of the concentration of free radical myocardial mitochodria in state 4 respiration, a sample of mitochondria was obtained in state 4, the reaction was stopped by liquid nitrogen as soon as possible, and the measurement was made by ESR spectrometry (JES-ME 3X ESR spectrometer, Japanese Electron Optics Laboratory Co.). ESR intensity was estimated from the maximum deflection of the ESR signals of the sample in comparison to the standard signals of manganese chloride inserted in the same resonance cavity of the ESR spectrometer. The details of this method have been reported previously (Suzuki, 1975).

RESULTS

In the intact canine myocardial mitochondria, after the addition of sodium succinate, an ESR signal was observed; the g value was 2.003. The free radical concentration changed at the different respiratory states of mitochondria; it was markedly increased in state 4 respiration after the addition of sodium succinate and markedly decreased in state 3 respiration after the addition of ADP. In this study, the free radical concentration in state 4 respiration was used as an indicator for the evaluation of the oxidative phosphorylation system of mitochondria (Figure 1.).

In Table 1, the free radical concentration in state 4 respiration of myocardial mitochondria, isolated 60 min after intravenous injection of Intralipid and heparin in normal dogs, was compared to that of normal, control mitochondria. In the high FFA group, the free radical concentration in state 4 respiration averaged 6.2 ± 0.04, indicating a significant decrease in comparison to 7.2 ± 0.05 in the normal control ($p < 0.05$).

In the group with high FFA, the respiratory control index (RCI) of the mitochondria was 2.50 ± 0.25, significantly lower than the normal control 3.72 ± 0.26 ($p < 0.01$) (Table 1).

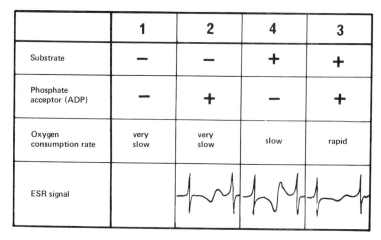

	1	**2**	**4**	**3**
Substrate	−	−	+	+
Phosphate acceptor (ADP)	−	+	−	+
Oxygen consumption rate	very slow	very slow	slow	rapid
ESR signal				

Figure 1. Free radical concentration of myocardial mitochondria at the different respiratory states. The free radical concentration was markedly increased in state 4 respiration after the addition of sodium succinate. In state 3 respiration, addition of ADP had a depressing effect. ESR = electron spin resonance spectrometer.

Figure 2 shows the rise of plasma FFA during intravenous infusion of 1.0 μg/kg/min of noradrenaline in normal dogs and the inhibitory effect of nicotinic acid and its analog (Nicomol; 2,2,6,6-tetrakis (nicotinoyloxymethyl) cyclohexanol). Nicotinic acid and Nicomol significantly inhibited the rise of plasma FFA.

Table 2 shows the clinical data for the antiarrhythmogenic effects of the nicotinic acid analog (Nicomol). Seven males and 10 females (a total of 17 patients) were studied. Review of background disease revealed hypertension in seven patients, ischemic heart disease in 10, and diabetes mellitus in four. In each case, in addition to the same drugs administered up to the time of Nicomol administration, 600–1,200 mg of Nicomol were added to compare the frequency of arrhythmia appearance before and after administration of this drug. As shown

Table 1. Free radical concentration in state 4 respiration and respiratory control index of myocardial mitochondria isolated from control and high plasma FFA canine hearts

Group	Number in experiment	Free radical concentration in state 4 respiration	Respiratory control index
Control	5	0.72 ± 0.05	3.72 ± 0.26
High plasma FFA	5	0.62 ± 0.04	2.50 ± 0.25
		($p < 0.05$)	($p < 0.01$)

Results are the mean ± S.E.M.

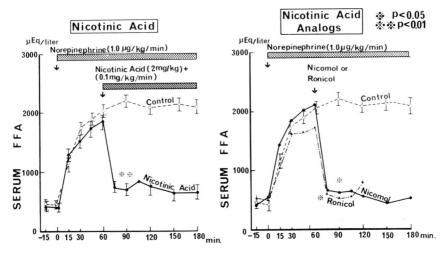

Figure 2. Serum free fatty acid concentrations in anesthetized dog under the influence of norepinephrine and subsequent addition of infusion of nicotinic acid or Nicomol. Norepinephrine infusion (1.0 μg/kg/min) for 3 hr. Nicotinic acid, one dose at 1 hr (2.0 mg/kg), and infusion started at 1 hr (0.1 mg/kg/min). Nicomol, one dose at 1 hr (20 mg/kg).

in Table 2, excellent results, with disappearance of arrhythmia, were seen in seven patients, and good results, with a decrease of arrhythmia, were seen in four, indicating a positive effect in 11 cases (64.7%).

DISCUSSION

It is well known that almost all provoking factors of arrhythmia in ischemic heart disease, such as catecholamine, mental stress, caffeine, smoking, high-fat diet, and exercise, etc., may elevate the level of plasma FFA. It has been shown

Table 2. Antiarrhythmic effect of Nicomol in patients

	Number of patients	Disappearance of arrhythmia	Diminished arrhythmia	No response
Supraventricular tachycardia	4	2	0	2
Atrial fibrillation	3	2	0	1
Atrial flutter	1	1	0	0
Supraventricular extrasystoles	2	1	1	0
Ventricular extrasystoles	6	1	3	2
Ventricular tachycardia	1	0	0	1
Total	17	7	4	6

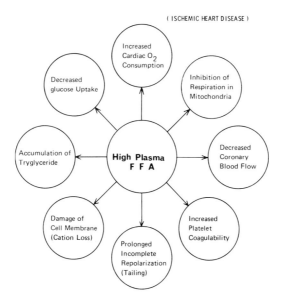

Figure 3. Diagrammatic representation of the mechanism of provocation of arrhythmia by high plasma FFA level in ischemic heart as it is corrently understood.

that high plasma FFA levels may be arrhythmogenic to ischemic heart (Kurien, Yates, and Oliver, 1969), but the mechanism of such arrhythmogenic effect remains to be elucidated.

Figure 3 illustrates the mechanism of provocation of arrhythmia by the high plasma FFA level in ischemia heart as it is currently understood. This mechanism may be outlined as follows:

1. Because FFA increases oxygen consumption by the myocardium, high plasma FFA level further stimulates myocardial hypoxia.

2. As the energy source of ischemic heart, glucose is required for anaerobic metabolism. Glucose uptake by the myocardium, however, is inhibited by the high plasma FFA level.

3. In ischemic heart, excess FFA cannot be oxidized and is therefore stored in the myocardium as triglyceride.

4. Cations disappear from the myocardium as a result of detergent effects on the cell membrane by the high plasma FFA level in the blood (Kurien and Oliver, 1970).

5. There are still many points to be clarified as to the electrophysiological mechanism of the arrhythmogenic effect of high plasma FFA, but Elzbieta *et al.* (1975) have reported that FFA has a shortening effect on the duration of transmembrane action potentials.

6. Excess FFA facilitates platelet aggregation and causes thrombosis (Hoak, Warner, and Conner, 1967).

7. Coronary blood flow is decreased (Severeid and Long, 1969).

8. Mitochondrial respiration of the myocardium is inhibited by high plasma FFA (Björntorp, Ellis, and Bradford, 1964).

In this study, the effect of high plasma FFA level on the function of the oxidative phosphorylation system of myocardial mitochondria was studied by means of electron spin resonance (ESR) spectrometer, as stated above. High plasma FFA level caused a decrease of the free radical concentration of myocardial mitochondria in state 4 respiration. These results closely resembled those seen after 1 and 2 hr of myocardial ischemia and those seen in mitochondria with added dinitrophenol acting as an uncoupler of oxidative phosphorylation *in vitro* (Kakizawa, 1977).

These results suggest that high plasma FFA may have an uncoupling effect on oxidative phosphorylation in myocardial mitochondria, and that it may play an important role in the arrhythmogenic effect on ischemic heart.

The action of β-blockers to inhibit FFA release from adipose tissue is well known. β-Blockers, however, inhibit FFA release that has been stimulated by catecholamine but not by ACTH or growth hormone.

Nicotinic acid, on the other hand, is said to inhibit the release of FFA from adipose tissue stimulated by 1) catecholamine, 2) ACTH, or 3) growth hormone plus dexamethazone (Fain, Galton, and Kovacev, 1966) However, in addition to the potent inhibitory action on FFA release, nicotinic acid also has the well known vascular effect of causing a flash, so that an administration of a large dose can create problems.

In light of these results, in addition to the widely practiced use of coronary vasodilators and β-blockers, a supplemental use of an inhibitor for the rapid rise of plasma FFA should be considered in the treatment of ischemic heart disease.

REFERENCES

BJÖRNTORP, P., ELLIS, H. A., and BRADFORD, R. H. 1964. Albumin antagonism of fatty acid effects on oxidation and phosphorylation reaction in rat liver mitochondria. J. Biol. Chem. 239:339–344.

CARLSON, L. A., and ORÖ, L. 1962. The effect of nicotinic acid on the plasma free fatty acids. Demonstration of a metabolic type of sympathicolysis. Acta Med. Scand. 172: 641–645.

CHANCE, B., and HAGIHARA, B. 1963. Intracellular respiration. Phosphorylating and non-phosphorylating oxidation reactions. The 5th Int. Cong. Biochem. Pergamon Press, Macmillan Co., New York. p. 3.

ELZBIETA, W. D., MARIA, C., ANDRZEJ, B., and BOHDAN, L. 1975. Influence of sodium palmitate on the cellular action potential of the left ventricle of isolated perfused guinea-pig heart. Acta Physiol. Pol. 26:1–11.

FAIN, J. N., GALTON, D. J., and KOVACEV, V. P. 1966. Effects of drugs on the lipolytic action of hormones in isolated fat cells. Mol. Pharmacol. 2:237–247.

HOAK, J. C., WARNER, E. M., and CONNER, W. E. 1967. Platelets, fatty acids, and thrombosis. Circ. Res. 20:11–17.

HOAK, J. C., WARNER, E. M., and CONNER, W. E. 1972. Effects of acute free fatty acid mobilization on the heart. *In* E. Bajusz and G. Rona (eds.), Recent Advances in Cardiac Structure and Metabolism. Vol. 1: Myocardiology, pp. 127–135. University Park Press, Baltimore.

KAKIZAWA, N. 1977. Studies on free radical formation and respiratory function of heart mitochondria in experimental coronary occlusion. J. Jpn. Coll. Angiol. 17:505–513.

KURIEN, V. A., and OLIVER, M. F. 1970. A metabolic cause for arrhythmias during acute myocardial hypoxia. Lancet 18:813–815.

KURIEN, V. A., YATES, P. A., and OLIVER, M. F. 1969. Free fatty acids, heparin, and arrhythmias during experimental myocardial infarction. Lancet 26:185–187.

SEVEREID, L., CONNOR, W. E., and LONG, J. P. 1969. The depressant effect of fatty acid on the isolated rabbit heart. Proc. Soc. Exp. Biol. Med. 131:1239–1243.

SUZUKI, Y. 1975. Studies on the free radicals in myocardial mitochondria by electron spin resonance (ESR) spectrometry: Studies on experimental infarction dogs. Jpn. Circ. J. 39:683–691.

Mailing address:
N. Yamazaki, M.D.,
Third Department of Internal Medicine,
Hamamatsu Medical University, 3600-Honda-Cho, Hamamatsu (Japan).

Recent Advances in Studies on
Cardiac Structure and Metabolism, Volume 12
Cardiac Adaptation
Edited by T. Kobayashi, Y. Ito, and G. Rona
Copyright 1978 University Park Press Baltimore

X-RAY MICROANALYSIS OF MITOCHONDRIAL CALCIUM

H. D. SYBERS

Department of Pathology, Baylor College of Medicine,
Houston, Texas, USA

SUMMARY

X-ray microanalytical techniques using wavelength dispersive (WDS) and energy dispersive spectrometry (EDS) indicate that Ca^{2+} is present in intramitochondrial granules which occur in myocardial cells following irreversible ischemic injury. Preliminary results using tissue prepared for routine electron microscopy suggest that the degree of calcium binding that occurs in the mitochondria increases with increased duration of ischemia. Free ions are leached out of the tissue during processing; hence, the role of ion redistribution in producing myocardial necrosis cannot be elicited from a study of this nature. However, with continued progress in the development of techniques of tissue preparation, x-ray spectrometry may provide a means of assessing quantitative ion alterations that occur during ischemia.

INTRODUCTION

The role of ions in the function of contractile cells has been investigated extensively with a wide variety of techniques. It is well known that the cations (sodium, potassium, and calcium) are intimately involved in excitation-contraction and that agents which inhibit their movements into or out of the cell disrupt normal contractile activity.

Redistribution of ions occurs during a number of pathological conditions during which the excitation-contraction phenomenon also is disturbed (Urbanek *et al.,* 1975). The onset of myocardial ischemia results in cessation of contraction and a rapid decrease in ATP levels within a short time. Several studies using biochemical, histochemical, and tissue fractionation techniques indicate that redistribution of ions coincides with these alterations. Jennings and his coworkers (Jennings *et al.,* 1965, 1969, 1974) have shown in myocardial ischemia that densities are formed within the mitochondria at approximately the time when irreversible changes occur in the cell, and, with the aid of microincineration, studies have shown that some of these densities appear to be composed of calcium phosphate (Shen and Jennings, 1972). Fleckenstein and his workers (Fleckenstein *et al.,*

This work was supported by NHLI Grant 19147-01.

1975; Janke *et al.*, 1975) studying noncoronarogenic myofiber necrosis induced by isoproterenol injection, have hypothesized that excessive mitochondrial calcium accumulation is a principal cause of the fiber necrosis. Lehr and his coworkers (Lehr, Chau, and Irene, 1975), however, have suggested that magnesium loss from the mitochondria, rather than calcium overload, is the mechanism responsible for the production of necrotic lesions. Thus, it seems that while the exact mechanism involved is debatable, a good deal of evidence exists that suggests that ion redistribution within the cell may play a significant role in the production of necrotizing lesions.

One of the major difficulties in evaluating the role of cation shifts in the production of fiber necrosis has been the inability to detect and quantitate the concentration of ions within the organelles under *in vivo* conditions. The studies which have been cited all rely on measurements in tissues and cells that have been subjected to procedures that would in themselves result in a reduction or redistribution of the ions. Recently, however, with the advent of electron probe techniques coupled with x-ray spectrometry, it has been possible to analyze specific organelles or structures within the cell (Coleman and Terepka, 1972; Sjostrom and Thornill, 1974; Somlyo *et al.*, 1974), and it is anticipated that further refinement of these techniques will permit a quantitative evaluation of ion shifts.

The appearance of dense intramitochondrial granules containing calcium phosphate after 30–40 min of ischemia (Jennings *et al.*, 1965, 1969, 1974; Shen and Jennings, 1972) indicates that binding of calcium and phosphorus occurs and that this bond is strong enough to resist leaching during preparation for electron microscopy. Thus, it may be possible to employ tissue that has been routinely prepared for electron microscopy to determine whether or not binding of calcium occurs progressively with the increased duration of ischemic injury.

MATERIALS AND METHODS

The tissues examined in these studies were derived from dog and rabbit and were analyzed with both wavelength and energy dispersive analytical techniques. Basic experimental methods were common to all. The animals were anesthetized with pentobarbitol sodium (30 mm/kg) and respiration was maintained via endotracheal intubation on 95% O_2/5% CO_2 with a Harvard animal respirator. After left thoractotomy, the anterior descending coronary artery was ligated for varying periods of time before sacrifice (60 min to 28 hr). The hearts were fixed by retrograde coronary perfusion with 3.5% glutaraldehyde in 0.1 M cocadylate buffer at pH 7.3. Small pieces of tissue (1 X 2 X 2 mm) from the left ventricle were removed and fixed for an additional 4 hr before post-fixation in 1% osmium tetroxide. The tissue was dehydrated through ethanol and embedded in araldite. Thick sections (1 μm) were stained with toluidine blue for orientation.

Thin sections were stained with uranyl acetate and lead citrate and examined with a transmission electron microscope. Sections of 600 Å and 1,000 Å were put on Formvar carbon-coated grids for microanalysis.

Wavelength Dispersive Microanalysis

Sections of approximately 1,000 Å were examined in an ETEC Autospec wavelength dispersive spectrometer (WDS) using pentaerythritol (PET) crystals. The specimens were analyzed using the scanning transmission mode (STEM) as a primary electron probe. The sections were examined at a 30° tilt with an accelerating voltage of 30 kV and specimen current of 1.5 na for a count time of 200 sec. Beam conditions were maintained constant throughout the acquisition of data. Recordings were made for peak count (P) with the WDS set for calcium $K\alpha$ (1.549 Å). Background was determined by offsetting the crystal from the calcium position to 1.599 Å. Peak to background determinations were made from four representative mitochondria in each of four specimens of 60-min, 5-hr, 24-hr, and 28-hr duration of ischemia.

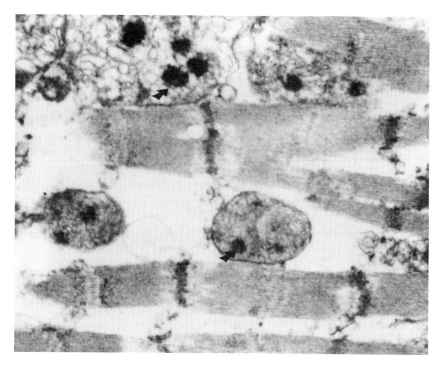

Figure 1. Twenty-four-hour infarct: numerous dense precipitates (arrows) within the mitochondria. Transmission electron micrograph of a 600-Å section. × 25,100.

Energy Dispersive Analysis

Other samples prepared in a similar manner were examined in an EDAX energy dispersive spectrometer (EDS) attached to a Philips 301 electron microscope. The spot size was reduced to analyze a 3,000 Å area with a specimen current of 40 μa at a 30° tilt and an 80-kV accelerating voltage. Peak to background readings were obtained from mitochondria containing granules, mitochondria without granules, and contractile material. Background readings were obtained by focusing on a clear area of the Formvar carbon-coating.

Similar analyses were conducted using a JEOL 100 C with a Kevex 5100 energy dispersive spectrometer. Both the STEM and TEM modes were utilized as a primary electron probe.

In a single specimen of a 24-hr infarct, four mitochondria without granules were analyzed for calcium and five granules containing mitochondria were analyzed at a 60-kV accelerating voltage in an AEI CORA energy dispersive analytical system.

RESULTS

Routine TEM of control tissue revealed a normal ultrastructure, while that of ischemic regions showed changes of myocardial infarction characterized by intracellular edema, swelling, and disruption of myofibrils with margination of nuclear chromatin. Prominent, densely staining granules were present in mitochondria as early as 1 hr after onset of ischemia and were seen more frequently in later stages when most of the mitochondria contained multiple large granules (Figure 1).

Table 1. WDS analysis of calcium in mitochondria

Specimen	Control			1 hr			5 hr			24 hr			28 hr		
	P	B	P–B	P	B	P–B	P	B	P–B	P	B	P–B	P	B	P–B
1	66	36	30	83	59	24	91	56	35	161	80	81	115	58	57
2	68	54	14	96	64	32	103	55	48	125	67	58	127	42	85
3	50	36	14	86	56	30	92	52	40	145	54	91	122	53	69
4	50	48	2	81	51	30	81	55	26	128	78	50	125	44	81
Average P–B		15			29			37.25			70			73	

P = peak counts over 200 sec; B = background counts over 200 sec; P–B = difference in counts between P and B.

WDS analysis of mitochondria in normal and infarcted cells revealed the presence of calcium. Peak to background ratios were higher in specimens that had been subjected to prolonged ischemia than in the normal control tissue, but some calcium could be identified in all mitochondria examined (Table 1).

EDS analysis of myofibrils revealed no noticeable calcium peaks, and mitochondria without granules were not distinguishable from background determinations (Figures 2 and 3). Large copper, osmium, and lead peaks were present in all specimens, reflecting the staining procedures and the use of copper grids in this study. A calcium peak was invariably found in mitochondrial granules (Figure 4). Table 2 represents results from four mitochondria without granules and five granule-containing mitochondria from a 24-hr infarct examined in an AEI CORA with energy dispersive spectrometry. Mitochondria with granules in all cases

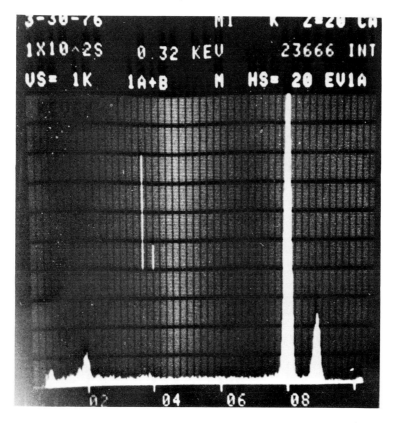

Figure 2. EDS analysis of myofilaments. Note absence of calcium peak (long vertical bar).

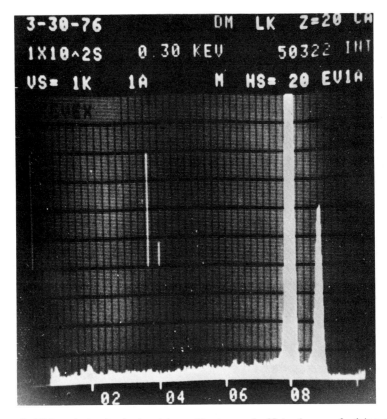

Figure 3. EDS analysis of mitochondrion without granule. Note absence of calcium peak (long vertical bar).

revealed calcium, while, in those without granules, Ca^{2+} levels were indistinguishable from background determinations. Figures 5 and 6 illustrate a typical specimen before and after microanalysis.

DISCUSSION

The results of this study, while preliminary, clearly indicate the feasibility of employing electron probe techniques in the qualitative study of cation binding that may occur during myocardial infarction. The ability to focally analyze a small area within a cell and at the same time to visualize the ultrastructural appearance of that area before and after analysis provides a potential means of assessing structure-function relationships which was heretofore not possible.

It must be kept in mind that these studies do not indicate *total* calcium concentrations because free ions were leached from the cell during processing for

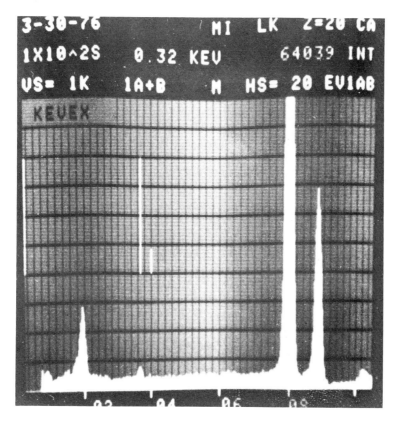

Figure 4. EDS analysis of mitochondrion containing granules. Note calcium peak (long vertical bar).

electron microscopy (Sjostrom and Thornell, 1974). Hence, only those that were *bound in vivo* would be expected to remain *in situ*. Furthermore, a knowledge of whether or not all of the bound ions continue to remain bound during processing is crucial to assuming that a quantitative analysis is even possible. At present we have no direct evidence to indicate whether or not this assumption is correct.

No attempt was made in this study to derive a truly quantitative analysis of calcium concentration but rather to employ a semiquantitave approach to ion shifts. By comparing total counts in mitochondria containing granules to total counts in mitochondria without granules, or to contractile filaments, it is possible to determine the direction of ion shifts during various periods of ischemia. A consistent relationship between the presence of intramitochondrial granules and a calcium peak was observed in all cases, regardless of whether EDS or WDS was employed for the analysis. While the sample size is much too small to provide definitive conclusions, there was a trend toward higher peak to

Table 2. Calcium in mitochondria with dense bodies compared to mitochondria without dense bodies in 24-hr infarct (EDS analysis)

Specimen	Mitochondria with granules				Mitochondria without granules			
	P	B	P–B	Integral count under peak	P	B	P–B	Integral count under peak
1	76	33	43	173	0	0	0	3
2	88	49	39	117	0	0	0	0
3	62	30	32	112	0	0	0	0
4	60	31	29	53	0	0	0	14
5	55	34	21	163				

Analysis performed by AEI CORA at a 60-kV accelerating voltage.

background counts in mitochondria containing granules which roughly paralleled the duration of ischemia. Interpretation of these data is, however, complicated by the fact that not all mitochondria in an injured cell develop dense granules. In these mitochondria without granules, peak to background ratios for calcium are not larger than those in the contractile filaments, and frequently no calcium peak can be identified.

These data suggest that, for proper interpretation of the significance of mitochondrial calcium binding on the cell, a number of additional factors need to be determined. The most important of these is the determination of *total* intramitochondrial calcium concentration. If this is known, it may be possible to ascribe a cause-effect relationship to calcium overload and the development of intramitochondrial granules. *In vitro* studies employing isolated mitochondria suggest that formation of calcium-phosphate granules and the form in which they precipitate can be modulated by various concentrations of Mg^{2+} (Sordahl and Silver, 1975). If methods can be devised for determining total intraorganelle calcium, similar manipulations may be feasible in intact animals that may aid our understanding of processes associated with the development of irreversible injury.

The major remaining hurdle to be overcome in employing electron probe techniques for the study of free ion concentration involves tissue preparation. Evidence from several laboratories (Appelton, 1974; Sjostrom and Thornell, 1974; Somlyo, 1975) suggests that cryoultramicrotomy followed by freeze-drying of the thin sections may be an acceptable method for tissue preparation. Further development of these techniques is currently underway.

Adequate sampling of the tissue is of major importance, because it has been shown that not all cells within an ischemic region will be affected to the same

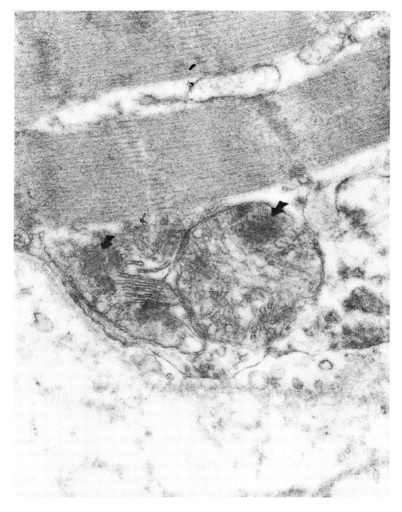

Figure 5. Twenty-four-hour infarct: mitochondrion containing granules before analysis (arrows). × 91,000.

degree, and even within an injured cell not all mitochondria develop granules (Cox *et al.,* 1968). The problem of adequate tissue sampling may be minimized by employing an experimental model such as that described by Jennings, Wartman, and Zudyk (1957) in which a relatively homogeneous infarct results in the posterior papillary muscle following circumflex coronary occlusion.

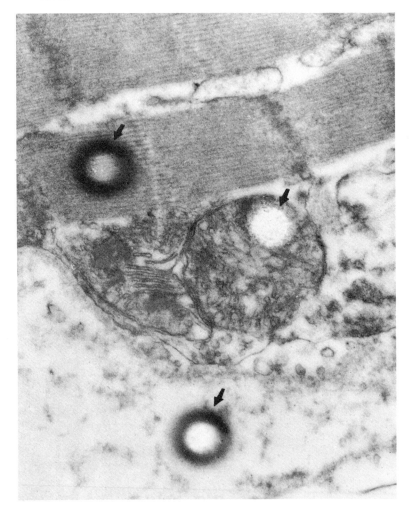

Figure 6. Twenty-four-hour analysis. Note spot size of analyzed area in mitochondrion, myofilaments, and background (arrows). × 81,000.

REFERENCES

APPELTON, T. C. 1974. A cryostat approach to ultra thin "dry" frozen sections for electron microscopy: A morphologic and x-ray analytical study. J. Microsc. 100:49–74.
COLEMAN, J. R., and TEREPKA, A. R. 1972. Electron probe analysis of the calcium distribution in cells of the embryonic chick chorioallantoic membrane. I. A critical evaluation of techniques. J. Histochem. Cytochem. 20:401–413.
COX, J. L., MCLAUGHLIN, V. W., FLOWERS, N. C., and HORAN, L. C. 1968. The

ischemic zone surrounding acute myocardial infarction: Its morphology as detected by dehydrogenase staining. Am. Heart J. 76:650–659.

FLECKENSTEIN, A., JANKE, J., DORING, H. J., and LEDER, O. 1975. Key role of Ca in production of noncoronarogenic myocardial necroses. A. Fleckenstein and G. Rona (eds.), Recent Advances in Cardiac Structure and Metabolism. Vol. 6: Pathophysiology and Morphology of Myocardial Cell Alteration, pp. 21–32. University Park Press, Baltimore.

JANKE, J., FLECKENSTEIN, A., HEIN, B., LEDER, O., SIGEL, H. 1975. Prevention of myocardial Ca overload and necrotization by Mg and K salts or acidosis. *In* A. Fleckenstein and G. Rona (eds.), Recent Advances in Cardiac Structure and Metabolism. Vol. 6: Pathophysiology and Morphology of Myocardial Cell Alterations, pp. 33–43. University Park Press, Baltimore.

JENNINGS, R. B., BAUM, J. H., and HERDSON, P. B. 1965. Fine structural changes in myocardial ischemic injury. Arch. Pathol. 79:135–143.

JENNINGS, R. B., SOMMERS, H. M., HERDSON, P. B., and KALTENBACH, J. P. 1969. Ischemic injury of myocardium. Ann. N.Y. Acad. Sci. 156:61–78.

JENNINGS, R. B., and GANOTE, C. E. 1974. Structural changes in myocardium during acute ischemia. Circ. Res. 35:156–172.

JENNINGS, R. B., WARTMAN, W. B., and ZUDYK, Z. E. 1957. Production of an area of homogeneous myocardial infarction in the dog. Arch. Pathol. 63:580–585.

LEHR, D., CHAU, R., and IRENE, S. 1975. Possible role of magnesium loss in the pathogenesis of myocardial fiber necrosis. *In* A. Fleckenstein and G. Rona (eds.), Recent Advances in Cardiac Structure and Metabolism. Vol. 6: Pathophysiology and Morphology of Myocardial Cell Alterations, pp. 95–109. University Park Press, Baltimore.

SHEN, A. C., and JENNINGS, R. B. 1972. Myocardial calcium and magnesium in acute ischemic injury. Am. J. Pathol. 67:417–440.

SJOSTROM, M., and THORNELL, L. E. 1974. Preparing sections of skeletal muscle for transmission electron analytical microscopy (TEAM) of diffusable elements. J. Microsc. 103:101–112.

SOMLYO, A. V., SILCOX, J., and SOMLYO, A. P. 1975. Electron probe analysis and cryoultramicrotomy of cardiac muscle: Mitochondrial granules. *In* G. W. Bailey (ed.), 33rd Annual Proceedings Electron Microscopy Society of American, pp. 532–533. Claitor's Publishing Division, Baton Rouge.

SOMLYO, A. P., SOMLYO, A. V., DEVINE, C. E., PETERS, P. D., and HALL, T. A. 1974. Electron microscopy and electron probe analysis of mitochondrial cation accumulation in smooth muscle. J. Cell Biol. 61:723–742.

SORDAHL, L. A., and SILVER, B. B. 1975. Pathological accumulation of calcium by mitochondria: Modulation by magnesium. *In* A. Fleckenstein and G. Rona (eds.), Recent Advances in Cardiac Structure and Metabolism. Vol. 6: Pathophysiology and Morphology of Myocardial Cell Alterations, pp. 85–93. University Park Press, Baltimore.

URBANEK, E., VASKU, J., BEDNARIK, B., PRASLICKA, M., and POSPISIL, M. 1975. Electrolyte changes in myocardial injury. *In* A. Fleckenstein and G. Rona (eds.), Recent Advances in Studies on Cardiac Structure and Metabolism. Vol. 6: Pathophysiology and Morphology of Myocardial Cell Alterations, pp. 43–58. University Park Press, Baltimore.

Mailing address:
Harley D. Sybers, M.D., Ph.D.,
Department of Pathology, Baylor College of Medicine,
Texas Medical Center, Houston, Texas 77030 (USA).

Recent Advances in Studies on
Cardiac Structure and Metabolism, Volume 12
Cardiac Adaptation
Edited by T. Kobayashi, Y. Ito, and G. Rona
Copyright 1978 University Park Press Baltimore

ELEMENTAL COMPOSITION OF ISCHEMIC MYOCARDIUM DETERMINED BY X-RAY MICROANALYSIS

M. ASHRAF and C. M. BLOOR

Department of Pathology, University of California, San Diego,
School of Medicine, La Jolla, California, USA

SUMMARY

Elemental composition of ischemic myocardium was attempted with x-ray microanalysis. Energy dispersive spectrum exhibited calcium $K\alpha$ and phosphorus $K\alpha$ peaks from mitochondrial deposits, and Ca $K\alpha$ peaks from nucleus, contraction bands, and Z lines of the ischemic myocardial cell. Ca and P contents were confirmed with wavelength dispersive spectrometers. Mg was present in the mitochondrial deposits which lacked Ca. This study suggests a formation of phosphate salt of Ca at different intracellular sites and also of Mg with mitochondrial deposits.

INTRODUCTION

Myocardial cell death follows coronary artery occlusion as a result of a combination of factors, including defective energy metabolism, uncontrolled cell swelling, and excessive intracellular accumulation of calcium (Brachfeld, 1973; Kloner *et al.*, 1974). The electron microscope studies of ischemic myocardium show that the electron-dense deposits appear within the cells, particularly in the mitochondria, the nucleus, and the perinuclear zones. These have been associated with abnormal accumulation of certain ions (Shen and Jennings, 1972; Buja *et al.*, 1976; Ashraf, Sybers, and Bloor, 1976). Precise chemical analysis of these areas is difficult because of the lack of reliable histochemical techniques.

The recent application of the energy dispersive spectrometer (EDS) and the wavelength dispersive spectrometer (WDS) with the electron microscope has permitted simultaneous analysis of biological specimens for elements and correlation of their location in the subcellular organelles (Chandler, 1973; Russ, 1974). In spite of the recent uses of EDS and WDS in biological specimens, problems still remain to be solved in preparing tissue to preserve the intracellular

This work was supported by Research Grant HL 18122 and Contract HL 17682 from the United States Public Health Service.

elements that tend to leach or dislocate during the electron microscopic procedures.

In this study we attempted to determine the elemental composition of ischemic myocardium with EDS and WDS.

MATERIALS AND METHODS

Two canine hearts were rendered ischemic by ligating the anterior descending artery for 24 hr and were perfused with 3.5% buffered glutaraldehyde, pH 7.3. Small pieces (1 mm^3) were cut and either processed as such or post-fixed with 1.5% osmium tetroxide for electron microscopy. The tissue blocks were dehydrated in ethanol and embedded in araldite. Some pieces were prepared according to the calcium precipitation technique as previously described (Ashraf, Sybers, and Bloor, 1976).

Semithin sections about 1500 Å thick were cut with an ultramicrotome and put on copper or titanium grids and coated with about a 200 Å layer of carbon. These were analyzed in the Etec scanning electron microscope (SEM) attached to a Kevex 5100 silicon (Lithium-drifted) EDS and Etec scanning Autospec WDS using pentaerythritol and rubidium acid phthalate crystals. The tissue was examined at a tilt of 45° and at an accelerating voltage of 25 or 40 kV and a specimen current of 1 or 6 na. The electron probe was checked periodically to prevent drifting of the beam. All analyses were made with the EDS for 400 sec or longer, and readings of 100 sec were made for peak count with the WDS tuned to magnesium $K\alpha$, calcium $K\alpha$, and phosphorus $K\alpha$ lines.

RESULTS

Ischemia produced several morphological changes in the cardiac cells, as demonstrated in Figures 1 and 2.

No elemental peaks in the energy dispersive spectrum were seen in the normal cells that were processed either routinely for electron microscopy or with the calcium precipitation technique. A few readings for the calcium contents of two mitochondria, two sarcoplasmic reticula (SR), nine junctional sarcoplasmic reticula (JSR), and one nucleus were taken with WDS. Average calcium $K\alpha$ peak/background ratios of 1.1:1, 1.7:1, 1.3:1, and 1.1:1 for mitochondria, SR, JSR, and nucleus, respectively, were obtained.

The energy dispersive spectrum from the mitochondrial granules showed a calcium $K\alpha$ peak at 3.60 keV (Figure 3), and other peaks originated from grid and electron microscope parts. The phosphorus and osmium peaks, which overlapped, were sorted out with WDS (Figure 4) or with EDS using non-osmicated tissue. Calcium and phosphorus contents in the intramitochondrial granules were confirmed with WDS. Electron-dense deposits from 10 different

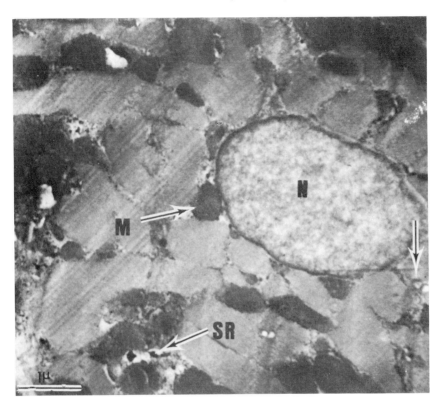

Figure 1. Scanning transmission electron micrograph (STEM) of a normal myocardial cell treated with oxalate to preserve the distribution of calcium. Electron dense precipitate is seen in the mitochondria (M), free sarcoplasmic reticulum (SR), junctional SR (arrow), and nucleus (N). × 16,000.

mitochondria were analyzed. Average calcium $K\alpha$ and phosphorus $K\alpha$ peak/background ratios were 1.5:1 and 7.5:1, respectively. In some mitochondrial deposits, peak/background ratio for calcium or phosphorus was less than 1.0, indicating an absence of both elements.

Because there was no indication of elements other than calcium and phosphorus in the EDS spectrum of mitochondrial deposits, no time-consuming effort was made in the WDS for the search of other ions, with the exception of magnesium, which was present in two of the four deposits analyzed. The average peak/background ratio was 1.6:1.

EDS spectra similar to mitochondrial granules were obtained from the nucleus (Figure 5), contraction bands, Z lines, and lysosomes. A single reading of contraction band, nucleus, Z line, and lysosomes for calcium counts with WDS showed a peak/background ratio of more than 2.0, while phosphorus peak/back-

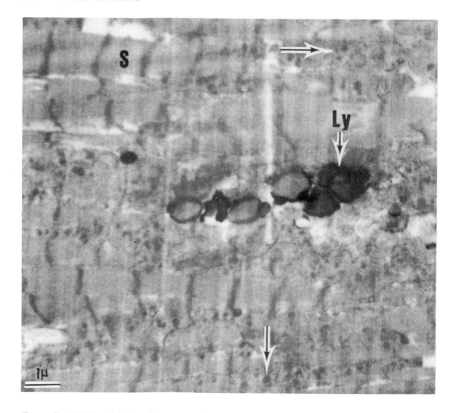

Figure 2. STEM of ischemic myocardium. Mitochondria containing intramitochondrial granules (arrow) are shown. Ly = lysosome; S = sarcomere. × 9,500.

ground ratio was slightly better than 1.0, except lysosome background counts, which exceeded the peak counts.

DISCUSSION

The results of these observations show that the elemental composition of the ischemic myocardial cells can be determined by EDS and WDS on tissue routinely embedded in epoxy. The rationale of feasibility and reliability for detecting certain ions is based upon the fact that some elements form chemical complexes with others at several intracellular sites of these abnormal cells. These electron-dense deposits or complexes are fairly stable during tissue treatments and can be analyzed for their chemical composition. On the other hand, spectral peaks of all naturally ocurring ions in the similarly processed normal tissue are indistinguishable from the background. The preservation of some of these ions

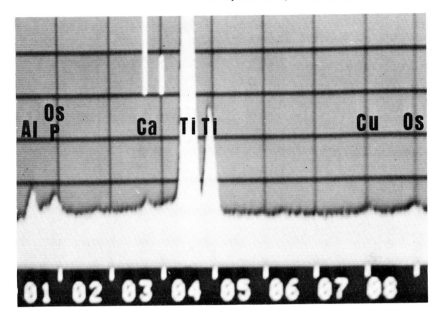

Figure 3. Energy dispersive spectrum of mitochondrial granule displaying calcium peak at 3.60 keV. The other peaks originated from the grid and its holder and osmium. Osmium and phosphorus peaks with similar energy levels are observed at approximately 2 keV. Partly reproduced from Ashraf, Sybers, and Bloor (1976) with publisher's permission.

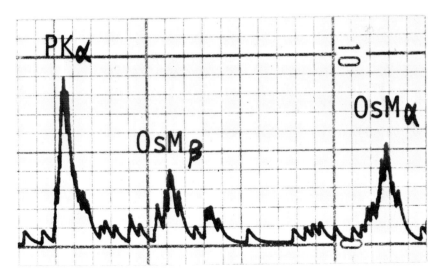

Figure 4. Wavelength spectrum of intramitochondrial granule shows phosphorus and osmium peak emission.

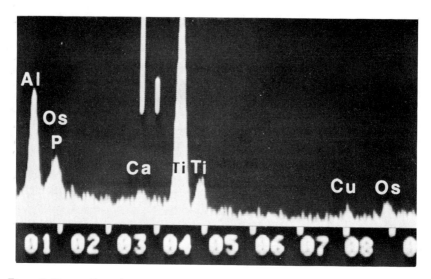

Figure 5. Energy dispersive spectrum of ischemic myocardial cell nucleus showing calcium peak at 3.60 keV. Phosphorus and osmium peaks also are visible.

can be slightly improved by precipitating them histochemically before aldehyde fixation (Mizuhira, 1973; Ashraf, Sybers, and Bloor, 1976). Cryoultramicrotomy is the most suitable method for preserving ions and estimating diffusable ions (Sjostrom and Thornell, 1975). Cryosectioning, therefore, seems to be the best approach for accurately describing elements within an area.

During myocardial ischemia, the ionic shifts are accompanied by several ultrastructural changes. Most visible are those in the mitochondria, which swell within a half-hour of coronary artery occlusion and develop electron-dense bodies, which are calcium phosphate, as determined by microincineration (Shen and Jennings, 1972) and x-ray microanalysis (Buja *et al.,* 1976; Ashraf, Sybers, and Bloor, 1976). Although Jennings' and Buja's groups have reported that calcium phosphate is only present in the granular or spicular-like inclusions of mitochondria associated with the transient ischemia, or at the peripheral zone of permanent ischemia, we have found it also is common in permanent ischemia. With the SEM we were unable to differentiate between the two types of mitochondrial inclusions analyzed in the sections that were 1500 Å thick because of its poor resolving power. In addition to calcium and phosphorus in the intramitochondrial deposits, magnesium also was found in association with phosphorus only, suggesting either formation of phosphate salt of calcium or of magnesium in the granules. Further evaluation of these limited observations, which were made on tissue prepared suboptimally for analysis, is required to gain total elemental information on transient or permanent ischemia.

The association of phosphorus and calcium with abnormally condensed nuclear chromatin material may be significant to the process of cell injury. Similarly, formation of contraction bands in some ischemic cells may be caused by an excessive accumulation of excess calcium and phosphorus over the sarcomeres as indicated by electron probe analysis and because of a reduced ability of sarcoplasmic reticulum to sequester calcium from the sarcoplasm. During permanent ischemia the source of excess calcium in the mitochondria and other intracellular sites appears to be from within the cells. Calcium, an important ion for muscle contraction, is thus particularly associated with the mitochondria, sarcoplasmic reticulum, and sarcomeres. When cell contraction ceases because of anoxia, this calcium appears to aggregate or redistribute and is trapped by inorganic phosphate that is released at sites of ATPase activity (Plattner, 1975) and excessive breakdown of ATP. This phenomenon is particularly visible in the mitochondria where phosphorus counts were far greater than in other areas of the cell. Thus, the appearance of calcium or magnesium phosphate precipitates seems to be a sign of irreversible cell injury (Trump and Arstila, 1971; Shen and Jennings, 1972).

REFERENCES

ASHRAF, M., SYBERS, H. D., and BLOOR, C. M. 1976. X-ray microanalysis of ischemic myocardium. Exp. Mol. Pathol. 24:435–440.

BRACHFELD, N. 1973. Myocardial metabolic dysfunction following infarction. In E. Corday and H. Swan (eds.), Myocardial Infarction, pp. 26–38. Williams and Wilkins Co., Baltimore.

BUJA, L. M., DEES, J. H., HARDING, D. F., and WILLERSON, J. T. 1976. Analytical electron microscopic study of mitochondrial inclusions in canine myocardial infarcts. J. Histochem. Cytochem. 24:508–516.

CHANDLER, J. A. 1973. Recent developments in analytical electron microscopy. J. Microsc. 98:359–378.

KLONER, R. A., GANOTE, C. E., WHALEN, D. A., and JENNINGS, R. B. 1974. Effect of a transient period of ischemia on myocardial cells. II. Fine structure during the first few minutes of reflow. Am. J. Pathol. 74:399–422.

MIZUHIRA, V. 1973. Demonstration of the elemental distribution in biological tissues by means of the electron microscope and electron probe x-ray microanalyzer. Acta Histochem. Cytochem. 6:44–52.

PLATTNER, H. 1975. Ciliary granule plaques: Membrane intercalated particle aggregates associated with Ca^{2+}-binding sites in Paramecium. J. Cell Sci. 18:257–269.

RUSS, J. C. 1974. X-ray microanalysis in the biological sciences. J. Submicrosc. Cytol. 6:55–79.

SHEN, A. C., and JENNINGS, R. B. 1972. Myocardial calcium and magnesium in acute ischemic injury. Am. J. Pathol. 67:417–440.

SJOSTROM, M., and THORNELL, L. E. 1975. Preparing sections of skeletal muscle for transmission electron analytical microscopy (TEAM) of diffusable elements. J. Microsc. 103:101–112.

TRUMP, B., and ARSTILA, A. 1971. Cell injury and cell death. In M. F. LaVia and R. B. Hill (eds.), Principles of Pathobiology, pp. 9–95. Oxford University Press, New York.

Mailing address:
M. Ashraf, Ph.D.,
Department of Pathology, M-012,
University of California, San Diego, School of Medicine, La Jolla, California 92093 (USA).

Recent Advances in Studies on
Cardiac Structure and Metabolism, Volume 12
Cardiac Adaptation
Edited by T. Kobayashi, Y. Ito, and G. Rona
Copyright 1978 University Park Press Baltimore

ULTRASTRUCTURAL FEATURES OF DISEASED HUMAN ATRIAL MUSCLE CELLS

H. MITSUI, K. KAWAMURA, K. ISHIZAWA,
M. OMAE, and C. KAWAI

Third Division, Department of Internal Medicine
Kyoto University, Faculty of Medicine, Kyoto, Japan

SUMMARY

Left atrial myocardial tissues, excised at the time of surgery from 30 Japanese patients, were studied using light and electron microscopy and the freeze-fracture technique. All had mitral valvular disease, and, in 22 (74%) patients, atrial fibrillation also was present. In all patients, most of the left atrial cardiocytes were hypertrophied and surrounded by various amounts of fibrous tissue. Degenerative alterations included large masses of lipofuscin granules and lamellar bodies, disorganized myofibrils, widened Z-line material, selective loss of thick filaments, and prominent tubules of sarcoplasmic reticulum. A high incidence of tubular aggregates was observed in 70% of the cases. Such alterations were seen more often in the mitral regurgitation group as compared to the mitral stenosis group. Atrial cardiocytes were found to be more susceptible to disease processes, such as rheumatic fever and subsequent pressure and/or volume overloading, than ventricular cardiocytes. Human atrial cardiocytes may be utilized in future cytopathological studies to study the effect of processes leading to cardiocyte hypertrophy and degeneration.

INTRODUCTION

Electron microscopic observations have been reported on the cytopathological changes of the ventricular myocardium of patients with various heart diseases (Legato, 1970; Maron and Ferrans, 1974; Maron, Ferrans, and Roberts, 1975a, 1975b). By contrast, the ultrastructural studies on atrial myocardium in the diseased human heart (Kawamura *et al.,* 1969; Roy, Dorais, and Morin, 1972; Fenoglio and Wagner, 1973; Mitsui *et al.,* 1975) are limited. There are, however, a considerable number of comprehensive descriptions concerning the atrial myocardium of experimental animals in normal and pathophysiological conditions (Rona, Chappel, and Kahn, 1962; Simpson and Rayns, 1968; Hibbs and Ferrans, 1969; McNutt and Fawcett, 1969; Forssmann and Giradier, 1970; Berger and Rona, 1971a, 1971b; Dusek, Boutet, and Rona, 1973; Sommer and Waugh, 1976).

The present work was an attempt to determine the incidence of a wide variety of fine structural alterations encountered in hypertrophied and degenerated atrial cardiocytes in patients with mitral valve disease and then to compare these findings with observations of diseased ventricular cardiocytes.

MATERIALS AND METHODS

Left atrial tissues were obtained from 30 Japanese patients with mitral valvular diseases at the time of open-heart surgery. These patients comprised two groups: 1) 20 patients with mitral stenosis (11 with predominantly pure mitral stenosis, five with aortic regurgitation, and four with tricuspid regurgitation), 14 of whom had atrial fibrillation (70%), and 2) 10 patients with mitral regurgitation (five with predominantly pure mitral regurgitation and five with additional tricuspid regurgitation), in eight of whom atrial fibrillation also was present (80%). A total of 30 patients were clinically diagnosed as having mitral valvular diseases, presumably of rheumatic origin. Patients included eight males and 22 females, the youngest being a 17-year-old boy with mitral regurgitation, and the oldest a 49-year-old housewife with mitral stenosis. The average age, at the time of operation, of those with mitral stenosis and mitral regurgitation was 37.4 and 26.3 years, respectively. The time interval from the probable onset of rheumatic fever to the operation ranged from six months to 35 years, while that from the onset of congestive heart failure to the operation was from six months to 15 years. Cardiothoracic ratio and mean pulmonary capillary wedge pressure or mean left atrial pressure also ranged from 48 to 86% and from 7 to 30 mm Hg, respectively.

All freshly excised tissues were processed immediately for routine light and electron microscopic examination, and some for freeze-fractured cardiac muscle cell preparation.

RESULTS

In all tissues examined by light microscopy, the majority of atrial cardiac muscle cells was found hypertrophied to a great extent. Transverse diameters of these cells ranged from 7.5 to 80.2 μm, while the average values in individual cases were from 18 to 34 μm. In the histopathological studies, active rheumatic lesions were seldom observed, while varying degrees of fibrosis were almost always present, particularly in older patients with mitral stenosis.

Electron microscopic observation of atrial cardiac muscle cells disclosed a wide variety of ultrastructural features of hypertrophy and degeneration. These features, however, differed in extent and severity from one block to another, from one cell to another, and even between different regions of the cell in the same patient (Figures 1, 2, and 6). Freeze-fracture and etching techniques demonstrated, to some extent, the relationship among the subcellular membrane systems (Figure 3) and provided an *en face* view of the gap junction (Figure 12).

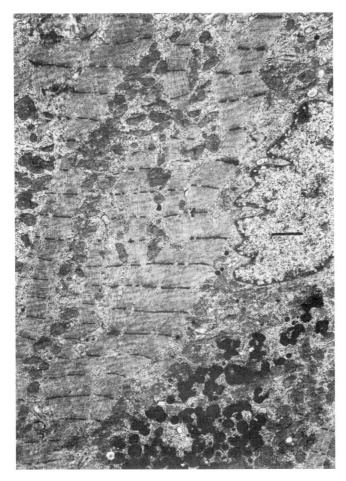

Figure 1. A hypertrophied left atrial cardiocyte from a 47-year-old female patient with severe mitral stenosis and atrial fibrillation. Note the typical appearance of fine structural components: nucleus, mitochondria, Golgi complexes, rough ER, free ribosomes, glycogen granules, lipofuscin bodies, lysosomes, atrial specific granules, compact myofibrils with somewhat widened Z lines, and moderately dilated T tubules. × 8,400. Calibration bar indicates one μm for all figures.

Hypertrophied atrial cardiocytes (Figure 1) with increased compact myofibrils in register also showed different grades of early degenerative changes: increased lipofuscin granules, slightly expanded Z lines, myofibril disarray, hyperplastic Golgi complexes, and rough endoplasmic reticulum (ER), as well as an accumulation of glycogen granules.

The most severely affected atrial cardiocytes (Figure 2) revealed such subcellular changes as a decrease in the number of myofibrils, an extensive accumula-

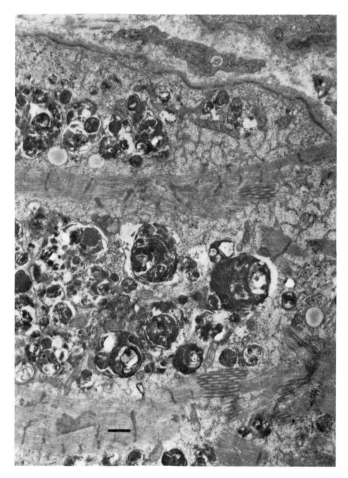

Figure 2. Left atrial cardiocyte with severe degenerative changes from the same patient as in Figure 1. Note the extensive lipofuscin bodies and lamellar complexes, the decreased number of myofibrils with myofibrillar lysis, the proliferation of sarcoplasmic reticulum in lacework, the entangled cytofilaments, the decreased population of mitochondria, and the appearance of tubular aggregates along the longitudinal axis of myofibrils. Even in this advanced stage of degeneration, polysomes and ribosomes (upper left) are evident, whereas atrial specific granules are rare. × 6,200.

tion of glycogen granules, lipofuscin bodies, and lamellar complexes, a fairly large sarcoplasmic area free of myofibrils with profuse proliferation of sarco-tubules (Figure 5), large masses of abnormal Z-line material (Figures 4 and 8), thickened basement membrane (Figures 2 and 5), selective loss of thick myofilaments (Figure 6), an entangled meshwork of cytoskeletal filaments approximately 100 Å in diameter (Figure 5), and tubular aggregates (Figure 2, 6, 9, and

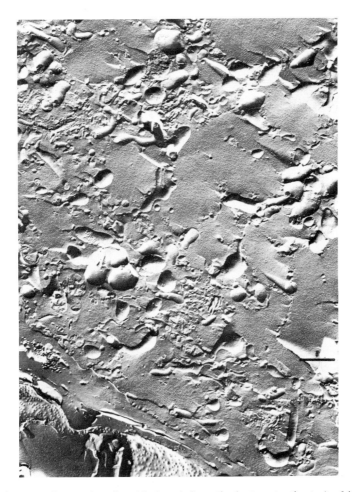

Figure 3. Freeze-fractured replica (shadowed from the bottom to the top) of left atrial cardiocyte from a 49-year-old female with mitral stenosis and atrial fibrillation. In the lower left, there is a capillary, then interstitial space with collagen fibers broken off; in the upper middle, a cardiocyte fractured and cleaved almost perpendicularly to the long axis of myofibrillar arrangements. The finest granulations represent broken off thick and thin myofilaments. Mitochondria are demonstrated as convex or concave large domes when cleavage runs along their outer membranes, or in forms that reveal their interior and their cristae when they are fractured. Large tubular structures with branchings and dilations appear to be transverse tubules, while the smaller and slender tubules represent sarcoplasmic reticulum, which in some regions show a close association with Golgi complexes. Numerous micropinocytotic vesicles or caveolae also are evident along the sarcolemma and capillary endothelial cell. An opening of a T tubule to extracellular space (lower left), comparable in its dimension to that of pinocytotic vesicles, is noted. × 9,600.

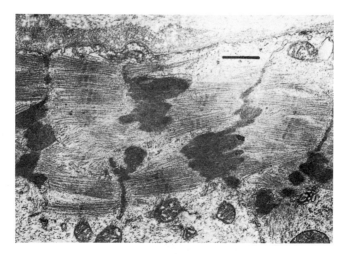

Figure 4. Portion of a cardiac muscle cell from a 41-year-old patient with combined mitral stenosis, regurgitation, and atrial fibrillation. Expanded Z lines, disorganized sarcomeres, and tubular aggregation (lower right in cross-section) are observed in addition to Z tubules and a small number of dwarf mitochondria. × 10,000.

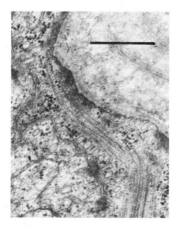

Figure 5. Portion of a moderately degenerated cardiocyte from the same patient as in Figure 1, showing subsarcolemmal dense plaques and corresponding focal thickenings of basal lamina that give an impression of the "hemidesmosomes" of epithelial cells. Disorganized thin filaments appear to be inserted into these subsarcolemmal plaques, the electron density of which appears to be identical to that of Z-line material. × 17,500.

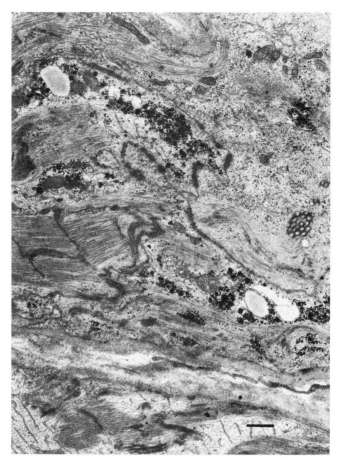

Figure 6. Four cardiocytes, from the same patient as for Figure 1, showing various stages of degeneration. In the lower cardiocyte with moderate to advanced degeneration, myofibrillar lysis, proliferating sarcotubules, entangled and whorled cytofilaments, and tubular aggregation are noted. The cell in the middle left appears in a stage of early degeneration with compact myofibrils and widened Z-line material extending over one sarcomere length, while cells in the middle right and upper region show a greatly advanced stage of degeneration characterized by myofibrillar disarray and tubular aggregates. × 7,500.

10). These features of severely degenerated cardiocytes appeared in patients with either mitral stenosis or mitral regurgitation, who had a prolonged clinical course and/or intractable congestive heart failure.

In atrial cardiocytes with lesser degrees of ultrastructural alterations, focal thickening of Z lines was fairly common with an accumulation of Z-line-like material in the subsarcolemmal region (Figures 4, 6, and 7). These subsarco-

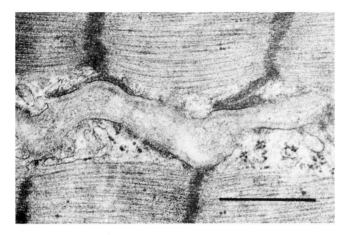

Figure 7. Portion of two atrial cardiocytes from a 30-year-old female patient with mitral regurgitation and atrial fibrillation. Subsarcolemmal plaques in continuity with somewhat widened Z lines. × 2,600.

lemmal plaques were frequently located directly opposite the focal thickenings of basement membrane (Figures 5 and 7). Proliferation of Z-line material into adjacent sarcomeres (Figures 2, 6, and 8) also was noted, associated with myofibrillar lysis; thick myofilaments were reduced in number, while the thin myofilaments were relatively increased (Figure 8). These thin filaments could not always be distinguished from leptofilaments of cytoskeleton (Virágh and

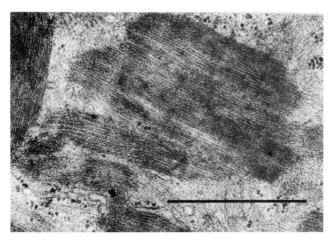

Figure 8. High power view of expanded Z-line material extending in different directions in a left atrial cardiocyte from a 27-year-old female with mitral stenosis. Note fine parallel striations at regular intervals of 200 Å. These expanded Z lines with striation and with continuous disorganized thin filaments are almost invariably flanked with sarcotubules. × 38,000.

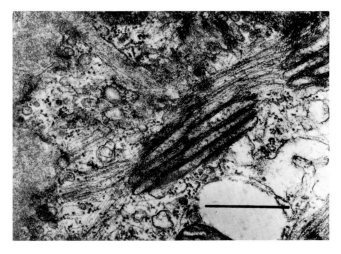

Figure 9. Portion of a moderately degenerated cardiocyte from a 41-year-old male with mitral stenosis and atrial fibrillation. Note tubular aggregates with adjacent proliferating sarcotubules. × 23,000.

Challice, 1969) and also were frequently observed beneath the subsarcolemmal plaques (Figure 5) and in association with intercalated discs (Figures 6 and 13).

Another remarkable feature was the presence of tubular aggregates in 70% of the cases (Figures 2 and 6). This structure was in close proximity to adjacent disorganized myofibrils and dilated sarcotubules (Figures 9 and 10). Although its appearance was not influenced by the presence or absence of atrial fibrillation, it

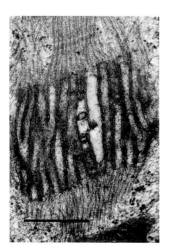

Figure 10. A tubular aggregation intervenes between successive sarcomeric pattern; their localization corresponds to that of Z lines. × 18,000.

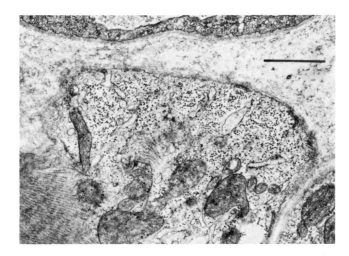

Figure 11. Portion of a left atrial cardiocyte from a 26-year-old female with mitral regurgitation and atrial fibrillation. A small tubule in the upper left region opens to the extracellular space, suggesting a T tubule in its development. Rough-surfaced endoplasmic reticulum is in the vicinity. × 17,000.

appeared to be related to the severity and duration of the pathophysiological conditions.

Another striking feature in these atrial cardiocytes was the formation of caveolae of the sarcolemma (Figures 2 and 11), similar infoldings were noted at the nonspecialized regions of intercalated discs (Figures 12 and 13) and dilated T tubules. In some cases, these caveolae were continuous with tubular invaginations of sarcolemma (Figure 11), suggesting the early formation of T tubules lacking basement membrane (Ishikawa, 1968). The formations of caveolae or micropinocytosis also may contribute to an increase in the effective surface area of these degenerated cells. Although the openings of T tubules to the sarcolemmal surface could not be distinguished from the caveolae by thin-sectioning, the results obtained by the application of freeze-replica to these cells did to some extent support the hypothesis that caveolae may be regarded as T-tubule precursors.

Small dwarfed, elongated, and irregularly shaped mitochondria increased in number where myofibrils had been lost. Morphologically, such mitochondria almost invariably had densely packed intact cristae. Giant mitochondria were occasionally apparent close to the nucleus. A close, membrane-to-membrane contact was observed at the outer mitochondrial membrane (Figure 14). A correlation between atrial fibrillation and dehiscence of the intercalated disc could not be established (Kawamura and James, 1971). In most cases, the intercalated disc appeared normal; dehiscence was observed rarely at the non-

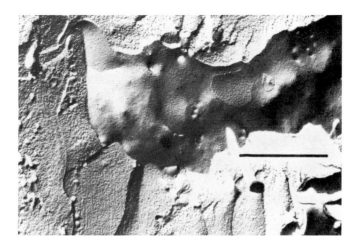

Figure 12. Freeze-fractured and etched replica (shadowed from the bottom to the top) of two adjacent cardiocytes from the same patient as in Figure 3. Extracellular space is seen on the left, and a two-dimensional display of an intercalated disc is in the middle portion. *En face* view of a gap junction is clearly evident. Also noted are micropinocytotic vesicles at the nonspecialized region of the disc. × 26,000.

specialized contact area (Figure 15). In one patient with mitral regurgitation as a result of an acutely perforated mitral cusp, dissociation occurred at the fasciae adherentes. Atrial specific granules appeared to decrease in number according to the extent of cellular degeneration, while dilated T tubules were frequently encountered (Figure 16).

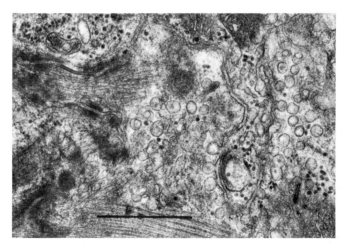

Figure 13. Intercalated disc with extensive convolution and profuse pinocytotic vesicles from the same patient as for Figure 1. × 26,000.

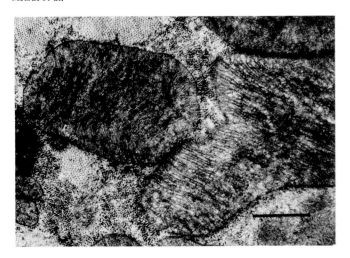

Figure 14. Giant mitochondria as large as 8 μm possessing densely packed cristae. Note the intimate membrane-to-membrane contact (from a 40-year-old male patient with mitral stenosis and atrial fibrillation). × 15,600.

DISCUSSION

It is generally accepted that the fine structural heterogeneity of atrial cardiocytes is related to their various functions (Berger and Rona, 1971a, 1971b). The somewhat hyperplastic Golgi complexes and rough ER, as well as the expanded Z lines, and their continuity with subsarcolemmal dense plaques suggesting early degeneration, also may be present in normal atrial cardiocytes of the rat (Hibbs

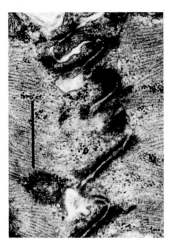

Figure 15. Dissociations at the nonspecialized region of an intercalated disc; same patient as for Figure 8. × 18,000.

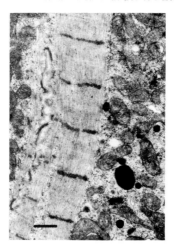

Figure 16. Portion of a hypertrophied cardiocyte from a 40-year-old male patient with mitral stenosis and aortic regurgitation but without atrial fibrillation. Note the "T-tubule" courses along the myofibril, forming couplings with the sarcoplasmic reticulum, and the atrial-specific granules, lysosomes, and small pleomorphic mitochondria. × 6,500.

and Ferrans, 1969) and of the cat (McNutt and Fawcett, 1969). Furthermore, widened Z lines related to sarcomerogenesis have been reported in hypertrophying cardiocytes (Bishop and Cole, 1969; Legato, 1970), as well as in degenerating cells, together with streaming and clumping of Z lines (Maron, Ferrans, and Roberts, 1975b). For these reasons, it is difficult to evaluate some of the subcellular alterations seen in diseased human atrial cardiocytes.

The wide spectrum of ultrastructural alterations, as seen in this study, has rarely been demonstrated in human atrial myocardium from patients with mitral valvular disease (Kawamura *et al.*, 1969; Roy, Dorais, and Morin, 1972; Fenoglio and Wagner, 1973). While quite identical observations were made in ventricular cardiocytes from patients with aortic valvular disease (Maron, Ferrans, and Roberts, 1975a, 1975b), degenerative changes in the atrial cardiac muscle described herein were more common. As our patients with mitral regurgitation were relatively younger and have had a shorter clinical course before surgery than do those patients with mitral stenosis, the hemodynamic effect subsequent to volume-overloading on the myocardium appears to be more potent than that of pressure-overloading. This interpretation is in agreement with findings of Maron, Ferrans, and Roberts concerning aortic valvular diseases.

Tubular aggregates were first reported in the human atrial myocardium by Kawamura *et al.* (1969), briefly mentioned by Roy, Dorais, and Morin (1972), described in more detail by Mitsui *et al.* (1975), and recently discussed by Thiedemann and Ferrans (1976). Maron and Ferrans (1974) observed identical structures in ventricular cardiac muscle cells in severely diseased human ventricles. Tubular aggregates have never been reported in experimental animals in association with myocardial hypertrophy and degeneration. The higher incidence of tubular aggregation in human atrial cardiocytes as compared to that noted in ventricular cardiac muscle cells indicates the possibility that this adaptive or degenerative response may be associated with a rather low grade of cellular organization of atrial cardiocytes or their fine structural heterogeneity. The functional significance of this structure, however, remains to be elucidated. The intimate association of tubular aggregates with proliferating sarcoplasmic reticulum and disorganized myofibrils with expanded Z-line material suggests that this structure may represent mismatched assembly or patchwork of contractile filaments subsequent to pathological conditions; atrial fibrillation by uncoordinated contraction of high frequency in different portions of a single cell may be an important initiating condition.

In hypertrophying and degenerating atrial cardiocytes, it appeared that T tubules were laid down *de novo* as a consequence of intense activity of micropinocytosis or caveolation of the sarcolemma (Ishikawa, 1968; Forssmann and Giradier, 1970). With respect to atrial specific granules, numerous comprehensive studies have been conducted (Bencosme and Berger, 1971) without any definitive conclusion as to their functional role. This study suggests that the number of these granules appeared to be directly proportional to the grade of hyperplastic Golgi complexes.

The observations concerning diseased human atrial cardiocytes made herein provide a model for future studies on the cytopathological aspects of human heart disease.

Acknowledgment Thanks are due to M. Ohara, Kyoto University, for assistance in preparing this manuscript.

REFERENCES

BENCOSME, S. A., and BERGER, J. M. 1971. Specific granules in mammalian and non-mammalian vertebrate cardiocytes. In E. Bajusz and G. Jasmin (eds.), Functional Morphology of the Heart. S. Karger, Basel.

BERGER, J. M., and BENCOSME, S. A. 1971. Fine structural cytochemistry of granules in atrial cardiocytes. J. Mol. Cell. Cardiol. 3:111–124.

BERGER, J. M., and RONA, G. 1971a. Functional and fine structural heterogeneity of atrial cardiocytes. *In* E. Bajusz and G. Jasmin (eds.), Functional Morphology of the Heart, pp. 540–590. S. Karger, Basel.

BERGER, J. M., and RONA, G. 1971b. Fine structure of extra-nodal transitional cardiocytes in rat left atrium. J. Mol. Cell. Cardiol. 2:181–185.

BISHOP, S. P., and COLE, C. R. 1969. Ultrastructural changes in the canine myocardium with right ventricular hypertrophy and congestive heart failure. Lab. Invest. 20: 219–229.

DUSEK, J., BOUTET, M., and RONA, G. 1973. Ultrastructural changes in isoproterenol-induced atrial necrosis. *In* E. Bajusz and G. Rona (eds.), Recent Advances in Studies on

Cardiac Structure and Metabolism. Vol. 2: Cardiomyopathies, pp. 423–432. University Park Press, Baltimore.

FENOGLIO, J. J., Jr., and WAGNER, B. M. 1973. Studies in rheumatic fever. VI. Ultrastructure of chronic rheumatic heart disease. Am. J. Pathol. 73:623–636.

FORSSMANN, W. G., and GIRADIER, L. 1970. A study of the T system in rat heart. J. Cell Biol. 44:1–19.

HIBBS, R. G., and FERRANS, V. J. 1969. An ultrastructural and histochemical study of rat atrial myocardium. Am. J. Anat. 124:251–280.

ISHIKAWA, H. 1968. Formation of elaborate networks of T system tubules in cultured skeletal muscle with special reference to the T system formation. J. Cell Biol. 38:51–66.

KAWAMURA, K., and JAMES, T. N. 1971. Comparative ultrastructure of cellular junctions in working myocardium and the conduction system under normal and pathologic conditions. J. Mol. Cell. Cardiol. 3:31–60.

KAWAMURA, K., MITSUI, H., HAYASHI, K., NOHARA, Y., TAKAYASU, M., HIGASA, Y., KOIE, H., TSUSHIMI, K., and ABE, H. 1969. Electron microscope studies of the human heart. III. The left atrial myocardium in mitral valvular diseases. Jpn. Circ. J. 33(abstr.):1141.

LEGATO, M. J. 1970. Sarcomerogenesis in human myocardium. J. Mol. Cell. Cardiol. 1:425–437.

McNUTT, N. S., and FAWCETT, D. W. 1969. The ultrastructure of cat myocardium. II. Atrial Muscle. J. Cell Biol. 42:46–67.

MARON, B. J., and FERRANS, V. J. 1974. Aggregates of tubules in human cardiac muscle cells. J. Mol. Cell. Cardiol. 6:249–264.

MARON, B. J., FERRANS, V. J., and ROBERTS, W. C. 1975a. Myocardial ultrastructure in patients with chronic aortic valve disease. Am. J. Cardiol. 35:725–739.

MARON, B. J., FERRANS, V. J., and ROBERTS, W. C. 1975b. Ultrastructural features of degenerated cardiac muscle cells in patients with cardiac hypertrophy. Am. J. Pathol. 79:387–434.

MITSUI, H., KAWAMURA, K., ISHIZAWA, K., OMAE, M., and KAWAI, C. 1975. "Tubular Aggregates" in human atrial myocardial cells. J. Clin. Electron Microscopy 8:311–312.

RONA, G., CHAPPEL, C. I., and KAHN, D. S. 1962. The pathogenesis of atrial infarction. Experimental data. Am. J. Pathol. 41:455–466.

ROY, P. E., DORAIS, J., and MORIN, P. J. 1972. Les foyers de nécrose intracellulaire focale dans le muscle cardiaque humain. Ann. Anat. Pathol. (Paris) 17:39–51.

SIMPSON, F. O., and RAYNS, D. G. 1968. The relationship between the transverse tubular system and other tubules at the Z disc level of myocardial cells in the ferret. Am. J. Anat. 122:193–208.

SOMMER, J. R., and WAUGH, R. A. 1976. The ultrastructure of the mammalian cardiac muscle cell—with special emphasis on the tubular membrane systems. Am. J. Pathol. 82:192–232.

THIEDEMANN, K. U., and FERRANS, V. J. 1976. Ultrastructure of sarcoplasmic reticulum in atrial myocardium of patients with mitral valvular disease. Am. J. Pathol. 83:1–38.

VIRÁGH, S., and CHALLICE, C. E. 1969. Variations in filamentous and fibrillar organization, and associated sarcolemmal structures, in cells of the normal mammalian heart. J. Ultrastruct. Res. 28:321–334.

Mailing address:
H. Mitsui, M.D.,
Third Division, Department of Internal Medicine,
Kyoto University, Faculty of Medicine,
Kyoto 606 (Japan).

Cardiomyopathies

Recent Advances in Studies on
Cardiac Structure and Metabolism, Volume 12
Cardiac Adaptation
Edited by T. Kobayashi, Y. Ito, and G. Rona
Copyright 1978 University Park Press Baltimore

CHARACTERIZATION OF MYOSIN FROM PATIENTS WITH ASYMMETRIC SEPTAL HYPERTROPHY

B. J. MARON, V. J. FERRANS, and R. S. ADELSTEIN

Cardiology Branch and the Section of Pathology,
National Heart and Lung Institute,
National Institutes of Health, Bethesda, Maryland, USA

SUMMARY

Human cardiac myosin isolated from operatively obtained samples of ventricular septum and left ventricular free wall of patients with asymmetric septal hypertrophy (ASH) was compared, with respect to structural and enzymatic properties, to myosin isolated from hearts of patients without heart disease. The following parameters were studied: 1) activation of myosin ATPase activity by K^+-EDTA and Ca^{2+}, 2) molecular weight of the heavy and light chains of myosin as determined by electrophoretic migration in SDS-polyacrylamide gels, and 3) ability to form bipolar aggregates at low ionic strength, as examined by electron microscopy. No difference was present in any of these parameters between human cardiac myosin from patients with ASH and from patients without heart disease. Thus, the genetic defect present in patients with ASH is not expressed in the particular structural and functional characteristics of myosin evaluated in this study.

INTRODUCTION

Asymmetric septal hypertrophy (ASH, hypertrophic cardiomyopathy) is a genetically determined cardiac disease that is transmitted as an autosomal dominant trait (Clark, Henry, and Epstein, 1973) and is characterized by disproportionate thickening of the ventricular septum with respect to the left ventricular free wall (Clark, Henry, and Epstein, 1973). Hypertrophied and bizarrely-shaped cardiac muscle cells arranged in a disorganized fashion are the characteristic histological feature of the ventricular septum of virtually all patients with ASH (Ferrans, Morrow, and Roberts, 1972; Maron *et al.,* 1974). These disorganized cardiac muscle cells presumably are a morphological expression of the genetic defect in ASH (Maron *et al.,* 1974). Disorganized cardiac muscle cells are widely distributed in the left ventricular free wall of patients without outflow obstruction, but are rarely present in the ventricular free walls of patients with obstruction (Maron *et al.,* 1974).

With these morphological observations in mind, the present study was undertaken to determine whether the biochemical and structural characteristics of myosin isolated from the ventricular septum of patients with obstructive ASH differ from those of myosin isolated from the left ventricular free wall of the same patients or from the left ventricle of patients without heart disease.

MATERIALS AND METHODS

Patient Selection and Clinical Data

The biochemical studies reported in this chapter are based on analyses of myocardium obtained from 14 patients with obstructive ASH and from four patients without heart disease. The clinical diagnosis of ASH was confirmed in each of the 14 patients by cardiac catheterization, by echocardiography (Clark, Henry, and Epstein, 1973) and at operation. The age of the patients ranged from 20 to 71 years (average 42); seven were men and seven were women. Each of the four patients used as controls in this study died of noncardiac diseases and had no evidence of heart disease at necropsy.

Selection of Tissue

In each patient with ASH, myocardium was taken at the time of left ventricular myotomy-myectomy. This tissue (0.5–2.7 g) was resected from the cephalad portion of the left side of the ventricular septum. Biopsies (0.2–0.5 g) of the left ventricular free wall were taken in six patients. Tissue from the four patients without heart disease was obtained from the left ventricular free wall, 6–20 hr after death.

Preparation of Actomyosin

Each gram of muscle was suspended in 2 ml of an ice-cold extracting buffer containing 15 mM Tris (hydroxy methyl) amino methane hydrochloride (Tris-HCl) (pH 7.5), 0.5 M KCl, 1 mM ethylenediaminetetraacetate (EDTA), and 5 mM dithiothreitol (DTT) and was homogenized for 1 min. The homogenized muscle was suspended in the same extracting buffer for an additional 10 min. The extract was sedimented at $24{,}000 \times g$ for 10 min. The supernatant was decanted, the concentration of KCl was lowered to 0.1 M by dilution with an ice-cold solution of 1 mM EDTA, and the pH was adjusted to 6.3. This solution was sedimented and the resulting precipitate of cardiac actomyosin was resuspended in a volume of the extracting buffer sufficient to provide a protein concentration of 8–12 mg/ml at pH 7.3.

Purification of Myosin

$MgCl_2$ and ATP were added to preparations of cardiac actomyosin to a final concentration of 5 mM each, at pH 7.3. Two fractions were then obtained from the actomyosin by the addition of saturated ammonium sulfate (0–30% and 30–50% saturation). Final purification of myosin was obtained by chromatography of the 30–50% ammonium sulfate fraction on a 1.9 × 82-cm column of Sepharose 4B equilibrated with a solution containing 15 mM Tris-HCl buffer (pH 7.5), 0.5 M KCl, 1 mM EDTA, and 5 mM DTT. The resulting fractions of effluent volume were assayed for ATPase activity (Adelstein, Pollard, and Kuehl, 1971). The fractions with peak ATPase activity were pooled for characterization of myosin ATPase activity (in the presence of EDTA, Ca^{2+}, or Mg^{2+}) and for gel electrophoresis.

Gel Electrophoresis

Polyacrylamide-SDS gel electrophoresis was performed by the method of Fairbanks, Steck, and Wallach (1971). Electrophoresis was performed on 40–80-μg protein samples for about 90 min. The gels were stained with Coomassie brilliant blue.

Determination of ATPase Activity of Myosin

The ATPase activity of myosin was determined in the four patients without heart disease and in 12 of the 14 patients with ASH. Assays were performed at $37°C$ in the presence of 0.5 M KCl and 2 mM ATP, in addition to either 2 mM EDTA, 10 mM $CaCl_2$, or 5 mM $MgCl_2$. Inorganic phosphate production was determined by a modification of the method of Martin and Doty (1949). Molecular weights of proteins were determined by polyacrylamide-SDS gel electrophoresis according to the method of Weber and Osborn (1969).

Preparation of Bipolar Aggregates of Myosin Molecules

Aliquots of purified myosin were diluted either slowly by dialysis (18 hr) against a buffer containing 10 mM Tris-HCl (pH 7.0), 0.1 M KCl, 1 mM $MgCl_2$, and 2.5 mM DTT, or diluted rapidly by addition of four volumes of water. After dilution, the protein solution was negatively stained with 1% uranyl acetate by the method of Huxley (1963) and examined with an electron microscope.

RESULTS

Myosin ATPase Activity

Data on the myosin ATPase activities of specimens analyzed in this study are summarized in Table 1. The K^+-EDTA-activated ATPase activity in 12 specimens of ventricular septum from patients with ASH (mean 1.5 ± 0.3 μmol of inorganic phosphate released per mg of protein per min) did not differ significantly from that obtained in patients without heart disease (mean 1.4 ± 0.1). Furthermore, the K^+-EDTA-activated myosin ATPase activity in four specimens of left ventricular free wall from patients with ASH (mean 1.4 ± 0.6 μmol of inorganic phosphate released per mg of protein per min) did not differ significantly from that of myosin from the ventricular septum of the same patients (1.6 ± 0.4). In

Table 1. ATPase activity of myosin from patients with ASH and from patients without heart disease

| Condition | Number of patients | Specific activity[a] | | | K+-EDTA-ATPase Ca2+-ATPase ratio (mean) |
		K+-EDTA-ATPase (mean ± S.D.)	Ca2+-ATPase (mean ± S.D.)	Mg2+-ATPase	
ASH					
Ventricular septum	12	1.5 ± 0.3	0.3 ± 0.1	< 0.01	5.0
LV free wall[b]	4	1.4 ± 0.6	0.3 ± 0.3	< 0.01	5.0
Normal	4	1.4 ± 0.1	0.3 ± 0.1	< 0.01	4.5

[a]Expressed in μmol of inorganic phosphate released per mg of protein per min.
[b]Includes left ventricular apex in three patients and the left ventricular posterior papillary muscle in one patient.
LV = left ventricular.

320

all specimens of myosin, Ca^{2+}-activated ATPase activity was significantly lower than K$^+$-EDTA-activated ATPase activity (Table 1).

Polyacrylamide-SDS Gel Electrophoresis

Polyacrylamide-SDS gel electrophoresis was performed on preparations of cardiac actomyosin, purified myosin, or both, from patients with ASH and from patients without heart disease (Figures 1–3). Preparations of actomyosin showed a characteristic pattern of bands (Figure 1) that included: 1) a band at 200,000

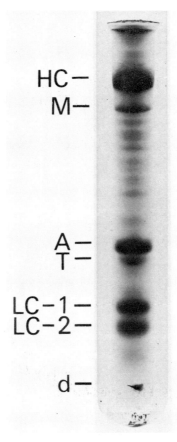

Figure 1. Pattern of peptide bands obtained from actomyosin prepared from the ventricular septum of a 71-year-old woman with obstructive ASH. 5% polyacrylamide-1% SDS gel. Electrophoretic migration was from top to bottom. HC = heavy chain of myosin; M = M-protein; A = actin; T = tropomyosin; LC-1 = light chain of myosin (molecular weight of 25,000 daltons); LC-2 = light chain of myosin (molecular weight of 20,000 daltons); d = tracking dye. (Reprinted with permission of the American Heart Association (Maron, Ferrans, and Adelstein, 1977).)

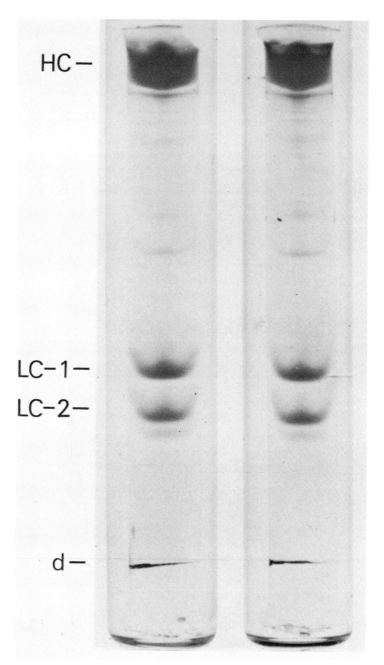

Figure 2. Patterns of peptide bands of purified human cardiac myosin after electrophoresis in 7.5% polyacrylamide-1% SDS gels. Left: preparation from ventricular septum of a 62-year-old man with obstructive ASH. Right: preparation from left ventricular free wall of a patient without heart disease. Electrophoretic migration was from top to bottom. HC = heavy chain of myosin; LC-1 = light chain of myosin (molecular weight of 25,000 daltons); LC-2 = light chain of myosin (molecular weight of 20,000 daltons); d = tracking dye. Trace amounts of other proteins, that were not identified, also are present in both gels. (Reprinted with permission of the American Heart Association (Maron, Ferrans, and Adelstein, 1977).)

daltons representing the heavy chains of myosin, 2) a band at 25,000 daltons and a band at 20,000 daltons representing the two different light chains of myosin, and 3) bands representing other contractile proteins including M-protein (molecular weight 165,000 daltons), actin (44,000 daltons), and tropomyosin (subunit 35,000 daltons). Polyacrylamide-SDS gel electrophoresis of purified preparations of myosin showed only the heavy and light chains of myosin (Figure 2). The patterns of bands in polyacrylamide-SDS gels (using preparations

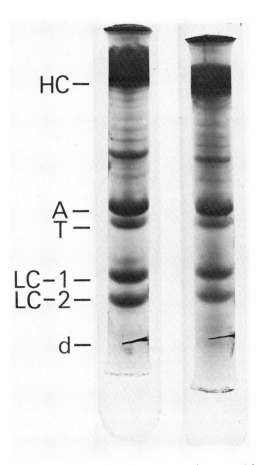

Figure 3. Patterns of peptide bands obtained from actomyosin prepared from a 55-year-old man with obstructive ASH. 7.5% polyacrylamide-1% SDS gels. Left: preparation from ventricular septum. Right: preparation from left ventricular free wall. Electrophoretic migration was from top to bottom. HC = heavy chain of myosin; A = actin; T = tropomyosin; LC-1 = light chain of myosin (molecular weight of 25,000 daltons); LC-2 = light chain of myosin (molecular weight of 20,000 daltons); d = tracking dye. Other relatively indistinct bands, that were not definitively identified, also were present. (Reprinted with permission of the American Heart Association (Maron, Ferrans, and Adelstein, 1977).)

of actomyosin or purified myosin) were similar for the ventricular septum and the left ventricular free wall of patients with ASH (figure 3) and for the left ventricular free wall of patients without heart disease (Figure 2).

Bipolar Aggregates of Myosin Molecules

Bipolar aggregates of myosin molecules formed when the ionic strength of purified preparations of cardiac myosin was lowered from a concentration of 0.5 M KCl to 0.1 M KCl (Figure 4). These aggregates ranged from 4,000 Å to 1 μm in length and from 100 to 300 Å in width. They often showed a bare central shaft area. Lateral projections were, however, prominent at the ("tufted") ends of the aggregates (Figure 4A, B, E, and F). Bipolar aggregates with these features were most commonly observed when the ionic strength of the purified myosin solution was rapidly lowered. When the ionic strength of the purified myosin solution was slowly lowered, the aggregates were generally longer and more spindle-shaped (Figure 4C and D). There were no apparent differences in the morphological features of aggregates of myosin molecules formed in preparations from patients with ASH or from patients without heart disease.

DISCUSSION

The results of this study show that myosin from the ventricular septum of patients with obstructive ASH and myosin obtained from the left ventricular free wall of patients with ASH or patients without heart disease do not differ significantly in the following parameters: 1) ATPase activity, 2) molecular weights of the myosin subunits, as determined by electrophoresis in polyacrylamide-SDS gels, and 3) morphological features of bipolar aggregates of myosin molecules. Our investigation represents the first detailed biochemical study of purified human cardiac myosin from patients with ASH. In agreement with the findings of others (Klotz *et al.*, 1975), we also have shown that purified myosin, with preservation of ATPase activity, can be obtained from normal human cardiac muscle for up to 20 hours after death. It was of concern to us initially that myosin isolated from hearts obtained postmortem would be degraded and oxidized to such an extent that it would be unsuitable for comparison with myosin isolated from operatively obtained specimens. However, using the procedures outlined in this study, myosin that showed no evidence of proteolysis or oxidation of sulfhydryl groups was purified from postmortem tissue. The absence of significant proteolysis was confirmed by the fact that little or no degraded myosin was evident after electrophoresis of myosin in SDS-polyacrylamide gels (see Figure 2). Furthermore, the ratio of the K^+-EDTA-activated myosin ATPase activity to the Ca^{2+}-activated myosin ATPase activity was the same for myosin isolated from postmortem tissue of patients without heart

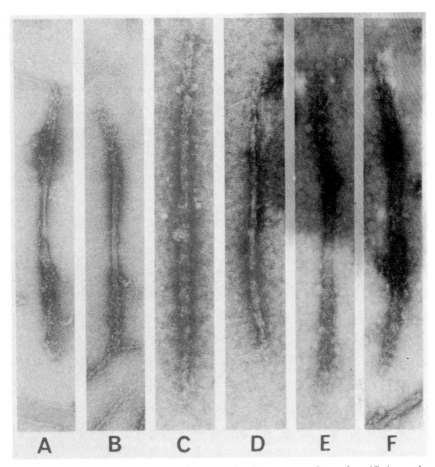

Figure 4. Bipolar aggregates of myosin molecules from preparations of purified myosin. From ventricular septum of a 28-year-old woman with obstructive ASH (A–D) and from left ventricular free wall from a patient without heart disease (E and F). Magnification X 150,000 for each micrograph. A and B: bipolar aggregates, formed when the concentration of KCl is rapidly lowered from 0.5 M to 0.1 M, have characteristic bare central zone, irregular lateral projections along the rest of the shaft, and tufted ends. C: Longer, spindle-shaped aggregate, formed when concentration of KCl is slowly reduced from 0.5 M to 0.1 M by dialysis. D: Shorter, spindle-shaped aggregate without bare central zone or projections, formed when concentration of KCl is slowly reduced from 0.5 M to 0.1 M by dialysis. E and F: Bipolar aggregates with bare central zone and irregular lateral projections along the remainder of the shaft, formed when the concentration of KCl is rapidly reduced from 0.5 M to 0.1 M. (Reprinted by permission of the American Heart Association, Inc. (Maron, Ferrans, and Adelstein, 1977).)

disease and from operatively obtained specimens from patients with ASH. This finding indicated that oxidation of sulfhydryl groups did not occur in our preparations, because oxidation usually results in an increase in the Ca^{2+}-activated myosin ATPase activity and a decrease in the K^+-EDTA-activated myosin ATPase activity (Katz, 1970).

REFERENCES

ADELSTEIN, R. S., POLLARD, T. D., and KUEHL, W. M. 1971. Isolation and characterization of myosin and two myosin fragments from human blood platelets. Proc. Natl. Acad. Sci. USA 68:2703–2707.

CLARK, C. E., HENRY, W. L., and EPSTEIN, S. E. 1973. Familial prevalence and genetic transmission of idiopathic hypertrophic subaortic stenosis. N. Engl. J. Med. 289: 709–714.

FAIRBANKS, G., STECK, T. L., and WALLACH, D. F. H. 1971. Electrophoretic analysis of the major polypeptides of the human erythrocyte membrane. Biochemistry 10: 2606–2617.

FERRANS, V. J., MORROW, A. G., and ROBERTS, W. C. 1972. Myocardial ultrastructure in idiopathic hypertrophic subaortic stenosis. A study of operatively excised left ventricular outflow tract muscle in 14 patients. Circulation 45: 769–792.

HUXLEY, H. E. 1963. Electron microscope studies on the structure of natural and synthetic protein filaments from striated muscle. J. Mol. Biol. 7:281–308.

KATZ, A. M. 1970. Contractile proteins of the heart. Physiol. Rev. 50:63–158.

KLOTZ, C., AUMONT, M. C., LEGER, J. J., and SWYNGHEDAUW, B. 1975. Human cardiac myosin ATPase and light subunits. A comparative study. Biochim. Biophys. Acta 386:461–469.

MARON, B. J., FERRANS, V. J., and ADELSTEIN, R. S. 1977. Isolation and characterization of myosin from subjects with asymmetric septal hypertrophy. Circ. Res. 40: 468–473.

MARON, B. J., FERRANS, V. J., HENRY, W. L., CLARK, C. E., REDWOOD, D. R., ROBERTS, W. C., MORROW, A. G., and EPSTEIN, S. E. 1974. Differences in distribution of myocardial abnormalities in patients with obstructive and nonobstructive asymmetric septal hypertrophy (ASH): Light and electron microscopic findings. Circulation 50:436–446.

MARTIN, J. B., and DOTY, D. M. 1949. Determination of inorganic phosphate. Modification of isobutyl alcohol procedure. Anal. Chem. 21:965–967.

WEBER, K., and OSBORN, M. 1969. Reliability of molecular weight determinations by dodecyl sulfate-polyacrylamide gel electrophoresis. J. Biol. Chem. 244:4406–4412.

Mailing address:
Barry J. Maron, M.D.,
Cardiology Branch, National Heart and Lung Institute,
Building 10, Room 7B–15, Bethesda, Maryland 20014 (USA).

Recent Advances in Studies on
Cardiac Structure and Metabolism, Volume 12
Cardiac Adaptation
Edited by T. Kobayashi, Y. Ito, and G. Rona
Copyright 1978 University Park Press Baltimore

INTERRELATION OF LEFT VENTRICULAR FUNCTION AND MYOCARDIAL ULTRASTRUCTURE AS ASSESSED BY ENDOMYOCARDIAL BIOPSY: COMPARATIVE STUDY OF HYPERTROPHIC AND CONGESTIVE CARDIOMYOPATHIES

M. SEKIGUCHI, K. HAZE, M. HIROE,
S. KONNO, and K. HIROSAWA

Heart Institute of Japan,
Tokyo Women's Medical College,
Tokyo, Japan

SUMMARY

Fifty-eight patients with idiopathic cardiomyopathy, 38 with hypertrophic cardiomyopathy, and 20 with congestive cardiomyopathy underwent left ventriculography, and 13 parameters of left ventricular function were assessed. The hemodynamics were correlated with the ultrastructural features and with the patients' prognoses.

Of these 58 cases, 43 underwent myocardial biopsy from either the right and/or the left ventricle. Myocardial ultrastructure was evaluated both qualitatively and quantitatively along two dimensions, an ultrastructural pathology index with 13 parameters and a contractility failure index, composed of a cluster of six of the 13. Eight of the 13 dimensions of left ventricular function studies differentiated hypertrophic and congestive cardiomyopathy at a significant level. Death rate was significantly high in congestive cardiomyopathy (53%), while, in hypertrophic cardiomyopathy, only one death was recorded.

Ejection fraction and mean circumferential shortening rate, the two dimensions of systolic power failure, were significantly reduced in congestive cardiomyopathy and highly correlated with severe pathology as indicated by the ultrastructural pathology index and the contractility failure index.

In conclusion, six ultrastructural dimensions, i.e., myofibrillar fragmentation, swollen mitochondria with cristolysis, widened intercalcated discs, deposition of abnormal substances, cellular edema, and swollen capillaries are cogent indicators of pathology and are contributing factors in systolic pump failure.

INTRODUCTION

Since endomyocardial biopsy was developed in 1962 by Konno (Konno, Sekiguchi, and Sakakibara, 1971), it has proved to be a safe and dependable method

This work was supported by a grant from the Japanese Ministry of Health and Welfare for the study of cardiomyopathy.

for establishing diagnosis, as well as for assessing the disease condition of patients with cardiomyopathy (Sekiguchi and Konno, 1969; Sekiguchi, 1974, in preparation).

Idiopathic cardiomyopathy has been classified in two groups, i.e., hypertrophic and congestive cardiomyopathy (HCM and COCM), by cardiologists (Goodwin and Oakley, 1972). However, the correlative study of hemodynamics, myocardial pathology, especially as assessed by ultrastructural techniques, and patient prognosis has not been attempted.

Therefore, this survey was conducted to determine the most effective way of discriminating between hypertrophic and congestive cardiomyopathy by the integrated analysis of the ultrastructural investigation of the myocardium, left ventricular function studies, and the patients' prognoses. We have investigated more than 200 cases of myocardial biopsy, taken according to the method of Konno by electron microscope.

MATERIALS AND METHODS

In this study, biopsied myocardial specimens from both the right and left ventricles in 35 cases of hypertrophic and 35 cases of congestive cardiomyopathy were subjected to our battery of analytic procedures. For the control study, biopsied mycardium from various kinds of congenital and valvular heart diseases (40 cases) was ultilized.

The salient features, which consist of 13 ultrastructural findings and which were evaluated as being of equal importance, were assigned a quantitative value such as +++(3), ++(2), +(1), and –(0). By adding the values, a score specific to the severity of each disease category was obtained.

The 13 features, or parameters, were: 1) mitochondriosis, 2) mitochondrial change, 3) fragmentation and sparsity of myofibrils, 4) myofibrillar changes, 5) myofibrillar disarray, 6) changes in tubular structure, 7) increase in dense bodies and/or myelin figures, 8) increase in deposition of glycogen and/or other substances, 9) widening of the intercalated discs, 10) increase in RER and/or ribosomes, 11) cellular edema, 12) capillary edema, and 13) others, such as nuclear deformity.

The resulting pathological indices, aligned in order of decreasing magnitude, were as follows (Sekiguchi, in preparation): 1) idiopathic congestive cardiomyopathy (10.9), 2) idiopathic hypertrophic cardiomyopathy (9.0), 3) primary pulmonary hypertension (9.0), 4) tetralogy of Fallot (8.0), 5) mitral stenosis (7.0), 6) patent ductus arteriosus with pulmonary hypertension (5.4), 7) pulmonary stenosis (4.8), 8) ventricular septal defect (4.0), and 9) atrial septal defect (3.0).

RESULTS AND DISCUSSION

It seemed that in cases of congenital heart disease with secondary hypertrophy of cardiac muscle cells, such as pulmonary stenosis, the ultrastructural pathology score was less important. We think that it may represent rather well the conspensatory stage of hypertrophy as suggested by Meerson (1965).

In order to visibly link the qualitative findings described below with these numerical or quantitative indices, Figure 1 was constructed.

In both HCM and COCM, mitochondriosis, mitochondrial change, myofibrillar fragmentation and sparsity, and other changes such as Z band changes were commonly found. In HCM, increase in glycogen deposition and disarray of myofibrils in the myocytes were more frequently observed, while, in COCM, widened intercalated discs, deposition of abnormal substances, cellular edema, and swollen capillaries were more commonly present.

The interrelation of left ventricular function and the myocardial ultrastructure, as assessed by endomyocardial biopsy, also was investigated. Fifty-eight patients with idiopathic cardiomyopathy, 38 with hypertrophic, and 20 with congestive cardiomyopathy, underwent left ventriculography, and 13 parameters of left ventricular function were assessed (Dodge *et al.,* 1960; Gorlin *et al.,* 1964; Kasser and Kennedy, 1969; Feild *et al.,* 1973). Ten parameters were useful in this study for differentiating COCM from HCM, e.g., end-systolic wall thickness, end-diastolic volume, end-systolic volume, ejection fraction, mean circumferential shortening rate (Gorlin *et al.,* 1964), mean systolic tensile force, stroke work index, stroke index, left ventricular mass, and the ratio of mass to end-diastolic

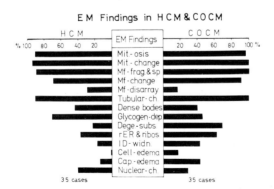

Figure 1. Incidence of electron microscopic parameters in hypertrophic (HCM) and congestive (COCM) cardiomyopathies. Mit. = mitochondrial; Mf = myofibrillar; frag. & sp = fragmentation and sparsity; ch. = change; Dege.-subs. = degenerative substance; widn. = widening.

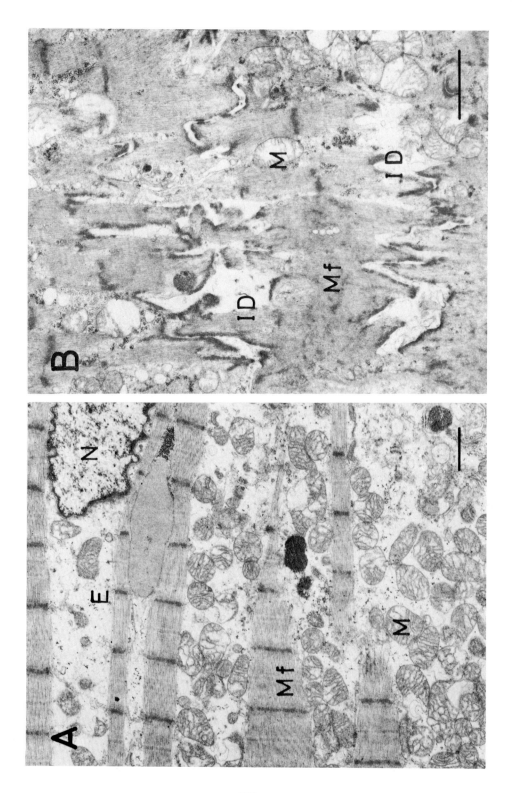

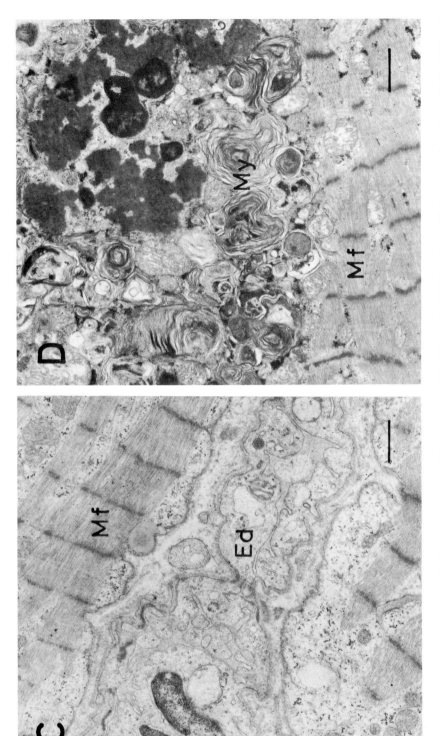

Figure 2. Examples of ultrastructural findings that may contribute to contractility failure. A: Cellular edema (E), fragmentation of myofibrils (Mf), and swelling of mitochondria (M) with cristolysis. × 12,000. B: Widening of the intercalated disc (ID). × 19,200. C: Capillary edema. × 12,000. D: Deposition of degenerative substances, in this case, myelin figures (My). × 12,000. Bars in each picture indicate 1 μm.

volume. The results of the ejection time index, left ventricular end-diastolic pressure, and cardiac index did not discriminate the two groups.

Of the total 43 cases, 33 patients underwent right ventricular biopsies, exclusively, and 10 had left ventricular biopsies exclusively, while in 10 both left- and right-sided biopsies were performed.

Biopsy specimens were evaluated quantitatively along two dimensions. The first was an index of pathology as assessed ultrastructurally using the parameters as described above, and the other was a contractility failure score composed of only six of the 13 dimensions. Artifacts were avoided by careful evaluation (Ferrans *et al.*, 1973). Those cases that showed marked interstitial fibrosis by light microscopy were excluded in order to eliminate other factors that might contribute to impaired ventricular function.

The six parameters were (Figure 2): 1) fragmentation of myofibrils, 2) swelling of mitochondria with cristolysis, 3) widening of the intercalated discs, 4) cellular edema, 5) capillary edema, and 6) deposition of degenerative substances. These six were selected as representing a contractility index because they apparently contributed to reduced contractile ability. Four separate grades of severity (+++, ++, +, −) also were applied to each of these parameters.

Figure 3 shows the results of a study that compared the myocardial ultrastructure in congestive and hypertrophic cardiomyopathies along two dimensions. It is to be noted that, of the 10 patients who died, one had HCM, and nine had COCM.

In the HCM group, 10 of the 26 cases (38%) had a total score exceeding 10. In the COCM group, by contrast, 12 of the 17 cases (70%) exceeded this level and nine of the 12 cases are known to have died.

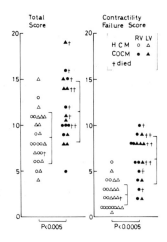

Figure 3. Severity of myocardial ultrastructural changes in hypertrophic and congestive cardiomyopathies.

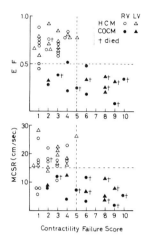

Figure 4. Relationship between left ventricular function and myocardial ultrastructure, which is assessed by contractility failure score. Total score: Calculated by the quantitative evaluation of 13 ultrastructural findings (see text). Contractility failure score: Calculated by the quantitative evaluation of six ultrastructural findings (see text and Figure 2). RV = right ventricular biopsy; LV = left ventricular biopsy; EF = ejection fraction; MCSR = mean circumferential shortening rate.

The contractility failure score showed a more obvious difference, that is, a score exceeding five occurred in 12 out of the 17 cases, and eight of the 12 died within the follow-up period of up to eight years.

As the ejection fraction (EF) and mean circumferential shortening rate (MCSR) gave the most representative results in this study, they are demonstrated in Figure 4.

Those cases that can be classified under 0.5 of EF showed a high contractility failure score and a high mortality rate. These cases numbered 10 out of 15, that is, they amounted to 67% as contrasted to only 2 out of the 26 (8%) in HCM.

The approach outlined in this chapter is still unrefined because of a host of measurement problems and because issues of validity and interrater (the rating among various investigators) reliability remain to be solved. Because the results were favorable and indicative, it is hoped that this study will aid others in their conceptualization and understanding of the cardiomyopathies.

Acknowledgment The authors extend their appreciation to Miss Barbara Levene who made the necessary English corrections.

REFERENCES

DODGE, H. T., SANDLER, H., BALLEW, D. W., and LORD, J. D. 1960. The use of biplane angiography for the measurement of left ventricular volume in man. Am. Heart J. 60: 762–776.

FEILD, B. J., BAXLEY, W. A., RUSSEL, R. O., HOOD, W. P. JR., HOLT, J. H., DOWLING, J. T., and RACKLEY, C. E. 1973. Left ventricular function and hypertrophy in cardiomyopathy with depressed ejection fraction. Circulation 4:1022–1031.

FERRANS, V. J., MASSUMI, R. A., SHUGOLL, G. I., ALI, N., and ROBERTS, W. C. 1973. Ultrastructural studies of myocardial biopsies in 45 patients with obstructive or congestive cardiomyopathy. *In* E. Bajusz and G. Rona (eds.), Recent Advances in Studies on Cardiac Structure and Metabolism. Vol. 2: Cardiomyopathies, pp. 231–272. University Park Press, Baltimore.

GOODWIN, J. F., and OAKLEY, C. M. 1972. The cardiomyopathies. Brit. Heart J. 34:545–552.

GORLIN, R., ROLETT, E. L., YURCHAK, P. M., ELLIOT, W. C., LANE, F. J., and LEVY, R. H. 1964. Left ventricular volume in man measured by thermodilution. J. Clin. Invest. 43:1203–1221.

KASSER, I. S., and KENNEDY, J. W. 1969. Measurement of left ventricular volumes in man by single-plane cineangiocardiography. Invest. Radiol. 4:83–90.

KONNO, S., SEKIGUCHI, M., and SAKAKIBARA, S. 1971. Catheter biopsy of the heart. Radiol. Clin. North Am. 9:491–510.

MEERSON, F. Z. 1965. A mechanism of hypertrophy and wear of the myocardium. Am. J. Cardiol. 15:755–760.

SEKIGUCHI, M., and KONNO, S. 1969. Histopathological differentiation employing endomyocardial biopsy in the clinical assessment of primary myocardial disease. Jpn. Heart J. 10:30–46.

SEKIGUCHI, M. 1974. Electron microscopical observations of the myocardium in patients with idiopathic cardiomyopathy using endomyocardial biopsy. J. Mol. Cell. Cardiol. 6:111–122.

SEKIGUCHI, M. Ultrastructural study of myocardial hypertrophy utilizing endomyocardial biopsy. In preparation.

Mailing address:
Morie Sekiguchi, M.D.,
Heart Institute of Japan, Tokyo Women's Medical College,
10 Kawada-cho, Shinjuku-ku, Tokyo, 162 (Japan).

Recent Advances in Studies on
Cardiac Structure and Metabolism, Volume 12
Cardiac Adaptation
Edited by T. Kobayashi, Y. Ito, and G. Rona
Copyright 1978 University Park Press Baltimore

ROLE OF ACETALDEHYDE IN THE PATHOGENESIS
OF ALCOHOLIC CARDIOMYOPATHY

M. NAGANO, S. KAGEYAMA, M. SHIMIZU,
N. SAITO, S. ANAZAWA, and S. TOMIZUKA

Department of Internal Medicine, The Jikei University
School of Medicine, Tokyo, Japan

SUMMARY

Rats given both ethanol and tolbutamide showed decreased oxidative phosphorylation of the myocardial mitochondria as compared with rats given only ethanol. There were no differences in ethanol consumption and blood ethanol levels between the two groups. The concentration of acetaldehyde tended to be higher in rats given both ethanol and tolbutamide than in rats given ethanol alone. It is concluded that acetaldehyde plays a more important role in the production of alcoholic cardiomyopathy than does ethanol itself.

INTRODUCTION

Cardiomyopathy is sometimes seen in chronic alcoholic patients, and it has been reported that, in experimental animals, chronic alcohol intake can cause myocardial damage, especially the disturbance of mitochondria. However, whether it is caused by ethanol itself, its metabolites, or other factors remains to be elucidated. We investigated the pathogenesis of alcoholic cardiomyopathy by determination of enzyme activities and oxidative phosphorylation of mitochondria of rat myocardium. Rats were given ethanol and the oral hypoglycemic agent, tolbutamide, which has an Antabuse effect, or acetaldehyde dehydrogenase inhibitor, in order to induce a high concentration of acetaldehyde in the blood.

MATERIALS AND METHODS

The experiment was carried out in four groups of 4-week-old male Wistar rats. Ethanol and tolbutamide were given freely in drinking water as the rats' only liquid intake. Group A was given 10% ethanol, Group B, 200 mg/liter of tolbutamide, and Group C, 10% ethanol and 300 mg/liter of tolbutamide. The control group was given water. The dose of tolbutamide per kg body weight was equivalent to the therapeutic dose for humans. Rats were fed a commercial laboratory diet. There was no difference in body weight increase among the groups. The average intake of ethanol in Groups A and C was 700 mg/100 g body weight/day. The average intake of tolbutamide in Groups B and C was 2.0 mg/100 g body weight/day. The following enzymes of the left ventricular muscle were measured between the 8th and the 20th week after beginning ingestion of the following drugs: 1) in glycolysis, HK, PFK, ALD, α-GPDH, GAPDH, Enolase, PK, and LDH, 2) in the trichoracetic (TCA) cycle, NADP-ICDH, and MDH, 3) in the pentose phosphate (PPh) cycle, G-6-PDH and 6-PGDH, and 4) of transaminases, GOT and GPT. Between the 26th and the 36th week, mitochondria of rat myocardium were obtained by the procedure as previously described (Nagano *et al.*, 1975).

RESULTS

Enzymes

The enzyme activities that were determined are illustrated in Figures 1, 2, 3, and 4. Group C, which was given both ethanol and tolbutamide, showed an 18% increase in the activity of HK, compared to the control group. There were no statistically significant changes in other enzymes among groups.

Oxidative Phosphorylation of Mitochondria

The ADP/O ratios and the respiratory control indices (RCI), with succinate and glutamate as the substrates, are illustrated in Figures 5 and 6. When succinate was the substrate, Group C showed a 17% decrease in ADP/O ratio and a 23% decrease in RCI, compared to the control group; Group A showed a 10% decrease in ADP/O ratio, compared to the control group. When glutamate was the substrate, Group C showed a 15% decrease in ADP/O ratio, compared to the control group.

DISCUSSION

There were no statistically significant changes in enzyme activities and oxidative phosphorylation of mitochondria among Groups A, B, and the control. In other words, rats given either ethanol or tolbutamide alone showed no significant changes, except that rats given only ethanol showed a decreased ADP/O ratio when succinate was the substrate.

On the other hand, there was decreased oxidative phosphorylation in rats given both ethanol and tolbutamide. With succinate as the substrate, the ADP/O ratio was decreased by 17% and the RCI was decreased by 23%. With glutamate as the substrate, the ADP/O ratio was decreased by 15%. Inhibition of oxidative phosphorylation, observed in ethanol-fed animals, was attributed to the direct

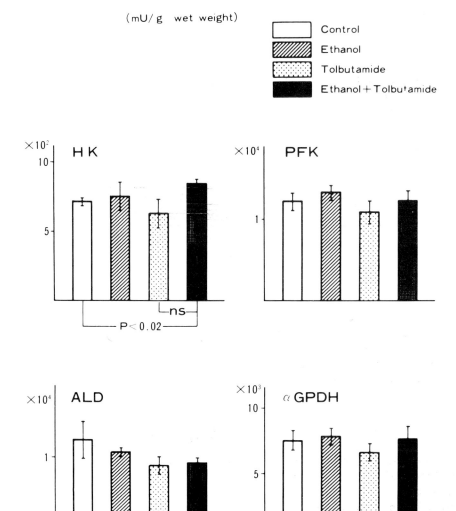

Figure 1. Enzyme activities in glycolysis (1).

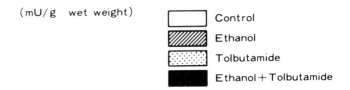

(mU/g   wet weight)

☐ Control
▧ Ethanol
⬚ Tolbutamide
■ Ethanol+Tolbutamide

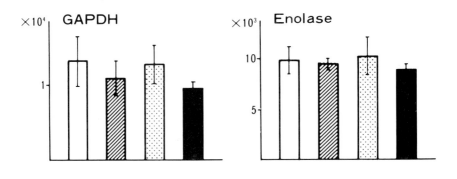

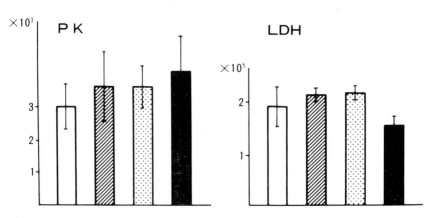

Figure 2. Enzyme activities in glycolysis (2).

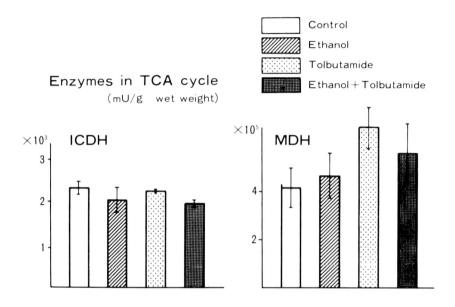

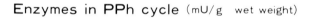

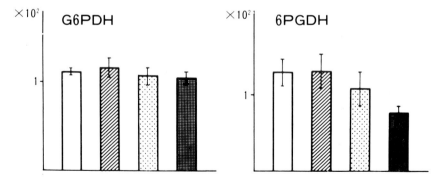

Figure 3. Enzyme activities in the tricarboxylic acid (TCA) cycle and the pentosephosphate (PPh) cycle.

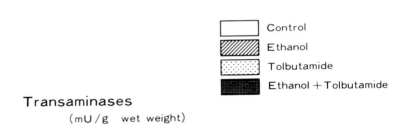

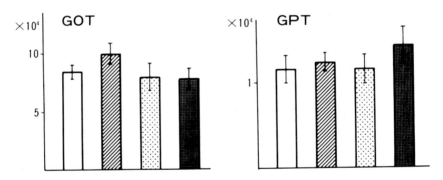

Transaminases

(mU / g   wet weight)

Figure 4. Enzyme activities of transaminases.

toxic effect of ethanol on the myocardium. However, in our experiment, there was no difference in either ethanol consumption or blood ethanol levels between rats given ethanol alone and rats given both ethanol and tolbutamide. The concentration of acetaldehyde in the blood tended to be higher in rats given both ethanol and tolbutamide than in rats given ethanol alone. These data suggest that acetaldehyde plays a more important role in the production of alcoholic cardiomyopathy than ethanol itself.

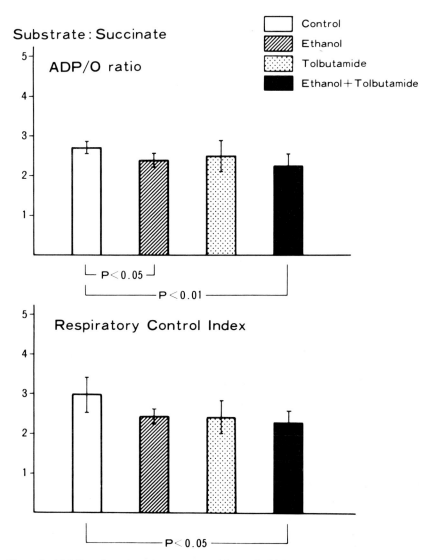

Figure 5. ADP/O ratio and respiratory control index (RCl) in mitochondria with succinate as the substrate.

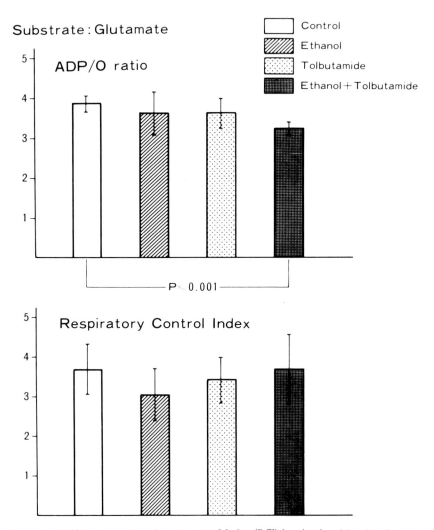

Figure 6. ADP/O ratio and respiratory control index (RCl) in mitochondria with glutamate as the substrate.

REFERENCES

CERERBAUM, A. I., and RUBIN, E. 1975. Molecular injury to mitochondria produced by ethanol and acetaldehyde. Fed. Proc. 34:2045–2051.

NAGANO, M. 1974. Myokardstoffwechsel bei experimenteller Hypertonie. Jikeikai Med. J. 21(suppl.):73–81.

NAGANO, M., MOCHIZUKI, S., KOGURE, T., KOSUGA, T., SAITO, N., and TOMIZUKA, S. 1975. Oxidative phosphorylation in mitochondria isolated from stressed rat heart. *In* P. E. Roy and P. Harris (eds.), Recent Advances in Studies on Cardiac Structure and Metabolism. Vol. 8: The Cardiac Sarcoplasm, pp. 293–300. University Park Press, Baltimore.

PACHINGER, O. M., TILLMANNS, H., MAO, J. C., FAUVEL, F. M., and BING, R. J. 1973. The effect of prolonged administration of ethanol on cardiac metabolism and performance in the dog. J. Clin. Invest. 52:2690–2696.

Mailing address:
M. Nagano, M.D.,
Department of Internal Medicine, The Jikei University School of Medicine,
Nishi-Shinbashi, Minato-ku, Tokyo (Japan).

Recent Advances in Studies on
Cardiac Structure and Metabolism, Volume 12
Cardiac Adaptation
Edited by T. Kobayashi, Y. Ito, and G. Rona
Copyright 1978 University Park Press Baltimore

LOWERING OF BLOOD ACETALDEHYDE LEVELS– A POSSIBLE APPROACH TO PREVENTION OF ALCOHOLIC CARDIOMYOPATHY

C. S. ALEXANDER,[1] H. T. NAGASAWA,
E. G. DEMASTER, and D. J. W. GOON

Medical Research Laboratories, Veterans Administration
Hospital, and the Departments of Medicine and Medicinal
Chemistry, University of Minnesota, Minneapolis, Minnesota, USA

SUMMARY

Based on the assumption that circulating acetaldehyde (AcH) is cardiotoxic, D-penicillamine was administered to dogs given alcohol orally, or given AcH intravenously. Paralleling the increase in plasma norepinephrine (NE) and epinephrine (E) induced by AcH infusion, hemodynamic measurements showed a positive inotropic response with increase in pulse, blood pressure, left ventricular contractility, and cardiac output. Infusion of D-penicillamine abruptly lowered circulating levels of AcH and catecholamines, which was accompanied by an appropriate hemodynamic response.

INTRODUCTION

The etiology of alcoholic cardiomyopathy is unknown. In assessing the debilitating effect of chronic alcohol ingestion on the heart, the evidence suggests that acetaldehyde (AcH), the first metabolite of ethanol metabolism, is the toxic agent. AcH elicits many actions not shown by ethanol, e.g., it inactivates coenzyme A (Ammon, Estler, and Heim, 1971), produces acute hemodynamic effects on the isolated mammalian heart (James and Bear, 1967; Gailis and Verdy, 1971), induces catecholamine release from adrenergic neurons (Walsh, Hollander, and Truitt, 1969), alters biogenic amine metabolism (Davis et al., 1967), condenses with biogenic amines (Davis and Walsh, 1970), and inhibits myocardial protein synthesis (Schreiber, Oratz, and Rothschild, 1974). In addition, inhibitors of aldehyde dehydrogenase (AldDH) precipitate the well known Antabuse-like symptoms.

This work was supported in part by a program grant from the Veterans Administration and in part by USPHS Grant 1–R01–00663.

[1] Deceased.

Ethanol metabolism occurs primarily in the liver, whereas the heart, which contains little alcohol dehydrogenase (ADH) (Forsyth, Nagasawa, and Alexander, 1976; Raskin and Sokoloff, 1972), does not metabolize ethanol to any significant extent. Thus, the level of circulating blood AcH may be a primary etiological factor when considering the adverse effect of alcohol on the heart. AcH blood levels recently have been shown to be higher in the alcoholic than in the nonalcoholic after an acute dose of alcohol (Korsten *et al.*, 1975).

One possible approach to the prevention of alcoholic cardiomyopathy is to reduce the level of circulating AcH. In previous reports, we have shown that D-penicillamine, a sulfhydryl amino acid derived from penicillin, 1) diverts part of the AcH generated during ethanol metabolism to urinary excretory pathways in the rat by condensing with ethanol-derived AcH and producing 2,5,5-tri-methylthiazolidine-4-carboxylic acid (TTCA) (Nagasawa *et al.*, 1975) and 2) lowers ethanol-derived circulating blood AcH levels (Nagasawa *et al.*, 1977). The present study examines the effect of D-penicillamine infusion on blood AcH and catecholamine levels and on various hemodynamic parameters in the anesthetized dog.

MATERIALS AND METHODS

Fifteen large mongrel and beagle dogs were studied; five received 4 g/kg of ethanol, six received bolus AcH, and four received AcH by I.V. infusion. Dogs receiving AcH were anesthetized with pentobarbital (30 mg/kg). Catheters were positioned in the pulmonary artery, aorta, left ventricle, femoral artery, and left and right foreleg veins. Blood samples for catecholamine and AcH determinations were drawn from the femoral artery. AcH and D-penicillamine were infused in the left and right foreleg veins, respectively, using Harvard pumps. The hemodynamic parameters measured were heart rate, pulmonary arterial (PA) pressure, aortic pressure, left ventricular end-diastolic pressure (LVEDP), and cardiac output (CO).

Plasma catecholamines were assayed using a radiometric enzyme procedure (Passon and Peuler, 1973) and blood AcH was determined by a head-space gas chromatographic assay (Cohen, MacNamee, and Dembiac, 1975). Urine was collected over 5 g of Na_2CO_3, and the TTCA metabolite was isolated and identified as previously described (Nagasawa *et al.*, 1975).

RESULTS

The sequence of metabolic reactions described in this study is shown in Figure 1. The first two steps involved in the metabolism of ethanol are the oxidations of ethanol to AcH and AcH to acetate, catalyzed by ADH and AldDH, respectively. D-Penicillamine diverts AcH from its normal metabolic fate via a nonenzymatic

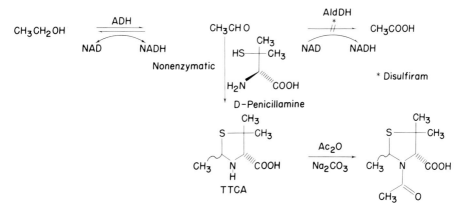

Figure 1. Reaction scheme showing the diversion of ethanol-derived metabolic AcH by D-penicillamine.

condensation reaction yielding TTCA, which is excreted in the urine (Nagasawa *et al.,* 1975). TTCA is usually *N*-acetylated during the work-up procedure to permit chromatographic separation of TTCA from the other urinary metabolites.

Our first attempts at examining the effect of AcH on catecholamine blood levels and on various hemodynamic parameters were conducted by administering either ethanol orally or AcH by bolus I.V. injection. In trial experiments, we found that 4 g/kg of ethanol, a dose selected to produce anesthesia, resulted in vomiting. We therefore switched to administering AcH by bolus injection, which did produce the desired hemodynamic response. The duration of the response, however, was not sufficiently long for cardiac output determinations. This could only be accomplished by giving AcH by continuous infusion, a procedure that enabled the maintenance of a near steady-state level of circulating AcH.

The results of two dog experiments using I.V. AcH and D-penicillamine infusion are shown in Figures 2 and 3. The rate of AcH infusion was increased until a 20% rise in pulse or blood pressure was observed. This was associated with increased pulmonary arterial (PA) pressure, LVdP/dt, and cardiac output, presumably as a direct consequence of elevated epinephrine (E) and norepinephrine (NE) levels. D-Penicillamine infusion was then initiated either after an interruption of AcH infusion (Figure 2) or during continuous AcH infusion (Figure 3). In both dogs, D-penicillamine infusion strikingly decreased the circulating AcH, E, and NE blood levels. The hemodynamic response appropriately paralleled the falling levels of AcH and catecholamines. The AcH-induced hemodynamic responses also were reversed by propranolol (2 mg/kg, I.V.; data not shown).

TTCA, as its *N*-acetylated derivative, was isolated from the urine of dogs receiving ethanol orally and D-penicillamine by infusion (Figure 4). Similarly,

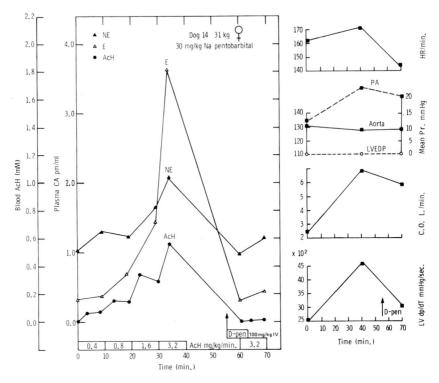

Figure 2. Effect of D-penicillamine on AcH and catecholamine blood levels and on various hemodynamic parameters during *discontinuous* infusion of AcH in an anesthetized dog.

TTCA was identified in the urine of three human volunteers given D-penicillamine and consuming 1 g/kg of ethanol in the form of vodka.

DISCUSSION

The diversion of ethanol-derived AcH from its normal metabolic pathway to TTCA following the administration of D-penicillamine was first demonstrated in the rat (Nagasawa *et al.,* 1975). Although the amount of ethanol-derived AcH converted to TTCA is not large enough to influence the overall rate of ethanol metabolism (Nagasawa *et al.,* 1977), the present demonstration that D-penicillamine lowers AcH levels even when continuously infused may be of great significance. If D-penicillamine were to divert only this *circulating* acetaldehyde to innocuous excretory metabolites, the heart, which contains little ADH (Raskin and Sokoloff, 1972; Forsyth, Nagasawa, and Alexander, 1976) and thus is exposed to circulating AcH, might be protected from AcH toxicity.

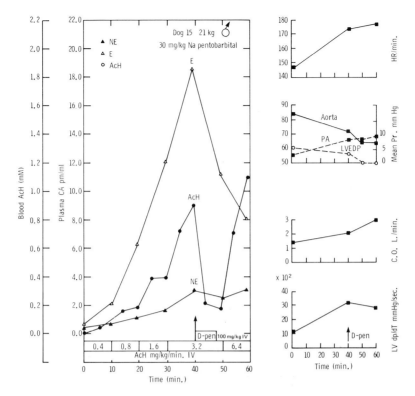

Figure 3. Effect of D-penicillamine on AcH and catecholamine blood levels and on various hemodynamic parameters during *continuous* infusion of AcH in an anesthetized dog.

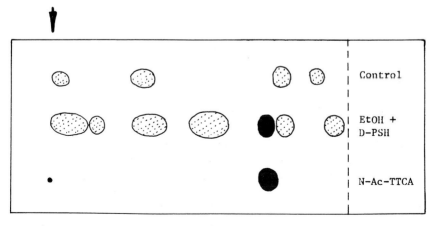

Figure 4. Thin-layer chromatogram (TLC) of ethyl acetate extracts of acetylated urine from control and ethanol-plus-D-penicillamine (D-PSH)-treated beagle dog. The arrow and dotted line denote origin and solvent front, respectively.

We have demonstrated in dogs that the acute positive hemodynamic response to AcH infusion (caused by releasing NE and E into the circulation) could be reversed by I.V. infusion of D-penicillamine. The chronic interstitial fibrosis that is found in alcoholic cardiomyopathy may be the result of repeated inotropic stimulation by catecholamines released by AcH. Whether or not cardiomyopathy can be prevented by agents that sequester AcH in the manner described with D-penicillamine remains to be demonstrated.

REFERENCES

AMMON, H. P. T., ESTLER, C-J., and HEIM, F. 1971. Effect of alcohol and acetaldehyde on coenzyme A. *In* M. K. Roach, W. M. McIsaac, and P. J. Creaven (eds.), Biological Aspects of Alcohol, pp. 185–211. University of Texas Press, Austin.

COHEN, G., MacNAMEE, D., and DEMBIAC, D. 1975. Elevation of blood acetaldehyde by pargyline during ethanol administration. Biochem. Pharmacol. 24:315–316.

DAVIS, V. E., BROWN, H., HUFF, J. A., and CASHEW, J. L. 1967. Ethanol-induced alterations of norepinephrine metabolism in man. J. Lab. Clin. Med. 69:787–799.

DAVIS, V. E., and WALSH, M. J. 1970. Alcohol, amines, and alkaloids: A possible biochemical basis for alcohol addiction. Science 167:1005–1007.

FORSYTH, G. W., NAGASAWA, H. T., and ALEXANDER, C. S. 1976. Ethanol metabolism by the rat heart and alcohol dehydrogenase activity. Can. J. Biochem. 54:539–545.

GAILIS, L., and VERDY, M. 1971. The effect of ethanol and acetaldehyde on the metabolism and vascular resistance of the perfused heart. Can. J. Biochem. 49:227–233.

JAMES, T. N., and BEAR, E. S. 1967. Effects of ethanol and acetaldehyde on the heart. Am. Heart J. 74:243–255.

KORSTEN, M. A., MATSUZAKI, S., FEINMAN, L., and LIEBER, C. S. 1975. High blood acetaldehyde levels after ethanol administration. N. Engl. J. Med. 292:386–389.

NAGASAWA, H. T., GOON, D. J. W., CONSTANTINO, N. V., and ALEXANDER, C. S. 1975. Diversion of ethanol metabolism by sulfhydryl amino acids. D-Penicillamine-directed excretion of 2,5,5-trimethyl-D-thiazolidine-4-carboxylic acid in the urine of rats after ethanol administration. Life Sci. 17:707–714.

NAGASAWA, H. T., GOON, D. J. W., DEMASTER, E. G., and ALEXANDER, C. S. 1977. Lowering of ethanol-derived metabolic acetaldehyde in rats by D-penicillamine. Life Sci. 20:187–194.

PASSON, P. G., and PEULER, J. D. 1973. A simplified radiometric assay for plasma norepinephrine and epinephrine. Anal. Biochem. 51:618–631.

RASKIN, N. H., and SOKOLOFF, L. 1972. Enzymes catalyzing ethanol metabolism in neural and somatic tissue of the rat. J. Neurochem. 19:273–282.

SCHREIBER, S. S., ORATZ, M., and ROTHSCHILD, M. A. 1974. Alcoholic cardiomyopathy. II. The inhibition of cardiac microsomal protein synthesis by acetaldehyde. J. Mol. Cell. Cardiol. 6:207–213.

WALSH, M. J., HOLLANDER, P. B., and TRUITT, E. B., JR. 1969. Sympathomimetic effects of acetaldehyde on the electrical and contractile characteristics of isolated left atria of guinea pigs. J. Pharmacol. Exp. Ther. 167:173–186.

Mailing address:
H. T. Nagasawa, Ph.D.,
Medical Research Laboratories, Veterans Administration Hospital,
Minneapolis, Minnesota 55417 (USA).

Recent Advances in Studies on
Cardiac Structure and Metabolism, Volume 12
Cardiac Adaptation
Edited by T. Kobayashi, Y. Ito, and G. Rona
Copyright 1978 University Park Press Baltimore

IS THERE A CALCIUM-CAUSED DEFECT OF OXIDATIVE PHOSPHORYLATION IN CARDIOMYOPATHIC HAMSTER HEARTS?

K. WROGEMANN, E. NYLEN, and M. C. BLANCHAER

Department of Biochemistry, Faculty of Medicine,
University of Manitoba, Winnipeg, Manitoba, Canada

SUMMARY

Mitochondria from cardiomyopathic hamster hearts have elevated calcium levels, which may cause a defect of oxidative phosphorylation in a small fraction of them. Using a combination of dual labeling and density-gradient centrifugation, it was not possible to isolate such an abnormal fraction. However, cardiomyopathic mitochondria are more susceptible to damage by calcium *in vitro,* suggesting that an abnormal fraction does exist nevertheless.

INTRODUCTION

Our extensive work on cardiomyopathic hamsters and the findings of others made us postulate the sequence of events of the pathogenesis illustrated in Figure 1. Accordingly, mitochondria are damaged by an excessive influx of calcium into the cell and the resultant lack of energy initiates a vicious cycle of mitochondrial calcium overloading and energy lack that leads ultimately to cell necrosis. We have found such a calcium-caused defect of oxidative phosphorylation in BIO 14.6 hamsters (Wrogemann, Jacobson, and Blanchaer, 1973). By density gradient centrifugation we have shown that only a fraction of all mitochondria is calcium loaded. This agrees well with histological findings of focal necrosis (Mezon, Wrogemann, and Blanchaer, 1974). Studies with calcium-deficient diets or calcium-antagonistic drugs by Jasmin and Solymoss (1975) and Lossnitzer *et al.* (1975) seem to support the causal relationship between mitochondrial calcium damage and cell necrosis indicated in Figure 1. However, while we have been able to show a calcium-caused mitochondrial defect in skeletal muscle (Wrogemann *et al.,* 1975), the ability to prevent necrosis by calcium-antagonistic drugs appears to be restricted to heart muscle (Jasmin and Solymoss, 1975). Our attempts to demonstrate the calcium-caused defect of oxidative phosphorylation in cardiomyopathic hearts have been unsuccessful to date, although mitochondrial calcium levels in hearts are significantly elevated.

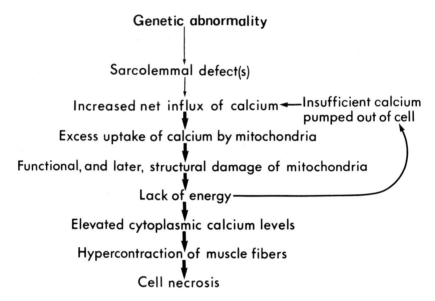

Figure 1. Sequence of events postulated for the occurrence of cell necrosis in cardiomyopathic hamsters.

(Wrogemann, Blanchaer, and Jacobson, 1972; Wrogemann *et al.,* 1975). In this chapter, further attempts to elicit a small population of abnormal, calcium-loaded organelles that could underly the occurrence of focal necrosis in the hearts of BIO 14.6 hamsters are described.

MATERIALS AND METHODS

Cardiomyopathic hamsters were of strain BIO 14.6, available from the Trenton Experimental Laboratory Animal Company, Bar Harbor, Maine, USA. Mitochondria were studied as described previously (Wrogemann, Blanchaer, and Jacobson, 1972; Wrogemann, Jacobson, and Blanchaer, 1973). Isolated mitochondria were fractionated by sucrose density-gradient centrifugation (Mezon, Wrogemann, and Blanchaer, 1974). In dual labeling studies, hamsters were injected intraperitoneally with 170–250 μCi of [U-^{14}C]leucine or 680–1,000 μCi of [4,5-^{3}H]leucine. The counting data were analyzed and plotted by a special computer program (Wrogemann *et al.,* in preparation).

RESULTS AND DISCUSSION

Heart mitochondria at all stages of the cardiomyopathy show no defect in oxidative phosphorylation (Wrogemann, Blanchaer, and Jacobson, 1972). However, the *in situ* levels of calcium in mitochondria isolated under conditions of minimal calcium movement (Thakar, Wrogemann, and Blanchaer, 1973) are significantly elevated at 7 ± 1 and 13 ± 2 nmol of calcium/mg of protein in 14 normal and 14 BIO 14.6 hamsters, respectively. This elevation of calcium could uniformly affect all organelles or may stem from a small fraction of mitochondria with excessive levels of calcium, as we postulate in Figure 1. Such a fraction can be isolated from skeletal muscle of BIO 14.6 hamsters by density-gradient centrifugation (Mezon, Wrogemann, and Blanchaer, 1974). However, with heart mitochondria this method showed no abnormal fraction (data not shown). We therefore hoped to increase the sensitivity of this technique by labeling proteins of normal and cardiomyopathic (dystrophic) hamsters with [³H]- and [¹⁴C] leucine, respectively, *in vivo,* isolate mitochondria in one preparation from the combined tissues, and subject them to a single density gradient. Any slight difference in sedimentation of the organelles would then become apparent as a

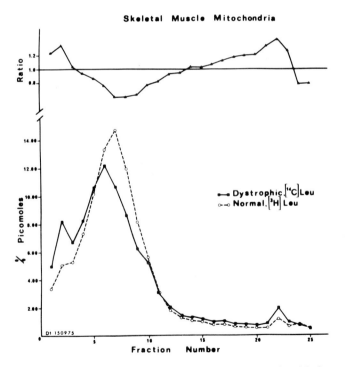

Figure 2. Fractionation on a 35–45% w/w sucrose gradient of mitochondria from a mixture of normal and dystrophic skeletal muscle labeled with [³H]- and [¹⁴C] leucine, respectively. Data show percentage of incorporated picomoles of leucine and the ratio of [¹⁴C]/[³H] for each gradient fraction. Calcium in the input mixture: 31 nmol/mg of mitochondrial protein.

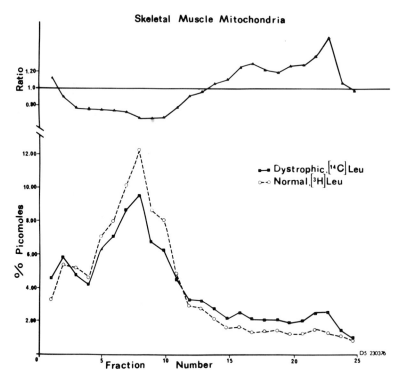

Figure 3. Fractionation of skeletal muscle mitochondria from a normal and dystrophic hamster subjected to one hour of swimming. Calcium in the input mixture: 133 nmol/mg of mitochondrial protein. Other conditions as in Figure 2.

deviation from unity of the ratio of [^{14}C]leucine over [^{3}H]leucine. Figure 2 shows that this approach indicates, as expected, a clear tendency of mitochondria from dystrophic skeletal muscle to sediment at a higher density, i.e., a higher fraction number. Analysis of calcium showed that the organelle content of this ion is indeed higher in the lower part of the gradient (data not shown). However, heart mitochondria showed no differential sedimentation pattern between normal and cardiomyopathic animals.

According to our working hypothesis (Figure 1 and Wrogemann and Pena, 1976), the additional drain on energy by heavy exercise should aggravate the mitochondrial calcium overloading. Figure 3 shows that after one hour of swimming the abnormal sedimentation pattern in skeletal muscle becomes more pronounced as a consequence of much higher calcium levels. However, this again is not apparent in heart mitochondria from the same animals (Figure 4).

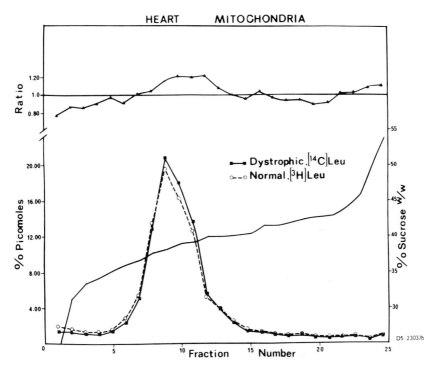

Figure 4. Fractionation of heart mitochondria from a normal and dystrophic hamster subjected to one hour of swimming. Calcium concentration in the input mixture: 2.1 nmol/mg of mitochondrial protein. Other conditions as in Figure 2.

To see whether or not heart mitochondria would show, at least, a calcium-caused defect *in vitro,* oxidative phosphorylation was studied in the presence of increasing amounts of calcium in the test medium (Figure 5). Qualitatively, the heart mitochondria behave like skeletal muscle organelles (Wrogemann, Jacobson, and Blanchaer, 1973), i.e., both normal and dystrophic organelles accumulate calcium with a concomitant decline in respiratory control until mitochondria become uncoupled. At this time, they are unable to retain both calcium and magnesium, and they lose the ions into the medium. However, it is noteworthy that dystrophic mitochondria become uncoupled at lower calcium levels and also show a tendency to lose magnesium before they become totally uncoupled. This finding warrants further investigation because it is compatible with our concept that the isolated mitochondria indeed represent a mixture containing a small population that is calcium-damaged.

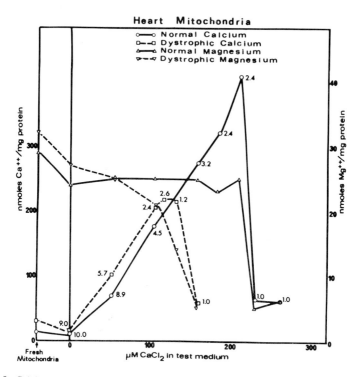

Figure 5. Calcium and magnesium levels and respiratory control ratios of heart mitochondria assayed in the presence of increasing concentrations of calcium in the test medium. The respiratory control ratios appear beside the points for calcium.

REFERENCES

JASMIN, G., and SOLYMOSS, B. 1975. Prevention of hereditary cardiomyopathy in the hamster by Verapamil and other agents. Proc. Soc. Exp. Biol. Med. 149:193–198.
LOSSNITZER, K., JANKE, J., HEIN, B., STAUCH, M., and FLECKENSTEIN, A. 1975. Disturbed myocardial calcium metabolism: A possible pathogenic factor in the hereditary cardiomyopathy of the Syrian hamster. *In* A. Fleckenstein and G. Rona (eds.), Recent Advances in Cardiac Structure and Metabolism. Vol. 6: Pathophysiology and Morphology of Myocardial Cell Alterations, pp. 207–217. University Park Press, Baltimore.
MEZON, B. J. WROGEMANN, K., and BLANCHAER, M. C. 1974. Differing populations of mitochondria isolated from normal and dystrophic hamster skeletal muscle. Can. J. Biochem. 52:1024–1032.
THAKAR, J. H., WROGEMANN, K., and BLANCHAER, M. C. 1973. Effect of ruthenium red on oxidative phosphorylation and the calcium and magnesium content of skeletal muscle mitochondria of normal and BIO 14.6 dystrophic hamsters. Biochim. Biophys. Acta 314:8–14.
WROGEMANN, K., BLANCHAER, M. C., CORBY, P., and PENA, S. D. J. "SCINT II," an

improved Fortran IV program for the analysis of data from dual-labelled liquid scintillation samples. In preparation.

WROGEMANN, K., BLANCHAER, M. C., and JACOBSON, B. E. 1972. Oxidative phosphorylation in cardiomyopathic hamsters. Am. J. Physiol. 222:1453–1457.

WROGEMANN, K., BLANCHAER, M. C., THAKAR, J. H., and MEZON, B. J. 1975. On the role of the mitochondria in the hereditary cardiomyopathy of the Syrian hamster. *In* A. Fleckenstein and G. Rona (eds.), Recent Advances in Cardiac Structure and Metabolism. Vol. 6: Pathophysiology and Morphology of Myocardial Cell Alterations, pp. 231–241. University Park Press, Baltimore.

WROGEMANN, K., JACOBSON, B. E., and BLANCHAER, M. C. 1973. On the mechanism of a calcium associated defect of oxidative phosphorylation in progressive muscular dystrophy. Arch. Biochem. Biophys. 159:267–278.

WROGEMANN, K., and PENA, S. D. J. 1976. Mitochondrial calcium overload: A general mechanism for cell necrosis in muscle diseases. Lancet 1:672–673.

Mailing address:
Dr. K. Wrogemann,
Department of Biochemistry, Faculty of Medicine,
University of Manitoba, Winnipeg, Manitoba R3E 0W3 (Canada).

Recent Advances in Studies on
Cardiac Structure and Metabolism, Volume 12
Cardiac Adaptation
Edited by T. Kobayashi, Y. Ito, and G. Rona
Copyright 1978 University Park Press Baltimore

ADENYLATE CYCLASE, CYCLIC NUCLEOTIDE PHOSPHODIESTERASE, AND PHOSPHORYLASE ACTIVITY OF CARDIOMYOPATHIC HAMSTER HEARTS

S. J. SULAKHE, B. L. RUSSELL, and P. V. SULAKHE

Department of Physiology, College of Medicine,
University of Saskatchewan, Saskatoon, S7N 0W0, Canada

SUMMARY

Activities of adenylate cyclase in homogenates were reduced, whereas those of phosphodiesterases were elevated in hearts of myopathic hamsters (BIO 82.62). Affinities for either Mg^{2+} or ATP of cyclase were unaffected in myopathy. Ca^{2+} stimulation of particulate phosphodiesterases was not observed in myopathy. Although the cardiac phosphorylase content was reduced at the advanced stages of myopathy, $-AMP/+AMP$ ratios remained similar to those found in normal hearts.

INTRODUCTION

Earlier, we reported that NaF-stimulated adenylate cyclase activities in myopathic hearts were reduced and that β-adrenergic amine stimulation of this enzyme was abolished at advanced stages of cardiomyopathy (Sulakhe and Dhalla, 1972). In this chapter, we describe the changes in the activities of adenylate cyclase, cyclic nucleotide phosphodiesterase, and phosphorylase in myopathic hearts of Syrian hamsters (BIO 82.62) of various ages.

MATERIALS AND METHODS

Normal and myopathic Syrian hamsters (BIO 82.62) were obtained from the Trenton Experimental Laboratory Animal Company, Bar Harbor, Maine, USA. Enzyme assays and isolation of fractions were performed as have been described previously (St. Louis and Sulakhe, 1976; Sulakhe et al., 1976). Phosphorylase activities in perfused (Langendorff) hearts were determined by the method to be reported elsewhere (Sulkhe and Sulakhe, in preparation).

This work was supported financially by the Saskatchewan Heart Foundation and the Muscular Dystrophy Association of Canada and America.

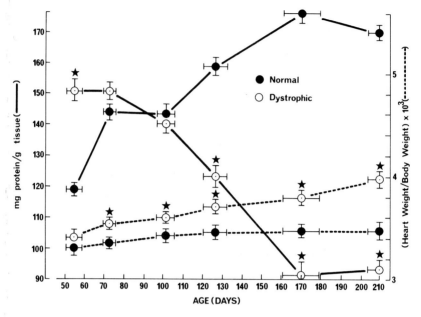

Figure 1. Cardiac protein content and heart weight/body weight ratios in normal and myopathic Syrian hamsters (BIO 82.62) of various ages.

RESULTS

Figure 1 shows that the cardiac protein content was reduced significantly while heart weight/body weight ratio was elevated in older myopathic hamsters compared to age-matched control animals. The content of adenylate cyclase, assayed as basal, epinephrine-, and NaF-stimulated activity, also was significantly lower in myopathic hearts (Figure 2). It is interesting to note that adenylate cyclase content was slightly higher in younger myopathic hamsters. The change in adenylate cyclase was mainly caused by the change in the specific activity of the enzyme in cell-free preparations isolated from myopathic hearts of all age groups. The change in the affinity for ATP, even at very advanced stages of myopathy, could not be detected (Figure 3); similarly, affinities for Mg^{2+} were unaffected. In other studies, about 80–90% of the cyclase activity was found to be particulate in normal and myopathic hearts of 40–200-day-old animals.

In contrast to cyclase, cyclic nucleotide phosphodiesterase activity is present mainly in the soluble cytoplasm, although about 20% of the total activity is particulate in hamster hearts. As the myopathic process advances, a greater portion of the total phosphodiesterase is present in the soluble fraction with a concomitant loss in the particulate enzyme activity. It is of interest to note that

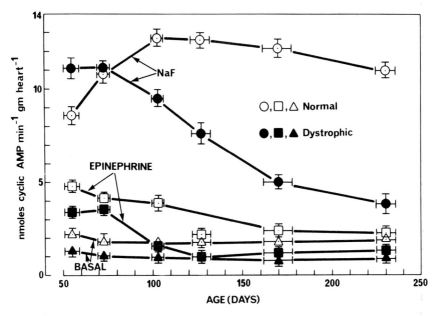

Figure 2. Adenylate cyclase activities in normal and myopathic hearts. For adenylate cyclase assay, 0.8 mM [α-^{32}P] ATP and 10 mM $MgCl_2$ were present. When added, epinephrine was 100 μM and NaF was 8 mM.

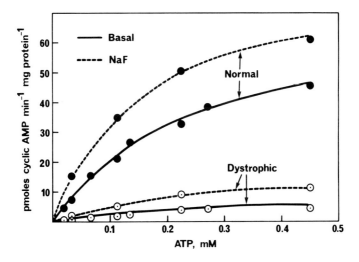

Figure 3. Adenylate cyclase activities in hearts of normal and myopathic hamsters (240 days old). For assay, see Figure 2.

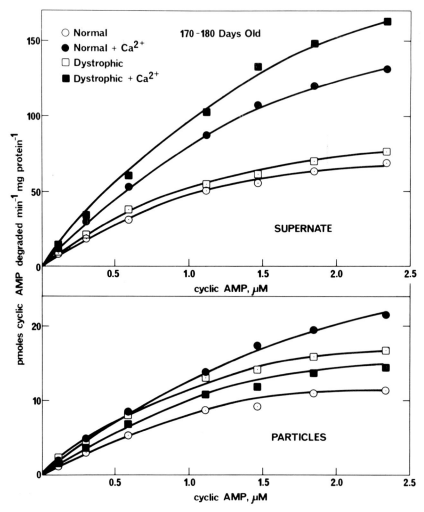

Figure 4. cAMP phosphodiesterase activity in washed particles and supernatant fractions assayed at lower substrate concentrations. Phosphodiesterase assay contained 5 mM Mg^{2+} and 5 mM EGTA. When present, $CaCl_2$ was 5.10 mM.

Ca^{2+} stimulation of the particulate phosphodiesterase (either with cAMP or cGMP as substrate), which is seen in normal hearts, is not observed in the myopathic hearts. These results are shown in Figures 4, 5, and 6. Note that both high and low K_m phosphodiesterases are present in the washed particles and supernatant fractions of normal and myopathic hearts. The homogenate phosphodiesterase activities in myopathic hearts, however, were elevated compared to normal levels.

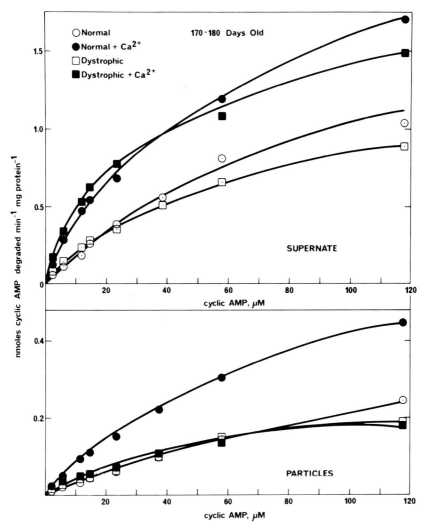

Figure 5. cAMP phosphodiesterase activity in washed particles and supernatant fractions assayed at higher substrate concentrations. Assay conditions similar to those described under Figure 4.

As expected, phosphorylase *a* content of myopathic heart was reduced in advanced stages of the disease; however, the ratios (−AMP/+AMP) were similar to those seen in normal heart (of all ages tested). It also was noted that the ratios increased from 0.06 ± 0.01 and 0.075 ± 0.01 (45 days old) to 0.17 ± 0.02 and 0.16 ± 0.02 (173 days old) in normal and myopathic hearts, respectively, and thereafter plateaued at that level.

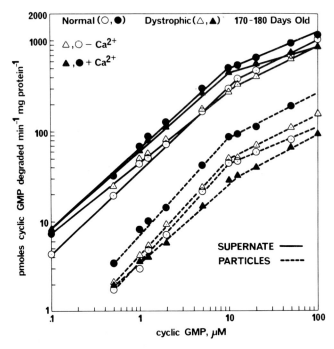

Figure 6. cGMP phosphodiesterase activity in washed particles and supernatant fractions assayed at different substrate concentrations. Assay conditions similar to those described under Figure 4.

DISCUSSION

Concerning the metabolism of cyclic nucleotides in myopathy, the following observations were made: 1) reduced adenylate cyclase in advanced stages of myopathy associated with reduction in the NaF stimulation, as well as β-adrenergic amine stimulation, of the enzyme; 2) no detectable change in the affinities of the cyclase for ATP or Mg^{2+}, as well as in the subcellular distribution of the cyclase; 3) elevated phosphodiesterase activities in homogenates and supernatants; 4) lack of Ca^{2+} stimulation of the particulate diesterase.

In another strain of myopathy (UM-X7.1), reduced adenylate cyclase activities in hearts of 150-day-old hamsters were reported recently by Harrow *et al.* (1975). However, change in the phosphodiesterase (low affinity) was not observed. Cardiac cAMP content was elevated in younger myopathic animals and was reduced in older animals compared to the normal counterparts (Harrow *et al.*, 1975).

Although an abnormal metabolism of cyclic nucleotide is observed in myopathic hearts, it is not clear whether or not it contributes to the pathogenesis of the disease. Future studies are needed to understand the mechanism(s) responsible for the reported alterations in the cyclic nucleotide synthesis and the degradation, which undoubtedly are secondary to the primary genetic defect in this model.

REFERENCES

HARROW, J. A. C., SINGH, J. N., JASMIN, C., and DHALLA, N. S. 1975. Studies on adenylate cyclase-cyclic AMP system of the myopathic hamster (UM-X7.1) skeletal and cardiac muscles. Can. J. Biochem. 53:1122–1127.

ST. LOUIS, P. J., and SULAKHE, P. V. 1976. Adenylate cyclase, guanylate cyclase and cyclic nucleotide phosphodiesterases of guinea pig cardiac sarcolemma. Biochem. J. 158:535–541.

SULAKHE, P. V., and DHALLA, N. S. 1972. Adenyl cyclase activity in failing hearts of genetically myopathic hamsters. Biochem. Med. 6:471–482.

SULAKHE, S. J., and SULAKHE, P. V. 1976. Phosphorylase activities in myopathic heart and skeletal muscle. In preparation.

SULAKHE, P. V., SULAKHE, S. J., LEUNG, N. L., ST. LOUIS, P. J., and HICKIE, R. A. 1976. Guanylate cyclase: Subcellular distribution in cardiac muscle, skeletal muscle, cerebral cortex and liver. Biochem. J. 157:705–712.

Mailing address:
P. V. Sulakhe, Ph.D.,
Department of Physiology, College of Medicine,
University of Saskatchewan, Saskatoon S7N 0W0 (Canada).

Recent Advances in Studies on
Cardiac Structure and Metabolism, Volume 12
Cardiac Adaptation
Edited by T. Kobayashi, Y. Ito, and G. Rona
Copyright 1978 University Park Press Baltimore

DIFFERENTIAL RESPONSES OF CANINE MYOSIN ATPase ACTIVITY AND TISSUE GASES IN THE PRESSURE-OVERLOADED VENTRICLE DEPENDENT UPON DEGREE OF OBSTRUCTION: MILD VERSUS SEVERE PULMONIC AND AORTIC STENOSIS

J. WIKMAN-COFFELT, T. KAMIYAMA,
A. F. SALEL, and D. T. MASON

Section of Cardiovascular Medicine,
Department of Medicine, University of California, Davis,
School of Medicine, Davis, California, USA

SUMMARY

Mild pulmonic stenosis, induced in dogs by banding the pulmonary artery, elevated right ventricular peak systolic pressure to 60% above the control and elevated right ventricular K^+- and Ca^{2+}-activated myosin ATPase activities. In contrast, severe pulmonic stenosis, which elevated right ventricular peak systolic pressure to 300% above the control, did not produce an increase in myosin enzymatic ATPase V_{max} values but caused a decrease in myosin activity. Mild aortic stenosis, induced by banding the ascending aorta, forcing a transaortic pressure gradient of 25 mm Hg, caused an elevation in left ventricular myosin ATPase, whereas severe aortic banding, brought about by creating a transaortic pressure gradient of 55 mm Hg, never caused an elevation in left ventricular myosin enzymatic V_{max} values, but, like severe pulmonic banding, caused a decrease in K^+- and Ca^{2+}-activated myosin activities. Normal left ventricular myosin V_{max} values in μmol of PO_4/mg·min at $37°C$ were: K^+ = 2.84 ± 0.22, and Ca^{2+} = 0.97 ± 0.14. For right ventricular myosin they were: K^+ = 2.15 ± 0.16, and Ca^{2+} = 0.74 ± 0.10. Analyses of tissue gases, based on mass spectrometry data, showed that the hypertrophied ventricles had an elevated tissue pCO_2 and an elevation in the cGMP/cAMP ratio.

INTRODUCTION

The force and the velocity of cardiac contraction are largely governed by the rate at which myosin hydrolyzes ATP (Oscar *et al.,* 1971; Vitali-Mazza *et al.,*

This work was supported in part by Research Program Project Grants HL 14780 and AMDD 16716 from the National Institutes of Health, Bethesda, Maryland, and by a Research Grant from the California Chapter of the American Heart Association.

1972). Therefore, myosin was analyzed in a series of experiments in which a pressure overload was produced either by pulmonic or aortic banding of dogs for varying lengths of time.

MATERIALS AND METHODS

Mild and severe aortic stenoses were induced by banding the ascending aorta as described previously (Wikman-Coffelt *et al.*, 1976). Severe systolic pressure overload of the right ventricle was induced by using an inflatable Jacobson cuff (Wikman-Coffelt *et al.*, 1975c); mild banding of the pulmonary artery has been described elsewhere (Wikman-Coffelt *et al.*, 1975a). Purification of canine myocardial myosin and analyses of myosin ATPase activity were described in earlier reports (Wikman-Coffelt *et al.*, 1975b). To obtain myosin from cardiac ventricles, only the free wall of the chambers was used; the septum was not analyzed. Tissue gases were monitored with a mass spectrometer (Brantigan, Gott, and Martz, 1972) using teflon membranes as catheters. Membranes were inserted through a small incision in the epicardial surface and gently pushed into position so that the membrane dissected its own way through the myocardial fibers to reside at a depth of 1−2 mm below the surface.

RESULTS AND DISCUSSION

In the studies reported in this chapter, the molecular function of purified canine cardiac myosin is expressed with Ca^{2+} and with K^+ as the activator cations; activities are expressed in enzymatic V_{max} values as μmol of PO_4 released in a mg of myosin per min. Right ventricular myosin was approximately 30% lower in ATPase activity as compared to left ventricular myosin with either K^+ or CA^{2+} as the activator cation (Figure 1). With NH_4^+ as the activator cation, all myosin ATPase activities were the same. A close correlation existed between the ATPase activity of myosin and the structure of myosin. No differences could be determined in the electrophoresis patterns between left and right ventricular myosins (Wikman-Coffelt *et al.*, 1975b). It was noted, however, that there were more light chains relative to heavy chains in right ventricular canine myosin (Wikman-Coffelt *et al.*, 1975b), and that the number of Ca^{2+} binding sites was nearly twice as great in right ventricular myosin as in left ventricular myosin (Brantigan, Gott, and Martz, 1972; Wikman-Coffelt *et al.*, 1976).

Myosin was analyzed in a series of experiments in which a pressure overload, produced either by pulmonic or aortic banding, was imposed on dogs for varying lengths of time. When the banding was mild, such as in mild aortic stenosis with the peak systolic pressure gradient being approximately 25 mm Hg, myosin elevated in its enzymatic V_{max} values. Myosin enzymatic function peaked five weeks post-operatively and returned to near normal values 16 weeks after

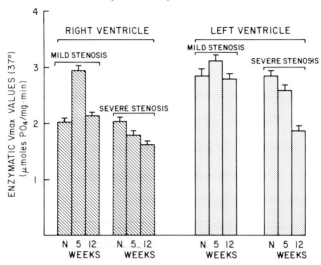

Figure 1. Myosin enzymatic V_{max} values for normal canine right and left ventricular myosin. Average V_{max} values for K^+-, Ca^{2+}-, and NH_4^+-activated right and left ventricular myosins are shown. Each bar represents six animals. The incubation was carried out at $37°C$ for 5 min. Substrate was added before the addition of myosin to stabilize the enzyme at this incubation temperature. Mean values of V_{max} (± S.E.M.) are shown. For mild aortic stenosis in dogs, the ascending aorta was banded, affecting a transaortic peak systolic pressure gradient of 25 mm Hg. For severe aortic stenosis, a transaortic peak systolic pressure gradient of 50 mm Hg was created by banding the ascending aorta as described earlier (Wikman-Coffelt *et al.,* 1976). Severe pulmonic stenosis was performed by using the Jacobson cuff and increasing right ventricular peak systolic pressure to >60 mm Hg. Mild pulmonic stenosis was performed by banding the pulmonary artery and elevating right ventricular peak systolic pressure to 45 mm Hg.

surgery (Figure 1) (Wikman-Coffelt *et al.,* 1975, 1976). When aortic banding was severe, affecting a peak systolic transaortic pressure gradient of 50 mm Hg, myosin decreased in activity and continued to decrease until the animals were in congestive heart failure (Figure 1). The left ventricular enzymatic V_{max} values by 16 weeks post-operatively declined to those similar to the normal right ventricle. Associated with a decrease in myosin enzymatic V_{max} values in the severely pressure-overloaded left ventricle, there were more light chains relative to heavy chains present in myosin and a greater number of calcium-binding sites (Brantigan, Gott, and Martz, 1972; Wikman-Coffelt *et al.,* 1976), thereby simulating normal right ventricular myosin.

When excess pressure was placed on the right ventricle by banding the pulmonary artery in dogs, alterations also occurred in myosin enzymatic

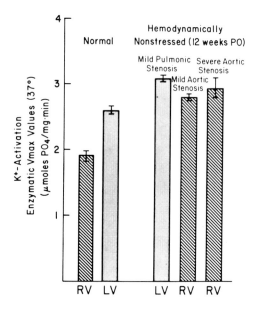

Figure 2. Myosin enzymatic V_{max} values and surgical interventions are as described in Figure 1. Values shown are for myosins from the hemodynamically nonstressed ventricles. PO = postoperative.

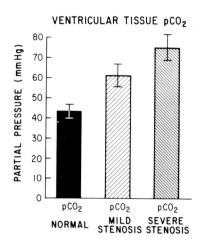

Figure 3. Ventricular tissue gases in mild and severe stenosis in dogs. Intramyocardial gas tensions are expressed in mm Hg and were analyzed using the mass spectrometer described by Brantigan, Gott, and Martz (1972).

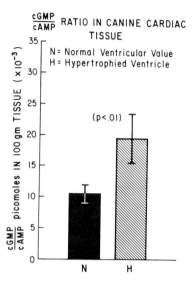

Figure 4. The cyclic nucleotides, cAMP and cGMP, were quantified by a radioimmunoassay (Schwarz/Mann). Tissue was prepared for quantification as described in the Schwarz/Mann radioimmunoassay kit. Values are based on 100 mg of tissue $\times$ 10^{-3}. Normal cAMP levels were 1.52 ± 0.39 pmol per mg of tissue. Normal cGMP values were 14.18 ± 5.83 pmol per gm of tissue.

activity. If banding was mild, thereby increasing right ventricular peak systolic pressure 60% above normal, myosin rose in its activity, peaked in enzymatic V_{max} values by five weeks post-operatively, and returned to near normal values of right ventricular myosin 16 weeks after surgery (Figure 1) (Wikman-Coffelt *et al.*, 1975a). If pulmonary banding was severe, thereby increasing right ventricular peak systolic pressure 300% above normal, myosin decreased in enzymatic V_{max} values (Figure 2). If the animals displayed clinical manifestations of heart failure, both ventricular myosins had a depressed ATPase activity.

In addition, the mass spectrometer (Furuse, Brawey, and Gott, 1973) was employed to measure stressed myocardial tissue pCO_2 and pO_2. It was noted that, related to cardiac hypertrophy, there was a significant increase in tissue

Table 1. cGMP/cAMP ratio

	LV	RV
Hypertrophied tissue	2.82	0.97
	($p < .01$)	($p < .01$)
Normal values	0.74	0.60

Values are placed on 100 mg of tissue $\times$ 10^{-3}.

pCO_2 (Figure 3). Associated with hypertrophy, in general, there also was an increase in the cGMP/cAMP ratio (Figure 4 and Table 1). No significant alterations in myosin activity were observed earlier than 3 weeks after stenosis. It appeared that alterations observed in myosin activity were the result of newly synthesized myosin associated with cellular changes in muscle energetics. Formation of free carbon dioxide is secondary to the production of lactate and a shift in the myocardial bicarbonate buffer system (Brantigan, Gott, and Martz, 1972). The fall in intracellular pH that can be induced by glycolysis, causing an elevation in tissue pCO_2, may be of great importance in determining the eventual fate of ischemic tissue and also may be responsible for cellular alterations leading to changes in the type of myosin synthesized.

REFERENCES

BRANTIGAN, J. W., GOTT, V. I., and MARTZ, M. N. 1972. A teflon membrane for measurement of blood and intramyocardial gas tensions by mass spectroscopy. J. Appl. Physiol. 32:276–282.

FURUSE, A., BRAWEY, R., and GOTT, V. 1973. Effects of isoproterenol, L-norepinephrine and glucagon on myocardial gas tensions in animals with coronary artery stenosis. J. Thorac. Cardiovasc. Surg. 65:815–824.

OSCAR, H. L., BING, S. M., BARRY, L. F., and HERBERT, J. L. 1971. Mechanical properties of rat cardiac muscle during experimental hypertrophy. Circ. Res. 28:234–245.

VITALI-MAZZA, L., ANVERSA, P., TEDESCHI, F., MASTANDREA, R., MAVILLA, V., and VISIOLI, O. 1972. Ultrastructural basis of acute left ventricular failure from severe acute aortic stenosis in the rabbit. J. Mol. Cell. Cardiol. 4:661–671.

WIKMAN-COFFELT, J., FENNER, C., COFFELT, J. R., SALEL, A., KAMIYAMA, T., and MASON, D. T. 1975a. Chronological effects of mild pressure overload on myosin ATPase activity in the canine right ventricle. J. Mol. Cell. Cardiol. 7:219–224.

WIKMAN-COFFELT, J., FENNER, C., SMITH, A., and MASON, D. T. 1975b. Comparative analyses of the kinetics and subunits of myosin from canine skeletal muscle and cardiac tissue. J. Biol. Chem. 250:1257–1262.

WIKMAN-COFFELT, J., FENNER, C., WALSH, R., SALEL, A., KAMIYAMA, T., and MASON, D. T. 1975c. Comparison of mild vs severe pressure overload on the enzymatic activity of myosin in the canine ventricles. Biochem. Med. 14:139–146.

WIKMAN-COFFELT, J., WALSH, R., FENNER, C., KAMIYAMA, T., SALEL, A., and MASON, D. T. 1976. Effects of severe hemodynamic pressure overload on the properties of canine left ventricular myosin: Mechanism by which myosin ATPase activity is lowered during chronic increased hemodynamic stress. J. Mol. Cell. Cardiol. 8:263–270.

Mailing address:
Joan Wikman-Coffelt, Ph.D.,
Section of Cardiovascular Medicine, Department of Medicine,
University of California, Davis, School of Medicine, Davis, California 95616 (USA).

Recent Advances in Studies on
Cardiac Structure and Metabolism, Volume 12
Cardiac Adaptation
Edited by T. Kobayashi, Y. Ito, and G. Rona
Copyright 1978 University Park Press Baltimore

MYOCARDIAL METABOLISM OF SPONTANEOUSLY HYPERTENSIVE RAT

N. SAITO, S. ANAZAWA, T. KOGURE,
M. KOSUGA, and M. NAGANO

Department of Internal Medicine, The Jikei University,
School of Medicine, Tokyo, Japan

SUMMARY

Oxidative phosphorylation of myocardial mitochondria isolated from spontaneously hypertensive rats (SHR) was determined polarographically. The concentrations of high-energy phosphate compounds, the concentrations of intermediate metabolites, and the activities of the enzymes within the metabolic systems of glycolysis, the pentose phosphate (PPh) cycle, and the tricarboxylic acid (TCA) cycle of the myocardium of SHR were determined.

The gradual development of cardiac hypertrophy was observed in SHR in comparison with normotensive Wistar rats. There were no significant differences in the function of oxidative phosphorylation of the mitochondria, in concentrations of high-energy phosphate compounds and carbohydrate metabolites, or in activities of glycolytic enzymes between SHR and normotensive Wistar rats.

INTRODUCTION

The authors have reported previously that no difference exists between the function of myocardial mitochondria obtained from hypertrophied heart of Goldblatt rats and that from chronic, pressure-overloaded heart (Nagano *et al.,* 1975). In the present study, the authors investigated the function of myocardial mitochondria and other myocardial metabolic activities of the hypertrophied hearts in spontaneously hypertensive rats (SHR) bred by Okamoto and his coworkers in Japan (Okamoto and Aoki, 1963).

MATERIALS AND METHODS

SHR were fed on a commercial laboratory diet and given tap water. The systolic blood pressure was measured indirectly by the tail-water plethysmographic method. The whole heart of male SHR, bred from 6 to 50 weeks, was prepared under urethane anesthesia and artificial respiration and then isolated by thoracotomy.

The mitochondria were isolated from the whole heart by the method of Chance and Hagihara (1961), incubating the myocardium for 3 min with

373

10,000 PUN of Nagarse® proteinase. ADP/O ratio and respiratory control index (RCI) were calculated from the curve obtained by charting the changes in mitochondrial oxygen consumption determined polarographically, with succinate as the substrate.

The concentrations of high-energy phosphate compounds, creatine phosphate (CP), ATP, ADP, and AMP were determined for the whole heart. The concentrations of the glycolytic intermediate metabolites and the metabolites of the TCA cycle (F-1,6-DP, α-GP, triose-P, pyruvate, lactate, oxalacetate, and malate) were determined enzymologically. The activities of the enzymes of glycolysis (HK, PFK, aldolase, α-GPDH, GAPDH, enolase, PK, and LDH), the pentose phosphate (PPh) cycle (G-6-PDH, P-6-GDH), the tricarboxylic acid (TCA) cycle (ICDH, MDH), and the transaminases (GOT, GPT) also were determined.

RESULTS

The blood pressure in SHR rose gradually from the seventh week after birth, and heart weight/body weight ratio was increased from the fifteenth week, as reported by Okamoto and coworkers (1963). ADP/O ratio and respiratory control index (RCI) of the mitochondria isolated from SHR are indicated in Figures 1 and 2. No significant differences were seen in the changes in ADP/O ratio and RCI during the evolution of cardiac hypertrophy. Similarly, no significant differences were seen in the concentrations of high-energy phosphate compounds (CP, ATP, ADP, and AMP) (Figure 3), nor in the glycolytic intermediate metabolites (Figure 4).

The enzyme activities of glycolysis, the PPh cycle, the TCA cycle, and the transaminases are indicated in Figures 5 and 6. The results were similar to those of normotensive Wistar rats, with the exceptions of low activity of enolase and high activity of hexokinase in SHR.

DISCUSSION

The SHR bred by Okamoto and Aoki are famous world-wide as experimental animal models for studying human essential hypertension. According to Takatsu and Kashii (1972), in SHR the increase in blood pressure is seen from the seventh week after birth, and the heart weight/body weight ratio, in comparison with the normotensive Wistar rats, increases from the fifteenth week after birth. Morphologically, it has been reported that, from the fifteenth week on, the mitochondria increased in number and size and showed a lack of uniformity in distribution, as well as changes indicating degeneration. The sarcoplasmic reticula also increased in number. During one year of observation the myocardial cell became hypertrophied to adapt to the pressure overload.

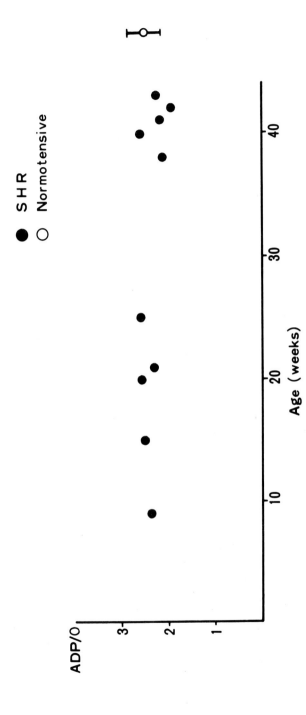

Figure 1. ADP/O ratio of mitochondria isolated from myocardium of SHR.

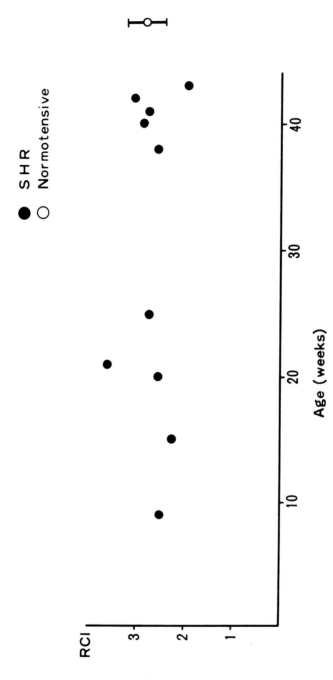

Figure 2. Respiratory control index (RCI) of mitochondria isolated from myocardium of SHR.

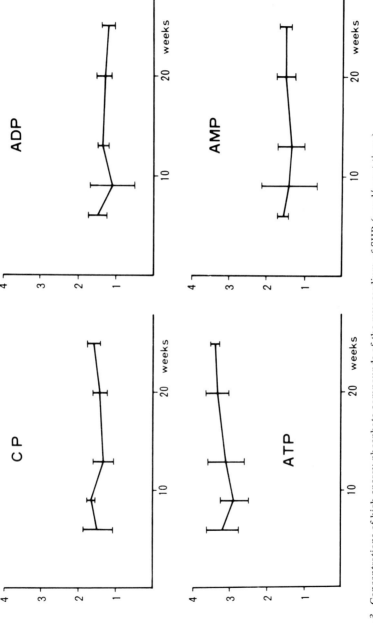

Figure 3. Concentrations of high-energy phosphate compounds of the myocardium of SHR (μmol/g wet tissue).

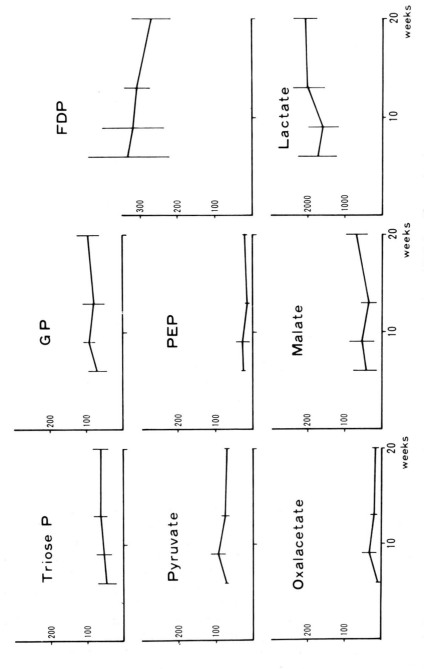

Figure 4. Concentrations of glycolytic intermediate metabolites of the myocardium of SHR (nmol/g wet tissue).

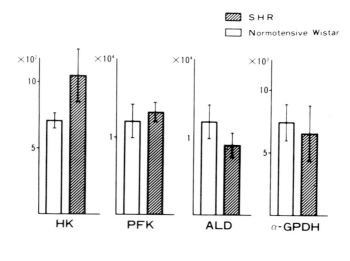

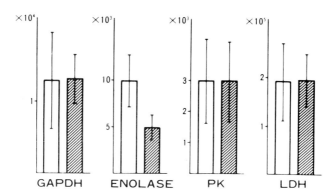

Figure 5. Enzyme activities of the myocardium (1) of SHR (mU/g wet weight).

Many investigators have reported that most, if not all, stimuli that lead to hypertrophy involve increase oxygen consumption and ATP utilization. However, in the present study, there were no significant differences in the function of oxidative phosphorylation of the mitochondria, in the concentrations of high-energy phosphate compounds and carbohydrate metabolites, and in the activities of glycolytic enzymes between the myocardium of normotensive Wistar rats and the hypertrophied myocardium of SHR.

In comparison with the function of the oxidative phosphorylation of the mitochondria isolated from hypertrophied heart, it has been reported that there were no significant differences between SHR and Goldblatt renovascular hypertensive rats (Nagano, 1974). While, in Goldblatt renovascular hypertensive rats,

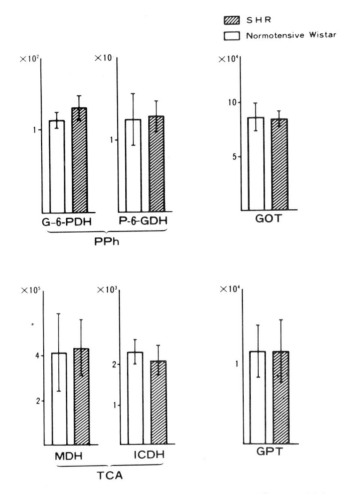

Figure 6. Enzyme activities of the myocardium (2) of SHR (mU/g wet weight).

an acceleration of the PPh cycle was indicated, no such acceleration was found in the SHR.

In Goldblatt renovascular hypertensive rats, the elevated cardiac work and myocardial hypertrophy are caused by the rapid development of hypertension, which results in the failure of adaptation of the myocardial metabolism. On the other hand, it is considered that the myocardial hypertrophy of the SHR is associated with sufficient metabolic adaptation to the chronic pressure overload obtained from slowly progressing hypertension.

It is concluded that these findings in the SHR provide evidence that a constitutional, mild pressure overload might be involved in a regulatory adaptation mechanism maintaining the energy source for cardiac work.

REFERENCES

CHANCE, B., and HAGIHARA, B. 1961. Techniques for the application of polarography to mitochondrial respiration. Biochem. Biophys. Acta 46:134–142.

NAGANO, M. 1974. Myokardstoffwechsel bei experimenteller Hypertonie. Jikeikai Med. J. 21(suppl.):73–81.

NAGANO, M., MOCHIZUKI, S., KOGURE, T., KOSUGA, M., SAITO, N., and TOMIZUKA, S. 1975. Oxidative phosphorylation in mitochondria isolated from stressed rat heart. *In* P. Roy and P. Harris (eds.), Recent Advances in Studies on Cardiac Structure and Metabolism. Vol. 8: The Cardiac Sarcoplasm, pp. 293–300. University Park Press, Baltimore.

OKAMOTO, K., and AOKI, K. 1963. Development of a strain of spontaneously hypertensive rats. Jpn. Circ. J. 39:282–293.

TAKATSU, T., and KASHII, C. 1972. Cardiac hypertrophy in spontaneously hypertensive rats. *In* K. Okamoto (ed.), Spontaneous Hypertension, Its Pathogenesis and Complications, pp. 166–172. Igaku Shoin, Tokyo; Springer-Verlag, New York.

Mailing address:
N. Saito, M.D.,
The Third Department of Internal Medicine, the Jikei University School of Medicine, Nishi-shimbashi, Minatoku, Tokyo 105 (Japan).

Recent Advances in Studies on
Cardiac Structure and Metabolism, Volume 12
Cardiac Adaptation
Edited by T. Kobayashi, Y. Ito, and G. Rona
Copyright 1978 University Park Press Baltimore

REDUCED RESPONSE OF
CARDIAC NOREPINEPHRINE RELEASE
TO ISOMETRIC HANDGRIP EXERCISE IN HEART FAILURE

T. HANEDA, Y. MIURA, K. MIYAZAWA,
T. SATO, K. SHIRATO, T. HONNA,
T. NAKAJIMA, T. ARAI, K. KOBAYASHI,
H. SAKUMA, K. YOSHINAGA, and T. TAKISHIMA

Department of Internal Medicine, Tohoku University,
School of Medicine, Sendai, Japan

SUMMARY

In order to evaluate the relation of cardiac norepinephrine (NE) release to left ventricular function, blood was taken simultaneously from the coronary sinus (CS) and the aorta (A) in 19 patients with heart diseases, at rest and during isometric handgrip exercise (IHG) at 30% of their maximal contraction. Plasma NE was analyzed by Renzini's THI method. The concentrations of plasma NE at rest were 397 ± 66 (S.E.M.) ng/liter in CS and 292 ± 50 in A. IHG significantly increased NE to 578 ± 88 in CS and to 462 ± 85 in A ($p <$ 0.001). Estimated NE release from the heart ($\Delta NE = NE_{CS} - NE_A$) correlated inversely to left ventricular end-diastolic pressure at rest ($r = -0.520$, $p < 0.05$) and during IHG ($r = -0.689$, $p < 0.01$). The changes in ΔNE induced by IHG correlated to the slope of the left ventricular function curve ($r = 0.618$, $p < 0.01$). It is concluded that the response of cardiac NE release to exercise is reduced in patients with depressed cardiac function.

INTRODUCTION

Cardiac norepinephrine (NE) stores have been shown to be reduced in human and in experimental animals with congestive heart failure (Chidsey *et al.,* 1963, 1964, and 1965; Spann *et al.,* 1965). Reduced chronotropic and inotropic responses to sympathetic nerve stimulation also have been reported in animals with congestive heart failure (Covell, Chidsey, and Braunwald, 1966). These facts suggest that the compensatory mechanism mediated by cardiac catecholamine might be disturbed in the failing heart. However, it has not been demonstrated whether or not the release of NE from the heart is impaired in patients with depressed cardiac function. The present study was undertaken to evaluate the relation of cardiac NE release to left ventricular (LV) function in patients with heart diseases.

MATERIALS AND METHODS

Studies were performed with 19 patients who underwent cardiac catheterization without any premedication. Eleven of the patients were male and eight were female, ages 16–70 with a mean age of 37. No sympatho-mimetic or -lytic medication was given to them for at least four weeks before the study. Clinical diagnosis was cardiomyopathy in six cases, mitral and aortic insufficiency in three, mitral stenosis in two, functional murmur in two, essential hypertension in four, anemia in one, and pulmonary arteriovenous (A-V) fistula in one. LV and aortic pressures were measured by an 8F Cordis pigtail catheter with a Statham P_{23} db pressure transducer. Cardiac output was determined by the indicator dilution method using indocyanine green dye. A 9F Gensini catheter was introduced through the femoral vein into the coronary sinus (CS) for blood sampling and flow measurement. Coronary sinus blood flow (CSBF) was measured with a continuous dye-injection technique reported previously (Ishikawa et al., 1972). Ten ml of blood for plasma NE assay was withdrawn simultaneously from CS and the aorta (A). After control measurements, patients were asked to perform isometric handgrip exercise (IHG) at 30% of their maximal contraction for 3 min. Hemodynamic measurements and blood samplings were repeated during the last minute of exercise.

LV stroke-work index (LVSWI) was calculated from the formula:
$$\text{LVSWI} = \text{SIX (LVSP} - \text{LVEDP)} \times 1.36/100$$
where, SI = stroke index (ml/M^2),
LVSP = LV systolic pressure (mm Hg),
LVEDP = LV end-diastolic pressure (mm Hg), and
LV function curve was constructed from the changes in LVSWI and LVEDP.

Plasma NE concentration was analyzed with Renzini's THI method. In our laboratory, the minimal sensitivity of this method is 0.25 ng/aliquot of plasma. To confirm the reproducibility and the recovery rate of the whole procedure, three control plasma specimens containing a known amount of NE were involved in every assay. The difference (ΔNE) between plasma NE concentrations in CS (NE_{CS}) and in A (NE_A) was used as a tentative index for determining the extent of NE release from the cardiac tissue.

RESULTS

Hemodynamic values and plasma NE_{CS} and NE_A at rest and during IHG are summarized in Table 1. Plasma NE_{CS} was significantly greater than NE_A at rest ($p < 0.001$). IHG increased both NE_{CS} and NE_A significantly ($p < 0.001$) in parallel with the augmentation of hemodynamic parameters. However, individual

Table 1. Hemodynamic parameters and plasma norepinephrine (NE) levels of coronary sinus (CS) and coronary artery (A) in 19 patients

	At rest		During IHG	
Heart rate (beats/min)	84	± 4	98	± 7
Mean aortic pressure (mm Hg)	102	± 3	123	± 4
Cardiac index (liter/min/M^2)	3.91 ±	0.23	4.33 ±	0.29
LVEDP (mm Hg)	15	± 2	22	± 3
LVSWI (g m/M^2)	81.1	± 8.2	94.6	± 10.7
CSBF (ml/min/M^2)	94	± 7	124	± 12
NE in CS (ng/liter)	397	± 66	578	± 88
NE in A (ng/liter)	292	± 50	462	± 85

Values represent the mean ± S.E.M.

IHG = isometric handgrip exercise; LVEDP = left ventricular end-diastolic pressure; LVSWI = left ventricular stroke work index; CSBF = coronary sinus blood flow.

NE concentrations in CS and in A failed to correlate significantly to heart rate, mean aortic pressure, cardiac index. LVEDP, LVSWI, and CSBF at both stages. During IHG, ΔNE (NE$_{CS}$ − NE$_A$) increased in patients without depressed LV function, e.g., those with functional murmur and mitral stenosis (from 60 to 232 ng/liter, on the average, and from 358 to 645 ng/liter, respectively). In contrast, these values decreased in patients with depressed LV function, e.g., those with

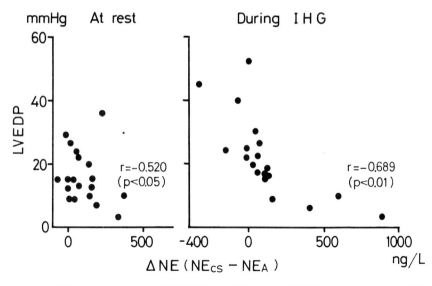

Figure 1. Relationship between ΔNE (NE$_{CS}$ − NE$_A$) and LVEDP at rest and during IHG (isometric handgrip exercise).

cardiomyopathy and mitral and aortic insufficiency (from 42 to −6 ng/liter and from 128 to −76 ng/liter, respectively). The ΔNE inversely correlated to LVEDP at rest, and this relation became more evident during IHG (Figure 1). The changes in ΔNE induced by IHG correlated significantly to the slope of LV function curve ($r = 0.618$, $p < 0.01$). There was no significant correlation between the changes in ΔNE and those in CSBF induced by IHG.

DISCUSSION

In the resting patients studied, no significant relation was found between NE_{CS} and hemodynamic parameters, while ΔNE inversely correlated to LVEDP. Isometric exercise induces an increase in aortic pressure so that LV function can be evaluated from the relationship between changes in LVSWI and LVEDP (Helfant, De Villa, and Meister, 1971; Kivowitz *et al.*, 1971). In this study, IHG induced a significant elevation of NE_{CS} and NE_A in parallel with the hemodynamic augmentation. This finding suggests that sympathetic nerve stimulation plays an important role in hemodynamic changes during exercise. The inversed correlation that was found between ΔNE and LVEDP at rest became more evident during IHG.

The changes in ΔNE induced by IHG correlated to the slope of LV function curve, demonstrating the decline of ΔNE in patients with a shallow slope of LV function curve. This decline of ΔNE values can be attributed to either the decreased cardiac NE release or the increased NE removal through the coronary vascular bed. In the failing heart, however, the increased NE removal does not seem the major cause of the decline of ΔNE values, because Spann *et al.* (1965) have demonstrated that NE uptake in the cardiac tissue is reduced in experimental failing heart. It is also unlikely that the changes in ΔNE were influenced by the changes in coronary flow or chronotropic state because there was no relationship between the changes in ΔNE and the increase in CSBF or heart rate during IHG. These facts, therefore, lead us to conclude that the decreased ΔNE observed in patients with depressed cardiac function represents the decreased cardiac NE release.

REFERENCES

CHIDSEY, C. A., BRAUNWALD, E., MORROW, A. G., and MASON, D. T., 1963. Myocardial norepinephrine concentration in man: Effects of reserpine and of congestive heart failure. N. Engl. J. Med. 269:653–658.

CHIDSEY, C. A., BRAUNWALD, E., and MORROW, A. G. 1965. Catecholamine excretions and cardiac stores of norepinephrine in congestive heart failure. Am. J. Med. 39: 442–451.

CHIDSEY, C. A., KAISER, G. A., SONNENBLICK, E. H., SPANN, J. F., JR., and BRAUNWALD, E. 1964. Cardiac norepinephrine stores in experimental heart failure in the dog. J. Clin. Invest. 43:2386–2393.

COVELL, J. W., CHIDSEY, C. A., and BRAUNWALD, E. 1966. Reduction of the cardiac response to postganglionic sympathetic nerve stimulation in experimental heart failure. Circ. Res. 19:51–56.

HELFANT, R. H., De VILLA, M. A., and MEISTER, S. G. 1971. Effect of sustained isometric handgrip exercise on left ventricular performance. Circulation 44:982–993.

ISHIKAWA, K., MIYAZAWA, K., TSUIKI, K., MATSUNAGA, A., HANEDA, T., KATORI, R., and NAKUMURA, T. 1972. Measurement of coronary sinus blood flow by dye dilution technique in man. J. Lab. Clin. Med. 79:75–84.

KIVOWITZ, C., PARMLEY, W. W., DONOSO, R., MARCUS, H., GANZ, W., and SWAN, H. J. C. 1971. Effects of isometric exercise on cardiac performance: The grip test. Circulation 44:994–1002.

SPANN, J. F., JR., CHIDSEY, C. A., POOL, P. E., and BRAUNWALD, E. 1965. Mechanism of norepinephrine depletion in experimental heart failure produced by aortic constriction in the guinea pig. Circ. Res. 17:312–321.

Mailing address:
Takashi Haneda, M.D.,
The First Department of Internal Medicine, Tohoku University, School of Medicine, Seiryo Cho, Sendai (Japan).

ENZYME CHANGES
IN
MYOCARDIAL INJURY

Recent Advances in Studies on
Cardiac Structure and Metabolism, Volume 12
Cardiac Adaptation
Edited by T. Kobayashi, Y. Ito, and G. Rona
Copyright 1978 University Park Press Baltimore

EXPERIMENTAL STUDY ON ENZYME DISTRIBUTION AND ITS RELATION TO MYOCARDIAL ISCHEMIC CHANGES FOLLOWING CORONARY CIRCULATORY DISTURBANCES

Y. NOHARA,[1] I. YAMASAWA,[1] S. KONNO,[1] K. SHIMIZU,[1]
H. IWANE,[1] C. IBUKIYAMA.[1] and A. HARA[2]

[1] Department of Internal Medicine,
Tokyo Medical College, Tokyo, Japan
[2] Third Department of Internal Medicine,
Faculty of Medicine, Kyoto University, Kyoto, Japan

SUMMARY

Coronary artery ligation of canine heart was performed to investigate the relationship between the lactate dehydrogenase (LDH) pattern in myocardium and the distribution of coronary flow, especially in the early stage of ligation and after reperfusion. In the myocardium of normal dogs, the LDH pattern was similar in the left ventricle, the interventricular septum, and the right ventricle; the average LD5:LD4 ratio was 1.1, 1.2, and 1.2, respectively, and consisted mainly of heart type. In the left and right auricles, however, the ratios were 0.3 and 0.2, respectively, lacking heart type. In the left ventricle, LD5:LD4 ratio in the subendocardium was different from that in the subepicardial layer. Blood flow distribution in canine myocardium was investigated by the fluorescent pattern on the cut surface of heart, in which 10% fluorescein sodium was injected into the cavity. By this method the evolution of the ischemic area from the endocardial layer to the epicardial side following coronary artery ligation and the effect of reperfusion on the ischemic area were clarified. Electron microscopic studies indicated that loss of mitochondrial function may account for the irreversibility of myocardial cell alteration. A new method for studying enzyme localization in tissues was introduced for studying LDH isoenzyme distribution in normal and injured myocardium.

INTRODUCTION

The authors, on the basis of patterns of lactate dehydrogenase (LDH) and its isoenzymes, have previously classified angina pectoris in four categories (Nohara, 1968; Yamasawa, 1973; Nohara *et al.*, 1974). In this study, from the data obtained by coronary ligation of canine heart, the relationship between the LDH pattern in myocardium and the distribution of coronary blood flow, especially in the early stage of ligation and after reperfusion, was examined.

MATERIALS AND METHODS

Dogs weighing 8—20 kg were used. Cabaud-Wroblewski's (1958) method for LDH measurement and for agar-agarose gel electrophoresis, modified by Wieme (1959) and Yoshida and Kitamura (1967) for LDH isoenzymes, was used. Five peaks of LDH activity were designated as LD5, LD4, LD3, LD2, and LD1, according to the degree of migration (from greatest to least, respectively) to the anodal side.

RESULTS

LDH and Its Isoenzymes in Normal Canine Myocardium

Various sections of canine heart were homogenized and its supernatants were used for LDH isoenzyme determination. In the left ventricle, the interventricular septum, and the right ventricle, the average LD5:LD4 ratios were 1.1, 1.2, and 1.2, respectively, and consisted mainly of heart type. In contrast, in the left and right atrial myocardium, the average LD5:LD4 ratios were 0.3 and 0.2, respectively, not containing the heart-type isoenzyme. In the left ventricular myocardium, the LD5:LD4 ratio in the subendocardial layer was different from that of the subepicardial myocardium, i.e., the former was 1.12 and the latter was 0.9, in average value (Figure 1). These findings suggest that the metabolic process may be different in the ventricular and atrial myocardium, as well as in the subendocardial and subepicardial ventricular myocardium.

Coronary Blood Flow and ECG Findings
following Coronary Artery Ligation and after Reperfusion of Canine Heart

The ligation was performed just above the second bifurcation of the anterior descending branch of the left coronary artery, setting the electrode (ca. 5 X 5 mm) on the mid portion of the occluded area. After ligation of various durations, 10% fluorescein sodium (10 ml) was injected instantaneously, and 30 sec after injection the heart was removed and frozen. A cross-sectional surface of the frozen heart was observed under ultraviolet light. By studying the fluorescence pattern of the cross-sectional surface, blood flow distribution was investigated (Figure 2).

Hearts from controls and cases of ligation for 5 min, 10 min, 20 min, 6 hr, and 10 hr were compared. In the cases of 5-min ligation, fluorescent defect in the occluded region of the myocardium, indicating ischemic area, was only found occasionally. Ligation, lasting for 10 min, 20 min, 6 hr, and 10 hr, resulted in more prominent area that was devoid of fluorescence, expanding from the endocardial side to the subepicardial myocardium. Surface ECG in the mid portion of the occluded area revealed ST elevation beginning approximately 1—2 min after ligation and reaching maximal value after approximately 5—30 min.

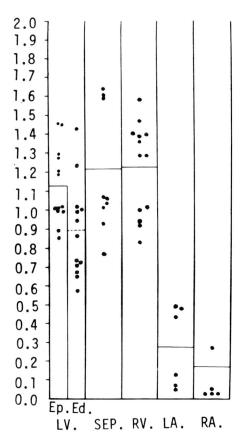

Figure 1. LD5:LD4 in heart muscle extracts. LV. = left ventricle; Ep. = epicardial side; Ed. = endocardial side; SEP. = ventricular septum; RV. = right ventricle; LA. = left atrium; RA. = right atrium.

Following the release of coronary ligation, fluorescein sodium was injected to investigate the coronary blood flow distribution:

1. In the case of 10-min ligation, followed by a gradual release to 80% stenosis in 10 min, a fluorescent defect pattern was found to be reduced from the epicardial side to the endocardial layer, and the ECG showed a gradual decrease of ST-segment elevation.

2. In the case of 10-min ligation, followed by a gradual release to 60% stenosis in 25 min, the fluorescent pattern was found to be entirely normal, and ST-segment elevation was found only exceptionally.

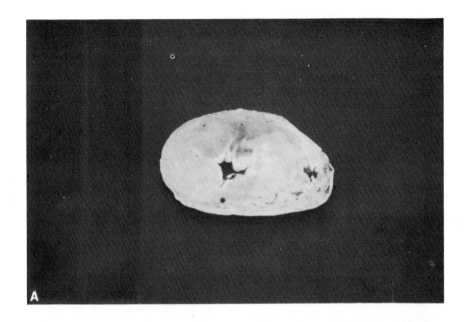

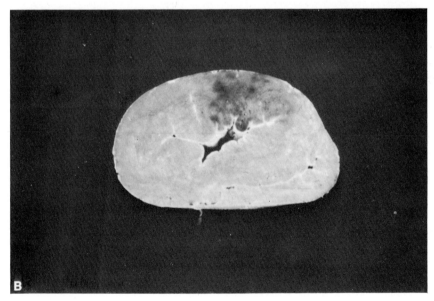

Figure 2A and B.

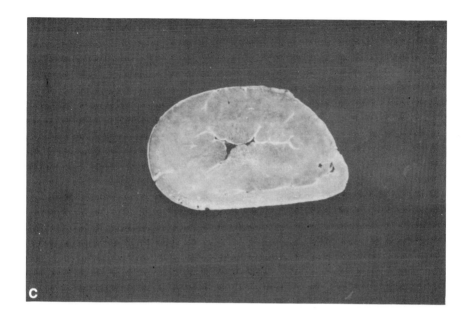

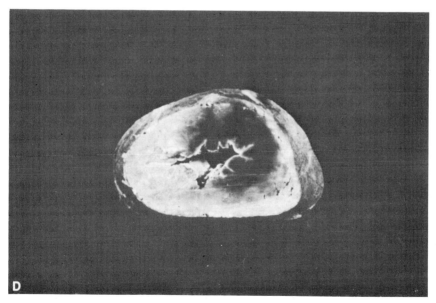

Figure 2C and D.

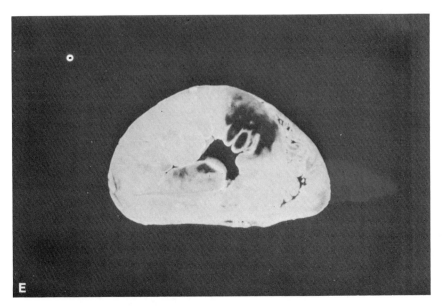

Figure 2A–E. Fluorescent pattern on the cut surface of frozen canine heart in which 10% fluorescein sodium was injected. The fluorescent defect represents absence of blood flow. A = 10-min ligation; B = 10-min ligation, followed by reperfusion in 10 min (ca. 20% coronary flow); C = 10-min ligation, followed by reperfusion in 25 min (40% coronary flow); D = 6-hr ligation; E = 10-hr ligation, followed by reperfusion.

3. Comparing 6-hr ligation and 10-hr ligation, followed by reperfusion for 1.5 min, the latter case showed a reduced area of fluorescent defect. In all these experiments no ST-segment depression was observed on the ECG.

Histochemical Findings and Electron Microscopic Findings of the Enzymes in Myocardium Following Coronary Ligation and Subsequent Reperfusion

The most prominent histochemical finding was a focal decrease of phosphorylase activity 5 min after ligation. Periodic-acid-Schiff (PAS) and succinate dehydrogenase (SDH) stains and LDH reaction were increased in a late stage of ligation. As to the electron microscopic findings, in the case of 5-min ligation, there was a decrease of mitochondrial matrix density and glycogen granules were decreased in the sarcoplasma (Figure 3); these changes were more pronounced following 30-min ligation; endoplasmic reticulum became distended. In the case of 30-min ligation and 5-hr release, mitochondria were recovered close to the control findings; however, the dilatation of endoplasmic reticulum still persisted. Mitochondria were recovered insufficiently in 60-min ligation and 5-hr release.

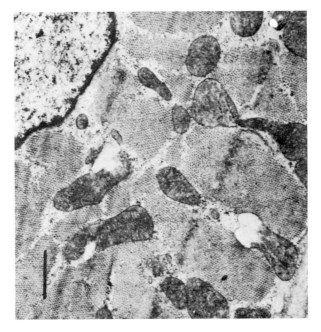

Figure 3. Electron microscopic findings of canine heart muscle following ligation for 5 min. There is a loss of mitochondrial cristae and matrix density, and a decrease of glycogen granules in some parts of the sarcoplasm.

A New Method to Clarify the Localization of LDH Isoenzymes in the Tissue Section

This new method is similar to the histochemical method, by which localization of the examined material in the tissue is clarified by chemical method. It consists of clarifying the localization of LDH isoenzymes in the tissue by electrophoresis, and the principle of this new method lies in the following procedure: 1) After examined tissue is frozen, the filter paper is placed firmly on the cross-sectional surface of the frozen tissue, and 2) as a result the enzyme molecules on the cut surface are reabsorbed in the surface layer of the filter paper; 3) then, the filter paper is treated as usual by LDH isoenzyme examination method by paper electrophoresis. The details of this method are given in *Acta Histochemica et Cytochemica* (Yamasawa and Nohara, in press).

The pattern of LDH isoenzymes on the cross-sectional surface of kidney, heart, and liver by this method are shown in Figure 4. These examples show the characteristic localization of LDH isoenzymes in each organ as naturally situated. While this method offers new avenues in heart research by investigating

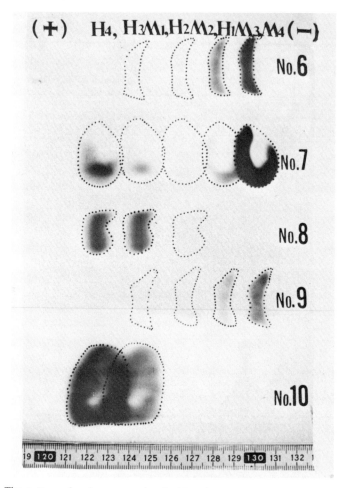

Figure 4. The pattern of various organs by the histochemical electrophoresis method. Nos. 6 and 7 = Kidney; Nos. 8 and 10 = Heart; No. 9 = Liver.

LDH isoenzymes in myocardium, many points remain unsolved at the present time.

REFERENCES

CABAUD, P., and WROBLEWSKI, F. 1958. Colorimetric measurement of lactic de-
    hydrogenase activity of body fluids. Am. J. Clin. Pathol. 30:234.
COHEN, L., DJORDJEVICH, J., and ORMISTE, V. 1964. Serum lactic dehydrogenase
    isoenzyme patterns in cardiovascular and other diseases, with particular reference to
    acute myocardial infarction. J. Lab. Clin. Med. 64:355.
NOHARA, Y. 1968. Enzymatic investigation of intermediate form of angina pectoris. Jpn.
    J. Med. 7:201.

NOHARA, Y., YAMASAWA, I., HARA, A., KUMAGAYA, T., and TAKAYASU, M. 1974. Variant form of angina pectoris with special reference to serum lactate dehydrogenase isoenzymes with some histological findings. The Seventh World Congress of Cardiology, Sept., 1974, Buenos Aires, Argentina.

PRINZMETAL, M., KENNAMER, R., MERLISS, R., WADA, T., and BOR, N. 1959. Angina pectoris. 1. A variant form of angina pectoris. Preliminary report. Am. J. Med. 27:375.

WIEME, R. J. 1959. An improved technique of agar-gel electrophoresis on microscope slides. Clin. Chim. Acta 4:317.

YAMASAWA, I. 1973. Serum enzyme patterns in acute ischemic heart diseases with special reference to LDH isoenzymes in intermediate types of ischemic heart disease, fresh myocardial infarction, and cardiogenic shock. Jpn. Circ. J. 37:507.

YAMASAWA, I., and NOHARA, Y. A new method for geometrical demonstration of LDH isoenzymes—Histochemical electrophoresis. Acta Histochem. Cytochem. In press.

YOSHIDA, M., and KITAMURA, M. 1967. LDH isoenzyme. Jpn. Clin. Pathol. Special No. 12:96.

Mailing address:
Y. Nohara, M.D.,
Department of Internal Medicine, Tokyo Medical College,
6-7-1, Nishi-shinjuku, Shinjuku-ku, Tokyo, Japan 160

Recent Advances in Studies on
Cardiac Structure and Metabolism, Volume 12
Cardiac Adaptation
Edited by T. Kobayashi, Y. Ito, and G. Rona
Copyright 1978 University Park Press Baltimore

THE INFLUENCE OF PLASMA VOLUME CHANGES
ON ENZYMATIC ESTIMATION OF INFARCT SIZE

S. A. G. J. WITTEVEEN,[1] S. J. SMITH,[2]
G. BOS,[2] and W. Th. HERMENS[3]

[1] Department of Cardiology, Leiden, [2] Department of Medicine, Rotterdam, and
[3] Medical Faculty, Maastricht, The Netherlands

SUMMARY

In 18 patients, myocardial injury was estimated by mathematical analysis of the rise in plasma activity of α-hydroxybutyrate (α-HBDH) dehydrogenase as observed by multiple sampling after admission. This enzyme represents the lactate dehydrogenase isoenzymes LDH_1 and LDH_2. Changes in plasma volume were assessed by determining hematocrit values at the same time as the enzyme activities. Infarct size was expressed in IU/liter of plasma and in grams of heart muscle per liter of plasma (g/liter). Significant changes in plasma volume, reflected in hematocrit changes, occurred (average 12%): 10 patients without pulmonary edema showed an average change of 7%; for the group of eight patients with pulmonary edema, the change was 17%. When calculated infarct size was not correlated for plasma volume changes, a significant overestimation occurred (11.7%, range 0.7–29.7%). In the subgroup of patients with pulmonary edema the mean overestimation was 15.8%, and, in patients without pulmonary edema, the mean overestimation was 8.5%. It is concluded that plasma volume changes after an acute myocardial infarction have to be taken into account when infarct size is calculated on the basis of plasma enzyme levels.

INTRODUCTION

The determination of plasma enzyme levels for quantitative purposes after an acute myocardial infarction in man has been practiced for several years now (Witteveen, Hermens, and Hemker, 1970; Witteveen et al., 1970; Sobel et al., 1972; Norris, 1975). Its main value lies in the fact that a reasonable estimate can be made of the extent of the infarcted area, an important factor in the prognosis of the individual patient. It also provides the physician with a basis for comparing the effects of certain therapeutic interventions (Hermens et al., 1975). In this way, differences in relatively small groups of patients can be discerned. However, certain drugs, which are increasingly used in the coronary care unit today, clearly influence the hemodynamic status of the patient, e.g., β-adrenergic blockers, diuretics, and blood-pressure lowering agents. This implies that the plasma volume in that patient cannot be considered constant.

This study was undertaken to calculate the effect of changes in plasma volume on infarct quantitation and to assess whether or not corrections must be made to compensate for these changes.

MATERIALS AND METHODS

Eighteen patients with acute myocardial infarction were studied. The diagnosis was established by a history of chest pain, electrocardiographic changes, and elevations of the blood levels of creatine phosphokinase (CPK), glutamic oxalo-acetic transaminase (GOT), lactate dehydrogenase (LDH), and α-hydroxy-butyrate dehydrogenase (α-HBDH). Patients with chronic illness and patients who developed an acute illness other than their myocardial infarction during the period of the study were excluded.

Treatment consisted of bedrest, oxygen by nasal catheter, anticoagulant therapy (fenprocoumon), and furosemide given intravenously, if pulmonary edema occurred. Pulmonary edema was considered to be present if moist rales were heard, which were rated as mild (+), moderate (++), or severe (+++), and if the roentgenogram showed signs of pulmonary congestion.

α-HBDH was used for infarct quantification, representing more or less the cardiospecific isoenzymes LDH_1 and LDH_2. Blood samples for α-HBDH were taken every eight hours during the first three days and, thereafter, progressively less frequently. Samples in which the plasma showed hemolysis were discarded. α-HBDH was determined according to the method of Rosalki and Wilkinson (1964). Hematocrit was determined by the cyanide method (Kampen and Zijlstra, 1961).

Analysis of Data

Data were analyzed using a two-compartment model with time dependent intravascular volume $V_i(t)$ and extravascular volume $V_e(t)$ (for details see Smith *et al.*, 1976). The total amount of enzyme released into the circulation at time $t(A(t))$ is given by the equation:

$$A(t) = V_i(t)C_i(t) + V_e(t)C_e(t) + K_o \int^t V_i(\tau)C_i(\tau)d\tau \qquad (1)$$

where $C_i(t)$ and $C_e(t)$ are the intra- and extravascular activities of time t. K represents the elimination constant. To calculate the enzyme release caused by the infarction, $C_i(t)$ and $C_e(t)$ are corrected by subtracting the normal plasma activities C_{lim}:

$$\overline{C}_i(t) = C_i(t) - C_{lim} ; \overline{C}_e(t) = C_e(t) - C_{lim}$$

To express the total enzyme release per liter plasma $Q_{(t)}$, the following formula is used:

$$Q(t) = \frac{A(t)}{V_i(t)} = \overline{C}_i(t) + \frac{V_e(t)}{V_i(t)} \cdot \overline{C}_e(t) + K_o \int^t \frac{V_i(\tau)}{V_i(t)} \overline{C}_i(\tau)d\tau \qquad (2)$$

$Q(t)$ reaches its final value after the enzyme release from the infarcted area has stopped (between 40 and 75 hr after the acute event).

When t becomes large, normal values C_{lim} are again obtained and the equation (2) reduces to:

$$Q(t = large) = K_o \int^t \frac{V_i(\tau)}{V_i(t)} C_i(\tau)d\tau \qquad (3)$$

$Q(t)$ was calculated at $t = 200$ because plasma volume changes occur mainly during the first 200 hr.

The correction factors, that are necessary to take into account the changes in plasma volume, $V_i(\tau)/V_i(t)$, were calculated by using the following formula:

$$\frac{V_i(t)}{EV} = \frac{100 - H(t)}{H(t)} \qquad (4)$$

where EV is the total red cell volume and $H(t)$ is the hematocrit as a percentage.

Because EV can be considered constant one obtains:

$$\frac{V_i(\tau)}{V_i(t)} = \frac{(100 - H(\tau)) \cdot H(t)}{(100 - H(t)) \cdot H(\tau)} \qquad (5)$$

Using the $H(t)$ values that were determined from the blood samples that were used for α-HBDH determinations $Q(t)$ could be calculated using the correction of equation (5).

RESULTS

In 10 patients, the clinical course was uncomplicated; eight patients had signs of pulmonary edema and were treated with furosemide. In patients with pulmonary edema, total enzyme release per liter of plasma ranged from 212–758 IU/liter; in the edema group the range was from 495–1,463 IU/liter.

Plasma volumes were reflected in the hematocrit changes, which are shown in Figure 1. In general a decrease in hematocrit occurred from the time of admission until 200 hr, after which time leveling off was apparent. This decrease was 12% for the whole group, 17% for the group with pulmonary edema, and 7% for the group without pulmonary edema.

In Table 1 the relevant data are given for all patients. When enzyme values before and after correction for plasma volume changes are compared, important

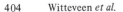

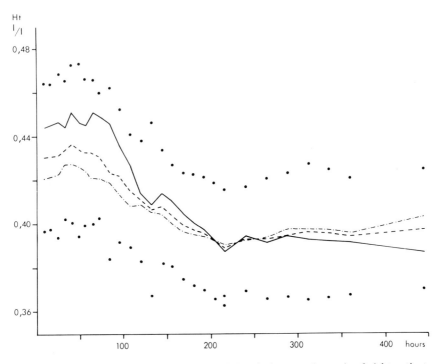

Figure 1. Time course of mean hematocrit of the whole group (– – –), of eight patients with pulmonary edema (——), and of ten patients without pulmonary edema (–·–). Standard deviation of the whole group is indicated in the figure.

differences can be seen: the average overestimation of the uncorrected values was 11.7%. Especially in the group with pulmonary edema, a marked overestimation was found ranging from 7.5–29.7% (mean 15.8%).

Figure 2 shows the effect of the correction for plasma volume on the total calculated enzyme release per liter in a patient with edema.

CONCLUSIONS

It is clear from these data that grave errors in infarct quantitation of plasma enzyme levels can be made, if the plasma volume after the infarction is treated as a constant. Particularly in patients with complications that must be treated vigorously, the influence of plasma volume changes is apparent. Therefore, it is concluded that, especially in clinical trials in which therapeutic interventions are made that can easily influence the hemodynamics, these plasma volume changes must be taken into account when calculating infarct size from blood enzyme levels.

Table 1. Comparison of enzyme levels before and after correction for plasma volume changes

Patient number	Pulmonary edema rales	x-ray (stage)	Furosemid therapy	Total enzyme release (IU/liter) uncorrected	corrected	Overestimation of uncorrected values (%)
1	−	−	−	354	351	− 0.7
2	−	−	−	483	458	− 5.2
3	−	−	−	666	652	− 2.2
4	−	−	−	489	466	− 4.6
5	−	−	−	873	758	−13.1
6	−	−	−	330	317	− 3.8
7	−	−	−	486	469	− 3.5
8	−	−	−	445	384	−13.7
9	−	−	−	265	212	−20.0
10	−	−	−	487	396	−18.6
11	+	II	+	549	495	− 9.7
12	+	I	−	1,194	1,104	− 7.5
13	++	III	+	1,129	859	−23.9
14	++	III	+	1,128	993	−11.9
15	++	II	+	1,234	1,064	−13.7
16	+	I	−	863	607	−29.7
17	+	II	+	797	656	−17.7
18	−	II	+	1,675	1,463	−12.6

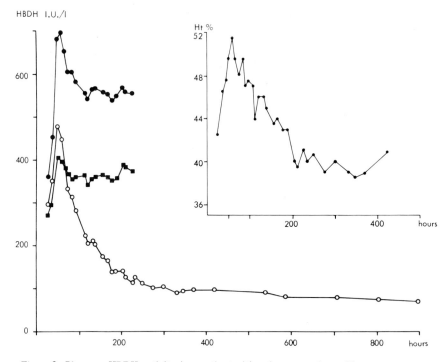

Figure 2. Plasma α-HBDH activity in a patient with pulmonary edema. Plasma curve = ○—○; uncorrected calculated total enzyme release = ●—●; corrected calculated total enzyme release = ■—■. The insert shows the time course of hematocrit in this patient.

REFERENCES

HERMENS, W. Th., WITTEVEEN, S. A. G. J., HOLLAAR, L., HEMKER, H. C. 1975. Effect of a thrombolytic agent (urokinase) on necrosis after acute myocardial infarction. *In* P. E. Roy and G. Rona (eds.), Recent Advances in Studies on Cardiac Structure and Metabolism. Vol. 10: The Metabolism of Contraction, page 319. University Park Press, Baltimore.

KAMPEN, E. J. VAN, and ZIJLSTRA, W. G. 1961. Standardization of hemoglobinometry II. The hemoglobin-cyanide method. Clin. Chim. Acta 6:538.

MESZAROS, W. I. 1973. Lung changes in left heart failure. Circulation 47:859.

NORRIS, R. M., WHITLOCK, R. M. L., BARRATT-BOYES, C., SMALL, C. W. 1975. Clinical measurement of infarct size. Circulation 51:614.

ROSALKI, S. B., and WILKINSON, J. H. 1964. Serum α-hydroxybutyrate dehydrogenase in diagnostics. JAMA 189:61.

SMITH, S. J., BOS, G., HAGEMEIJER, F., HERMENS, W. Th., WITTEVEEN, S. A. G. J. 1976. Influences of changes in plasma volume on quantitation of infarct size in man by means of plasma enzyme levels. J. Mol. Med. 1:199.

SOBEL, B. E., BRESNAHAN, G. F., SHELL, W. F., YODER, R. D. 1972. Estimation of infarct size in man and its relation to prognosis. Circulation 46:640.

WITTEVEEN, S. A. G. J., HERMENS, W. Th., HEMKER, H. C. 1970. Quantitation of myocardial infarction in man by elevation of plasma enzyme levels. Abstract VIth World Congress of Cardiology. Cardiovasc. Res. 4:326.
WITTEVEEN, S. A. G. J., HERMENS, W. Th., HEMKER, H. C., HOLLAAR, L. 1970. Quantitation of enzyme release from infarcted heart muscle. *In* J. H. de Haas, H. C. Hemker, and H. A. Snellen (eds.), Ischaemic Heart Disease. Leiden University Press, Leiden, The Netherlands.

Mailing address:
S. A. G. J. Witteveen, M.D.,
Department of Cardiology, University Hospital,
Leiden (The Netherlands).

Recent Advances in Studies on
Cardiac Structure and Metabolism, Volume 12
Cardiac Adaptation
Edited by T. Kobayashi, Y. Ito, and G. Rona
Copyright 1978 University Park Press Baltimore

CHANGES IN PURINE NUCLEOSIDE CONTENT IN HUMAN MYOCARDIAL EFFLUX DURING PACING-INDUCED ISCHEMIA

W. J. REMME, J. W. De JONG, and P. D. VERDOUW

Catheterization Department and Cardiochemistry,
Thoraxcenter and Department of Biochemistry I,
Erasmus University, Rotterdam, The Netherlands

SUMMARY

Pacing-induced myocardial ischemia in 18 patients resulted in an increase of coronary sinus hypoxanthine levels from 1.20 ± 0.18 μM during control to 2.41 ± 0.52 μM ($p < 0.025$) during pain. In addition, early lactate production occurred frequently before angina was noted. Neither hypoxanthine nor lactate levels changed in seven nonanginal patients, nor were significant alterations in potassium, inorganic phosphate, glucose, or oxygen saturation found in all patients. Myocardial hypoxanthine production seems a useful indicator of ischemia in the human heart.

INTRODUCTION

Alterations in the lactate extraction pattern reflecting increased anaerobic glycolysis have been used in various studies of the human heart to identify the degree of ischemia. However, the usefulness of lactate determinations alone has been questioned, and, recently, the simultaneous measurement of additional biochemical markers of myocardial ischemia has been re-emphasized (Brachfeld, 1976). During the early phase of myocardial ischemia, adenosine triphosphate concentration decreases progressively with the subsequent accumulation of adenosine diphosphate and adenosine monophosphate. An increased purine nucleoside concentration in canine heart within seconds of coronary artery occlusion also has been reported (Olsson, 1970). These nucleosides readily pass the intact myocardial cell membrane, and determination of their concentrations in the venous effluent may provide insight into the severity of myocardial ischemia. Thus, adenosine release in the human heart during pacing-induced ischemia has been shown (Fox *et al.,* 1974). In porcine heart, ischemia is reflected very well by both inosine and hypoxanthine production (De Jong and Goldstein, 1974; De Jong, Remme, and Verdouw, 1976; Verdouw, De Jong, and Remme, 1978). This study was undertaken to investigate the usefulness of inosine and/or hypoxanthine as early and sensitive biochemical markers of human myocardial ischemia.

MATERIALS AND METHODS

Twenty-five patients evaluated for coronary artery disease were catheterized without premedication after an overnight fast. A 7F Zucker bipolar pacing catheter was positioned just inside the coronary sinus orifice for pacing, and an 8F Dallons-Telco tipmicromanometer catheter was placed in the left ventricle for pressure recording. Catheters also were used for simultaneous blood sampling.

Pacing Procedure

Control measurements were taken in duplicate. Pacing was then started with a heart rate 10 beats higher than sinus rhythm. Every 2 min the pacing rate was raised by 10 beats/min until anginal pain or atrioventricular block occurred. Every 4 min simultaneous arterial and coronary sinus blood samples were drawn until pain or block occurred. Pacing was then continued for another 1–2 min to allow for last blood sampling during pacing (P_3). Subsequently, 5 and 10 min after pacing, blood was sampled again for determinations during recovery (R_1 and R_2, respectively). Data obtained during control (C), the last three sampling periods during pacing (P_1, P_2, and P_3, respectively), and during R_1 and R_2 are given below.

Biochemical Measurements

During each sampling, 1.5 ml of blood were quickly transferred into 1.5 ml of ice-cold 8% $HClO_4$, shaken and kept frozen until determinations. Determinations included lactate assay with a Technicon AutoAnalyzer II (Apstein *et al.,* 1970) and inosine and hypoxanthine determinations (Olsson, 1970). Approximately 2.5 ml of blood were collected for the assay of glucose, potassium, and inorganic phosphate on the AutoAnalyzer. Oxygen saturation was determined on a hemoreflectometer.

RESULTS

Eighteen patients, mean age 47.9 ± 1.4 years, developed anginal pain during pacing (anginal group A). Mean age of the nonanginal patients (NA) was 43.4 ± 2.1 years. The heart rates during C, P_1, P_2, P_3, R_1, and R_2 (Table 1) were not different for A and NA.

Lactate

Results are shown in Figure 1. The arterial levels in both groups remained constant throughout the study. In NA, lactate extraction remained unchanged during pacing. In A, venous levels rose progressively during pacing with a significant increase already occurring during P_2 ($p < 0.02$). However, only

Table 1. Heart rates and changes in glucose, oxygen, potassium, and inorganic phosphate during control, pacing, and recovery periods

	Heart rate	Glucose (% extr.)[a]	Oxygen (% extr.)	Potassium (A–CS mM)[b]	Inorganic phosphate (AnCS mM)
Group A[c]					
C	78 ± 4	2.3 ± 0.8	60 ± 2	−0.13 ± 0.05*	−0.01 ± 0.02
P_1	110 ± 4	−1.2 ± 2.7	62 ± 2	−0.35 ± 0.06	−0.04 ± 0.01*
P_2	123 ± 5	1.5 ± 1.0	59 ± 2	−0.33 ± 0.10	−0.01 ± 0.01
P_3	133 ± 4	2.0 ± 1.1	58 ± 2	0.18 ± 0.10*	−0.04 ± 0.1
R_1	77 ± 4	3.2 ± 1.4	61 ± 2	−0.07 ± 0.08	0.00 ± 0.01
R_2	77 ± 5	0.6 ± 1.7	61 ± 2	−0.34 ± 0.10	0.01 ± 0.01
Group NA[d]					
C	70 ± 3	0.6 ± 2.8	66 ± 1	−0.51 ± 0.12	−0.04 ± 0.03
P_1	107 ± 4	2.3 ± 1.9	62 ± 2	−0.24 ± 0.19	0.01 ± 0.03
P_2	129 ± 5	0.6 ± 1.5	60 ± 1	−0.45 ± 0.07	−0.02 ± 0.01
P_3	143 ± 7	0.9 ± 1.5	58 ± 2	−0.16 ± 0.15	−0.01 ± 0.01
R_1	73 ± 4	−0.6 ± 2.5	59 ± 2	−0.05 ± 0.12	−0.02 ± 0.03
R_2	75 ± 3	−2.9 ± 3.0	61 ± 2	−0.23 ± 0.13	0.00 ± 0.04

[a] % extr. = percentage extraction ($\frac{A-CS}{A} \times 100\%$).

[b] A–CS = arterial–coronary sinus difference.
[c] A = patients who developed anginal pain.
[d] NA = nonanginal patients.
*$p < 0.05$ (A v. NA).
Values are means ± S.E.M.

during the last pacing period were venous levels of A and NA significantly different (0.78 ± 0.08 and 0.49 ± 0.04 mM, respectively; $p < 0.025$). Venous levels in A equaled arterial levels during R_1 and were back to control values during R_2.

Hypoxanthine

Results are given in Figure 2. Stable and equal arterial levels were found in A and NA during the study. In NA, venous levels also were constant and of the same magnitude as the corresponding arterial levels. There was a progressive increase in venous levels of A during pacing, which became significantly different from C during P_3 (from 1.20 ± 0.18 to 2.41 ± 0.52 μM, $p < 0.025$). Venous hypoxanthine levels during P_3 in A and NA also were different ($p < 0.05$). Venous levels of A gradually returned to control values during the recovery phase.

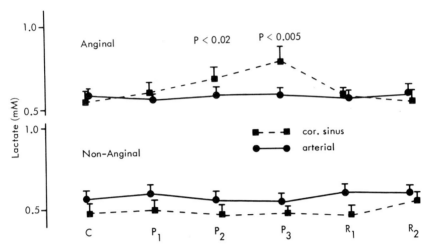

Figure 1. Arterial and coronary sinus levels of lactate in anginal and nonanginal patients during control, pacing, and recovery. Alterations are found in venous lactate levels in the anginal group with significant elevations during P_2 and P_3 ($p < 0.02$ and $p < 0.005$, respectively) compared to control (C). During angina (P_3), venous levels were different in both groups ($p < 0.05$).

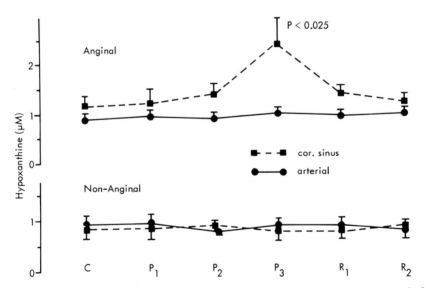

Figure 2. Arterial and coronary sinus levels of hypoxanthine in anginal and nonanginal patients during control, pacing, and recovery. Progressive rise in venous levels in the anginal group with significant elevation during P_3 ($p < 0.025$) compared to control were found. During angina (P_3), venous levels were different in both groups ($p < 0.05$).

Inosine

Levels were too small for reliable determinations.

Glucose, Potassium, Inorganic Phosphate, Oxygen Saturation

Values are given in Table 1. Changes were very small, and neither of these metabolites showed sufficient alterations during pacing to provide any discriminant value between ischemic and nonischemic patients.

DISCUSSION

These data show an early change from lactate extraction to production in the anginal group during pacing, often before angina was noted. In addition, increasing hypoxanthine release was shown during the course of pacing with significantly elevated venous levels during anginal pain.

It is concluded that, in addition to lactate, hypoxanthine seems useful as a biochemical marker of ischemia in the human heart. In this study, no appreciable alteration in arterial and venous levels of the other metabolites was noted during ischemia.

REFERENCES

APSTEIN, C. S., PUCHNER, E., and BRACHFELD, N. 1970. Improved automatic lactate determination. Anal. Biochem. 38:20–34.

BRACHFELD, N. 1976. Characterization of the ischemic process by regional metabolism. Am. J. Cardiol. 37:467–473.

De JONG, J. W., and GOLDSTEIN, S. 1974. Changes in coronary venous inosine concentration and myocardial wall thickening during regional ischemia in the pig. Circ. Res. 35:111–116.

De JONG, J. W., REMME, W. J., and VERDOUW, P. D. 1976. Myocardial arteriovenous difference in carbohydrates, purine nucleosides, and electrolytes following occlusion and release of pig coronary artery. Am. J. Cardiol. 37(abstr.):130.

FOX, A. C., REED, G. E., GLASSMAN, E., KALTMAN, A. J., and SILK, B. B. 1974. Release of adenosine from human hearts during angina induced by rapid atrial pacing. J. Clin. Invest. 53:1447–1457.

OLSSON, R. A. 1970. Changes in content of purine nucleoside in canine myocardium during coronary occlusion. Circ. Res. 26:301–306.

VERDOUW, P. D., De JONG, J. W., and REMME, W. J. 1978. Hemodynamic and metabolic changes caused by regional ischemia in porcine heart. In G. Rona and Y. Ito (eds.), Recent Advances in Studies on Cardiac Structure and Metabolism. Vol. 12: Cardiac Adaptation, pp. 227–231. University Park Press, Baltimore.

Mailing address:
W. J. Remme, M.D.,
Laboratory for Experimental Cardiology, Erasmus University,
P.O. Box 1738, Rotterdam (The Netherlands).

Recent Advances in Studies on
Cardiac Structure and Metabolism, Volume 12
Cardiac Adaptation
Edited by T. Kobayashi, Y. Ito, and G. Rona
Copyright 1978 University Park Press Baltimore

NUCLEIC DNA AND RNA IN CARDIAC MUSCLE CELL OF EXPERIMENTAL MYOCARDIAL INFARCT

Y. YABE, Y. KASHIWAKURA, H. TANAKA, M. HASEGAWA,
A. TSUZUKU, and S. YOSHIMURA

First Department of Internal Medicine, Jikei University,
School of Medicine, Tokyo, Japan

SUMMARY

Myocardial infarction was produced in dogs, and the changes in nucleic acid synthetic activity were investigated quantitatively by microspectrophotometer in the myocardial cells as time progressed. DNA value, immediately after infarction, was greatly increased in comparison to that of the control group. At two weeks after infarction the value had increased to the highest level. After this point the value decreased, and, in 12 weeks, the mean value was back to the control level. Changes in RNA followed a pattern similar to DNA changes. The mechanism of the repair process of myocardial infarction was investigated.

INTRODUCTION

The extent and the prognosis of myocardial infarction are greatly influenced by the repair process of the infarct. A few reports are available on the analysis of metabolism of the anoxic myocardial cell. Yet many unclarified questions still remain regarding the details of the mechanism of the repair process. For example, past studies of the biochemical changes accompanying myocardial infarction are concerned mainly with the release of enzymes by myocardial muscles, reflecting processes of myocardial necrosis. On the other hand, the histochemical techniques contribute to the analysis of the biochemistry of evolving lesion; tissue repair is mostly revealed by collagen formation.

In order to clarify the repair process of the myocardial infarct, we studied nucleic acid synthesis considered to play the most important role in cell function by producing myocardial infarct in dogs and quantitatively investigating DNA and RNA synthetic activities of the myocardial cells.

MATERIALS AND METHODS

Myocardial infarct was produced in 50 mongrel dogs by ligating the left anterior descending coronary artery. The hearts were removed at 10 intervals following infarction, starting immediately after the ligature and continuing for 12 weeks. Specimens of myocardial tissues were taken from the infarcts and from the marginal area. The method employed for staining nucleic DNA was based on Feulgen reaction. In the reaction, hydrolysis is considered to be one of the most important factors. In the present study, 5 N HCl at room temperature was applied to obtain stability. The staining method for RNA was based on the Flax and Himes (1952) method using Azur B. The sections were treated by DNase and then stained in Azur B solution at 40°C for 3 hr. They were differentiated for 18 hr in butyl alcohol. Good stability was obtained (Figure 1). To measure the quantity of stained nucleic acid, an Olympas A4-type microspectrophotometer was used. Nucleic DNA was measured by two wavelength beams of 570 μm and 512 μm. On the other hand, RNA was measured by the use of beams, 590 μm and 503 μm (Figures 2 and 3). The relative values of DNA and RNA were calculated by Beer-Lambert's Law.

RESULTS

DNA and RNA values of normal lymphocytes were as follows (Figure 4): The mean value of DNA was 103.3, standard deviation (S.D.) was 22.7, and the histogram showed the mode at 2n, indicating a diploid pattern. This DNA value was established as the theoretical diploid value. The mean value of RNA was 132.7, and the histogram showed the mode at 145, distribution being limited to the left.

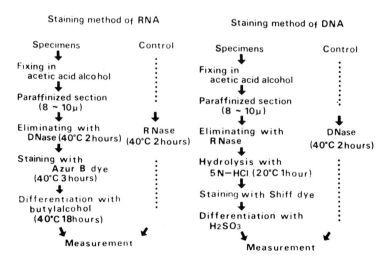

Figure 1. Staining methods of nucleic acid. Left: RNA staining based on the Flax and Himes method using Azur B. Right: DNA staining based on Feulgen reaction.

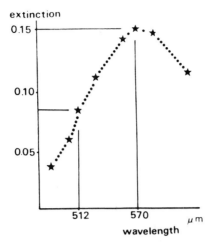

Figure 2. Standard absorption curve of Feulgen DNA.

DNA and RNA values of myocardial cells of the normal heart were as follows (Figures 4 and 5; Table 1): The mean value of DNA was 128.5, S.D. was 62.0, and the histogram showed a diploid pattern as with the normal lymphocytes. The mean value of RNA was 137.1 and the histogram showed the mode at 145.

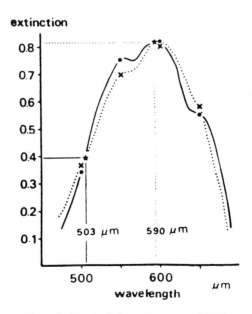

Figure 3. Standard absorption curve of RNA.

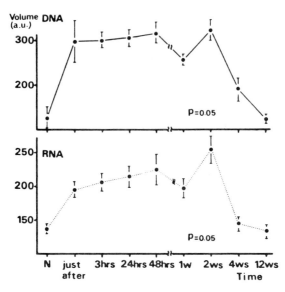

Figure 4. Histograms of the nucleic DNA and RNA in myocardial cells after infarction.

DNA and RNA values of myocardial cells after infarction were as follows (Figures 4 and 5; Table 1): Immediately after infarction the mean value of DNA was 305.8, S.D. was 127.3, and the mode showed an aneuploid state. The distribution was expanded and remarkably shifted to the right at 10n. The mean value of RNA was 194, and the mode was 175, distribution being shifted to the right. DNA and RNA values increased in 3 hr; in 24 hr, the mean value of DNA reached 310.0, S.D. was 87.3, the mode was at 5n, and the distribution was at 12n, showing clearly a hyperploid pattern. The mean value of RNA was 216.1, and the mode was 240; thus, distribution was shifted to the right and into higher range. In 48 hr, the DNA value reached 317.5, S.D. was 77.8, and the histogram showed polyploidization. The mean value of RNA was remarkably increased to 232.4. In one week, DNA and RNA values significantly decreased as compared to the values at 48 hr, but, in two weeks, the DNA value and S.D. reached the highest points, 323.9 and 103.3, respectively.

The histogram showed the mode at 6n and the distribution at 12n, the highest polyploidization. The mean value of RNA was 255.9, and the mode was at the far right at 260. RNA volume also was remarkably increased. However, in four weeks, DNA volume again was significantly decreased, showing the mode at 3n, and the distribution narrowed, clearly indicating a decrease in ploidy. In eight weeks, DNA and RNA volumes were further decreased, but DNA still retained its hyperdiploid pattern. In 12 weeks, the mean values of DNA and S.D. were greatly decreased to 105.5 and 53.5, respectively, and the histogram

Table 1. Nucleic acid content in myocardial cells of the experimental groups

| Material | Number of nuclei | Mode | DNA | | RNA |
			Distribution	Mean value (a.u.)	Mean value (a.u.)
normal	100	$2n^a$	2n–6n	128.5	137.2
immediately after occlusion	100	aneuploid	10n	305.8	194.5
3 hr after occlusion	100	4n	10n	306.9	204.5
24 hr	100	5n	12n	311.9	216.1
48 hr	100	5n	12n	317.5	232.4
1 week	100	4n	8n	262.4	186.7
2 weeks	100	6n	12n	323.3	255.9
4 weeks	100	3n	6n	180.4	150.2
12 weeks	100	2n	4n–6n	105.5	148.5

[a] 2n = diploid.

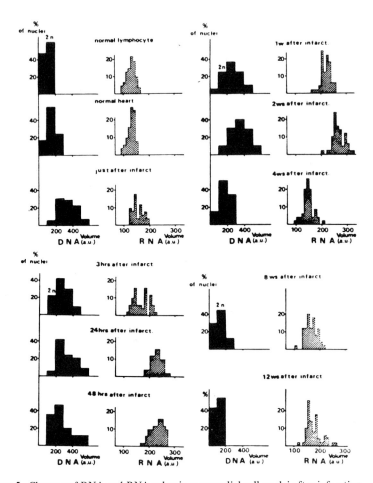

Figure 5. Changes of DNA and RNA value in myocardial cell nuclei after infarction.

showed a diploid pattern, as in the case of the control group. RNA volume again returned to the level of the control group, having a mean value of 150.2, and having the same mode and distribution as the control group.

DISCUSSION

As described in the introduction, in an analysis of the repair process, especially of the changes during the acute period, the most important factors to be considered are the direct influence of anoxia on the myocardial cells and the function of the individual cells. From this viewpoint, we tried to analyze the nucleic acid synthesis activity, as well as its metabolism, in each of the myocardial cells during the repair process.

As the first step, nucleic DNA and RNA of myocardial cells were stained at the same time. To do this we established a particular set of staining conditions, and we obtained technical stability (Flax and Himes, 1952). In previous reports from our group, quantitative determinations of nucleic DNA variation of myocardial cells in ischemic hearts by microspectrophotometer and autoradiography have been reported (Yoshimura et al., 1974, 1975). In addition to the DNA and RNA staining, measurement of nucleic acid was taken for each cell, not just an average, calculated by measuring the concentration of myocardium. In this manner, we eliminated the possibility of any contamination of the various cell populations.

In normal hearts the values of DNA and RNA were both extremely low, and the DNA histogram showed a diploid pattern similar to that of normal lymphocytes, suggesting that the DNA and RNA values of this cell population are almost constant. This finding also confirms the theory of Boivine and Vendrely (1946) concerning the constancy of DNA in highly matured cell populations.

The nucleic acid synthetic activity analysis, made immediately after infarction, indicates a remarkable increase of DNA and RNA values as compared to normal myocardial cells. This activation of DNA and RNA synthesis during the initial period following infarction was observed for 48 hr. In other words, the normal myocardial cells having stable nucleic synthesis developed into cells having activated nucleic acid synthetic activity during the acute period of infarction. This finding correlates to the activation of cell function subsequent to acute myocardial ischemia. Anoxia resulting from coronary obstruction seems to work as a cell growth promoter, as has been pointed out by Leblond (1964). Moreover, it is suggested from our study that this phenomenon causes the acceleration of the repair process of myocardial cells and, at the same time, contributes to the development of a resistant state against further damage to myocardial cells. Rona and Dusek also have reported that they observed a significant increase of glycogen and RNA content in the remote myocardium after infarction, which they considered to be the morphological equivalent of the increased myocardial resistance to a further insult, such as isoproterenol injury (Rona and Dusek, 1972).

In two weeks after coronary artery ligation, the values reached the highest level. The activation of DNA and RNA synthesis in each myocardial cell was augmented. The DNA histogram showed the highest polyploidization. This indicates that the cell population during this period would deviate greatly from the adjusting and controlling system characteristic of normal cardiac muscle cells and would possess the ability to proliferate and regenerate. Therefore, it is suggested that the repair process of myocardial cells after infarction reaches its peak during this period.

After four weeks, the DNA and RNA values clearly decreased. The activation of nucleic acid synthesis in each cell was lowered and was back to the level of the control group within 12 weeks. Particularly because DNA showed a diploid pattern, these cell populations are considered to be under the rule of a steady-state system.

The RNA activity of myocardial cells after infarction showed changes similar to those observed in the DNA synthetic activity. Therefore, it is considered that RNA receives the hereditary information from DNA, thus belonging to the messenger RNA group, and that RNA synthesis occurs at a quite rapid turnover.

Few studies have been undertaken to analyze nucleic acid in ischemic hearts. The study by Bing and Gudbjarnason (1968), using labeled precursors, showed an increase of nucleic acid and protein synthesis following infarction, as well as promotion of the reparative process and collagen formation, including the proliferation of fibroblasts. The results of our study on the connective tissue cells suggest a low activation of DNA synthesis as compared to that for the myocardial cells. Rona and Dusek also have reported that, in the remote myocardium and in the periphery of myocardial infarct, an increase of free ribosomes and rough endoplasmic reticulum, nucleic acid, and glycogen content, as well as an increase of enzymatic activities, such as glucose-6-phosphate dehydrogenase, in the myocardial tissues as compared to the connective tissues, occurred (Rona and Dusek, 1972).

REFERENCES

BING, R. J., and GUDBJARNASON, S. 1968. Metabolism of infarcted heart muscle during tissue repair. Am. J. Cardiol. 22:360–369.

BOIVINE, A., and VENDRELY, R. 1946. L'acide desoxyribonucleique du noyan cellulaire, depositaire des caracteres hereditaires; arguments dordre analytique. C. R. Acad. Sci. (Paris) 226:1061.

FLAX, M. H., and HIMES, M. H. 1952. Microspectrophotometric analysis of metachromatic staining of nucleic acid. Physiol. Zool. 25:297–311.

FUJII, K. 1973. A study on the development of intercoronary occlusion in dogs. Jikei Med. J. 88:1.

KASHIWAKURA, Y. 1975. A quantitative investigation of DNA content in smooth muscle cells of coronary collateral by the microspectrophotometric measurement. Jikei Med. J. 90:1–13.

LEBLOND, C. P. 1964. Classification of cell population on the basis of their proliferative behavior. Natl. Cancer Inst. Monogr. 14:119.

RONA, G., and DUSEK, J. 1972. Studies on the mechanism of increased myocardial resistance. In E. Bajusz and G. Rona (eds.), Recent Advances in Studies on Cardiac Structure and Metabolism. Vol. 1: Myocardiology, pp. 422–429. University Park Press, Baltimore.

TANAKA, H. 1976. A study on cell proliferation kinetics of coronary collateral vessels and myocardial muscles in ischemic heart. Jikei Med. J. 91:1–12.

YABE, Y. 1973. A study on the development of intercoronary anastomosis after experimental coronary occlusion in dogs. Jikei Med. J. 88:1–16.

YOSHIMURA, S., TSUZUKU, A., YABE, Y., et al. 1974. A study on kinetics of myocardial cell proliferation in ischemic heart. J. Jpn. Coll. Angiol. 14:381.

YOSHIMURA, S., TSUZUKU, A., YABE, Y., *et al.* 1975. A study on kinetics of myocardial cell proliferation in ischemic heart. J. Jpn. Coll. Angiol. 15:618.

Mailing address:
Dr. Yoshimasa Yabe,
First Department of Internal Medicine,
Jikei University School of Medicine,
3−19−18 Nishishinbashi, Minato-ku, Tokyo (Japan).

Recent Advances in Studies on
Cardiac Structure and Metabolism, Volume 12
Cardiac Adaptation
Edited by T. Kobayashi, Y. Ito, and G. Rona
Copyright 1978 University Park Press Baltimore

DOPAMINE-β-HYDROXYLASE ACTIVITY AFTER ACUTE MYOCARDIAL INFARCTION

K. OGAWA,[1] N. YAMAZAKI,[1] Y. SUZUKI,[1] N. KAKIZAWA,[1]
M. OKUBO,[1] Y. YOSHIDA,[1] T. NAKAMURA,[1] Y. WAKAMATSU,[1]
T. ITO,[1] H. SHIOZU,[1] M. BAN,[1] K. MIZUNO,[1]
T. KAMIKAWA,[1] and H. SASSA[2]

[1] Second Department of Internal Medicine, Nagoya University, School of
Medicine, Nagoya, Japan
[2] Ogaki City Hospital, Ogaki, Japan

SUMMARY

After acute myocardial infarction, serial serum dopamine-β-hydroxylase (DBH) activity was elevated in both high and low DBH subgroups. The observed increase in DBH activity on the first, second, and third days after acute myocardial infarction suggests an augmentation in sympathetic nervous system activity after acute myocardial infarction.

INTRODUCTION

Dopamine-β-hydroxylase (DBH), the enzyme that catalyzes the hydroxylation of dopamine to norepinephrine, is localized in the storage vesicles of the sympathetic nerves and in the chromaffine cells in the adrenal medulla; it is released from these sites along with norepinephrine (Geffen, Livett, and Rush, 1969). Studying the concentration of DBH in plasma appears to be a useful way to investigate sympathetic function (Weinshilboum and Axelrod, 1971).

On the other hand, the activity of the sympathoadrenergic system has been reported to be increased in patients with acute myocardial infarction; many authors have reported an increased concentration of catecholamines in both urine and plasma after myocardial infarction (Valori, Thomas, and Shillingford, 1967; Siggers, Salter, and Fluck, 1971). However, there has been no report on the activity of DBH after acute myocardial infarction. Therefore, in the present study, we determined the concentration of DBH in the serum of patients after acute myocardial infarction.

MATERIALS AND METHODS

Twenty-seven patients, admitted with acute myocardial infarction, were selected randomly for this study. Twenty-three patients were male and four were female. The age ranged from 42–70 years, with a mean age of 66 years. The diagnosis of acute myocardial infarction was made on the usual electrocardiographic criteria, together with an increase in the serum levels of myocardial enzymes. Blood samples were taken at the time of admission into the intensive care unit and, thereafter, they were collected for 10 days at the same time, early in the morning. The serum DBH activity was measured in duplicate on 10μliter aliquots of serum, according to the procedure of Nagatsu and Udenfriend (1972). Results were expressed as international units (IU), μmol of octopamines formed/min/liter of serum at 37°C. The Mann-Whiteney U test was used for statistical analysis (Siegel, 1956). All values were expressed as the mean ± S.E.M.

RESULTS

The serum DBH values were not distributed normally but were skewed to the right (Ogawa *et al.*, 1975). Accordingly, serial serum DBH activities after acute myocardial infarction were divided into two subgroups based on the degree of activity on the tenth day after acute myocardial infarction: 1) low DBH subgroup (0–25 IU) and 2) high DBH subgroup (25–50 IU).

Table 1 shows the mean DBH activity after acute myocardial infarction for 10 days. It was highest at the onset of acute myocardial infarction, decreased gradually for three days, and continued at approximately the same level for seven days thereafter.

Figure 1 shows serial serum DBH activity after acute myocardial infarction. The mean DBH activity of the high DBH subgroup of five patients with acute myocardial infarction was 43.3 ± 5.6 IU at the onset, 44.8 ± 8.8 on the second day, and 45.7 ± 6.8 on the third day; on the sixth day it decreased to 33.0 ± 5.1. Thus, the mean DBH activity on the first, second, and third days was significantly higher than that on the fifth, sixth, and seventh days after acute myocardial infarction in the high DBH subgroup ($p < 0.05$). The DBH activity of the low DBH subgroup of seven patients was 16.5 ± 2.4 at the onset, 16.6 ± 1.3 on the second day, and 15.3 ± 2.3 on the seventh day, definitely lower than that of the second day ($p = 0.05$).

DISCUSSION

The present investigation showed that serum DBH activities were increased at least for a few days after acute myocardial infarction. Many authors reported that there was more than one distribution pattern of serum DBH in their normal

Table 1. Serial DBH activity after acute myocardial infarction

Day after AMI [a]	1	2	3	4	5	6	7	8	9	10
Number of patients	12	17	21	12	13	9	12	13	8	6
DBH activity ± S.E.M.	27.3 ±4.6	23.3 ±3.6	19.7 ±2.9	21.0 ±3.9	19.1 ±3.4	19.6 ±4.1	17.6 ±4.0	20.9 ±4.2	13.2 ±2.0	15.0 ±4.4
Percentage change (%)	100	85.3	72.2	76.9	70.0	71.8	64.5	76.6	48.4	54.9

[a] AMI = acute myocardial infarction.

subjects (Weinshilboum *et al.,* 1973; Schanberg *et al.,* 1974; Ogawa *et al.,* 1975). Accordingly, our findings of serial serum DBH activities after acute myocardial infarction were divided into two subgroups depending on the degree of activity. The mean DBH activity was lower by 24% on the sixth day compared to its onset in the high DBH subgroup and also by 24% on the seventh day in the low DBH subgroup after acute myocardial infarction.

The biochemical indices of neuronal activity have been the determinations of plasma and urinary catecholamines or metabolites (Euler and Lishajko, 1961; Engelman, Portnoy, and Sjoerdsma, 1970). Increased levels of catecholamines in the urine after myocardial infarction have been reported by many authors

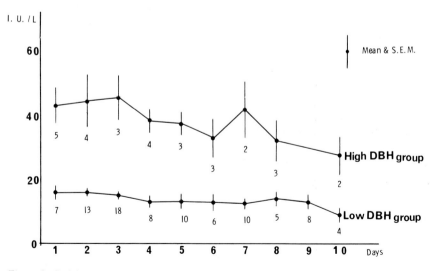

Figure 1. Serial serum DBH activity after acute myocardial infarction.

(Forssman, Harrsson, and Jensen, 1952; Valori, Thomas, and Shillingford, 1967), as have increased plasma catecholamine levels following myocardial infarction (Siggers, Salter, and Fluck, 1971; McDonald *et al.*, 1969). However, the potential significance of these observations has been lessened by recognition of the concept that urinary and plasma concentrations of catecholamines may be affected by variables other than adrenergic function, i.e., alternation of neuronal reuptake and storage, tissue metabolism, and renal clearance (Stone and De Leo, 1976). DBH, a catecholamine-synthesizing enzyme, is released with nor-epinephrine from the storage granules of sympathetic neurons. There is no known excretion and no reuptake, and plasma half-life appears to be much longer than that of catecholamine (Rush and Geffen, 1972).

Many animal and human studies support the hypothesis that plasma DBH activity provides a good index of sympathetic nervous system activity (Lamp-recht, Williams, and Kopin, 1973; Schanberg *et al.*, 1974). Although some investigators have suggested the DBH in plasma is not a satisfactory index of adrenergic function (Horwitz *et al.*, 1973; Noth and Mulrow, 1976), from the long plasma half-life of DBH and the small amount of soluble enzyme in vesicles relative to the large circulation pool of DBH, one may propose that DBH activity in plasma will best reflect catecholamine release during a prolonged period (Ross, Eriksson, and Hellstrom, 1974; Stone and De Leo, 1976).

In the present study, serum DBH activity increased significantly after acute myocardial infarction in both the high and low DBH subgroups. The observed elevation of DBH activity on the first, second, and third days after acute myocardial infarction suggests an early augmentation in sympathetic nervous system activity at the onset, and it coincides with the time of increased plasma catecholamines, of increased free fatty acids (FFA), and of life-threatening arrhythmia after acute myocardial infarction.

Acknowledgments   Many thanks to Professor T. Nagatsu for his valuable suggestions and discussions and to Miss K. Sano for her excellent technical assistance. Pargyline was obtained from Nippon Abbot K. K.

REFERENCES

ENGELMAN, K., PORTNOY, B., and SJOERDSMA, A. 1970. Plasma catecholamine concentrations in patients with hypertension. Circ. Res. 27(suppl.):141–146.
EULER, U. S., and LISHAJKO, F. 1961. Improved technique for the fluorometric estimation of catecholamines. Acta Physiol. Scand. 51:348–356.
FORSSMAN, O., HARRSSON, G., and JENSEN, C. C. 1952. The adrenal function in coronary thrombosis. Acta Med. Scand. 142:441–449.
GEFFEN, L. B., LIVETT, B. G., and RUSH, R. A. 1969. Immunological localization of chromogranins in sheep sympathetic neurons and their release by nerve impulses. J. Physiol. (Lond.) 204:58–59.
HORWITZ, D., ALEXANDER, R. W., LOVENBERG, W., and KEISER, H. R. 1973. Human serum dopamine-β-hydroxylase. Relationship to hypertension and sympathetic activity. Circ. Res. 32:594–599.

LAMPRECHT, F., WILLIAMS, R. B., and KOPIN, I. J. 1973. Serum dopamine-β-hydroxylase during development of immobilization induced hypertension. Endocrinology 92:953–956.

McDONALD, L., BAKER, C., BRAY, C., McDONALD, A., and RESTIEAUX, N. 1969. Plasma catecholamine after cardiac infarction. Lancet 2:1021–1023.

NAFTCHI, E. N., WOOTEN, F. G., LOWMAN, E. W., and AXELROD, J. 1974. Relationship between serum dopamine-β-hydroxylase activity, catecholamine metabolism and hemodynamic changes during paroxysmal hypertension in quadriplegia. Circ. Res. 35: 850–861.

NAGATSU, T., and UDENFRIEND, S. 1972. Photometric assay of dopamine-β-hydroxylase activity in human blood. Clin. Chem. 18:980–983.

NOTH, R. H., and MULROW, P. L. 1976. Serum dopamine-β-hydroxylase as an index of sympathetic nervous system activity in man. Circ. Res. 38:2–5.

OGAWA, K., YAMAZAKI, N., SUZUKI, Y., KAKIZAWA, N., YOSHIDA, M., OKUBO, M., YAMAMOTO, M., NAKAMURA, T., WAKAMATSU, Y., and ITO, T. 1975. The distribution pattern of serum dopamine-β-hydroxylase activity among normal Japanese subjects. IRCS Med. Sci. 3:589.

ROSS, S. B., ERIKSSON, H. E., and HELLSTROM, W. 1974. On the fate of dopamine-β-hydroxylase after release from the peripheral sympathetic nerves in the cat. Acta Physiol. Scand. 92:579–580.

RUSH, S. B., and GEFFEN, L. B. 1972. Radioimmunassay and clearance of circulating dopamine-β-hydroxylase. Circ. Res. 31:444–452.

SCHANBERG, S. M., STONE, R. A., KIRSHNER, N., GUNNELLS, J. C., and ROBINSON, R. R. 1974. Plasma dopamine-β-hydroxylase: A possible aide in the study and evaluation of hypertension. Science 185:523–525.

SIEGEL, S. 1956. Nonparametric Statistics for the Behavioral Sciences, pp. 116–127. McGraw-Hill, Kogakusha, Tokyo.

SIGGERS, D. C., SALTER, C., and FLUCK, D. C. 1971. Serial plasma adrenaline and noradrenaline levels in myocardial infarction using a new double isotope technique. Br. Heart J. 33:878–883.

STONE, R. A., and De LEO, J. 1976. Psychotherapeutic control of hypertension. N. Engl. J. Med. 294:80–94.

VALORI, C., THOMAS, M., and SHILLINGFORD, J. 1967. Free noradrenaline and adrenaline excretion in relation to clinical syndromes following myocardial infarction. Am. J. Cardiol. 20:605–617.

WEINSHILBOUM, R., and AXELROD, J. 1971. Serum dopamine-β-hydroxylase activity. Circ. Res. 28:307–315.

WEINSHILBOUM, R. M., RAYMOND, F. A., ELVEBACK, L. R., and WEIDMAN, W. H. 1973. Serum dopamine-β-hydroxylase activity; sibling-sibling correlation. Science 181: 943–945.

Mailing address:
Dr. Kouichi Ogawa,
The Second Department of Internal Medicine, Nagoya University,
School of Medicine, 65 Tsurumacho, Showaku, Nagoya (Japan).

Recent Advances in Studies on
Cardiac Structure and Metabolism, Volume 12
Cardiac Adaptation
Edited by T. Kobayashi, Y. Ito, and G. Rona
Copyright 1978 University Park Press Baltimore

RELEASE OF LYSOSOMAL ENZYMES
DURING ISCHEMIC INJURY OF CANINE MYOCARDIUM

M. G. GOTTWIK,[1] E. S. KIRK,[2] F. F. KENNETT,[3] and W. B. WEGLICKI[3]

[1] Department of Medicine, Harvard Medical School, Boston, Massachusetts, USA
[2] Division of Cardiology, Albert Einstein College of Medicine of Yeshiva University,
New York, New York, USA
[3] Department of Biophysics, Medical College of Virgina, Virginia School of Medicine,
Richmond, Virginia, USA

SUMMARY

The pathobiology of the process of myocardial injury during ischemia comprises a series of events that results in the release of lysosomal enzymes from their subcellular locations within the myocardium. We have developed a canine model of acute myocardial ischemia in which the anterior descending coronary artery is ligated, myocardial blood flow is measured using radioactive microspheres, and tissues from subendocardium and subepicardium are assayed for activity of lysosomal hydrolases: N-acetyl-β-glucosaminidase (NAG), β-glucuronidase (β-gluc), and acid phosphatase (AP). Particulate fractions of subendocardium revealed significant depletion of total acid hydrolases (NAG, β-gluc, and AP) after one and two hours of ischemia. In addition, after two hours of ischemia, the total activity of these three hydrolases in the subendocardial supernatant was decreased, correlating significantly with diminished myocardial blood flow (NAG: $r = 0.96$; β-gluc: $r = 0.95$; AP: $r = 0.75$). The diminished enzymatic levels in the supernatant suggested "washout" of the hydrolases that was more efficient in those ischemic areas that had higher myocardial flow (> 20% of control). These changes in distribution of lysosomal hydrolases indicate early involvement of these enzymes in the pathobiology of myocardial injury and demonstrate the dynamic relationship of "washout" of acid hydrolases with the degree of diminished blood flow.

INTRODUCTION

Recent cytochemical evidence has been reported that shows localization of activity of acid hydrolases in normal myocardium and depletion in the ischemic regions of the myocardium (Gottwik *et al.*, 1975; Hoffstein *et al.*, 1975). These very early changes in lysosomal hydrolases provide evidence of probable participation of these enzymes in the process of myocardial injury, because the enzymes are capable of hydrolyzing a number of components of the cell that are essential for normal function (Barrett, 1973).

This work was supported by grants from the National Institutes of Health, HL-19148-01, HL-11306 and HL-72-2953, and the American Heart Association, Inc., Massachusetts Chapter.

The use of radioactive microspheres to study the gradient of blood flow across the myocardial wall in normal and ischemic animals has provided a reliable baseline for correlation of these enzymatic changes with impaired flow (Domenech *et al.,* 1969; Becker, Fortuin, and Pitt, 1971). This technique has proved to be extremely useful in our studies of ischemia because it permits the performance of morphological and enzymatic assays on tissue for which the degree of diminished flow has been estimated (Gottwik *et al.,* 1975). This report outlines the way in which we have been able to correlate our analyses of tissue levels of acid hydrolases with the diminished volume of blood flow during periods of ischemia of one and two hours.

MATERIALS AND METHODS

Model of Ischemia

Dogs were anesthetized with pentobarbital sodium (27 mg/kg) before a left thoracotomy was performed for exposure of the left anterior descending coronary artery and for placement of a ligature on this artery (Gottwik *et al.,* 1975). After ligation of the artery, microspheres (15 μm in diameter and labeled with [85]Sr) were injected into the left atrium for a period of up to 30 sec while a reference sample was being obtained from the aorta. The calculation of blood flow to the subepicardium and subendocardium was made as described previously (Gottwik *et al.,* 1975).

Analysis of Tissue

At the end of 1 (14 animals) and 2 (8 animals) hr of ischemia, the normal and ischemic tissue was obtained and divided into subepicardial and subendocardial portions before homogenization in 0.15 M KCl, 0.005 M histidine at pH 7.0. Centrifugation of the above homogenate was performed to isolate a nuclear pellet (NP = 1,000 $\times$ g for 10 min), heavy lysosomal mitochondrial pellet (HL = 9,000 $\times$ g for 15 min), light lysosomal pellet (LL = 60,000 $\times$ g for 30 min), microsomal pellet (M = 120,000 $\times$ g for 30 min), and supernatant (S). A portion of the NP was used for counting the radioactivity of the microspheres, because these dense bodies (1.2 g/cc) sedimented in the NP fraction. Enzymatic assays for N-acetyl-β-glucosaminidase (NAG) (Woolen, Heyworth, and Walker, 1961), β-glucuronidase (β-gluc) (Gianetto and DeDuve, 1955), and acid phosphatase (AP) (Baggiolini, Hirsch, and DeDuve, 1969) were performed on each of the above fractions. Specific activities were calculated after the determination of protein (Lowry *et al.,* 1951); total activities were reported as μmol of activity/g wet weight of tissues. Cardiac catheters were positioned simultaneously in the coronary sinus and the coronary vein adjacent to the area of ischemia to allow measurement of NAG in the blood. Statistical evaluation was performed using Student's *t* tests for paired data, and $p < 0.05$ was considered to be significant (Snedecor and Cochran, 1967).

RESULTS AND DISCUSSION

The data for the subendocardial portion of the myocardium are presented because of the more profound ischemia compared to the subepicardium. Figure 1 depicts the alteration in total protein of all subendocardial fractions after 1 and 2 hr of ischemia. The M fraction contained only about 2% of the total protein of each sample, and thus the significant fall represents only a small absolute loss of protein. The significant loss of total protein in the supernatant at 2 hr is more important because this fraction contains more than 20% of the total protein of each sample of tissue.

Figures 2, 3, and 4 illustrate the changes in total subendocardial enzymatic activity for NAG, β-gluc, and AP at 1 and 2 hr of ischemia as percentages of the control. Levels of significance for each of the enzymes were calculated using total enzymatic activities (μmol/g wet weight) of normal and ischemic tissue. The data are presented as percentages for uniformity. In Figure 2 there is a loss of total subendocardial activity of NAG from NP, HL, LL, and M (the particulate fractions), with a significant increase in the S (supernatant) fraction at 1 hr, followed by a fall to near control levels at 2 hr. This may be interpreted as a shift of activity from a "bound" to a "soluble" distribution at 1 hr, with a loss of some of the accumulated "soluble" activity after 2 hr. In Figure 3 a similar redistribution of activity of β-gluc is noted at 1 hr for LL, M, and S fractions, followed by a loss of total S activity at 2 hr. In Figure 4 significant losses of total activity of AP are seen in the LL, M, and S fractions at 1 and 2 hr; the significant loss of activity of AP of the S fraction at 1 hr differs from the elevations seen for NAG and β-gluc at 1 hr. This may reflect a difference in the subcellular localization of this enzyme, as has been suggested (Lin and Fishman, 1972).

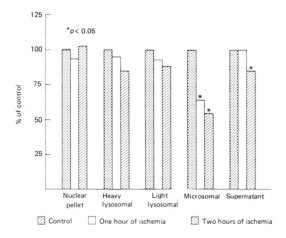

Figure 1. Changes in total protein of ischemic subendocardial fractions.

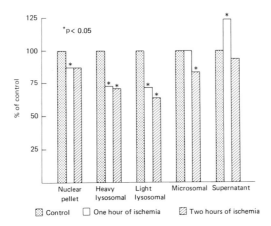

Figure 2. Changes in N-acetyl-β-glucosaminidase of ischemic subendocardial myocardium (total activity/fraction).

Table 1 presents the specific activities (μmol/mg/min) of NAG, β-gluc, and AP of the subendocardial myocardium after 2 hr of ischemia, and shows a concentration of NAG in the HL, LL, and S fractions, of β-gluc in the HL and S fractions, and of AP in the HL, LL, and S fractions. Significantly lower levels during ischemia are seen for NAG in the LL and M fractions, for β-gluc in the LL fractions, and for AP in the LL fractions. The only significant increase in specific activity was found for NAG in the S fraction. The presentation of total activity (Figures 2–4) provides more information concerning the quantities of enzyme in each fraction and allows an assessment of depletion of enzymatic activity caused by enhanced "washout" from permeable ischemic cells.

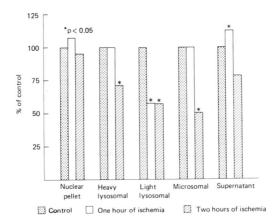

Figure 3. Changes in β-glucuronidase of ischemic subendocardial myocardium (total activity/fraction).

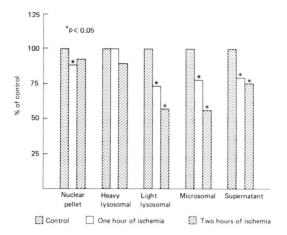

Figure 4. Changes in acid phosphatase of ischemic subendocardial myocardium (total activity/fraction).

Figure 5 is a correlation of changes in total enzymatic activity of the three hydrolases of the subendocardial S fraction with diminished myocardial flow after 2 hr of ischemia. It can be seen that these correlations of the S fraction are highly significant for NAG ($r = 0.96$) and β-gluc ($r = 0.95$) and less significant for AP ($r = 0.75$). The correlations for the 1-hr study (Gottwik *et al.*, 1975) were best for NAG in the HL fraction ($r = 0.90$) and for β-gluc and AP in the LL fractions ($r = 0.74$ and 0.54, respectively). At 2 hr, the correlations of these particulate fractions also were significant ($p < 0.05$, where $r = 0.60$ or greater) for NAG in HL ($r = 0.62$) and LL ($r = 0.75$), for c-gluc in HL ($r = 0.75$) and LL ($r = 0.79$), and for AP in HL ($r = 0.76$).

It should be noted in Figure 5 that there are three experiments in which the flow ranged from 10–20% of control. In these animals, catheterization of the coronary vein adjacent to the area of ischemia allowed estimation of elevated levels of NAG in the plasma that were 140% or more of control at 30 min and thereafter for up to 2 hr; the paired myocardial S fractions showed minimal depletion of NAG. The three experiments in which the flow to the ischemic area was less than 10% of control did not permit adequate sampling of the coronary vein because of the very small volume of venous flow; nevertheless, the subendocardial S fraction showed an average accumulation of total NAG. Finally, in the two experiments in which the flow was greater than 20% in the ischemic area, in spite of great depletion of NAG in the S fraction, the samples from the coronary vein did not show elevations of NAG attributable to dilution by the generous blood flow. In all of the above experiments, no elevations of NAG were seen in the coronary sinus samples. From these observations, we postulate a direct dependence of released myocardial soluble acid hydrolases on the degree of

Table 1 Specific activity of acid hydrolases of normal and ischemic subendocardial myocardium

Fraction	N-Acetyl-β-glucosaminidase			β-Glucuronidase			Acid phosphatase		
	Normal	Ischemic	p	Normal	Ischemic	p	Normal	Ischemic	p
NP	0.36	0.31	N.S.	0.10	0.13	N.S.	0.74	0.75	N.S.
HL	1.43	1.27	N.S.	0.49	0.46	N.S.	1.03	1.14	N.S.
LL	0.75	0.52	<0.02	0.23	0.21	<0.01	2.11	1.54	<0.05
M	0.25	0.42	<0.05	0.09	0.12	N.S.	0.60	0.62	N.S.
S	0.65	0.77	<0.01	0.37	0.34	N.S.	1.44	1.34	N.S.

NP = nuclear pellet; HL = heavy lysosomal mitochondrial pellet; LL = light lysosomal pellet; M = microsomal pellet; S = supernatant; p = significance.

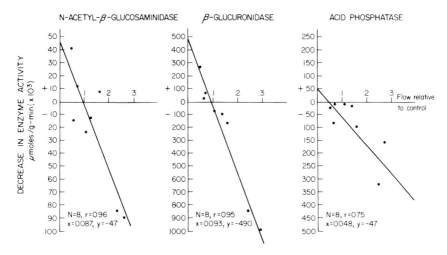

Figure 5. Correlation of acid hydrolases in the supernatant with the decrease of collateral flow after 2 hr of ischemia.

blood flow to the area. This unpredictable "washout" of enzymes in the clinical situation of ischemia would make the use of lysosomal hydrolases, as well as other enzymes, uncertain predictors of the amount of injury. In addition, where severe ischemia exists, the retention of "soluble" acid hydrolases may contribute to the "pathobiology of injury," while the "washout" of these hydrolases from areas of higher flow may be "protective."

REFERENCES

BAGGIOLINI, M., HIRSCH, J. G., and DeDUVE, C. 1969. Resolution of granules from rabbit heterophile leukocytes into district populations by zonal sedimentation. J. Cell Biol. 40:529–541.

BARRETT, A. J. 1973. Properties of lysosomal enzymes. *In* J. T. Dingle and H. B. Fell (eds.), Lysosomes in Biology and Pathology. American Elsevier Publishing Co., Inc., New York. Vol. 2: pp. 245–312.

BECKER, L. C., FORTUIN, J. F., and PITT, B. 1971. Effect of ischemia and acute anti-anginal drugs on the distribution of radioactive microspheres in the canine left ventricle. Circ. Res. 28:263–269.

DOMENECH, R. J., HOFFMAN, I. E., NOBLE, M. I. M., SAUNDERS, K. V., HENSON, J. R., and SUBIJANTO, S. 1969. Total and regional coronary blood flow measured by radioactive microspheres in conscious and anesthetized dogs. Circ. Res. 25:581–596.

GIANETTO, R., and DeDUVE, C. 1955. Tissue fractionation studies for comparative study of the binding of acid phosphatase, β-glucuronidase and cathepsin. Biochem. J. 59: 433–438.

GOTTWIK, M. G., KIRK, E. S., HOFFSTEIN, S., and WEGLICKI, W. B. 1975. Effect of collateral flow on epicardial and endocardial lysosomal hydrolases in acute myocardial ischemia. J. Clin. Invest. 56:914–923.

HOFFSTEIN, F. S., GENNARO, D. E., WEISSMAN, G., HIRSCH, J., STREUL, F., and FOX, A. C. 1975. Cytochemical localization of acid phosphatase activity in normal and ischemically injured dog myocardium. Am. J. Pathol. 79:193–206.

LIN, C. W., and FISHMAN, W. H. 1972. Microsomal and lysosomal acid phosphatase isoenzymes of mouse kidney: Characterization and separation. J. Histochem. Cytochem. 20:489–495.

LOWRY, O. H., ROSEBROUGH, N. J., FARR, A. L., and RANDALL, R. J. 1951. Protein measurement with the Folin phenol reagent. J. Biol. Chem. 193:265–275.

SNEDECOR, G. W., and COCHRAN, W. G. 1967. *In* Statistical Methods. 2nd Ed. Iowa State University Press, Ames, Iowa.

WOOLEN, J. W., HEYWORTH, P. G., and WALKER, P. G. 1961. Studies on glucosaminidase. Biochem. J. 78:111–116.

Mailing address:
W. B. Weglicki, Ph.D.,
Department of Biophysics, Medical College of Virginia,
Virginia School of Medicine, Richmond, Virginia (USA).

Recent Advances in Studies on
Cardiac Structure and Metabolism, Volume 12
Cardiac Adaptation
Edited by T. Kobayashi, Y. Ito, and G. Rona
Copyright 1978 University Park Press Baltimore

PEPSTATIN INHIBITION OF RAT MYOCARDIAL ACID PROTEASE

B. E. HOPKINS[1] and T. W. SMITH[2]

Cardiovascular Division, Peter Bent Brigham Hospital and
Harvard Medical School, Boston, Massachusetts, USA

SUMMARY

The protease inhibitor, pepstatin, inhibited acid protease in rat heart homogenates with a Ki of 7×10^{-11} M by a noncompetitive mechanism, but it had no effect on myocardial acid protease activity when given in high doses to intact animals. Exposure of heart slices to 10^{-7} M pepstatin for two hours also failed to produce demonstrable acid protease inhibition, suggesting that myocardial acid protease activity is unaffected by this potent inhibitor unless the integrity of the cell is disturbed.

INTRODUCTION

The role of myocardial acid protease in cellular protein turnover is uncertain (Goldberg and Dice, 1974; Rabinowitz, 1974), but activity of the enzyme has been found to increase with regression of cardiac hypertrophy (Wildenthal and Mueller, 1974). Pepstatin, a bacterial pentapeptide (Umezawa et al., 1970), is a potent inhibitor of brain acid protease (Marks, Grynbaum, and Lajtha, 1973) and of pepsin (Umezawa et al., 1970; Aoyagi et al., 1971), but it is relatively nontoxic in laboratory animals (Umezawa et al., 1970). If acid protease in the intact cell were to be inhibited by pepstatin, the enzyme's role in protein degradation might be further elucidated. Therefore, we examined the effects of pepstatin on rat myocardial acid protease both in homogenates and in intact cells.

This investigation was supported by United States Public Health Service Grant HL 18003.

[1] Dr. Hopkins was a Fellow of The Life Insurance Medical Research Fund of Australia and New Zealand.

[2] Dr. Smith is an Established Investigator of The American Heart Association.

MATERIALS AND METHODS

Acid Protease Assay

Hemoglobin was labeled with ^{14}C by reductive methylation using [^{14}C] formaldehyde (Rice and Means, 1971). Aliquots of enzyme were incubated for 15 min at 37°C in 1.0 ml of 0.5 M formate buffer, pH 4.0. The reaction was initiated by adding 10 μg of [^{14}C] hemoglobin (10^5 d.p.m.), stopped with 1.0 ml of unlabeled hemoglobin solution (1 mg/ml), 0°C, and 2 ml of 6% trichloracetic acid; the samples then were allowed to stand on ice for 10 min. After centrifuging the samples at 2,500 × g for 30 min, 1.0-ml aliquots of the supernatant were counted in a liquid scintillation counter. Counts released were a linear function of both time and enzyme protein concentration within the limits 5–60 min and 5–50 μg of protein, respectively, provided that less than 25% of the counts were released.

In Vivo Experiments

Five Sprague-Dawley male rats (200–250 g) were injected with pepstatin 5 mg/kg, I.P., 18 and 2 hr before death. An equal number were sham-injected. The animals were killed, their hearts quickly removed, and the isolated ventricles

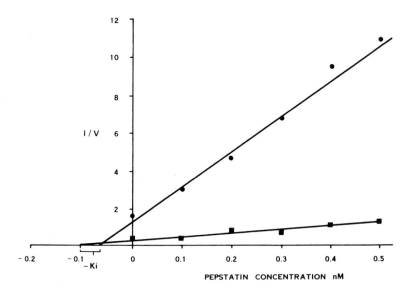

Figure 1. Plot of the reciprocal of acid protease reaction velocity at two different substrate concentrations. ●———● = [^{14}C] hemoglobin 1 μg·ml⁻¹; ■———■ = [^{14}C] hemoglobin 10 μg·ml⁻¹. The lines drawn were calculated by weighted, least squares analysis. Calculated intercepts on the abscissa are 0.060 ± 0.016 (S.D.) and 0.086 ± 0.150 for low and high substrate concentrations, respectively. The difference between intercepts is 0.026 ± 0.022, $p > 0.4$.

minced with scissors in a small amount of 20 mM Tris, 1 mM EDTA, pH 7.4. After homogenization (in 40 vol of buffer) with a Polytron PT-10 at a setting of 5.0, samples were assayed for protein (Lowry *et al.*, 1951). Triton X-100 was then added to 0.1% final concentration, and the mixture was allowed to stand for 1 hr at 0°C before being assayed for acid protease.

In Vitro Experiments

The hearts of six normal rats were removed, rinsed thoroughly with oxygenated (95% O_2/5% CO_2) Krebs-Ringer bicarbonate (KRB) solution, pH 7.4, containing 5 mM D-glucose, and the lateral left ventricular wall was dissected free. Mid-wall tissue slices then were made on a chilled Stadie-Riggs microtome moistened with buffer, and each slice (approximately 40 mg) was placed in 3.0 ml of KRB in a 25-ml Erlenmeyer flask and equilibrated with 95% O_2/5% CO_2. Pepstatin was added to half the flasks to a final concentration of 10^{-7} M, after which they were gently shaken for 2 hr at 37°C. Each slice was then removed, blotted gently, rinsed in 100 ml of fresh KRB for 10 sec, blotted again and then homogenized in 4.0 ml of water containing 0.1% Triton X-100. Aliquots containing 50 μg of protein were then assayed in triplicate for acid protease activity. To demonstrate that pepstatin persisted at the end of incubation, 20-μl aliquots of medium from each flask were added to a duplicate series of the same homogenates, and the protease assays were repeated.

RESULTS

Rat myocardial acid protease activity in homogenates was fully inhibited at pepstatin concentrations above 10^{-8} M. To delineate the inhibitory mechanism, the velocity of the reaction was measured at two different substrate concentrations in the presence of pepstatin concentrations varying from 10^{-10} M to 10^{-9} M. These data, plotted after Dixon (1953), are depicted in Figure 1. The Ki calculated by this method was 7 ± 1 (S.D.) $\times 10^{-11}$ M. The similarity of the intercepts on the abscissa in Figure 1 indicates that pepstatin inhibits the enzyme in a noncompetitive manner.

In rats receiving I.P. pepstatin, myocardial acid protease was not significantly different from that observed in sham-injected animals (12.8 ± 1.9 versus 13.1 ± 2.1 μg of hemoglobin lysed$\cdot$mg$^{-1}\cdot$hr^{-1}). Acid protease activity of left ventricle slices (Figure 2) was unchanged after a 2-hr exposure to 10^{-7} M pepstatin (12.1 ± 3.4 versus 11.6 ± 3.7 μg$\cdot$mg$^{-1}\cdot$hr^{-1}). However, upon the addition of a 1- to 50-dilution of the same media in which the slices were incubated to myocardial homogenates, acid protease activity was reduced by $96 \pm 10\%$ ($p < 0.001$). Acid protease activity in control slice homogenates did not change after the addition of their non-pepstatin-containing medium (12.7 ± 2.6 versus 12.1 ± 3.4 μg $\cdot$ mg^{-1} $\cdot$ hr^{-1}). Therefore, 2×10^{-9} M pepstatin markedly inhibited acid protease

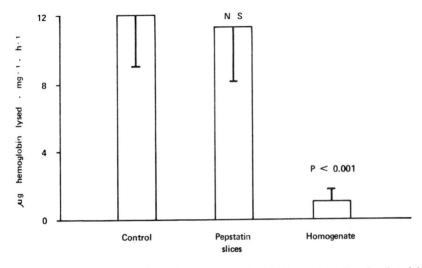

Figure 2. Acid protease activity in homogenates of rat left ventricle slices incubated in buffer (control) are compared with homogenates of slices incubated in 10^{-7} M pepstatin (pepstatin slices) and with the latter homogenates assayed in the presence of a 1- to 50-dilution of pepstatin-incubation medium (homogenate). Data for each group were obtained from slices of the same six rat ventricles. Triplicate protease assays were carried out on each of three slices from each animal in each group. Bars represent I.S.D.

in homogenates of tissue slices, despite a complete absence of reduction in activity after incubation of the intact slices in 10^{-7} M pepstatin.

DISCUSSION

The results of this study have demonstrated that pepstatin is a potent inhibitor of rat myocardial acid protease when added to heart homogenates. However, pepstatin has no effect on the enzyme in the intact animal when administered in doses which, if totally absorbed, could have produced tissue concentrations of pepstatin in excess of 10^{-7} M or about 1,000 times greater than the 50% inhibitory concentration demonstrated in homogenates. Because pepstatin is only sparingly soluble in water (Umezawa *et al.,* 1970), it could be postulated that poor absorption from the peritoneum accounted for these results. Data from incubation of tissue slices with pepstatin, however, indicate that this explanation cannot account for the results observed. It seems apparent that pepstatin cannot gain access to acid protease in intact myocardial cells. Whether the inhibitor cannot cross the cell membrane or the lysosomal membrane is not determined by these experiments. However, if means can be devised to facilitate access of pepstatin to acid protease within the lysosomes of intact cells in a concentration sufficient to inhibit the enzyme, definition of the latter's role in cellular protein turnover may be possible.

Pepstatin's inhibition of other proteases has been ascribed to various mechanisms (Umezawa *et al.,* 1970). In this study we have demonstrated that pepstatin's inhibition of rat myocardial acid protease resembled its effects on pepsin (Umezawa *et al.,* 1970) and on renin (Orth *et al.,* 1974) in being noncompetitive.

REFERENCES

AOYAGI, T., KUNIMOTO, S., MOROSHIMA, H., TAKEUCHI, T., and UMEZAWA, H. 1971. Effect of pepstatin on acid proteases. J. Antibiot. (Tokyo) 24:687–694.

DIXON, M. 1953. The determination of enzyme inhibitor constant. Biochem. J. 55: 170–171.

GOLDBERG, A. L., and DICE, J. F. 1974. Intracellular protein degradation in mammalian and bacterial cells. Ann. Rev. Biochem. 43:835–869.

LOWRY, O. H., ROSEBROUGH, N. J., FARR, A. L., and RANDALL, R. J. 1951. Protein measurements with the folinphenol reagent. J. Biol. Chem. 193:265–275.

MARKS, N., GRYNBAUM, A., and LAJTHA, A. 1973. Pentapeptide (pepstatin) inhibition of brain acid proteinase. Science 181:949–951.

ORTH, H., HACKENTHAL, E., LAZAR, J., MIKSCHE, U., and GROSS, F. 1974. Kinetics of the inhibitory effect of pepstatin on the reaction of hog renin with rat plasma substrate. Circ. Res. 35:52–55.

RABINOWITZ, M. 1974. Overview on pathogenesis of cardiac hypertrophy. Circ. Res. 35-II:3–11.

RICE, R. H., and MEANS, G. E. 1971. Radioactive labeling of proteins *in vitro.* J. Biol. Chem. 246:831–832.

UMEZAWA, H., AOYAGI, T., MORISHIMA, H., MATSUZAKI, M., HARADA, M., and TAKEUCHI, T. 1970. Pepstatin, a new pepsin inhibitor produced by Actinomycetes. J. Antibiot. (Tokyo) 23:259–262.

WILDENTHAL, K., and MUELLER, E. A. 1974. Increased cathepsin D activity during regression of thyrotoxic cardiac hypertrophy. Nature 249:478–479.

Mailing address:
Dr. Barry E. Hopkins,
Cardiology Research Laboratory, University Department of Medicine,
Perth Medical Centre, Nedlands, 6009 (Western Australia).

Recent Advances in Studies on
Cardiac Structure and Metabolism, Volume 12
Cardiac Adaptation
Edited by T. Kobayashi, Y. Ito, and G. Rona
Copyright 1978 University Park Press Baltimore

FEATURES OF LYSOSOMAL PROTEOLYTIC ENZYME ACTIVITY IN INFARCTED MYOCARDIUM

H. AKAGAMI, T. YAMAGAMI, N. SHIBATA, and S. TOYAMA

The Center for Adult Diseases, Osaka, Japan

SUMMARY

Myocardial infarction was produced in dogs to investigate the behavior of cardiac lysosomal enzymes; acid protease and β-glucuronidase activities were measured in whole myocardial homogenate and $30,000 \times g$ supernatant fractions.

Total activity of acid protease in the whole homogenate of the myocardium increased after 1 hr of infarction and showed maximal value after 6 hr, while in the $30,000 \times g$ supernatant fraction the activity began to increase after 3 hr and reached the maximal level by 24 hr.

Total β-glucuronidase activity in the whole homogenate decreased during the initial 3 hr after myocardial infarction and markedly increased after 12 hr. The activity in the $30,000 \times g$ supernatant fraction showed corresponding changes.

These findings that the increase in whole homogenate activity preceded that in the $30,000 \times g$ supernatant fraction may support the hypothesis that lysosomal enzymes may be newly synthesized and then solubilized in the infarcted myocardium.

INTRODUCTION

It has been reported that lysosomal enzymes from ischemic myocardium play an important role in ischemic heart injury (Hoffstein, Weissmann, and Fox, 1976). We have shown that acid protease released from infarcted myocardium is capable of degrading tissue proteins in injured myocardium. This chapter deals with the role of the lysosomal enzymes, acid protease, and β-glucuronidase in the infarcted myocardium. The possibility of synthesis of these enzymes in infarcted myocardium is discussed.

MATERIALS AND METHODS

Mongrel dogs weighing 5–8 kg were anesthetized with intravenous administration of pentobarbiturate, and the circumflex branch of the left coronary artery was ligated at the origin under artificial respiration with room air. Tissue from the left ventricle was removed at 1, 3, 6, 12, 24, and 48 hr and 6 days after infarction. Cardiac muscle was homogenized in 10 volumes of cold 0.25 M sucrose by a Teflon glass homogenizer. The homogenate was centrifuged at 700 X g for 30 min. All procedures were performed at 4°C.

The activities of acid protease and β-glucuronidase from the whole homogenate and from the 30,000 X g supernatant were assayed by the methods of Anson (1939) and Bergmeyer (1965), respectively.

RESULTS

Acid Protease

The total activity of acid protease in whole homogenate is shown in Figure 1. The amount of the activity in the control myocardium was 10.1 ± 1.9 mg of tyrosine/hr/g wet weight, while it increased to 48.1 ± 13.5 ($p<0.001$) and 95.5 ± 15.6 ($p < 0.001$) in the infarcted myocardium 1 hr and 3 hr after infarction, respectively. The activity levels were 87.5 ± 17.5 at 6 hr, 88.0 ± 15.1 at 12 hr, and 74.8 ± 8.6 at 24 hr after infarction. Two days after infarction, activity

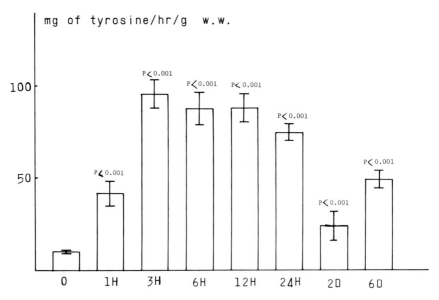

Figure 1. Total activity of acid protease in the whole homogenate. The incubation mixture in a final volume of 1.0 ml contained 0.15 ml of 0.1 M acetate buffer (pH 3.5), 0.1 ml of 1% Triton X-100, 0.05 ml of 4–5% bovine hemoglobin, and approximately 1.6 mg of whole homogenate protein in 0.25 M sucrose. The incubation was started by adding whole homogenate, only, at 37°C for 60 min and centrifuging the incubation tube at 2,000 rpm. Aliquots were removed from each tube, and assayed for phenol reagent positive material. (H = hour; D = day.)

declined to 24.0 ± 7.4 ($p < 0.001$), but it was still higher than the control level, and it increased again at 6 days after, to 44.9 ± 9.1 ($p < 0.001$).

The total activity of acid protease in the $30,000 \times g$ supernatant fraction is shown in Figure 2. In intact (control) myocardium, the activity was 3.1 ± 1.0 mg of tyrosine/hr/g net weight, and it increased to 4.1 ± 1.6, 7.2 ± 2.8, and 7.7 ± 2.2 at 1 hr, 3 hr, and 6 hr after infarction, respectively. There was no significant difference among the three groups. Twelve hrs after infarction, the activity increased to 36.5 ± 8.8 mg of tyrosine/hr/g wet weight ($p < 0.001$), and by 24 hrs it had further increased to the maximal level (55.5 ± 5.8, $p < 0.001$). Two days after infarction, the activity decreased to 15.2 ± 2.7 ($p < 0.001$, V.S. 24 hrs). Six days after infarction, it was 15.3 ± 4.2 (not significant V.S. 2 days).

β-Glucuronidase

As shown in Figure 3, total activities in the whole homogenate at 1 hr and 3 hr after infarction were 45.9 ± 6.9 and 58.1 ± 9.8 μg of phenolphthalein/hr/g wet weight, respectively, which were significantly lower than control levels (70.7 ± 1.4, $p < 0.001$). After 12 hr, the activity increased to 144.1 ± 2.8 ($p < 0.001$), and thereafter it increased continuously to the maximal level (443.0 ± 77.6, $p < 0.001$) at 6 days after infarction.

The time course of the activity in the $30,000 \times g$ supernatant fraction showed almost the same pattern as that of the whole homogenate (Figure 4).

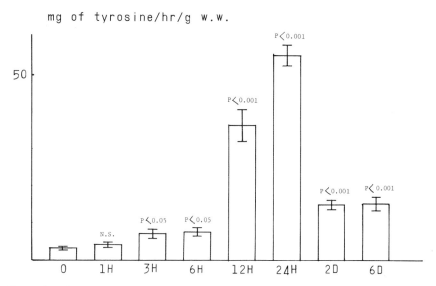

Figure 2. Total activity of acid protease in the soluble ($30,000 \times g$) fraction. For details of the assay system, see Figure 1.

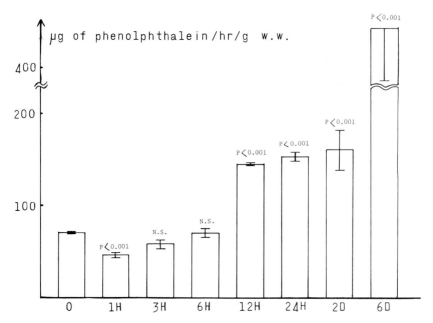

Figure 3. Total activity of β-glucuronidase in the whole hemogenate. The incubation mixture in a final volume of 1 ml contained 0.3 ml of 0.1 M citrate buffer (pH 4.5), 0.1 ml of 1% Triton X-100, 0.1 ml of 10 mM phenolphthalein monoglucuronide and approximately 1.6 mg of whole hemogenate protein in 0.25 M sucrose. The incubation was started by adding whole homogenate at 37°C for 1 hr, and the reaction was stopped by adding 1.0 ml of alkaline solution (Bergmeyer, 1965) and centrifuging the incubation tube at 2,000 rpm for 20 min. The optical density reading was 450 nm.

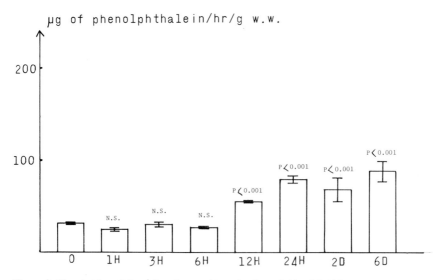

Figure 4. The total activity of β-glucuronidase in the soluble (30,000 $\times g$) fraction. For details of the assay system, see Figure 3.

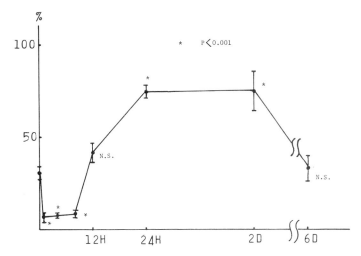

Figure 5. Ratio (or distribution) of total acid protease activity in the soluble (30,000 ×g) fraction of the activity in the whole homogenate.

The activity in intact myocardium was 31.5 ± 1.2 µg of phenolphthalein/hr/g wet weight, while a decline of activity occurred 1 hr after infarction (24.5 ± 4.1, $p < 0.001$) and an increase (54.8 ± 0.7) 12 hr after. There was no significant difference of activity among the values at 24 hr (79.6 ± 8.1), 2 days (68.3 ± 27.2), and 6 days (88.1 ± 21.0) after infarction.

Degree of Solubilization of the Enzymes

Figures 5 and 6 show the ratios, represented as percentages, of the activities in the 30,000 × g supernatant fraction to those in the whole homogenate after infarction. As shown in Figure 5, the acid protease activity ratio was 30.4 ± 7.1% in intact myocardium; it decreased at 1 hr (7.2 ± 4.5%, $p < 0.001$), 3 hr (7.8 ± 3.3%, $p < 0.001$), and 6 hr (8.7 ± 1.7%, $p < 0.001$) after infarction. Twelve hr after infarction, the ratio increased to 41.8 ± 10.2%; at 2 days after, it remained almost at the same level (67.2 ± 21.0%).

In the case of β-glucuronidase (Figure 6), the ratio in intact myocardium was 44.7 ± 2.4% and tended to increase 1 hr (53.1 ± 2.7%, $p < 0.001$) and 3 hr (52.3 ± 7.3%, $p < 0.05$) after infarction.

DISCUSSION

In this study, total activity of acid protease increased in both the whole homogenate and the soluble fractions of infarcted myocardium. This finding is compatible with a consideration that activation of lysosomal protcolytic en-

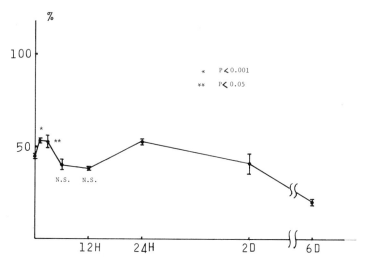

Figure 6. Ratio (or distribution) of total activity of β-glucuronidase in the soluble (30,000 ×g) fraction to the activity in whole homogenate.

zymes may contribute to ischemic myocardial injury. However, the pattern of release of acid protease after infarction was found to be different between the whole homogenate and the soluble fraction. The ratio of soluble fraction to total enzyme activity decreased in the early stages, but it increased 6 hr after infarction and then declined again after 2 days. These findings suggest that the enzyme is bound at the early stage to the infarcted myocardium and then is released as a soluble form from lysosomal granules, resulting in a rapid increment of its activity in the soluble fraction.

According to Wildenthal (1974), the myocardial cathepsin D content is influenced by metabolic disorders. Namely, it decreases rapidly in thyrotoxic cardiac hypertrophy and increases when thyrotoxicosis is corrected. Hinter-berger and Wollenberger (1976) also reported that protein synthesis was not totally blocked even in complete myocardial ischemia, but rather stimulated by some cofactors. Moreover, preliminary experiments in our laboratory showed that Daunorubicin, an inhibitor of protein synthesis, inhibited an increase of total acid protease activity in ischemic myocardium. Thus, it is considered that lysosomal enzymes are newly synthesized in infarcted myocardium.

The behavior of β-glucuronidase, the other lysosomal enzyme, in myocardial infarction was somewhat different from the case of acid protease, suggesting differences in character of these enzymes. That is, the enzyme activity did not increase at the early stage in the whole homogenate nor in the soluble fraction. However, the activity of β-glucuronidase was also found to be elevated 12 hr after infarction in both the whole homogenate and soluble fractions simultaneously.

REFERENCES

ANSON, M. L., 1939. The estimation of pepsin, trypsin, papain and cathepsin with hemoglobin. J. Gen. Physiol. 22:79.

BERGMEYER, H. U., 1965. Method of enzymatic analysis. Verlag Chemic. Academic Press, New York.

HINTERBERGER, U., and WOLLENBERGER, A., 1976. Protein synthesis in cell-free systems from totally ischemic rat myocardium. In P. Harris, R. J. Bing, and A. Fleckenstein (eds.), Recent Advances in Studies on Cardiac Structure and Metabolism. Vol. 7: Biochemistry and Pharmacology of Myocardial Hypertrophy, Hypoxia, and Infarction, pp. 341–347. University Park Press, Baltimore.

HOFFSTEIN, S., WEISSMANN, G., and FOX, A. C. 1976. Lysosomes in myocardial infarction: Studies by means of cytochemistry and subcellular fractionation with observations on the effects of methylprednisolone. In E. Braunwald (ed.), Protection of the Ischemic Myocardium. Am. Heart Assoc. Monograph No. 48:34–40.

WILDENTHAL, K., 1974. Increased myocardial cathepsin D activity during regression of thyrotoxic cardiac hypertrophy. Nature 249:478.

Mailing address:
Hirotaka Akagami, M.D.,
Department of Cardiovascular Disease, The Center for Adult Diseases, Osaka,
3-3, Nakamichi 1-chome, Higashinari-ku, Osaka 537 (Japan).

Recent Advances in Studies on
Cardiac Structure and Metabolism, Volume 12
Cardiac Adaptation
Edited by T. Kobayashi, Y. Ito, and G. Rona
Copyright 1978 University Park Press Baltimore

AUTOPHAGY IN CARDIAC MYOCYTES

H. D. SYBERS,[1] J. INGWALL,[2] and M. DeLUCA[2]

[1] Department of Pathology,
Baylor College of Medicine,
Houston, Texas, USA
[2] Department of Medicine and Biochemistry,
University of California, San Diego,
La Jolla, California, USA

SUMMARY

The fetal mouse heart (FMH) in organ culture continues to beat for a period of weeks, but degenerative changes occur. Electron microscopy revealed formation of autophagic vacuoles containing damaged organelles in some cells after the first day, indicating focal cytoplasmic injury. This process was accelerated by transient deprivation of oxygen and glucose followed by resupply of oxygen and glucose. FMHs were maintained for up to four hours in glucose-free media in an atmosphere of 95% N_2/5% CO_2 followed by resupply of O_2 and glucose. Twenty-four hours later, many cells recovered without residual injury. Many others revealed autophagic vacuoles ranging from those in which organelles were readily identified to those characteristic of residual bodies. It appears that focal injury stimulates the endoplasmic reticulum to enclose the damaged components, permitting localized lysosomal digestion without causing injury to the entire cell. Autophagy has not been emphasized as an important mechanism in transient ischemia in adult myocytes, but it may play a role in repair of sublethal injury. The FMH organ culture provides an excellent model for studying the sequential autophagic changes in a system in which these events can be accelerated.

INTRODUCTION

The ultrastructural manifestations of myocardial ischemia have been studied extensively in adult animals where it has been shown that the early changes that occur following coronary occlusion consist mainly of swelling of organelles and depletion of glycogen granules (Bryant, Thomas, and O'Neal, 1958; Caulfield and Klionsky, 1959; Jennings, Baum, and Herdson, 1965; Jennings *et al.,* 1969; Jennings and Ganote, 1974). These changes progress to a point at which irreversible injury has occurred. By this time, margination of nuclear chromatin is apparent, and mitochondria are swollen and often contain large, dense, calcium-phosphate precipitates (Shen and Jennings, 1972a). If blood is reperfused into the ischemic region, there is an acceleration of structural alterations

---

This work was supported by NHLI Grant 19147-01 and NHLI Contract 1-HL-81332.

and calcium uptake in those cells destined to undergo necrosis, while reversion of the cell cytoplasm to normal occurs in those that will recover (Herdson, Sommers, and Jennings, 1965; Shen and Jennings, 1972b). The question of whether or not focal cytoplasmic injury has occurred in the cells that recover, and, if so, in what manner these injured organelles are handled, has not been well studied.

A series of studies in which we employed fetal mouse hearts (FMH) maintained in organ culture under conditions which mimic ischemia, revealed many cellular alterations that are similar to those seen in adult ischemia (Sybers *et al.*, 1974, 1975; Ingwall *et al.*, 1975). Swelling of organelles, reduction in glycogen granules, increase in lipid vacuoles, and margination of nuclear chromatin were noted. These alterations did not occur as rapidly after glucose and oxygen deprivation as those seen in adult ischemia, and many of them could be reversed in some of the cells after as long as four hours of oxygen and glucose deprivation, suggesting some differences in the ability of fetal cells to sustain injury. Many of the cells that returned to a normal ultrastructural appearance revealed the presence of autophagic vacuoles containing degenerating organelles. Because similar findings have not been reported in adult ischemic injury, we have extended our observations to determine the sequence in which these changes occur and offer a speculation as to why autophagic vacuoles are not seen as often in adult tissue following ischemic injury.

MATERIALS AND METHODS

Intact beating hearts were obtained from 15- to 22-day-old fetal mice as previously described (Sybers *et al.*, 1975) and maintained on stainless steel grids in culture medium at an air (95% O_2/5% CO_2)-medium interface at $37°C$. Either minimum essential medium (MEM) or medium 199 and Earle's salt solution (Grand Island Biologicals) were used. All hearts were maintained in culture for at least 18 hr to allow stabilization before the experimental conditions were imposed.

Controls

The control hearts were maintained at $37°C$ in an environment of 95% O_2/5% CO_2 for periods of time that corresponded with those of the experimental groups.

Experimental: Deprivation of Glucose and Oxygen

Cultures were deprived of oxygen and glucose for periods of up to 4 hr at $37°C$. This deprivation was achieved by replacing the culture medium with argon- or nitrogen-saturated glucose-free MEM or Earle's salt solution and incubating the cultures in sealed culture jars continuously, or in some cases periodically flushing them with 95% N_2/5% CO_2. Oxygen content of the media was less than

5 mm Hg as determined with an Instrumentation Laboratories' gas analyzer. At the end of the experimental period, the hearts were rapidly fixed by immersion in 5% gluteraldehyde in phosphate buffer, pH 7.3, at 4°C. The atria were removed under a dissecting microscope, and tissue from the ventricles was minced and allowed to fix for 4 hr. After post-fixation in 1% osmium tetroxide and dehydration in acetone, the tissue was embedded in araldite for electron-microscopy. At least two blocks of tissue were selected randomly from each heart for examination. Thick sections (1 μm) were prepared and stained with toluidine blue and examined with the light microscope. Thin sections were cut and stained with uranyl acetate and lead citrate and examined in a Zeiss 9A electron microscope.

Experimental: Resupply of Glucose and Oxygen

In several of the hearts, oxygen and glucose were resupplied after the period of deprivation and were prepared for and examined with the electron microscope as described.

In four hearts, resupply of glucose and oxygen was begun after 1 hr of deprivation, and in another four hearts after 2 hr of deprivation. Two from each group were processed for electron microscopy after 1 and 2 hr of resupply. Two hearts were subjected to 3 hr and two hearts to 4 hr of deprivation, followed by a period of 24 hr of resupply of oxygen and glucose before preparing them for electron microscopy as above.

RESULTS

The myocytes from the control hearts that had been incubated in oxygenated media retained a normal ultrastructure in most of the cells (Figure 1); however, an occasional cell showed evidence of degenerative changes as previously described (Sybers et al., 1975).

The cells were oval to slightly elongated in shape, and the extent of development of the myofibrils was variable. In those cells with only sparsely developed fibrils, the thin filaments often appeared to arise from, or to be attached to, desmosomes. The nuclei were round to oval in shape and occupied a large proportion of the cell volume. The mitochondria were frequently elongated with irregular shapes. Abundant glycogen granules and ribosomes were present, and the Golgi apparatus was prominent. Tubular structures, thought to be sarcoplasmic reticulum, were found throughout the cytoplasm, but transverse tubules were found only when the myofibrils were well developed. The cell membranes had specialized regions with desmosomes and occasional tight junctions.

The hearts subjected to oxygen and glucose deprivation revealed progressive ultrastructural alterations as the duration of deprivation was increased.

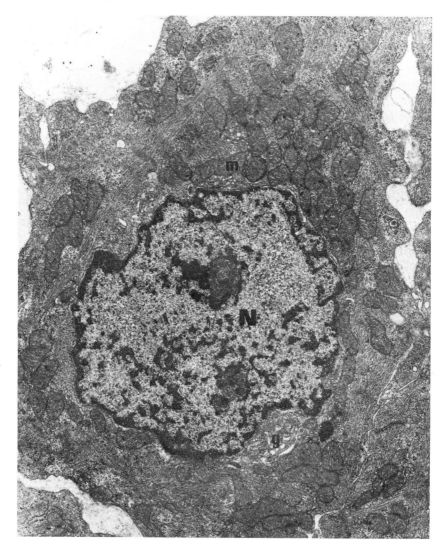

Figure 1. Normal Control. The nucleus (N) is relatively large and has evenly dispersed chromatin. Golgi apparatus (g) is prominent. Mitochondria (m) are normal. Myofilaments are well developed. × 12,420.

After 1 hr, most cells showed only minimal alterations, with mild swelling of mitochondria and often an increased number of lipid vacuoles. A slight decrease in glycogen granules was apparent in some of the cells, and a slight increase in the number of cells containing autophagic vacuoles occurred (Figure 2).

After 2–3 hr of deprivation, mitochondrial swelling with decreased matrix density was more apparent in most of the cells, but the presence of dense or

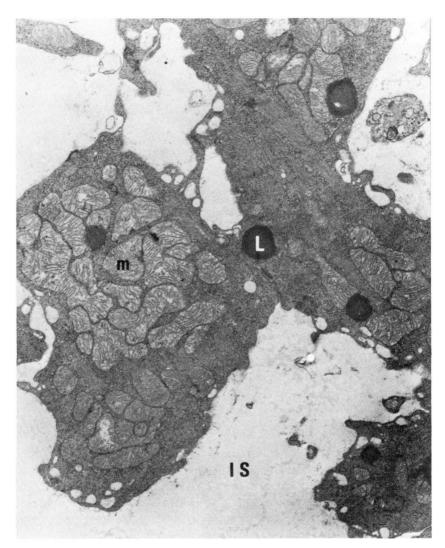

Figure 2. One hour of oxygen and glucose deprivation. There is a marked increase in interstitial space (IS). Lipid vacuoles (L) are prominent. Mitochondria (m) are swollen and have decreased matrix density. × 12,420.

flocculent intramitochondrial granules was rarely seen and, except for occasional cells after 2-hr nuclear alterations, was not severe. Structurally normal or nearly normal cells were still seen occasionally after 3 hr.

After 4 hr of glucose and oxygen deprivation, virtually all of the myocytes had undergone moderate to severe ultrastructural alterations with a marked decrease in glycogen granules, swelling and decreased matrix density in mitochondria, and myofibrillar disorganization. Margination of nuclear chromatin was present in most of the cells. Autophagic vacuoles were commonly seen. Sarcolemmal disruption was seen frequently, and cellular debris was often present in the interstitial spaces.

The hearts in which oxygen and glucose were resupplied following transient deprivation resumed beating and structural recovery occurred in many of the cells following periods of up to 4 hr of deprivation.

Resupply after 1 hr of deprivation resulted in a return toward normal in many of the cells; however, a marked increase in the presence of autophagic vacuoles was observed after the first hour of resupply. Many of these vacuoles contain structurally altered cellular components which are easily identified. Degenerating mitochondria, myofibrils, and glycogen granules are often seen surrounded by a single- or double-layered membrane. Occasional vacuoles contain densely stained osmiophilic residues. After 2 hr of resupply, there were fewer autophagic vacuoles present, and, of those, a relatively greater proportion were of the dense osmiophilic type.

When the cells were exposed to more severe injury as occurred after 3 or 4 hr of oxygen and glucose deprivation, resupply, as seen 24 hr later, revealed that many of the cells that had recovered contain residual bodies or lamellar bodies within their cytoplasm. Discrete organelles were seen less frequently within the autophagic vacuoles, suggesting that extensive degradation had occurred. The remainder of the cell cytoplasm and nucleus had returned to a normal ultrastructure except for an apparent decrease in myofilaments. As indicated previously, many cells had undergone necrosis when the period of injury was of 3- or 4-hr duration, but no attempt was made in this study to determine the relative proportion of cells that suffer irreversible damage as compared to those that may recover.

The sequence of autophagy from the early stages of sequestration of focally injured cytoplasm to degradation and residual body formation is shown in Figures 3–5.

DISCUSSION

The present study indicates that the formation of autophagic vacuoles for the sequestration, isolation, and degradation of damaged cytoplasmic components is a common reaction to injury in FMHs maintained in organ culture media. While they occur occasionally in the absence of interventions designed specifically to produce cell injury (Sybers et al., 1975), it is believed that their occurrence in these instances is a result of transient anoxia that occurs during dissection of the fetus.

Interventions that promote cell injury, such as deprivation of oxygen and glucose, elicit a marked increase in the number of cells that develop autophagic

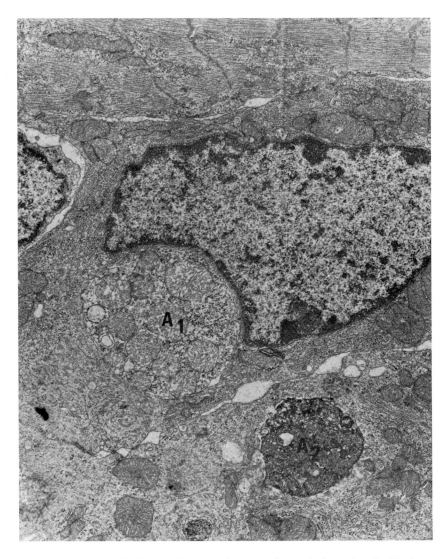

Figure 3.   Early autophagic vacuole. An early stage of vacuole formation (A_1) is shown containing mitochondria with decreased matrix density, tubules, and glycogen granules. A double membrane surrounds the vacuole. A later stage is shown in the periphery of an adjacent cell (A_2). $\times$ 12,420.

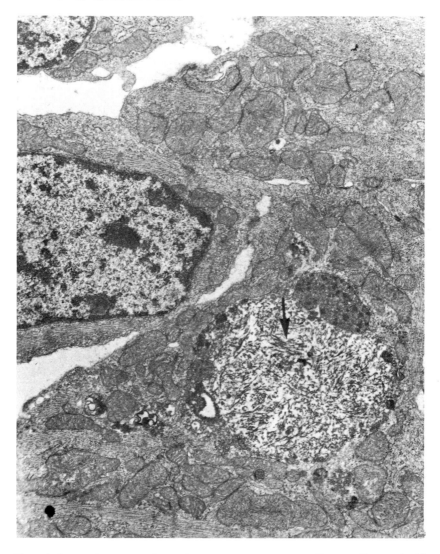

Figure 4. Intermediate stage of autophagic vacuoles. Some organelles are still recognized in this vacuole which contains fibrillar material (arrow) and mitochondria with dense intra-mitochondrial granules. Note the normal appearance of the remaining cell cytoplasm. × 12,420.

vacuoles. This response is readily observed in cells that have been resupplied with oxygen and glucose after a period of deprivation. The rapid increase following reoxygenation is in agreement with the studies of Shelburne, Arstila, and Trump (1973), who have shown that glucagon-induced autophagy in the liver is dependent upon adequate ATP levels. In previous studies with the FMH model we

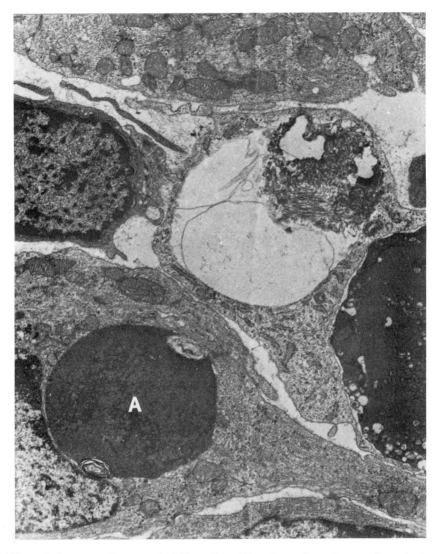

Figure 5. Late stage. Dense osmiophilic residues (A) make up the end stages of autophagic digestion. × 12,420.

have shown that ATP levels rapidly decrease following glucose and oxygen deprivation (Ingwall *et al.*, 1975).

The stimulus for formation of an autophagic vacuole and the organelles that are involved in their formation were not specifically determined in this study. However, their location in the periphery of the cell as well as in the perinuclear region indicates that the sarcoplasmic reticulum that is found in both locations is the most likely contributor. This is consistent with the study of Arstila and Trump (1968) in liver cells in which it was shown that enzymes that typify endoplasmic reticulum were found in the double-membrane system that encloses the autophagic vacuoles.

The presence of autophagic vacuoles in adult cells following transient ischemia has not been emphasized in previous reports (Herdson, Sommers, and Jennings, 1965; Jennings *et al.*, 1969). This suggests that it is not a common occurrence or that the vacuoles are less conspicuous in adult cells than in the FMH model. While the explanation for this difference may reside simply in the greater capacity of the FMH to withstand anoxic injury, other factors probably play a role. One of these may be the structural differences between adult and fetal cells. The fetal myocyte generally has an incompletely developed myofibrillar apparatus which has not yet assumed the closely packed parallel arrangement of fibrils that is seen in the adult myocyte. As such, the mitochondria and other membrane systems are often present as aggregates of organelles in close proximity to one another (Sheldon, Friedman, and Sybers, 1976). Focal injury to cytoplasmic components stimulates the formation of a membranous vacuole which, because of the proximity of the organelles, entraps adjacent, normal, or only slightly injured mitochondria and cytoplasmic components, occasionally including fragments of myofibrils. Once enclosed within the vacuole, lysosomal enzymes degrade all of the digestible components, leaving only the undigested materials as residual bodies. The adult cell with its parallel array of myofibrils tends to isolate the organelles from each other except in the relatively small perinuclear region. Consequently, focal injury affecting mitochondria may involve only one or two organelles in their interfibrillar location rather than the larger number as occurs in fetal cells. Myofibrillar engulfment is not readily achieved because of the length of the myofibers, because in the adult cell short, isolated segments of sarcomeres are not found unless severe injury has occurred. Consequently, the structural differences between adult and fetal cells may be important in the apparent differences in response to ischemic injury.

REFERENCES

ARSTILA, A. U., and TRUMP, B. F. 1968. Studies on cellular autophagocytosis. Am. J. Pathol. 53:687–733.

BRYANT, R., THOMAS, W. A., and O'NEAL, R. M. 1958. An electron microscopic study of myocardial ischemia in the rat. Circ. Res. 6:699–709.

CAULFIELD, J., and KLIONSKY, B. 1959. Myocardial ischemia and early infarction: An electron microscopic study. Am. J. Pathol. 35:489–523.

HERDSON, P. B., SOMMERS, H. M., and JENNINGS, R. B. 1965. A comparative study of the fine structure of normal and ischemic dog myocardium with special reference to early changes following temporary occlusion of a coronary artery. Am. J. Pathol. 46:367–386.

INGWALL, J. S., DeLUCA, M. A., SYBERS, H. D., and WILDENTHAL, K. 1975. Fetal mouse hearts: A model for studying ischemia. (ATP content/lysosomal enzymes/cardiac ultrastructure.) Proc. Natl. Acad. Sci. USA 72:2809–2813.

JENNINGS, R. B., BAUM, J. H., and HERDSON, P. B. 1965. Fine structural changes in myocardial ischemic injury. Arch. Pathol. 79:135–143.

JENNINGS, R. B., and GANOTE, C. E. 1974. Structural changes in myocardium during acute ischemia. Circ. Res. 35:156–172.

JENNINGS, R. B., SOMMERS, H. M., HERDSON, P. B., and KALTENBACH, J. P. 1969. Ischemic injury of myocardium. Ann. N.Y. Acad. Sci. 156:61–78.

SHELBURNE, J. D., ARSTILA, A. U., and TRUMP, B. F. 1973. Studies on cellular autophagocytosis. Am. J. Pathol. 73:641–670.

SHELDON, C. A., FRIEDMAN, W. F., and SYBERS, H. D. 1976. Scanning electron microscopy of developing cardiac myocytes. In Scanning Electron Microscopy/1976. Part V, pp. 631–636. IIT Research Institute, Chicago.

SHEN, A. C., and JENNINGS, R. B. 1972a. Myocardial calcium and magnesium in acute ischemic injury. Am. J. Pathol. 67:417–440.

SHEN, A. C., and JENNINGS, R. B. 1972b. Kinetics of calcium accumulation in acute myocardial ischemic injury. Am. J. Pathol. 67:441–452.

SYBERS, H. D., INGWALL, J., De LUCA, M., and NIMMO, L. 1975. Fetal mouse heart in organ culture. Lab. Invest. 32:713–719.

SYBERS, H. D., INGWALL, J., De LUCA, M., and ROSS, J., JR. 1974. Ultrastructure of fetal mouse hearts in organ culture: Effects of anoxia. In C. J. Arceneaux (ed.), Proceedings Electron Microscopy Society of America, 32nd Annual Meeting, pp. 30–31. Claitor's Publishing Division, Baton Rouge.

Mailing address:
Harley D. Sybers, M.D., Ph.D.,
Department of Pathology, Baylor College of Medicine,
Texas Medical Center, Houston, Texas 77030 (OSH).

Recent Advances in Studies on
Cardiac Structure and Metabolism, Volume 12
Cardiac Adaptation
Edited by T. Kobayashi, Y. Ito, and G. Rona
Copyright 1978 University Park Press Baltimore

cAMP ACTIVITY AND ISOPROTERENOL-INDUCED MYOCARDIAL INJURY IN RATS

B. BHAGAT,[1] J. M. SULLIVAN,[1] V. W. FISCHER,[1] E. M. NADEL,[1] and N. S. DHALLA[2]

[1] School of Medicine, St. Louis University, St. Louis, Missouri, USA
[2] School of Medicine, University of Manitoba, Winnipeg, Canada

SUMMARY

Isoproterenol-induced myocardial necrosis (ISO-MN) was obviated by the cardioselective β-blocker, practolol, suggesting that ISO-MN is caused by specific activation of myocardial β-adrenergic receptors. Because cAMP is the "second messenger" in such activation, enhanced activity of cAMP should aggravate ISO-MN. Pretreatment of rats with bretylium in various amounts, elicited no ill effects but enhanced the effects of ISO on the cAMP activity and also intensified the ISO-induced structural changes in the myocardium.

INTRODUCTION

Isoproterenol (ISO) activates myocardial β-adrenergic receptors (increased rate, force of contraction, and cardiac output) and acts on β-receptors in the vascular bed (vasodilation and decreased blood pressure). This drop evokes compensatory reflexes with increase in sympatho-adrenal activity. Decreased vagal tone and increased sympathetic activity augment the rate and force of cardiac contraction. The cardiac response to ISO is especially pronounced because both the reflex effects and the direct cardiac stimulant actions are in the same direction.

A large dose of ISO given to rats induces disseminated myocardial necrosis (MN) within 24 hours: electron microscopy reveals hypercontracted myofibrils, swollen mitochondria and intramitochondrial granular densities (Rona, Boutet, and Huttner, 1975). ISO-MN is obviated by pretreatment of rats with the β-adrenergic blocker dl-propranolol. ISO-MN is caused by β-adrenergic receptor stimulation because l-propranolol, but not d-propranolol, is effective. This study shows that practolol (cardioselective β-antagonist) blocked ISO-cardiac actions, ISO-myocardial hypertrophy, and ISO-MN, but enhanced blood pressure fall, suggesting that ISO-MN is mediated through specific activation of myocardial β-adrenergic receptors only.

RESULTS AND DISCUSSION

It is believed that enzyme adenylate cyclase, localized within plasma membranes, is an integral component of myocardial β-receptors. The enzyme has two subcomponents: receptor sites facing the cell exterior (recognizing relatively specific hormones) and catalytic sites facing the interior surface of the membrane (catalyzing cAMP synthesis from ATP). cAMP is degraded to 5'-AMP by the enzyme phosphodiesterase that is inhibited by methylxanthines. Interaction of ISO with β-receptors leads to activation of adenyl atelcyclase, enhancing cAMP synthesis. cAMP is responsible for ISO-actions in the body, including metabolic processes; cAMP is considered a "second messenger." Such "messenger" functions depend on its capacity to activate protein kinases. Activated kinases in turn interact with various enzymes or proteins by phosphorylation. For each action, cAMP activates a specific class of enzymes, with specialized proteins undergoing phosphorylation.

Because response to ISO is caused by activation of β-adrenergic receptors and because cAMP is the second messenger in such activation, any procedure enhancing cAMP synthesis should aggravate ISO-MN. When ISO (7.5 mg/kg, i.p.) was administered to rats, cAMP levels immediately increased. Within 5 min a fivefold increase in cardiac cAMP levels, sustained for 12 min, was observed, which then fell to initial levels, 30 min after ISO. Pretreatment with practolol (20 mg/kg, i.p.) 1 hr before ISO blocked ISO-induced increases in cAMP. Bretylium (25 mg/kg, i.p.) increased ISO-induced changes in cAMP (8- to 10-fold) (Figure 1). Practolol or bretylium had no effect on the basal level of cAMP. Whereas practolol blocked ISO-induced structural changes, bretylium intensified them. Bretylium, unlike practolol, blocked ISO-induced depletion of norepinephrine (Figure 2).

Electron microscopy of the myocardium, 7 hr after ISO, revealed subcellular alterations. Mitochondria showed a translucency of matrix with disarranged cristae. Bretylium alone elicited no ill effects. In combination with ISO, it produced severe ultrastructural changes not observed with ISO alone—myocardial foci of necroses were observed as well as accumulations of intramyocardial fat droplets, glycogen, and lysosomes (Figure 3).

Lehr *et al.* (1976) also have shown that prevention of cAMP breakdown by aminophylline led to pronounced aggravation of ISO-MN. The following observations may explain ISO-MN:

1. Challoner and Steinberg (1966) showed that catecholamine-induced lipolysis increased myocardial oxygen requirement, unrelated to myocardial mechanical activity. Thus, relative hypoxia caused by hyperlipidemia and hemodynamics contributes to ISO-MN.
2. Rona, Boutet, and Huttner (1975) demonstrated that altered sarcolemmal membrane permeability to macromolecules is crucial in ISO-MN.

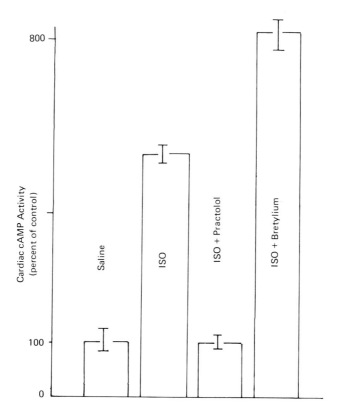

Figure 1. Effect of bretylium and practolol on ISO-induced changes in cardiac cAMP levels. Bretylium (25 mg/kg, i.p.) or practolol (20 mg/kg, i.p.) was injected 1 hr before saline (0.2 ml) or isoproterenol (ISO) (7.5 mg/kg, i.p.) injection. Rats were killed 5 min after the last injection. Results are mean ± S.E.M. of six rats.

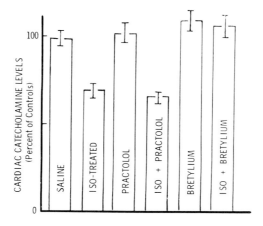

Figure 2. Effect of bretylium and practolol on ISO-induced depletion of cardiac catecholamines. The doses of drugs employed are the same as in Figure 1. Rats were killed 7 hr after saline or isoproterenol (ISO) injection and the results are mean ± S.E.M. of six rats. Bretylium and practolol when given alone had no effect on cardiac catecholamines.

467

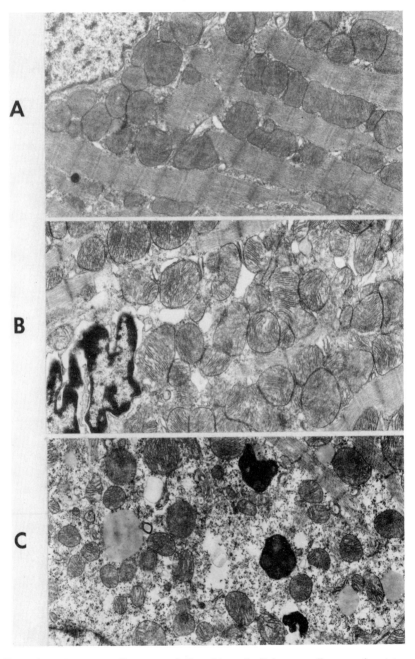

Figure 3. A: Rat myocardium—normal disposition of cellular organelles; uranyl acetate and lead citrate. × 13,000. B: rat myocardium 7 hr after ISO—note translucent mitochondrial matrix and deranged cristae; uranyl acetate and lead citrate. × 13,000. C: rat myocardium pretreated with bretylium 7 hr after ISO—focus of necrosis, characterized by accumulation of glycogen granules, fat droplets, and lysosomes, myofibrillar dissociation, and altered mitochondria; uranyl acetate and lead citrate. × 13,000.

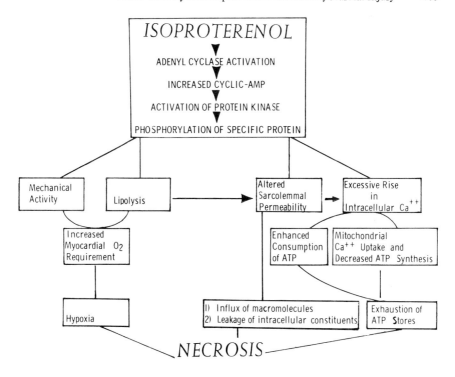

Figure 4. Events leading to myocardial necrosis.

3. Fleckenstein *et al.* (1975) proposed that ISO-induced excessive intracellular accumulation of free Ca^{2+} leads to rapid loss of high-energy phosphates that impair normal cell maintenance and exert a necrotizing effect upon the myocardium.

The triggering factor in relative hypoxia, altered membrane permeability, or Ca^{2+} overload is cAMP (Figure 4). Thus, severity of ISO-MN may be related to such increased levels.

REFERENCES

BHAGAT, B., SULLIVAN, J. M., and DHALLA, N. S. 1975. Alteration in norepinephrine pattern in the damaged myocardium in the rat. *In* A. Fleckenstein and G. Rona (eds.), Recent Advances in Studies on Cardiac Structure and Metabolism. Vol. 6: Pathophysiology and Morphology of Myocardial Cell Alterations, pp. 159–165. University Park Press, Baltimore.

CHALLONER, D. R., and STEINBERG, D. 1966. Effect of free fatty acid on the oxygen consumption of perfused rat heart. Am. J. Physiol. 210:280–286.

FLECKENSTEIN, A., JANKE, J., DORING, H. J., and LEDER, O. 1975. Key role of Ca in the production of noncoronarogenic myocardial necroses. *In* A. Fleckenstein and G.

Rona (eds.), Recent Advances in Studies on Cardiac Structure and Metabolism. Vol. 6: Pathophysiology and Morphology of Myocardial Cell Alterations, pp. 21–32. University Park Press, Baltimore.

LEHR, D., BLAIKCACK, R. G., BROWN, A., DAPSON, S. 1976. Pronounced aggravation of isoproterenol-induced myocardial necrosis by aminophylline. Fed. Proc. 35, 3 (abstr.): 124.

RONA, G., BOUTET, M., and HÜTTNER, I. 1975. Membrane permeability alterations as manifestation of early cardiac muscles cell injury. *In* A. Fleckenstein and G. Rona (eds.), Recent Advances in Studies on Cardiac Structure and Metabolism. Vol. 6: Pathophysiology and Morphology of Myocardial Cell Alterations, pp. 439–451. University Park Press, Baltimore.

Mailing address:
B. Bhagat,
School of Medicine, St. Louis University,
1402 South Grand Boulevard, St. Louis, Missouri 63104 (USA).

Recent Advances in Studies on
Cardiac Structure and Metabolism, Volume 12
Cardiac Adaptation
Edited by T. Kobayashi, Y. Ito, and G. Rona
Copyright 1978 University Park Press Baltimore

ELECTRON MICROSCOPIC STUDIES ON ATPase ACTIVITIES IN MYOCARDIAL INFARCTION

K. OZAWA,[1] T. KATAGIRI,[1] F. YOSHIDA,[1] H. NIITANI,[1] and Y. NAKAI[2]

[1] Third Department of Internal Medicine, and [2] Department of Anatomy,
Showa University School of Medicine,
Tokyo, Japan

SUMMARY

Comparative studies of the fine structural changes and histochemical examination of adenosine triphosphatase (ATPase) activity were performed in canine ischemic heart muscle cells following left coronary artery ligation. In the intact myocardial cells, the ATPase activities were observed most intensely in the sarcoplasmic reticulum (SR), particularly in the terminal cisternae (TC), and moderately around gap junctions of the intercalated discs and on myofilaments.

Ischemic cellular changes occurred three to 24 hours after coronary ligation and became severe after three to seven days. ATPase activities decreased at around 48 hours and also became weak at three to seven days. Two to three weeks after ligation, improvement of the fine structure and increase in ATPase activities were observed in the ischemic cells, suggesting recovery. ATPase activities in the ischemic cardiac cells appeared to be decreased in parallel with the process of the fine structural changes.

INTRODUCTION

The present study was undertaken in an attempt to elucidate by electron microscope the relationship between the fine structural changes and the ATPase activities as an index of cellular function in myocardial infarction.

MATERIALS AND METHODS

Thirty-five mongrel dogs, weighing 8–24 kg, were used in this study. The circumflex branch or the anterior descending branch of the left coronary artery was isolated and ligated under anesthesia with intravenous injection of pentobarbital sodium. The dogs were sacrificed from 15 min to 4 weeks after ligation.

This work was partially supported by a grant from the Ministry of Education, Science, and Culture.

The infarcted area was isolated immediately. For control, the noninfarcted left ventricular tissue was utilized. Tissue was minced into small blocks and prefixed in 2% glutaraldehyde buffered with 0.1 M Na-cacodylate (pH 7.4) and then immersed in the same solution overnight. Small blocks were sliced into 40 μm frozen sections and rinsed in 0.05 M Tris-maleate buffer (pH 7.4). Sections were incubated in the solution for ATPase reaction at 37°C for 30 min. The modified method of Wachstein and Meisel (1957) was employed by increasing the content of ATP to 5 mM while reducing the concentration of lead nitrate to 0.72 mM in the reaction medium. After incubation, the sections were rinsed briefly in the Tris-maleate buffer and then postfixed in 1% osmium tetroxide in 0.1 M Na-cacodylate buffer (pH 7.4). The sections were dehydrated in a graded series of ethanol and were embedded in Epon 812. Thin sections were cut with glass knives on a Porter-Blum microtome and examined with an Hitachi HS-9 electron microscope.

RESULTS

Left Ventricular Myocardial Cells in Normal Heart

ATPase activities were recognized most intensely in the terminal cisternae (TC) and moderately in the myofilaments (Figure 1) around gap junctions of the intercalated discs and in pinocytotic vesicles.

Infarcted Myocardial Cells

Fifteen minutes after ligation, ATPase activities in the ischemic myocardial cells were comparable to those in the noninfarcted area. From three to 24 hours after ligation, large, dense deposits appeared in the matrices of swollen mitochondria. Distribution and intensity of ATPase activity were mostly similar to those of intact cells. Two days after ligation, fine structural changes became severe. Sarcomeres were relaxed and myofilaments were disrupted. Intramitochondrial dense deposits increased in number and size. ATPase activities were not found on the myofilaments and around gap junctions, but were noted on a small remnant in the TC. From three days to one week, fine structural alterations were most severe. Myofibrils became dissociated and lost in places. Mitochondria showed typical degenerative features. Very faint reaction products were observed only in the SR on the Z lines (Figure 2A). From two to three weeks, improvement of fine structures occurred in the remaining cells in the ischemic focus, and ATPase reaction products were found slightly in TC and on the myofilaments (Figure 2B). The deposits increased in number with amelioration of fine structural changes. No reaction products were found in the mitochondria or in the nuclei.

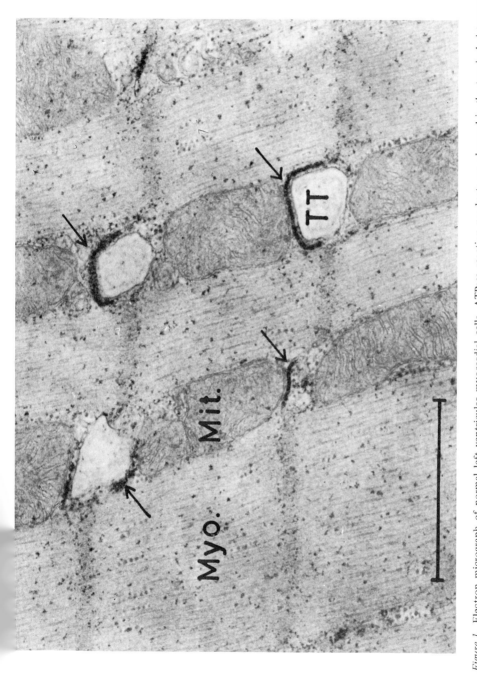

Figure 1. Electron micrograph of normal left ventricular myocardial cells. ATPase reaction products are observed in the terminal cisternae (arrows) and in the myofilaments (Myo.). TT = transverse tubules; Mit. = mitochondria. The bar indicates one micron. × 48,000.

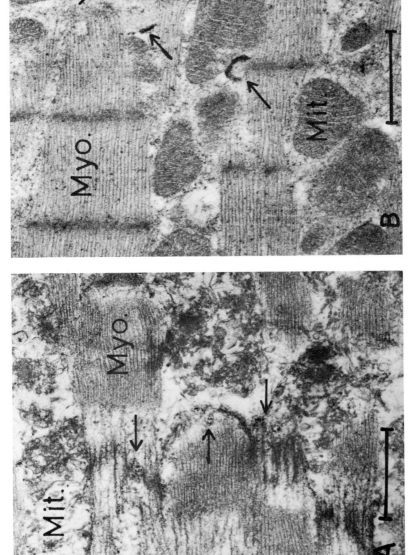

Figure 2. Electron micrographs of the infarcted myocardial cells. The bar indicates one micron. A: At seven days after coronary ligation, ATPase reaction products are seen in the sarcoplasmic reticulum (arrows) on the Z lines. Mitochondria (Mit.) show typical degenerative changes. Myo. = myofilaments. × 24,000. B: At 2 weeks, ATPase reaction products are observed in the terminal cisternae (arrows) and in the myofilaments (Myo.). Mit. = mitochondria. × 24,100.

DISCUSSION

In the normal myocardial cells, ATPase activity was usually observed in the TC, around gap junctions of intercalated discs, and on myofilaments. These findings were similar to the reports of Sommer and Spach (1964). In myocardial infarction, in agreement with previous papers (Jennings, Baum, and Herdson, 1965), the fine structural changes of the ischemic myocardium followed the duration of ischemia. Around three to seven days after coronary ligation, most necrotic ischemic cells have already been phagocyted by macrophages, and, at two to three weeks, the necrotic areas were replaced by connective tissue. The intensity of ATPase activity in the ischemic myocardial cells appeared to be decreased in parallel to the process of the degeneration. ATPase activity began to decrease at 24 to 48 hours after ligation and almost disappeared at around seven days; weak activities reappeared at two to three weeks.

Schwartz *et al.* (1972) reported that some ischemic cells could be viable in the dog ischemic heart. Both the fine structural improvement and reappearance of ATPase activities in the ischemic cells (at two to three weeks) probably indicate the recovery of the function in the surviving cells. By four weeks, the ATPase activities changed roughly in parallel to the fine structural recovery.

REFERENCES

JENNINGS, R. B., BAUM, J. H., and HERDSON, P. B. 1965. Fine structural changes in myocardial ischemic injury. Arch. Pathol. 79:135–143.

SCHWARTZ, A., WOOD, J. M., ALLEN, J. C., BORNET, E. P., ENTMAN, M. L., GOLD-STEIN, M. A., SORDAHL, L. A., SUZUKI, M., LEWIS, M., and LEVIS, R. M. 1972. Biochemical and morphological correlates of cardiac ischemia. Am. J. Cardiol. 32:46–61.

SOMMER, J. R., and SPACH, M. S. 1964. Electron microscopic demonstration of adenosine triphosphatase in myofibrils and sarcoplasmic membranes of cardiac muscle of normal and abnormal dogs. Am. J. Pathol. 44:491–505.

WACHSTEIN, M., and MEISEL, E. 1957. Histochemistry of phosphoatases at a physiologic pH. Am. J. Clin. Pathol. 27:13–23.

Mailing address:
K. Ozawa,
The Third Department of Internal Medicine, Showa University School of Medicine,
1-5-8 Hatanodai, Shinagawa-ku, Tokyo 142 (Japan).

CARDIAC
PROTECTION

Recent Advances in Studies on
Cardiac Structure and Metabolism, Volume 12
Cardiac Adaptation
Edited by T. Kobayashi, Y. Ito, and G. Rona
Copyright 1978 University Park Press Baltimore

MYOCARDIAL PROTECTION
DURING OPEN-HEART SURGERY:
PRESERVATION OF MYOCARDIAL METABOLISM
AND ULTRASTRUCTURE BY COLD CORONARY PERFUSION

A. NONOYAMA, K. KASAHARA, M. FUKUNAKA,
T. SATO, A. MASUDA,
S. KOTANI, and T. KAGAWA

Department of Thoracic Surgery, Kansai Medical
School, Moriguchi, Osaka, Japan

SUMMARY

Myocardial protection by means of selective, continuous coronary perfusion with cold oxygenated blood of low flow rate and of low perfusion pressure is an excellent procedure both clinically and experimentally. This method should be particularly useful in poor-risk patients, for whom a maximal preservation of the myocardium is imperative.

INTRODUCTION

Myocardial protection during open-heart surgery, more particularly during the cross-clamping of the aorta, has been attempted in several ways, but the best method for preserving the function, metabolism, and structural integrity of the myocardium has not been established yet.

Two years ago, we adopted the technique of selective, continuous coronary perfusion with cold oxygenated blood of low flow rate and of low perfusion pressure, and we have demonstrated, both clinically and experimentally, that this method is most effect for protecting the ischemic myocardium under aortic cross-clamping.

CLINICAL STUDY

Materials and Methods

This selective coronary perfusion is performed with oxygenated blood, chilled to approximately 10°C, which is supplied through the coronary perfusion line derived from the arterial line without the use of a coronary pump system. The cold blood is gained by immersing the coronary perfusion line in an ice-box without any support of a special heat exchanger.

Immediately after the cross-clamping of the aorta, the selective, continuous coronary perfusion is initiated by means of coronary arterial cannulation or aortic root perfusion.

The coronary perfusion is maintained at a flow rate of approximately 60 ml/min and a perfusion pressure of 100–150 mm Hg at a general hypothermia of about 30°C and a hematocrit of nearly 25%. This myocardial protection was performed for 15 patients, including nine patients with multiple valvular diseases who were intractable to medication because of severe myocardial damage. Time periods for cross-clamping of the aorta were 60–200 min (average 98 min).

In all cases, blood samples, for measuring oxygen concentration, lactate, and pyruvate before, during, and after the aortic cross-clamping, were taken from an arterial catheter and from that in the coronary sinus. In some cases, myocardial samples also were obtained for electron microscopy.

Results and Discussion

The myocardial temperature was maintained at 15°C in all cases during selective cardiac hypothermia. Even at a 15°C myocardial temperature, approximately 2 ml/min of oxygen were removed from the myocardium. Moreover, during hypothermic coronary perfusion, metabolism in the myocardium was satisfactorily maintained. Within the 60-min period of coronary perfusion, lactate production was negative, the lactate/pyruvate (L/P) quotient of the coronary sinus blood was maintained at about 15, the myocardial lactate extraction was positive, and the ΔEh, that is, the redox potential of the lactate and pyruvate system in the myocardium, also was positive, similar to that of the control value. During hypothermic coronary perfusion for over a period of 60 min, lactate production became positive, although it was low, and the myocardial lactate extraction reversed to negative, although it was within −10%. However, the redox potential remained positive, and the L/P quotient of the coronary sinus blood was within 15, which may indicate that anaerobic metabolism does not develop throughout the entire perfusion period.

After release of the aortic cross-clamping or after weaning from the pump-oxgenator, anaerobic metabolism was never demonstrated. These clinical results suggest that the metabolic process can continue with a hypothermic myocardium at approximately 15°C.

Electron microscopic study showed normal myocardium during hypothermic coronary perfusion. The ultrastructure of the papillary muscle of the right ventricle at 100 min after myocardial hypothermia during tricuspid valve replacement, e.g., the nucleus, mitochondria, and stainable glycogen, changed little when compared with the structure of the papillary muscle of the left ventricle at the beginning of coronary perfusion with cold blood during mitral valve replacement.

EXPERIMENTAL STUDY

Materials and Methods

Fifteen adult mongrel dogs, weighing 12–15 kg, were subjected to total body perfusion at a flow rate of 75 ml/kg/min, a hemodilution of 20–25% of hematocrit, and at a general hypothermia of about 30°C. The effects of a 2-hr period of continuous coronary perfusion with cold oxygenated blood (Group I) were compared with the effects of a continuous coronary perfusion with cold Ringer-lactate solution (Group II) and with the effects of a topical cooling with a cold, physiological sodium chloride solution (Group III).

In Group I, approximately 20 ml/min of cold oxygenated blood were perfused into the coronary artery through the aortic root cannula immediately after the aortic cross-clamping, and the myocardial temperature was maintained at 15°C in all areas of the myocardium. In Group II, 20–40 ml/min of a Ringer-lactate solution were perfused through the aortic root cannula, at a cooling to about 4°C and at a pressure of 100 cm H_2O; the myocardial temperature dropped to 10–15°C. However, a 10–15-ml/min perfusion of a Ringer-lactate solution did not reduce the temperature to below 15°C.

In all groups, blood samples from the arterial and coronary sinus were measured to evaluate the myocardial metabolism before, during, and after the aortic cross-clamping. Full-thickness samples of the left ventricular myocardium also were obtained. In an attempt to evaluate the distribution of coronary blood in each myocardial layer and to examine the viability of the capillary endothelial cells, a diaminobenzidine reaction test, with peroxidase as the tracer, was undertaken. Peroxidase was injected into the coronary artery at the end of a 2-hr period of myocardial hypothermia, and, immediately after the injection, an electron microscopic study was performed.

Results and Comment

In both Groups I and II, no temperature gradient was demonstrated for the various myocardial layers. In Group III, 20–40 ml/min of sodium chloride solution were poured over the surface of the myocardium, at a cooling to about 4°C and at a pressure of 100 cm H_2O. In this group, a temperature gradient of over 5°C between the subepicardial and the subendocardial layers of the myocardium was observed throughout the whole period of hypothermia.

In Group I, during hypothermic coronary perfusion, approximately 0.01 ml/min/g of the ventricular weight of oxygen was removed; lactate production was negative, and the redox potential was positive, although the L/P quotient of the coronary sinus blood showed high values. These findings suggested that the metabolic process would continue through the myocardial hypothermia as it did in the clinical cases.

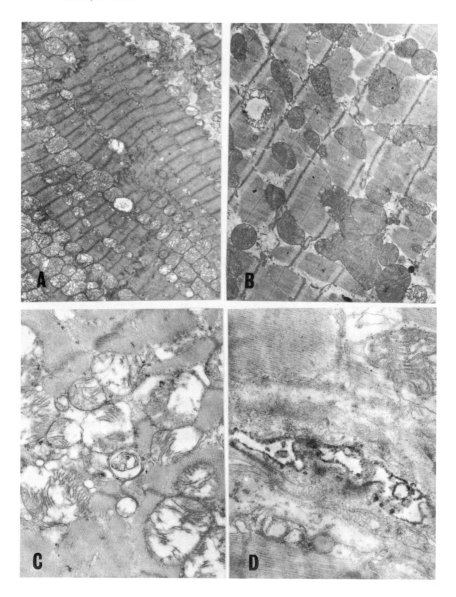

Figure 1. A: Myocardium at the end of a 2-hr period of coronary perfusion with cold blood (Group I); × 10,900. B: View after 2-hr myocardial hypothermia by means of coronary perfusion with cold Ringer-lactate solution (Group II); × 15,000. C: Inner layer of the myocardium at the end of a 2-hr period of topical cooling (Group III); × 17,000. D: Peroxidase is distributed uniformly at the level of coronary capillary endothelium within plasmalemmal vesicles. Endocardium in Group I (at the end of 2-hr coronary perfusion with cold blood); × 28,000.

After release of the aortic cross-clamping or after weaning from total body perfusion, no significant difference in left ventricular function was observed among the three groups. However, in Group I and in those of Group II in which the myocardial temperature was kept below $15°C$, the myocardial oxygen extraction was almost the same as the control value, lactate production was negative, and the myocardial lactate extraction and the redox potential were positive. These results indicated that myocardial metabolism may continue satisfactorily in these two groups. On the contrary, in Group III or in those of Group II in which the myocardial temperature was above $15°C$, the myocardial oxygen extraction fell below 15%, the lactate production was positive, the myocardial lactate extraction exceeded −10%, and the redox potential was negative. These results suggested that anaerobic metabolism may continue after release of the aortic cross-clamping and weaning from the cardiopulmonary bypass.

The electron microscopic observations correlated with the results of the biochemical findings. In Group I and in those of Group II in which the myocardial temperature was maintained below $15°C$, the structural integrity was well preserved during the cooling and even during the weaning from the cardiopulmonary bypass (Figures 1A and 1B). The myocardium was essentially normal in all layers, although the mitochondria were slightly swollen with some decrease in glycogen granules. On the contrary, in Group III, the ultrastructure showed a distinct abnormality in the inner layer of the myocardium, although, in the outer layer, the findings were comparable to those of Groups I and II. At the end of a 2-hr period of topical cooling, significant changes in nuclei, mitochondria, and myofibrils were observed along with a substantial decrease in stainable glycogen (Figure 1C). These changes tended to increase either when releasing the aortic cross-clamping or when weaning from the pump-oxygenator. At the rewarming period after the release of the aortic cross-clamping, the mitochondrial cristae were deformed with clearing of matrix and aggregation of nuclear chromatin, findings that may indicate irreversible cardiac muscle cell injury.

In Groups I and II, peroxidase could be observed in the capillary endothelium within plasmalemmal vesicles in the myocardial layers studied (Figure 1D). These results indicated that perfused cold blood may be uniformly distributed to maintain a perfect viability of the endothelium. However, there was a striking reduction of traces in Group III, in the subendocardial capillaries.

REFERENCES

BONNABEAU, R. C., VASKO, K. A., and LILLEHEI, C. W. 1972. The preservation of myocardial metabolism during cardiopulmonary bypass, In J. C. Norman (ed.), Cardiac Surgery, pp. 195–210. Appleton-Century-Crofts, New York.
ISOM, O. W., KUTIN, M. D., FALK, E. A., and SPENCER, F. C. 1973. Patterns of

myocardial metabolism during cardiopulmonary bypass and coronary perfusion. J. Thorac. Cardiovasc. Surg. 66:705–721.

STEMMER, E. A., McCART, P., STANTON, W. W., JR., THIBAULT, W., DEARDEN, L. S., and CONNOLLY, J. E. 1973. Functional and structural alterations in the myocardium during aortic cross-clamping. J. Thorac. Cardiovasc. Surg. 66:754–770.

TYERS, G. F. O., HUGHES, H. C., TODD, G. J., WILLIAMS, D. R., ANDREWS, E. J., PROPHET, G. A., and WALDHAUSEN, J. A. 1974. Protection from ischemic cardiac arrest by coronary perfusion with cold Ringer's lactate solution. J. Thorac. Cardiovasc. Surg. 67:411–418.

Mailing address:
Akira Nonoyama, M.D.,
Department of Thoracic Surgery, Kansai Medical School,
1-Fumizono-cho, Moriguchi-city, Osaka 570 (Japan).

Recent Advances in Studies on
Cardiac Structure and Metabolism, Volume 12
Cardiac Adaptation
Edited by T. Kobayashi, Y. Ito, and G. Rona
Copyright 1978 University Park Press Baltimore

MYOCARDIAL ENERGY METABOLISM AND PROTECTION OF HEART MUSCLE AT LOW TEMPERATURES

T. WATANABE, H. MURASHIGE, T. NAITO, S. SASSA,
S. TAKAHASHI, S. ASAZUMA, and I. HASHIMOTO

Department of Surgery, Kyoto Prefectural University
of Medicine, Kyoto, Japan

SUMMARY

It is very important to protect the myocardium during open-heart surgery. To provide this protection, a perfusate was made consisting chiefly of oxygenated cold Saviosol solution.

After the heart was arrested chemically by the injection of Young's solution and lidocaine following aortic cross-clamping, coronary perfusion was done by continuous gravity flow using our perfusate. Osmotic pressure of the perfusate was 390 mOSM and oxygenation was done by mixing with air.

Throughout the experiments, biopsies of the left ventricle were done at various intervals, and mitochondrial function was measured by polarography. The amount of high-energy phosphates and glycolytic metabolites and fine structural changes were examined. The electrolyte, the enzymes, the pO_2, pCO_2, and the pH of the perfusates in the arterial and venous sides were also measured.

In the perfused heart muscle at $10-20°C$, creatine phosphate was 2.85 μmol/g and ATP was 2.7 μmol/g even 6 hr later. The respiratory control rate of the heart mitochondria was over 4.0 and lactate was 267 mg% after 6 hr. According to our safety criteria, these values are sufficient to resuscitate the heart.

The merits of our myocardial protection are as follows:

1. Even hypertrophied heart muscle can be protected for 2–3 hr.
2. Intracardiac repair can be performed easily in a bloodless and flaccid state.
3. Our perfusion procedure is very simple and easily carried out.

We tried this method in clinical cases and obtained good results.

INTRODUCTION

Recently, surgical procedures in cases of heart disease have increased, making open-heart surgery of long duration necessary. In severe heart disease, the myocardium is already hypertrophic and is damaged before operation. Therefore, it is very important that the surgeon take active measures to protect the heart during open-heart surgery. For this purpose, a perfusate was made consisting chiefly of Saviosol solution, and coronary perfusion under cardiac arrest was

carried out. Myocardial preservation was examined from the aspect of myocardial energy metabolism in open-heart surgery, which we have been studying
for the past five years (Watanabe *et al.,* 1974a).

In this chapter, the changes in the heart muscle at various time intervals after
cardiac arrest and their influence on post-operative cardiac contraction at the
cellular and molecular levels (Watanabe *et al.,* 1974b) are reported. The results
of these fundamental studies should be of value in indicating what measures
should be taken during open-heart surgery.

MATERIALS AND METHODS

Mongrel dogs weighing 8–13 kg were used. The dogs were anesthetized with
pentobarbital. After the heart was arrested chemically by the injection of
Young's solution and lidocaine following aortic clamping, coronary perfusion
was done by continuous gravity flow using our own perfusate and by keeping
the heart in a flaccid state. The flow of the perfusate was 2.0 ml/kg/min;
perfusion pressure was 20–25 cm H_2O. By using various perfusates at a temperature of 5–40°C, the temperature of the heart muscle was kept at 10°C, 20°C,
and 37 °C. Osmotic pressure of the perfusate was 392 mOsм. Oxygenation was
done by bubbling with air.

The merits of our new perfusate are as follows: the electrolyte composition
is similar to the extracellular fluid, and it contains glucose and insulin as an
energy source, hydrocortisone as a membrane stabilizer, and potassium of 8
mEq/liter to prevent the consumption of ATP. Low molecular weight dextran
and heparin are combined for the maintenance of the microcirculation in the
myocardium. Perfusate pH is 8.1.

Throughout the experiments, biopsies of the left ventricle were done at
various intervals. The amount of high-energy phosphates and glycolytic metabolites and fine structural changes were examined. The electrolytes, the enzymes,
pO_2, pCO_2, and the pH of the perfusates in the arterial and venous sides also
were measured. The mitochondria of the heart muscle were divided by the
Chance-Hagihara method (Chance and Hagihara, 1963), and mitochondrial function was measured by polarography.

RESULTS

In the group with a heart muscle temperature of 20°C, the respiratory control
rate, state 3 respiration, and the phosphorylation rate of the nonperfused group
gradually declined with time. However, these values did not change in the
perfused group. In the nonperfused group at a heart temperature of 20°C, crea-

tine phosphates (CrP), and ATP values were markedly reduced, but lactic acid increased to level 16 times greater than the value at the moment of arrest 2 hr later. On the other hand, crP and ATP in the perfused group had hardly changed, and the lactate values were elevated only slightly after 2 hr.

The pO_2 and the pCO_2 differences between the arterial and venous sides were lowest when the heart muscle temperature was $10°C$ and highest when it was $37°C$. Because the pO_2 difference is in proportion to the oxygen supply in the tissues at a constant flow, the oxygen consumption is lowest in the $10°C$ group. The pH change between the arterial and venous perfusates was the same as the pO_2 difference.

CrP and ATP of the $37°C$ group declined markedly with time, while lactate increased markedly. However, changes in the values of the $10°C$ and $20°C$ groups were much smaller than those in the $37°C$ group.

In the perfused heart muscle at $20°C$, CrP was 2.85 $\mu mol/g$ and ATP was 2.7 $\mu mol/g$ even 6 hr later.

These values are high enough to resuscitate the heart. The lactate value was 267 mg% after 6 hr. Enzyme changes were almost never seen even after 6 hr of perfusion, and there also were no changes in the electrolytes.

Electron microscopic findings showed that there were no specific changes in the perfused group at $10°C$ and $20°C$ within 2 hr. After more than 2 hr in the nonperfused group with a heart muscle temperature of $20°C$, the mitochondrial matrix was greatly swollen, although the cristae had not yet been damaged. Glycogen granules were sparse, and the cytoplasm and the sarcoplasmic reticulum also were swollen. Separation between the cellular membrane and the myofibrils caused by the swelling of the cytoplasm was noted; but in the Z line the myofibrils were connected rather tightly.

In the perfused group at $20°C$ after 4 hr, glycogen granules still were found in great numbers around the mitochondria and in the interfibrillar spaces. Although the electron density of the mitochondrial matrix was slightly deteriorated, the cristae had not yet been damaged. Otherwise, the myofibrils were arranged regularly, and the sarcoplasmic reticula were not swollen.

In the subendocardium after 6 hr, glycogen granules were found in great numbers, but the electron density of the mitochondrial matrix decreased slightly after more than 4 hr. It should be emphasized that the same findings were obtained in the intermediate layers as in the subendocardium.

DISCUSSION

The effect of anoxia on the electromechanical activity of the heart muscle may be attributable to the reduced amount of ATP and to the dysfunction of the mitochondria (Ozawa et al., 1967) or the sarcoplasmic reticulum. During anaerobic glucose metabolism, the net yield of ATP from one molecule of glucose is only two molecules. During myocardial ischemia, there is a decrease in the glycogen, ATP, and CrP content of the heart. Under continuing hypoxic conditions, the inadequate amount of glucose does not provide enough energy to maintain biological function or heart muscle contraction at control levels.

Because the uptake of glucose in the heart is dependent upon extracellular glucose concentration, an increase of extracellular glucose should provide an increased amount of ATP through glycolysis.

Anoxic cardiac arrest, in combination with cardiopulmonary bypass, is extensively used in open-heart surgery. The success of open-heart surgery in severe cases depends to a large extent upon adequate protection of the myocardium during bypass. Failure to preserve the biochemical and morphological integrity of the cardiac cells during bypass can severely impair the functional recovery of the heart.

Cardiac surgeons have long desired to maintain a bloodless, flaccid heart for two to four hours during open-heart surgery without damage to the myocardium. Myocardial preservation has become one of the most important and difficult tasks in the field of cardiac surgery.

According to our fundamental research, it would be desirable for the cardiac cells to meet the following criteria: the amount of ATP should be at a level of more than 2.5 μmol/g; the respiratory control rate of the heart mitochondria should be over 4.0; intracellular pH should be over 6.7; pH values in the venous blood should be over 7.1; and the amount of lactate should be less than 400 mg/100 g. We have proved that our oxygenated perfusate containing glucose can maintain a relaxed heart muscle and, at the same time, provide enough myocardial energy metabolism at a heart temperature of 10–20°C for a period of 6 hr.

According to the Maloney Curve (Maloney and Nelson, 1975), a moderate myocardial depression can occur approximately 10 min after anoxic arrest at a heart temperature of 32°C and after approximately 44 min at 20°C. However, this curve can shift to the left side if the heart is hypertrophic or is in a state of ventricular fibrillation. On the contrary, if the heart is protected by the use of a membrane stabilizer or metabolic inhibitor, and by coronary perfusion, the curve can shift to the right side.

We tried this method on a 20-year-old male patient with ventricular septal defect and aortic insufficiency who underwent radical operation with cardiopulmonary bypass for 160 minutes. The aorta was clamped continuously for 134 minutes. The heart was completely bloodless and flaccid. Cardiac resuscitation was accomplished successfully without the use of inotropic drugs. No inotropic drugs were needed after operation. The post-operative course was very good. This perfusion method results in a greater right side shift of the curve.

CONCLUSIONS

Our coronary perfusion method, using oxygenated, modified Saviosol solution and maintaining myocardial energy metabolism for six hours at a heart temperature of $10-20°C$, provides myocardial protection.

REFERENCES

CHANCE, B., and HAGIHARA, B. 1963. Intracellular respiration: Phosphorylating and non-phosphorylating oxidation reactions. E. C. Slater (ed.). Pergamon Press, Oxford, p. 3.

MALONEY, J. V., JR., and NELSON, R. L. 1975. Myocardial preservation during cardiopulmonary bypass: An overview. J. Thorac. Cardiovasc. Surg. 70:1040–1050.

OZAWA, K., SETA, K., ARAKI, H., and HANDA, H. 1967. The effect of ischemia on mitochondrial metabolism. J. Biochem. 61:512–514.

WATANABE, T., TAKAHASHI, S., NAITO, T., SASSA, S., TORIYAMA, N., and HASHIMOTO, I. 1974a. Study on the energy metabolism of the myocardium during open heart surgery. J. Jpn. Surg. Soc. 75:396–399.

WATANABE, T., TAKAHASHI, S., NAITO, T., SASSA, S., MURASHIGE, H., TORIYAMA, N., ASAZUMA, S., and HASHIMOTO, I. 1974b. The correlation between metabolism and the contraction system of the myocardium in open-heart surgery. Jpn. Circ. J. 38:589–590.

Mailing address:
T. Watanabe, M.D.,
Department of Surgery, Kyoto Prefectural University of Medicine,
Kawaramachi, Hirokoji, Kamikyoku, Kyoto (Japan).

Recent Advances in Studies on
Cardiac Structure and Metabolism, Volume 12
Cardiac Adaptation
Edited by T. Kobayashi, Y. Ito, and G. Rona
Copyright 1978 University Park Press Baltimore

MYOCARDIAL METABOLISM DURING PROLONGED SELECTIVE HYPOTHERMIC CORONARY PERFUSION

S. HASHIMOTO, Y. KAWASHIMA, T. FUJITA, T. MORI,
H. TAKANO, H. YOKOTA, and H. MANABE

First Department of Surgery,
Osaka University Medical School,
Fukushima-ku, Osaka, Japan

SUMMARY

In the study discussed below, we assessed the myocardial protection provided by our method of selective hypothermic coronary perfusion. Using arterial and coronary venous blood samples, the following biochemical aspects of myocardial metabolism were calculated: 1) coronary arteriovenous (A-V) pH difference, 2) O_2 difference, 3) CO_2 difference, 4) respiratory quotient, 5) coronary A-V pyruvate difference, 6) lactate difference, 7) cardiac excess lactate, and 8) redox potential difference. Results indicate that, during coronary perfusion performed according to our method, metabolic changes are minimal and easily reversible shortly after coronary perfusion is terminated.

INTRODUCTION

The optimal method of myocardial protection during aortic valve surgery is still controversial (McGoon, 1975). Since 1967, we have performed selective hypothermic coronary perfusion on 88 patients. Among them, the longest coronary perfusion time with survival was 315 minutes, and the accompanying heart-lung bypass time was seven and one-half hours. We are now very satisfied with the results of our coronary perfusion method. In this chapter, the biochemical aspects of our selective hypothermic coronary perfusion are discussed.

MATERIALS AND METHODS

Figure 1 shows our method of coronary perfusion. The total coronary flow is 10% of the optimal body perfusion flow which is 2.0 liter/minM^2 for the adult patient. This total coronary flow is divided in two: 5/8 for the left and 3/8 for the right coronary artery. The temperature of coronary perfusion blood is maintained at 28°C, independent from that of body perfusion blood.

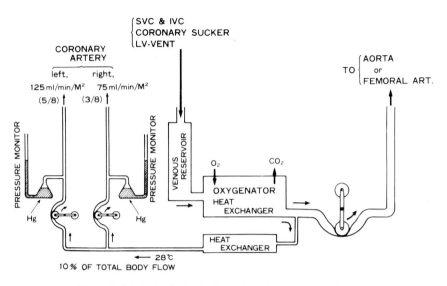

Figure 1. Method of selective hypothermic coronary perfusion.

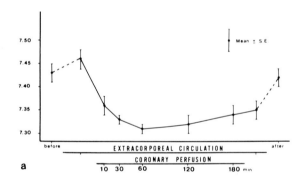

Figure 2a. Arterial pH during selective hypothermic coronary perfusion.

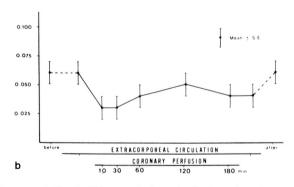

Figure 2b. Coronary A-V pH difference during selective hypothermic coronary perfusion.

492

In this study, the arterial and coronary venous blood was sampled at multiple points as follows: 1) before extracorporeal circulation, 2) soon after the beginning of extracorporeal circulation, 3) 10, 30, 60, 120, and 180 min after the commencement of coronary perfusion, 4) after the termination of coronary perfusion, and 5) after extracorporeal circulation. Blood gas was analyzed and the serum pyruvate and lactate contents were measured. From the results of these measurements, coronary arteriovenous (A-V) pH difference (Obeid *et al.*, 1972), O_2 difference (Moffitt, Rosevear, and McGoon, 1966), CO_2 difference, respiratory quotient, coronary A-V pyruvate difference, lactate difference, cardiac excess lactate (Huckabee, 1961), and redox potential difference (Gudbjarnason, 1962) were calculated.

RESULTS

The average arterial pH (Figure 2a) was 7.43 before extracorporeal circulation. It decreased after the initiation of coronary perfusion and remained around 7.30 to

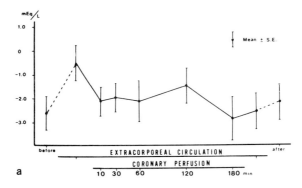

Figure 3a. Arterial BE during selective hypothermic coronary perfusion.

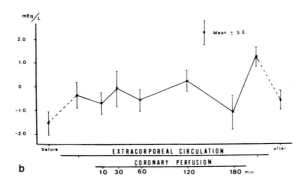

Figure 3b. Coronary A-V BE difference during selective hypothermic coronary perfusion.

7.35 during coronary perfusion. It went back to 7.42 after extracorporeal circulation. The coronary A-V pH difference (Figure 2b) was small throughout the study, well under 0.06.

The average arterial base excess (BE) (Figure 3a) was maintained within the normal range during coronary perfusion, -0.5 to -2.8 mEq/liter. The average coronary A-V BE difference (Figure 3b) remained mainly negative during the entire course of coronary perfusion, ranging from -1.1 to 0.3 mEq/liter.

The average coronary A-V O_2 difference (Figure 4a) was 9.7 vol% before extracorporeal circulation, and it decreased to 3.2–3.9 vol% during coronary perfusion. It recovered to 7.4 vol% after extracorporeal circulation was terminated. The coronary V-A CO_2 difference (Figure 4b) averaged 9.3 vol% before extracorporeal circulation, and it decreased to 2.9–3.5 vol% during coronary perfusion. It recovered to 7.3 vol% after extracorporeal circulation ended.

The myocardial respiratory quotient (Figure 5) was quite stable throughout the study and remained between 0.98 and 1.08.

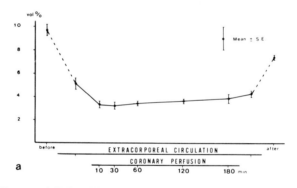

Figure 4a. Coronary A-V O_2 difference during selective hypothermic coronary perfusion.

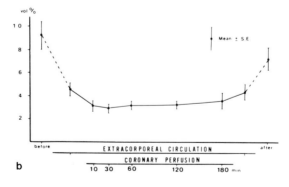

Figure 4b. Coronary V-A CO_2 difference during selective hypothermic coronary perfusion.

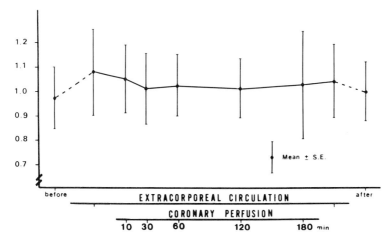

Figure 5. Myocardial respiratory quotient during selective hypothermic coronary perfusion.

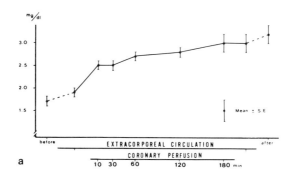

Figure 6a. Arterial pyruvate during selective hypothermic coronary perfusion.

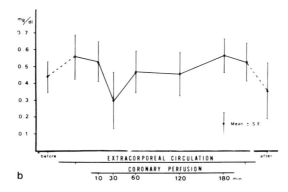

Figure 6b. A-V pyruvate difference during selective hypothermic coronary perfusion.

The content of arterial serum pyruvate (Figure 6a) was 1.7 mg/dl, on the average, before extracorporeal circulation, and it increased gradually to 3.0 mg/dl at 3 hr of coronary perfusion. It further increased to 3.2 mg/dl after cardiopulmonary bypass. The coronary A-V pyruvate difference was between 0.3 and 0.6 mg/dl throughout the study (Figure 6b).

The content of arterial serum lactate (Figure 7a) was 30.3 mg/dl at the beginning of the study, and the initiation of extracorporeal circulation brought it to a very high level, 57.7 mg/dl. The arterial serum lactate increased gradually during coronary perfusion, reaching 75.3 mg/dl by the end of study. The coronary A-V lactate difference (Figure 7b) averaged 4.5 mg/dl before extracorporeal circulation. During coronary perfusion, it decreased and ranged from −1.2 to 3.0 mg/dl; after extracorporeal circulation it recovered to 5.9 mg/dl.

The cardiac excess lactate (Figure 8a) was 0.3 mM/liter before extracorporeal circulation. At the beginning of the extracorporeal circulation, it in-

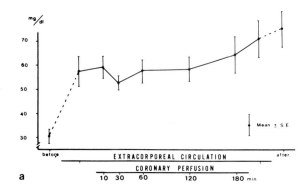

Figure 7a. Arterial lactate during selective hypothermic coronary perfusion.

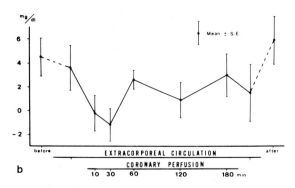

Figure 7b. Coronary A-V lactate difference during selective hypothermic coronary perfusion.

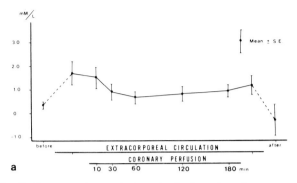

Figure 8a. Cardiac excess lactate during selective hypothermic coronary perfusion.

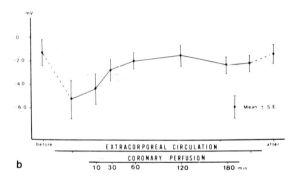

Figure 8b. Coronary redox potential difference during selective hypothermic coronary perfusion.

creased to 1.7 mM/liter, indicating a slight degree of hypoxia. During coronary perfusion, it ranged from 0.7 to 1.5 mM/liter, and it normalized to −0.3 mM/liter after extracorporeal circulation. The redox potential difference (Figure 8b) was −1.3 mV before extracorporeal circulation; at the beginning of extracorporeal circulation, it decreased to −5.3 mV, indicating a slight degree of hypoxia. During coronary perfusion, it ranged from −4.4 to −1.6 mV; at the end of extracorporeal circulation, it became −1.5 mV.

DISCUSSION

The low value of pH during coronary perfusion is attributable to the fact that the blood was sampled at 28°C and was measured at 37°C. These pH values return to the normal range after correction according to Rosenthal's temperature correction formula (Rosenthal, 1948). These results, i.e., that A-V pH difference was small and BE difference remained mainly negative, indicate that myocardial metabolism has no tendency toward hypoxia at any time during coronary perfusion, as far as an acid-base balance is concerned.

The low values of O_2 and CO_2 differences during coronary perfusion are mainly attributable to hypothermia and nonworking beating. These values are quite similar to those obtained in another group of patients who underwent extracorporeal circulation at $28°C$ without coronary perfusion. The stable respiratory quotient demonstrated that, during coronary perfusion, a good balance was maintained between the oxygen uptake and the carbon dioxide excretion of myocardial metabolism.

The amount of pyruvate extracted by the myocardium was statistically significant throughout the study. However, lactate was not actively extracted by the myocardium during coronary perfusion, although a significant uptake was present before and after extracorporeal circulation.

The results of the cardiac excess lactate and the redox potential difference show that myocardial metabolism tended to be anaerobic at the beginning of extracorporeal circulation, a condition attributed to the short period of anoxia during aortotomy and coronary cannulation. After the start of coronary perfusion, cardiac excess lactate and redox potential difference gradually improved and recovered to near normal by the end of the study.

CONCLUSION

The metabolic changes occurring during coronary perfusion with our method, described above, were minimal and easily reversible soon after the termination of coronary perfusion. This minimal change was based mainly on hypothermia and not on coronary perfusion per se. The results obtained in the present study indicate that the method of coronary perfusion we are utilizing is quite safe and reliable.

REFERENCES

GUDBJARNASON, S., HAYDEN, R. O., WENDT, V. E., STOCK, T. B., and BING, R. J. 1962. Oxidation-reduction in heart muscle. Theoretical and clinical considerations. Circulation 26:937–945.

HUCKABEE, W. E. 1961. Relationship of pyruvate and lactate during anaerobic metabolism. V. Coronary adequacy. Am. J. Physiol. 200:1169–1176.

McGOON, D. C. 1975. Myocardial preservation. Open discussion. J. Thorac. Cardiovasc. Surg. 70:1024–1029.

MOFFITT, E. A., ROSEVEAR, J. W., and McGOON, D. C. 1966. Myocardial metabolism during hypothermic coronary perfusion. Acta Anaesthesiol. Scand. (Suppl.) 23: 696–703.

OBEID, A., SMULYAN, H., GILBERT, R., and EICH, R. H. 1972. Regional metabolic changes in the myocardium following coronary artery ligation. Am. Heart J. 83: 189–196.

ROSENTHAL, T. B. 1948. The effect of temperature on the pH of blood and plasma *in vitro.* J. Biol. Chem. 173:25–30, 1948.

Mailing address:
S. Hashimoto, M.D.,
First Department of Surgery, Osaka University Medical School,
Fukushima-ku, Osaka (Japan).

Recent Advances in Studies on
Cardiac Structure and Metabolism, Volume 12
Cardiac Adaptation
Edited by T. Kobayashi, Y. Ito, and G. Rona
Copyright 1978 University Park Press Baltimore

EXPERIMENTAL STUDIES ON MYOCARDIAL METABOLISM OF CARBOHYDRATES AND LIPIDS IN SURFACE-INDUCED DEEP HYPOTHERMIA

H. SHIDA, M. MORIMOTO, K. INOKAWA, and J. TSUGANE

Second Department of Surgery, Faculty of Medicine,
Shinshu University, Asahi 3-1-1, Matsumoto, Nagano Prefecture, Japan

SUMMARY

In surface-induced deep hypothermia, metabolic acidosis resulting from lactacidemia was observed. In the hypothermic heart, the rate of reduction in the coronary arteriovenous (A-V) difference ratio of lactate, pyruvate, and nonesterified fatty acids (NEFA) was proportionately less than that of coronary flow and myocardial oxygen consumption, suggesting that lactate, pyruvate, and NEFA play important roles as energy fuels in the hypothermic heart. Myocardial metabolism of glucose was reduced; exogenous corticosteroids and ATP do not influence the myocardial metabolism of carbohydrates and lipids in the hypothermic heart.

INTRODUCTION

In the heart undergoing surface-induced deep hypothermia during open-heart surgery, metabolic acidosis resulting from lactacidemia is ordinarily observed, especially in the cooling phase. Moreover, it is supposed that the lactacidemia results from anaerobic glycolysis, caused by tissue hypoxia, and from the inability of the liver to metabolize an acidic metabolite (Shida, 1974). Therefore, under these situations, it is conceivable that the investigation of changes in myocardial metabolism constitutes one of the criteria upon which to evaluate hypothermia for open-heart surgery. This study was undertaken to investigate the myocardial metabolism of carbohydrates and lipids during hypothermia, by measuring the coronary arteriovenous difference of glucose, lactate, pyruvate, total fatty acids and nonesterified fatty acids (NEFA), and pyruvate dehydrogenase (PDH). In addition, the influence of high-dose administration of corticosteroids and ATP upon myocardial metabolism during hypothermia also was studied.

MATERIALS AND METHODS

Mongrel adult dogs were divided into three groups, with 5–7 dogs in each group:

Group I: No drug was administered.
Group II: 2 mg/kg of dexamethasone was administered intravenously.
Group III: 10 mg/kg of ATP-Na$_2$ was administered intravenously.

Ether anesthesia with autonomic blocking drugs and surface cooling was performed in the usual fashion in the clinical cases (Shida *et al.,* 1975). The average lowest temperature was approximately 23°C in the esophagus. Arterial blood was taken from the ascending aorta, and coronary sinus blood was taken by coronary cannulation or puncture. Blood gas, blood glucose, blood lactate, blood pyruvate, plasma total fatty acids, composition of total fatty acids, plasma NEFA, PDH by Wieland's method (Wieland, Patzelt, and Löffler, 1972), and coronary blood flow were measured before cooling and at as low as 23°C. Myocardial metabolism was evaluated by the coronary A-V difference ratio, indicating an uptake or a release of substances.

RESULTS

Blood pH and base excess showed a significant decrease at the lowest temperature. Namely, metabolic acidosis developed during hypothermia in each group. On the other hand, no significant change was observed in PaCo$_2$. In hypothermic anesthesia, FiO$_2$ was 100%, and ventilation was in the fashion of hyperventilation.

Coronary blood flow was reduced to approximately one half of the precooling level at the lowest temperature, showing a significant decrease ($p < 0.05$). Myocardial oxygen consumption, which was calculated by coronary blood flow, and coronary A-V oxygen difference also exhibited a significant decrease at 23°C, showing a reduction of approximately one-half of the precooling level. However, as mentioned above, in hypothermic ether anesthesia in a closed system, the PaO$_2$ level was extremely high. Therefore, to obtain an absolute value for myocardial oxygen consumption further investigations are necessary.

Blood glucose showed a significant increase at 23°C in each group. The hyperglycemia during hypothermia resulted from the suppression of insulin secretion, while it was suggested that the peripheral utilization of glucose was reduced. Coronary A-V glucose difference was as low as 1–6% even at 37°C, suggesting a very slight uptake in the cardiac muscle. At as low as 23°C, no significant change was observed. In Groups II and III, the same findings were observed. There were no special differences between them. Namely, it seemed that, during hypothermia, glucose was not utilized in the cardiac muscle as much as in the peripheral tissue.

A significant increase of blood lactate was observed at 23°C in each group. Namely, lactacidemia developed during hypothermia, resulting from anaerobic glycolysis and an inability of the liver to metabolize an acidic metabolite. Coronary A-V lactate difference was approximately 20% at the precooling, showing a definite utilization in the cardiac muscle. At 23°C, coronary A-V lactate difference decreased to approximately one-half of the precooling level; however, it still showed a definite uptake in the cardiac muscle. In Groups II and III, the same findings were observed. Therefore, it seems that high-dose exogenous corticosteroids and ATP do not influence myocardial lactate metabolism.

Each group showed a significant increase at 23°C in blood pyruvate as well as the change in lactate. From the aspect of myocardial pyruvate metabolism, coronary A-V pyruvate difference was more than 20% at the precooling, indicating a definite utilization of pyruvate. At as low as 23°C, coronary A-V pyruvate difference showed the same value as that of the precooling. This result suggests that pyruvate plays an important role as an energy source in cardiac muscle during hypothermia. As for the influence of corticosteroids and ATP upon myocardial pyruvate metabolism, no special differences among the three groups were recorded (Figure 1).

The active form of pyruvate dehydrogenase (PDH) in the cardiac muscle showed a decreasing trend at as low as 23°C, and the total activity also showed the same finding as the active form. However, there was no statistical difference between them. It was suggested that the stimulation of ATP production mediated by the tricarboxylic acid cycle from lactate and pyruvate as energy fuel in the cardiac muscle also might operate even during hypothermia (Figure 2).

Plasma total fatty acids showed a significant decrease at 23°C. As for the mechanism of decrease, it seemed that the accumulation of fatty acids in the

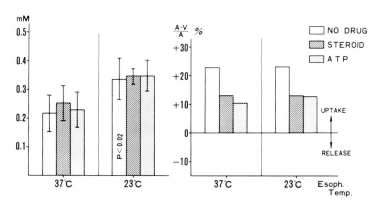

Figure 1. Changes of blood pyruvate and the coronary A-V difference ratio of pyruvate during hypothermia. Esoph. Temp. = temperature in the esophagus.

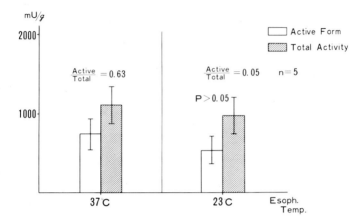

Figure 2. Changes of pyruvate dehydrogenase (PDH) activity in the cardiac muscle during hypothermia. Esoph. Temp. = temperature in the esophagus.

liver during hypothermia played an important role. On the other hand, with respect to myocardial metabolism of total fatty acids, coronary A-V difference showed less than 10% uptake at the precooling and at as low as 23°C, indicating no significant change.

Comparing the composition of total fatty acids of coronary arterial blood to that of coronary sinus blood at 37°C, no significant difference was noted between them. Furthermore, at as low as 23°C, there also was no significant difference between the two.

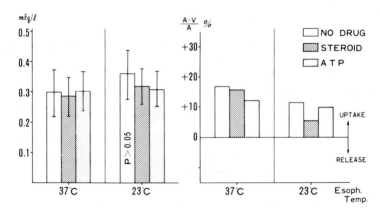

Figure 3. Changes of plasma nonesterified fatty acids (NEFA) and the coronary A-V difference ratio of NEFA during hypothermia. Esoph. Temp. = temperature in the esophagus.

Plasma NEFA showed no significant change at as low as 23°C in the condition without heparin in each group. As for myocardial metabolism of NEFA, the coronary A-V difference of NEFA showed approximately 15% uptake at the precooling in each group, while the coronary A-V difference of NEFA (except in the steroid group) still maintained more than 10% uptake at 23°C. Thus, it seems that NEFA also may operate as an important energy source during hypothermia, as do lactate and pyruvate (Figure 3).

DISCUSSION

As for the change of coronary blood flow and myocardial oxygen consumption associated with hypothermia, oxygen uptake by the myocardium is reduced as the temperature falls, and the rate of reduction in coronary flow is proportionately less than that for the entire body, indicating the greater need of the heart for oxygen (Edwards et al., 1954; Gerola, Feinberg, and Katz, 1959). In this study, the coronary A-V oxygen difference was unchanged at as low as 23°C because of hyperventilation of FiO_2 at 100%. Coronary blood flow was reduced to 46% of the normal, and oxygen uptake by the myocardium was reduced to 44% of the normal at 23°C.

In general, the heart normally uses many substances other than oxygen, such as glucose, lactate, pyruvate, and fatty acids for energy fuel. From the coronary A-V difference of lactate and pyruvate, lactate and pyruvate uptake by the myocardium at as low as 23°C was approximately more than 50% of the normal, although myocardial oxygen consumption was reduced to 44% of the normal. Moreover, PDH in the cardiac muscle showed no reduction at 23°C. Therefore, it seems that lactate and pyruvate play an important metabolic role in the hypothermic heart.

As for lipid metabolism in the cardiac muscle, fatty acids, especially NEFA, supposedly play an important role (Ballard et al., 1960; Bing, Danforth, and Ballard, 1960; Goto, 1962). Plasma NEFA showed a trend to slightly increase at as low as 23°C, indicating the decrease of peripheral utilization of NEFA, while the hypothermic heart still used NEFA as energy fuel as indicated by the coronary A-V difference of NEFA at 23°C.

In starvation, blood glucose decreases, while a compensatory increase of NEFA is observed, indicating a reverse correlation between blood glucose and plasma NEFA (Dole, 1956; Gordon and Cherkers, 1956). There is also a reverse correlation between glucose and NEFA with respect to myocardial metabolism (Goto, 1962). In hypothermia, blood glucose showed a significant increase, suggesting a decrease of utilization of glucose in the peripheral tissue and a suppression of insulin secretion. In the myocardial metabolism of glucose, the coronary A-V difference ratio of glucose was 1–6% before the cooling and 0–2%

at as low as 23°C. Namely, in this study, glucose uptake by the myocardium decreased at as low as 23°C.

From the standpoint that hypothermia is a condition of controlled shock, the influence of high doses of corticosteroids (Lillehei *et al.,* 1964) and ATP (Green and Stoner, 1950; Talaat, Massion, and Schining, 1964), which have such antishock effects as the improvement of microcirculation and the increase of cardiac output, upon carbohydrate and lipid metabolism of the whole body and cardiac muscle was studied. No definite effect of the administration of corticosteroids and ATP on myocardial metabolism of carbohydrates and lipids was observed.

REFERENCES

BALLARD, F. B., DANFORTH, W. H., NAEGLE, S., and BING, R. J. 1960. Myocardial metabolism of fatty acids. J. Clin. Invest. 39:717–723.

BING, R. J., DANFORTH, W. H., and BALLARD, F. B. 1960. Physiology of the myocardium. JAMA 172:438–444.

DOLE, V. P. 1956. A relation between non-esterified fatty acids in plasma and the metabolism of glucose. J. Clin. Invest. 35:150–154.

EDWARDS, W. S., TULUY, S., RUBER, W. E., SIEGEL, A., and BING, R. J. 1954. Coronary blood flow and myocardial metabolism in hypothermia. Ann. Surg. 139: 275–281.

GEROLA, A., FEINBERG, H., and KATZ, L. N. 1959. Myocardial oxygen consumption and coronary blood flow in hypothermia. Am. J. Physiol. 196:719–725.

GORDON, R. S., JR., and CHERKERS, 1956. Unesterified fatty acid in human blood plasma. J. Clin. Invest. 35:206–212.

GOTO, Y. 1962. The fatty metabolism in the heart muscle. Jpn. Circ. J. 26:121–127.

GREEN, H. N., and STONER, H. B. 1950. The present status of the adenine nucleotides in the bodily response to injury. Brit. Med. J. 2:805–809.

LILLEHIE, R. C., LONGERBEAM, J. K., BLOCH, J. H., and MANAX, W. G. 1964. The nature of irreversible shock. Ann. Surg., 160:682–710.

SHIDA, H. 1974. Pathogenesis and treatment of metabolic acidosis in open-heart surgery under surface-induced deep hypothermia. Jpn. J. Surg. 4:198–203.

SHIDA, H., MORIMOTO, M., SEKI, T., and INOKAWA, K. 1975. Metabolic changes in surface-induced deep hypothermia combined with cardiopulmonary bypass for cardiac surgery. Jpn. J. Surg. 5:73–83.

TALAAT, S. M., MASSION, W. H., and SCHINING, J. A. 1964. The effect of ATP administration in irreversible shock. Surgery 55:813–819.

WIELAND, O. H., PATZELT, C., and LÖFFLER, G. 1972. Active and inactive forms of pyruvate dehydrogenase in rat liver. Eur. J. Biochem. 26:426–433.

Mailing address:
Hiroshi Shida, M.D.,
Second Department of Surgery, Faculty of Medicine, Shinshu University,
Asahi 3-1-1, Matsumoto City, Nagano Prefecture (Japan).

Recent Advances in Studies on
Cardiac Structure and Metabolism, Volume 12
Cardiac Adaptation
Edited by T. Kobayashi, Y. Ito, and G. Rona
Copyright 1978 University Park Press Baltimore

PRESERVATION OF MYOCARDIAL MEMBRANE INTEGRITY IN THE EARLY PHASE OF ACUTE MYOCARDIAL ISCHEMIA

M. OKUDA[1] and A. M. LEFER

Department of Physiology, Jefferson Medical College,
Thomas Jefferson University, Philadelphia, Pennsylvania, USA

SUMMARY

Myocardial uptake of dexamethasone (Dex) or methylprednisolone (MP) was studied using tritiated tracers in isolated perfused cat hearts during acute myocardial ischemia. Considerable amounts of Dex and MP were incorporated into the plasma membranes in control, border-zone, and ischemic myocardium. Lesser amounts were bound to the remaining subcellular organelles. A gradient of the glucocorticoid uptake was observed decreasing from control myocardium to ischemic myocardium in all subcellular fractions. By the first hour of ischemia, the myocardial plasma membranes underwent marked depletion of activity of 5'-nucleotidase, a plasma membrane marker enzyme, indicating early loss of plasma membrane integrity in acute myocardial ischemia. The incorporation of Dex or MP into the plasma membranes resulted in a significant decrease in loss of 5'-nucleotidase activity of the plasma membranes in the border-zone and ischemic myocardium. The data provide direct evidence 1) to support a membrane stabilizing action of glucocorticoids, and 2) to focus on the plasma membranes as a potentially important site of protection during the early phase of acute myocardial ischemia.

INTRODUCTION

Pharmacological doses of synthetic glucocorticoids have been shown to protect myocardium against the spread of ischemic cellular damage (Barzilai *et al.,* 1972; Libby *et al.,* 1973; Morrison *et al.,* 1975). Recent studies have confirmed a significant decrease in release of membrane bound enzymes from ischemic myocardial tissue in the presence of glucocorticoids, suggesting that membrane stabilization is the mechanism of protective action of glucocorticoids (Spath, Lane, and Lefer, 1974; Spath and Lefer, 1975). However, none of these studies have provided direct evidence to support this concept. Moreover, there is lack of

Supported by Research Grant HL-17688 from The National Heart and Lung Institute of the NIH, USA.
[1] On leave of absence from the Department of Internal Medicine, National Defense Medical College, 500 Tokorosawa, Saitama Prefecture 359, Japan.

knowledge in such areas as myocardial uptake and the distribution of gluco-corticoids and their binding sites in myocardial cells, knowledge which is essential for the elucidation of glucocorticoid activity on myocardium.

The purposes of the present investigation were: 1) to study myocardial uptake of the glucocorticoids in both normal and ischemic myocardium, 2) to determine the subcellular distribution and binding loci in the myocardial cells, and 3) to correlate the glucocorticoid uptake to the preservation of membrane integrity in ischemic myocardium.

MATERIALS AND METHODS

Cat hearts of Langendorff preparations were used. The hearts were randomly divided into nonischemic and ischemic groups. In the ischemic group, the left anterior coronary artery was ligated and the artery was cut between ligatures to ensure total occlusion. Ischemic tissue was obtained from the area supplied by the occluded artery, and border-zone tissue was obtained from the adjacent area. In the nonischemic group, perfusion took place without coronary occlusion, and control samples of nonischemic myocardium were obtained. All hearts were perfused for 60 min by recirculation of 500 ml of Krebs-Henseleit solution containing tritiated glucocorticoid. The concentrations used were Dex 0.17 mM or MP 0.81 mM, which are equivalent to the doses of Dex 6 mg/kg body weight or MP 30 mg/kg body weight, respectively. After perfusion the hearts were flushed with 200 ml of ice-cold K-H solution via the aortic cannula to exchange the label in the extracellular fluid.

Homogenization of myocardial tissue and cellular fractionation were per-formed according to the method of Kidwai (1974) with minor modifications. The supernatant from 105,000-g centrifugation was designated as soluble frac-tion, S, and the pellet as particulate fraction, P. The latter was further fraction-ated by sucrose density-gradient ultracentrifugation. The formed bands were defined by their isopycnic densities and marker enzyme activities as: 1) F_1, plasma membranes, 2) F_2, light lysosomes and sarcoplasmic reticulum, 3) F_3 and F_4, light and heavy mitochondria, and 4) F_5, heavy lysosomes.

Metabolic states of the glucocorticoid in myocardial tissues were determined by extracting the compounds with methylene chloride and by subsequent identification on silica-gel thin layer chromatography (TLC) (Monder and Walker, 1970).

RESULTS AND DISCUSSION

In one hour, myocardial cellular uptake of [^{3}H]Dex and [^{3}H]MP in non-ischemic myocardium reached 0.9 ± 0.04 μM/g tissue and 1.5 ± 0.05 μM/g tissue, respectively (mean ± S.E.M.). The uptake in the border-zone tissue was not significantly lower than that in the nonischemic tissue. A significant decrease occurred in the uptake of both glucocorticoids by the ischemic myocardium (p < 0.001). Nevertheless, ischemic myocardium took up large amounts of the glucocorticoids (66–73% of the nonischemic). Because the supplying coronary artery was totally occluded, the data imply very high diffusion rates of the glucocorticoids in myocardial tissue and/or ample collateral coronary flow to the ischemic area.

In nonischemic myocardium, S/P ratios of the uptake were 7–10, indicating that a considerable portion of the total uptake was bound to the cellular particulate fractions. The S/P ratios increased significantly in ischemic myocardium as a result of membrane destruction and development of regional edema.

The myocardial tissues were found not to degrade glucocorticoids to any appreciable extent. With TLC, virtually 100% of the extracted radioactivity was identified as native steroids. Table 1 summarizes the absolute specific uptakes in each subcellular fraction expressed in nmol/mg of protein. The striking finding in nonischemic control tissue is the large uptake of glucocorticoids by the plasma membranes constituting 70–85% of the total particulate uptake for both steroids. The absolute uptake by plasma membranes was significantly lower in the border zone and in the ischemic tissue ($p < 0.01$). There was a progressively lower absolute uptake with each successive subcellular fraction ($F_1 > F_2 > F_3 > F_4 > F_5$) in all three areas.

Myocardial 5′-nucleotidase activity was exclusively recovered in the F_1 fraction, indicating that this fraction comprises most of the plasma membranes of the myocardial homogenates. In ischemic myocardium, the plasma membranes became significantly damaged, and the damage appeared to occur earlier than comparable changes in lysosomes. This was reflected in the very low specific activity of 5′-nucleotidase in the F_1 fraction obtained from the ischemic

Table 1. Distribution of ^{3}H-steroids in myocardial cell fractions

Fraction	Methylprednisolone (MP)			Dexamethasone (Dex)		
	C	B	I	C	B	I
F_1	38.0 ± 2.0	29.9 ± 2.7	21.7 ± 1.7	34.6 ± 3.2	18.2 ± 3.0	13.9 ± 2.1
F_2	8.6 ± 0.6	5.9 ± 0.5	3.6 ± 0.3	4.6 ± 1.0	4.9 ± 1.2	2.4 ± 0.6
F_3	3.8 ± 0.3	2.6 ± 0.3	1.4 ± 0.1	0.7 ± 0.1	0.8 ± 0.1	0.3 ± 0.1
F_4	2.3 ± 0.2	1.4 ± 0.1	0.7 ± 0.1	0.6 ± 0.1	0.7 ± 0.1	0.3 ± 0.1
F_5	1.3 ± 0.5	1.2 ± 0.4	0.7 ± 0.2	0.4 ± 0.2	0.9 ± 0.2	0.2 ± 0.1

All values are means expressed in nanomoles of glucocorticoid incorporated per mg of protein ± S.E.M. for eight hearts in each group. C = control area; B = border zone; I = ischemic area.

Table 2. Percent distribution of 5′-nucleotidase in supernatant and particulate fractions

| Type of preparation | Area | Percent Distribution | | p Value | |
		Supernatant	Particulate	From control	From same area in "no steroid" group
Control	C	0 ± 0	100 ± 0	—	—
Ischemic:	B	22.6 ± 7.3	77.4 ± 7.3	$p < 0.01$	—
No steroid	I	62.0 ± 10.7	38.0 ± 10.7	$p < 0.001$	—
Ischemic:	B	5.2 ± 4.2	94.8 ± 4.2	N.S.	$p < 0.05$
Dexa	I	34.2 ± 6.2	65.8 ± 6.2	$p < 0.001$	$p < 0.05$
Ischemic:	B	6.2 ± 4.2	93.8 ± 4.2	N.S.	$p < 0.05$
MP	I	33.4 ± 7.3	66.6 ± 7.3	$p < 0.01$	$p < 0.05$

All values are means ± S.E.M. of five hearts in each group.

myocardium (15 ± 0.6 U/mg of protein in normal myocardium, 5 ± 1.9 U/mg of protein in ischemic myocardium), and in the very high percentage of 5′-nucleotidase activity occurring in the supernatant of myocardial homogenates. As shown in Table 2, in the absence of glucocorticoids, 62% of the enzyme activity was found in the supernatant of the ischemic tissue and 23% of the activity in the border-zone supernatant. In the presence of glucocorticoids, this enzyme activity was only 33–34% and 5–6% of the total in the ischemic and border-zone supernatants, respectively.

Thus, the data provide essential information concerning myocardial uptake of Dex and MP and the mechanism of membrane stabilizing action of glucocorticoids that preserves plasma membrane integrity against the damaging effects of acute myocardial ischemia.

REFERENCES

BARZILAI, D., PLAVNICK, J., HAZANI, A. *et al.* 1972. Use of hydrocortisone in the treatment of acute myocardial infarction. Chest 61:488–491.

KIDWAI, A. M. 1974. Isolation of plasma membrane from smooth, skeletal, and heart muscle. Methods Enzymol. 31:134–144.

LIBBY, P. MAROKO, P. R., BLOOR, C. M. *et al.* 1973. Reduction of experimental myocardial infarct size by corticosteroid administration. J. Clin. Invest. 52:599–607.

MONDER, C., and WALKER, M. C. 1970. Interactions between corticosteroids and histones. Biochemistry 9:2489–2497.

MORRISON, J., MALEY, T., REDUTO, L. *et al.* 1975. Effect of methylprednisolone on predicted myocardial infarction size in man. Crit. Care Med. 3:94–102.

SPATH, J. A., JR., LANE, D. L., and LEFER, A. M. 1974. Protective action of methylprednisolone on the myocardium during experimental myocardial ischemia in the cat. Circ. Res. 35:44–51.

SPATH, J. A., JR., and LEFER, A. M. 1975. Effects of dexamethasone on myocardial cells in the early phase of acute myocardial infarction. Am. Heart J. 90:50–55.

Mailing address:
Dr. Minoru Okuda,
Associate Professor of Internal Medicine,
National Defense Medical College, 500 Tokorosawa,
Saitama Prefecture 359 (Japan).

Recent Advances in Studies on
Cardiac Structure and Metabolism, Volume 12
Cardiac Adaptation
Edited by T. Kobayashi, Y. Ito, and G. Rona
Copyright 1978 University Park Press Baltimore

TOLERANCE TO ISCHEMIA IN THE HUMAN HEART

JUTTA SCHAPER,[1] F. SCHWARZ,[2] and W. FLAMENG[3]

[1] Max-Planck-Institut für Physiologische u. Klinische Forschung
(W. G. Kerckhoff-Institut), D-6350 Bad Nauheim, West Germany
[2] Kerckhoff-Klinik Bad Nauheim, D-6350 Bad Nauheim, West Germany
[3] Department of Cardiovascular Surgery, University Gießen, D-6300 Gießen, West Germany

SUMMARY

The tolerance to ischemic cardiac arrest during open-heart surgery depends on the degree of hypertrophy and on the functional impairment of the heart. The angiographically determined muscle mass is a good indicator of the susceptibility of the myocardium to ischemic injury and of its ability to quickly restore myocardial structure upon reperfusion. Tissue from extremely hypertrophied hearts exhibited numerous degenerative alterations.

INTRODUCTION

In a recent study on the effect of ischemic cardiac arrest on myocardial ultrastructure in the human heart, it was observed that ischemia of 40-min duration is tolerated well, that 60 min of ischemia evokes severe myocardial damage and impairs the structural recovery during reperfusion, and that ischemic arrest of more than 60-min duration results in irreversible damage of large parts of the myocardium (Schaper *et al.,* 1977). It was obvious, however, that some hearts were more resistant to ischemic injury than were others, and the speed and degree of recovery during reperfusion varied greatly. This study represents an attempt to correlate the tolerance to ischemia in individual patients to the preoperative functional state of the heart, i.e., to the degree of hypertrophy and the performance of the left ventricle.

MATERIALS AND METHODS

Extensive clinical examinations, including left ventricular catheterization and cineangiography, were carried out on 12 patients (see Table 1) with aortic valve disease. Thereafter, all patients underwent surgery for aortic valve replacement under identical anesthesiological and surgical conditions. Cardiac arrest was induced by injection of a cold cardioplegic solution (Kirsch, Rodewald, and Kalmar, 1972) into the aortic root, and surgery was carried out on the nonbeat-

Table 1. Relationship between the muscle mass and the functional state of the heart and the ischemia tolerance, determined morphologically

Patient	Age	Diagnosis	Mm	EF	LVW I	Ischemia tolerance
Group A: Muscle mass < 200 g/m^2						
S.E.	67 yr	st. and reg.	163	84	46	+++
D.G.	19 yr	reg.	184	63	85	+++
H.E.	26 yr	reg.	141	62	103	+++
	mean value		163	69	78	good
Group B: Muscle mass 200–300 g/m^2						
S.A.	32 yr	st. and reg.	285	58	53	++
V.L.	62 yr	st. and reg.	259	54	38	+
E.E.	51 yr	ret.	275	61	39	+++
S.H.	37 yr	st.	283	82	53	+++
R.N.	31 yr	st.	295	47	35	++
	mean value		279	60	44	varying
Group C: Muscle mass > 300 g/m^2						
B.R.	41 yr	st.	334	62	43	++
A.D.	39 yr	reg.	301	25	24	+
G.G.	39 yr	reg.	583	18	16	+
S.G.	37 yr	st. and reg.	343	21	20	+
	mean value		390	31	26	reduced

With increasing Mm, a decrease in the functional parameters EF and LVWI and a reduction of the tolerance to ischemia are evident. There is no correlation between the type of aortic valve defect and the degree of functional impairment of ischemia tolerance.
Mm = muscle mass; EF = ejection fraction; LVWI = left ventricular work index.
Ischemia tolerance: +++ = good; ++ = slightly reduced; + = reduced.

ing, nonperfused heart under total cardiopulmonary bypass. In all patients, the heart was arrested for 40 min with a 10-min period of whole-body hypothermia.

Needle biopsies were taken from the anterior left ventricular wall before the induction of cardiac standstill, at the end of the ischemic interval, and 20 min after coronary reperfusion had started. The tissue was immediately fixed in cold 3% glutaraldehyde and processed in a routine procedure for electron microscopy. Examination of semithin sections revealed hypertrophied myocardial cells with increased width and length in all tissue samples. Multiple intercalated discs and other features, reported as being present in hypertrophied cells (Maron, Ferrans, and Roberts, 1975), were frequently observed.

RESULTS AND DISCUSSION

The relationship between the hemodynamic parameters and the tolerance to ischemia by ultrastructural criteria is demonstrated in Table 1. It is evident that in patients with a muscle mass below 200 g/m^2 and a rather good cardiac performance ischemic cardiac arrest is tolerated well, that there is no clear-cut correlation in the second group exhibiting a muscle mass of 200–300 g/m^2 and varying cardiac performance, and that the tolerance to ischemia in the group with a muscle mass above 300 g/m^2 and poor cardiac function is greatly reduced. It is also evident from this table that the tolerance to ischemia does not depend on the type of aortic valve defect but on the degree of hypertrophy and the impairment of cardiac function.

Figures 2–4 are typical examples of the different degrees of myocardial damage after ischemic injury. The micrographs are representative of the three groups described in Table 1. Figure 1 shows mitochondria from a control sample (before induction of ischemia) which demonstrate a satisfactory quality of fixation. Figures 2a and 2b show slightly injured mitochondria after ischemia (+++ in Table 1) and a quick structural recovery during reperfusion. In Figures 3a and 3b, moderate injury to mitochondria (++ in Table 1), followed by a slower restitution of the myocardial ultrastructure during reperfusion, is demonstrated. Severe mitochondrial injury (+ in Table 1) is illustrated in Figure 4a, while Figure 4b shows a very slow structural restoration after coronary reperfusion. It should be emphasized that all samples were taken after 40 min of ischemia or after a 20-min reperfusion period.

Differences in the reaction to ischemia between the epicardial and the endocardial layer could not be observed. This is easily explained by the fact that

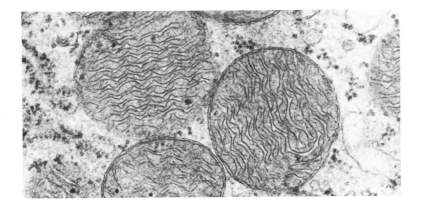

Figure 1. Good preservation of myocardial mitochondria by immersion fixation. Biopsy taken before induction of ischemia. × 48,000.

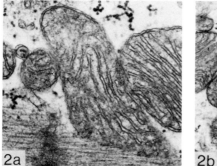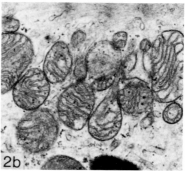

Figure 2a. Slight ischemic injury to mitochondria. × 48,000. *2b.* Nearly complete restoration of mitochondrial structure during reperfusion. × 20,400.

the perfusion for the entire heart had been interrupted and that the heart had been vented in order to relieve the intraventricular pressure, i.e., intramyocardial pressure gradients were absent.

During reperfusion the epicardial layer recovered more quickly from ischemic injury than the subendocardial tissue. Recovery in the subendocardial layer is delayed because of the limitation of myocardial perfusion by the increased intramyocardial pressure.

Tissue samples from the third group showed many ultrastructural alterations of severe hypertrophy and degeneration, such as Z-line changes, reduced amounts of contractile material, and irregularities in mitochondrial size, shape, and configuration. Abnormal distribution of nuclear chromatin, cytoplasmic inclusions in the nucleoplasm, and nuclear tubules were commonly observed. Many cells showed formation of myelin figures, increased amounts of T tubules

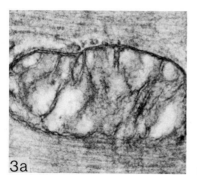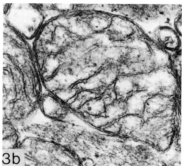

Figure 3a. Moderate ischemic injury to mitochondria. × 48,000. *3b.* Incomplete restitution of mitochondrial structure during reperfusion. × 39,000.

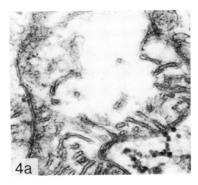 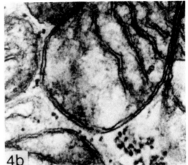

Figure 4a. Severe ischemic injury to mitochondria. × 48,000. *4b.* Mitochondria appear severely damaged, as after the ischemic period. × 60,000.

and sarcoplasmic reticulum, and large empty vacuoles. In the interstitial space, many very active fibroblast-like cells and an increased amount of cell debris, collagen, and elastic fibers were observed.

These changes occurred less regularly in the second group, and they were virtually absent in the first group, indicating that a positive correlation exists between the functional state of the heart and its ultrastructural characteristics, i.e., decreased cardiac function is usually accompanied by abnormalities in myocardial fine structure.

REFERENCES

KIRSCH, U., RODEWALD, G., and KALMAR, P. 1972. Induced ischemic arrest. Clinical experience with cardioplegia in open-heart surgery. J. Thor. Cardiovasc. Surg. 63: 121–130.

MARON, B. J., FERRANS, V. J., and ROBERTS, W. C. 1975. Ultrastructural features of degenerated cardiac muscle cells in patients with cardiac hypertrophy. Am. J. Pathol. 79:387–414.

SCHAPER, J., HEHRLEIN, F., SCHLEPPER, M., and THIEDEMANN, K-U. 1977. Ultrastructural alterations during ischemia and reperfusion in human hearts during cardiac surgery. J. Mol. Cell. Cardiol. 9:175–189.

Mailing address:
Jutta Schaper, M.D.,
Max-Planck-Institut für Physiologische u., Klinische Forschung
(W. G. Kerckhoff-Institut), D-6350 Bad Nauheim, Sprudelhof 11 (West Germany).

Recent Advances in Studies on
Cardiac Structure and Metabolism, Volume 12
Cardiac Adaptation
Edited by T. Kobayashi, Y. Ito, and G. Rona
Copyright 1978 University Park Press Baltimore

EFFECT OF PHYSICAL FITNESS ON MYOCARDIAL DAMAGE AND CIRCULATION AFTER MYOCARDIAL NECROSIS

M. AHMAD, M. TAJUDDIN, and M. TARIQ

Experimental and Metabolic Laboratory, Department of Medicine,
Aligarh Muslim University, Aligarh, India

SUMMARY

The effect of physical training (conditioning) on myocardial circulation and myocardial damage has been evaluated in experimental myocardial necrosis in albino rats. Conditioning was done by making the animals swim in a tank of water, thermostatically controlled at $32°$ $\pm 1°C$, 60 minutes daily, six days a week, for eight weeks. Myocardial necrosis was produced by subcutaneous injection of isoproterenol, 85 mg/kg body weight, on two consecutive days. Investigations included ECG (lead II), SGOT, SGPT, SLDH, SCPK, histopathology of the heart, and myocardial Rubidium 84 uptake. It was observed that, in conditioned animals, elevation of serum enzymes was less, incidence of cardiac arrhythmia was lower, myocardial damage was less marked, and myocardial circulation was better after myocardial necrosis in comparison to unconditioned animals. Less myocardial damage and lower incidence of cardiac arrhythmia are presumably associated with a better prognosis.

INTRODUCTION

Evaluation of physical training in the prevention of coronary heart disease (CHD) has attracted considerable interest during the past two decades. Physically active individuals have been observed to have a favorable status in terms of CHD incidence (Fox and Halkell, 1968; Paffenbarger *et al.*, 1970; Gyntelberg, 1973). Active rehabilitation of coronary patients by exercise (Brunner and Moshulam, 1969) and by supervised circuit training after myocardial infarction (Morgans and Buston, 1972) has been shown to decrease the incidence of reinfarction.

A comparison of metabolic changes after myocardial necrosis in fit (conditioned) and unfit (unconditioned) animals has shown that physically trained animals are likely to have less myocardial damage following ischemia (Tajuddin, Ahmad, and Tariq, 1974). However, the evaluation of myocardial circulation and of histopathological changes in the myocardium after experimental myocardial necrosis in the two groups would probably give a better indication of the beneficial effect of physical training.

The present study was undertaken to evaluate the effect of physical training on myocardial damage, cardiac arrhythmias, and myocardial circulation after isoproteronol-induced myocardial necrosis.

MATERIALS AND METHODS

Male albino rats weighing 100–150 g were selected for the study. Physical training (conditioning) involved making the animals swim 60 min per day for six days a week. The swimming program was continued for eight weeks before the induction of myocardial necrosis. The swimming tank was maintained at $32° \pm 1°C$ by a thermostatic device.

Myocardial necrosis was produced by subcutaneous injection of iso-proterenol, 85 mg/kg body weight, for two consecutive days.

The animals were divided into the following four groups:

Group I: Sedentary control; the animals were permitted normal cage activity.
Group II: Animals subjected to physical training.
Group III: Sedentary animals with isoproterenol-induced myocardial necrosis (SMN).
Group IV: Conditioned animals with isoproterenol-induced myocardial necrosis (CMN).

ECG (lead II) was recorded in each case after anesthetizing the animals with ether.

Serum transminases (SGOT) and (SGPT) were determined by the method of Reitman and Frankel (1957). Serum lactate dehydrogenase (LDH) was determined by the method of Wroblewski and La Due (1955), and serum creatine phosphokinase (CPK) was estimated by the method of Hughes (1962).

For histological examination, the heart tissue was fixed in 10% normal saline. Sections of 3 μm were cut and stained with hematoxylin and eosin.

Lesions were graded according to the following system (Rona et al., 1959):

Macroscopic lesions:
  Grade 0: No lesion.
  Grade 1: Mottling of the apex and distal parts of the left ventricle caused by intermingled pale and dark red streaks.
  Grade 2: Well demarcated necrotic area limited to the apex.
  Grade 3: Large infarct-like necrosis involving at least one-third of the left ventricle and extending to adjacent areas of the interventricular septum and of the right ventricle.
  Grade 4: Large infarct-like necrosis involving more than half of the left ventricle and interventricular septum, and extending to the distal portion of the right ventricle.

Microscopic lesions:

Grade 0: No lesion.

Grade 1: Focal lesions of the subendocardial portion of the apex or of the papillary muscle, composed of fibroblastic swelling or proliferation and accumulation of histiocytes.

Grade 2: Focal lesions extending over wider areas of the ventricle, with right ventricular involvement (lesions included edema, mottled staining, fragmentation, and segmentation of muscle fibers).

Grade 3: Confluent lesions of the apex and papillary muscles, with focal lesions involving other areas of the ventricles and auricles. The lesions included vacuolar and fatty degeneration, granular disintegration, hyalin necrosis of the muscle fibers, marked capillary dilatation with hemorrhages, extensive edema, occasionally with a mucoid component, causing sequestration of muscle fibers.

Grade 4: Confluent massive necrosis, with occasionally acute aneurysm or mural thrombi. The lesions were similar in character to those in Grade 3.

Myocardial circulation was evaluated in terms of Rubidium 84 uptake. Two μCi of Rubidium were injected through the jugular vein. The animal was sacrificed by decapitation 1 min after the injection. The heart was cut into fine sections that were counted in a scintillation counter.

RESULTS

Increase in SGOT was 143% above the normal value in SMN and 100% above in CMN. LDH levels increased by 103% and 66% in SMN and CMN, respectively. CPK elevation was 416% in SMN and 258% in CMN. Thus, there was significantly less increase in serum enzymes in the conditioned group after myocardial necrosis. SGPT elevation was, however, not significantly different in the two groups.

Macroscopic examination (Table 1) of the heart did not reveal any change (Grade 0) in five out of 10 rats in CMN as compared to SMN in which a Grade 0 change was observed only in one out of 10 hearts studied. Grade 1 change was present in one heart in SMN and in four animals in CMN. Grade 2 changes were observed in two hearts in SMN and in one heart in CMN. Three animals in SMN had Grade 3 changes and three animals had Grade 4 changes. Grade 3 and Grade 4 lesions were not observed in CMN.

Microscopic examination (Table 1) showed Grade 4 changes in 80% of the unconditioned animals as opposed to 30% in conditioned animals after myocardial necrosis. Two animals (20%) in the unconditioned group had Grade 3 changes, while six animals (60%) had Grade 3 changes in the conditioned group. One animal (10%) in the conditioned group had Grade 2 changes.

Table 1. Histopathological examination of the heart

	Macroscopic examination		Microscopic examination	
Grade	SMN[a] (No. of animals)	CMN[b] (No. of animals)	SMN (No. of animals)	CMN (No. of animals)
0	1 (10%)	5 (50%)	0	0
1	1 (10%)	4 (40%)	0	0
2	2 (20%)	1 (10%)	0	1 (10%)
3	3 (30%)	0	2 (20%)	6 (60%)
4	3 (30%)	0	8 (80%)	3 (30%)
Total number of animals	10	10	10	10

[a]SMN = Sedentary animals with isoproterenol-induced myocardial necrosis.
[b]CMN = Conditioned animals with isoproterenol-induced myocardial necrosis.

Thus, the macroscopic and microscopic examinations revealed less myocardial damage in conditioned animals after isoproterenol-induced myocardial necrosis than in unconditioned animals.

Rubidium 84 uptake study showed that conditioned animals (Group II) had better coronary circulation (Table 2). Rubidium 84 uptake by the heart was 150% in Group II animals (normal taken, 100%). After isoproterenol-induced myocardial necrosis, the uptake was 39.92% in CMN and 17.29% in SMN. It is evident from these findings that coronary circulation in CMN was twice that of SMN.

Electrocardiogram readings showed ST segment elevation, flat T waves, deep Q waves, bundle branch block, partial heart block, and complete heart block in different animals. Cardiac arrhythmia was observed in five out of 10 animals (50%) in SMN, whereas only two animals (20%) showed cardiac arrhythmia in CMN.

Table 2. Myocardial Rubidium 84 uptake

Group	Number of rats	Rubidium 84 uptake
Sedentary control	6	100.00%
Conditioned animals	6	150.00%
SMN[a]	6	17.23%
CMN[b]	6	35.98%

[a]SMN = Sedentary animals with isoproterenol-induced myocardial necrosis.
[b]CMN = Conditioned animals with isoproterenol-induced myocardial necrosis.

DISCUSSION

The value of physical activity as a preventive approach to coronary heart disease, although not conclusively proved, is widely accepted today as beneficial and prudent. However, its effect on the extent of myocardial damage and on the complications following myocardial infarction is yet to be evaluated.

The present study has shown that the rises in SGOT, LDH, and CPK were significantly lower in the conditioned group after isoproterenol-induced myocardial necrosis. Only SGPT did not reveal any significant difference between the two groups. Because the enzymatic changes parallel myocardial damage (La Due, Wroblewski, and Karmen, 1954), it can be concluded that the extent of myocardial damage is less severe in physically trained animals.

This assumption is supported by histological examination that showed less myocardial damage in the conditioned group. While Grade 0 damage, after macroscopic examination, was found in 10% of the rats in the unconditioned group, it was found in 50% of the animals in the conditioned group after myocardial necrosis. Microscopic examination showed Grade 4 changes in 80% of the unconditioned animals, while only 30% of the conditioned animals showed Grade 4 changes.

Although conditioning has been shown to improve myocardial circulation in normal animals (Stevenson *et al.,* 1964) the effect of conditioning on myocardial circulation after myocardial necrosis has not been evaluated. The present study suggests that myocardial circulation after isoproterenol-induced myocardial necrosis is better in conditioned animals than in unconditioned animals. It is noted that coronary circulation in CMN was twice that of SMN.

It is concluded from the present study that physically trained animals sustain less myocardial injury, have better circulation, and are less prone to cardiac arrhythmias. Because the disturbance in cardiac rhythm is an important determinant of the outcome of an ischemic attack, physically active persons are likely to have a more favorable prognosis after an attack of myocardial necrosis.

REFERENCES

BRUNNER, D., and MOSHULAM, N. 1969. Prevention of recurrent myocardial infarction by physical exercise. Isr. J. Med. Sci. 4:783–785.

FOX, S. M., and HALKELL, W. L. 1968. Physical activity and the prevention of coronary heart disease. Bull. N. Y. Acad. Med. 44:950–965.

GYNTELBERG, F. 1973. Physical fitness and coronary heart disease in Copenhagen males aged 40–59. II. Dan. Med. Bull. 20:105–112.

HUGHES, B. P. 1962. A method for the estimation of serum creatine kinase and its use in comparing creatine kinase and aldolase activity in normal and pathological sera. Clin. Chem. Acta 7:597–603.

La DUE, J. S., WROBLEWSKI, F., and KARMEN, A. 1954. SGOT activity in human acute transmural myocardial infarction. Science 120:497.

MORGANS, C. M., and BUSTON, W. M. 1972. Supervised circuit training after myocardial infarction. Physiotherapy 58:340–343.

PAFFENBARGER, R. S., LANGHLIN, M. R., GIMA, A. S., and BLACK, R. A. 1970. Work activity of longshoremen as related to deaths from coronary heart disease and stroke. New Eng. J. Med. 282:1109–1114.

REITMAN, S., and FRANKEL, S. 1957. A colorimetric method for the determination of serum glutamic oxalacetic and glutamic pyruvic transaminases. Am. J. Clin. Pathol. 28:57–63.

RONA, G., CHAPPEL, C. I., BALAZS, T., and GAUDRY, R. 1959. An infarct-like myocardial lesion and other toxic manifestations produced by isoproterenol in the rat. Arch. Pathol. 67:443.

STEVENSON, J. A. F., FELEKI, V., RECHNITZER, and BEATON, J. R. 1964. Effect of exercise on coronary tree size in the rat. Circ. Res. 15:265–269.

TAJUDDIN, M., AHMAD, M., and TARIQ, M. 1975. Effect of conditioning on myocardial metabolism after myocardial infarction. In P. E. Roy and G. Rona, Recent Advances in Studies on Cardiac Structure and Metabolism. Vol. 10: The Metabolism of Contraction, pp. 561–568. University Park Press, Baltimore.

WROBLEWSKI, R., and La DUE, J. S. 1955. Lactic dehydrogenase activity in blood. Proc. Soc. Exp. Biol. 20:210–213.

Mailing address:
Dr. M. Ahmad,
Experimental and Metabolic Laboratory, Department of Medicine,
Aligarh Muslim University, Aligarh (U.P.) (India).

Recent Advances in Studies on
Cardiac Structure and Metabolism, Volume 12
Cardiac Adaptation
Edited by T. Kobayashi, Y. Ito, and G. Rona
Copyright 1978 University Park Press Baltimore

PHARMACOLOGICAL PROTECTION OF HYPOXIC HEART

W. G. NAYLER, A. GRAU, and C. YEPEZ

Department of Medicine, Cardiothoracic Institute,
2 Beaumont Street, London, W1N 2DX, England

SUMMARY

The ability of β-adrenoceptor antagonists, with and without intrinsic sympathomimetic activity, and of verapamil to protect the heart against hypoxia-induced damage was investigated. Damage was quantitated in terms of a raised end-diastolic resting tension and creatine phosphokinase (CPK) release. The results indicate that both the d and the l isomers act differently, the l isomers preventing CPK release and the d isomers preventing the increase in resting tension.

INTRODUCTION

The primary event in myocardial infarction is a blockage or obstruction of the major vessels that normally supply a zone of tissue. A decreased blood flow is associated with a diminished rate of delivery of metabolic substrates and of oxygen to the affected area. This almost inevitably results in a variable degree of tissue hypoxia that in turn causes metabolic disturbances in the affected area. The result is a decreased rate of ATP production and a consequent fall in the tissue concentration of high-energy phosphate compounds. Hypoxia, therefore, is defined "as a situation which exists when coronary flow is maintained but the oxygen supply is insufficent to provide enough adenosine triphosphate to meet the prevailing energy requirements" (Williamson *et al.,* 1976). This disturbance in energy production leads to an alteration in the contractile state of the heart, the peak-developed tension being reduced and the end-diastolic tension increasing. Electrolyte shifts (Nayler, Grau, and Slade, 1976) also occur, there being a net gain in tissue Na^+ and Ca^{2+} and a loss of K^+. These changes in electrolyte composition in turn cause electrophysiological disturbances. Finally, structural lesions occur, especially in the mitochondria, plasma membranes, and contractile proteins (Figure 1). These structural lesions result in the appearance of various intracellular components, including creatine phosphokinase (CPK), in

These investigations were supported by grants from The British Heart Foundation and The Medical Research Council of Great Britain.

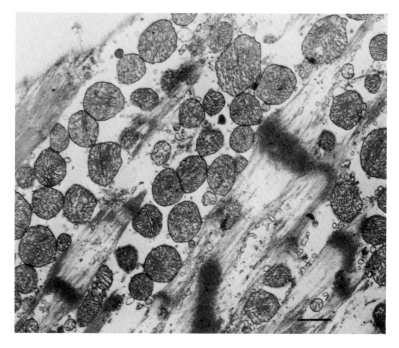

Figure 1. Longitudinal section of rat ventricular muscle perfusion fixed after 30-min perfusion under hypoxic (pO_2 < 6 mm Hg) conditions. Note swollen mitochondria, broken cell membrane and disorganized myofilaments. × 9,000.

the extracellular phase. In the present study we have used two of these parameters of hypoxia-induced damage—1) the rate of release of CPK and 2) the increase in end-diastolic resting tension—to compare, on a quantitative basis, the protection that various pharmacological agents may provide for the hypoxic heart.

MATERIALS AND METHODS

Isolated, Langendorff-perfused rabbit (New Zealand Whites) and guinea pig (Dunken Hartlen strain) hearts were used, as previously described (Nayler, Grau, and Slade, 1976), either as spontaneously beating or as electrically paced preparations. The experiments were performed at 37°C, and all of the hearts were perfused initially with Krebs-Henseleit buffer solution aerated with 95% O_2/5% CO_2. These conditions provide pO_2 values > 600 mm Hg. Developed tension was recorded by attaching a strain gauge to the apex of the left ventricle, the output from the strain gauge then being displayed on a Devices Multichannel recorder. Coronary flow was collected by timed collection and its CPK activity

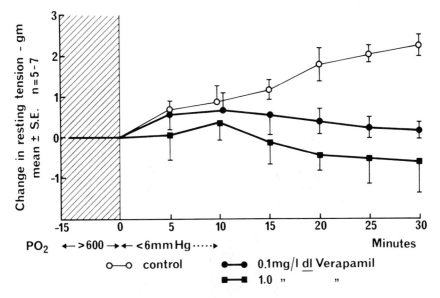

Figure 2. Effect of 0.1 and 1.0 mg/l *dl*-verapamil on the hypoxia-induced (pO$_2$ < 6 mm Hg) increase in end-diastolic resting tension. Each point is mean ± S.E.M. of five to seven experiments. Hypoxic perfusion was started at time zero.

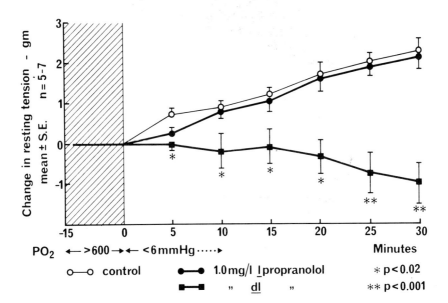

Figure 3. Effect of *dl*- and *l*-propranolol on the hypoxia-induced increase in end-diastolic resting tension. Hypoxic perfusion was started at time zero.

assayed spectrophotometrically (Nayler and Seabra-Gomes, 1976). Hypoxia was introduced, when required, by bubbling with 95% N_2/5% CO_2. This provided a pO_2 < 6 mm Hg.

RESULTS AND DISCUSSION

Figure 2 shows that the perfusion of isolated guinea pig hearts with hypoxic Krebs-Henseleit solution results in a steady increase in end-diastolic resting tension. This increase in end-diastolic tension could be prevented either by omitting Ca^{2+} from the extracellular phase or by adding the Ca^{2+}-antagonist drug, verapamil (Figure 2). This protective effect of verapamil appeared to be dose-dependent (Figure 2) and the *d* and *l* isomers were equipotent.

Figure 3 shows that *dl*-propranolol, which is a *β*-antagonist, also was effective in preventing hypoxia from causing a raised end-diastolic resting tension. *l*-Propranol (Figure 3), however, was not active, indicating perhaps that it was not

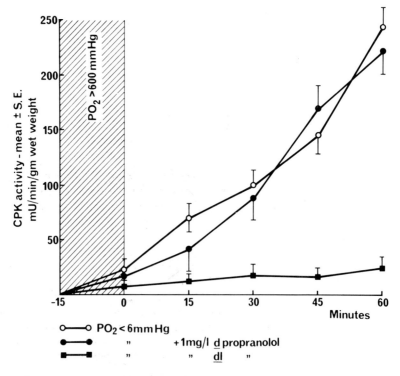

Figure 4. Effect of *d*- and of *dl*-propranolol on the hypoxia-induced release of CPK. Note that hypoxic perfusion was started at zero time. Each point is mean ± S.E.M. of six separate experiments.

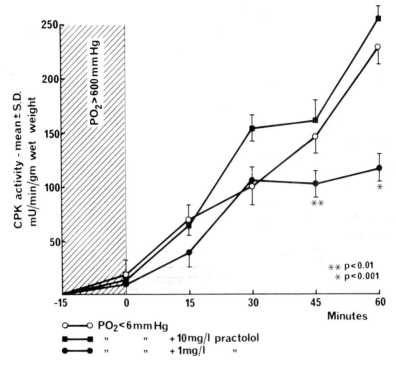

Figure 5. Effect of 1 mg/liter and 10 mg/liter of practolol on the release of CPK. Each point is the mean ± S.E.M. of six separate experiments in which the hypoxic perfusion was started at zero time.

the β-blocking activity of the *dl* racemer that was providing the protection. Subsequent studies confirmed that it was the *d* isomer that was the active component of the racemic mixture.

Hypoxia-Induced Release of CPK

Whereas it is the *d* isomer of propranolol (Figure 3) that prevents the hypoxic muscle from developing a raised end-diastolic resting tension, the data in Figure 4 show that the *d* isomer does not prevent the hypoxic muscle from releasing CPK. Similar results were obtained when the separate racemers of verapamil were used, i.e., the *d* isomer of verapamil failed to prevent the hypoxic muscle from releasing CPK, whereas the *l* isomer was effective.

Not all β-adrenoceptor antagonists are effective in preventing CPK release under these conditions. Thus, the results that are given in Figure 5 show that *dl*-practolol, a β-antagonist that has intrinsic sympathomimetic activity, can exacerbate the release.

In conclusion, we have shown that some, but not all, β-adrenoceptor antagonists can protect the hypoxic myocardium, and that both the *d* and the *l* isomers may be involved. β-Adrenoceptor antagonists that have intrinsic sympathomimetic activity may cause an exacerbation of the hypoxia-induced damage. *dl*-Verapamil, like *dl*-propranolol provides some protection, and, as with propranolol, both the *d* and the *l* isomers seem to be involved.

REFERENCES

NAYLER, W. G., GRAU, A., and SLADE, A. 1976. A protective effect of verapamil on hypoxic heart muscle. Cardiovasc. Res. 10:650–662.

NAYLER, W. G., and SEABRA-GOMES, R. 1976. The effect of methylpredisolone on hypoxic heart muscle. Cardiovasc. Res. 10:349–358.

WILLIAMSON, J. R., SCHAFFER, S. W., FORD, C., and SAFER, B. 1976. Contribution of tissue acidosis to ischemic injury in the perfused rat heart. Circulation 53:3, Suppl. 1:3–14.

Mailing address:
W. G. Nayler, D.Sc.,
Cardiothoracic Institute,
2 Beaumont Street, London W1N 2DX (England).

Recent Advances in Studies on
Cardiac Structure and Metabolism, Volume 12
Cardiac Adaptation
Edited by T. Kobayashi, Y. Ito, and G. Rona
Copyright 1978 University Park Press Baltimore

THE EFFECT OF NITROGLYCERIN, DIPYRIDAMOLE, AND PROPRANOLOL ON GLYCOGEN METABOLISM DURING CORONARY ARTERY LIGATION IN DOGS

K. ICHIHARA and Y. ABIKO

Department of Pharmacology, Asahikawa Medical College,
Asahikawa, Japan

SUMMARY

Ligation of one of the small branches of the canine left anterior descending coronary artery produced a typical anaerobic response in the region of myocardium that had been perfused by the ligated artery; the myocardial glycogen and phosphocreatine levels decreased, and the myocardial phosphorylase activity increased after coronary artery ligation. Pretreatment of the dogs with nitroglycerin or propranolol prevented or diminished the typical anaerobic response of the myocardium to coronary artery ligation, but the pretreatment with dipyridamole did not.

INTRODUCTION

It is generally accepted that myocardial ischemia causes the acceleration of glycogenolysis and the accumulation of intermediates of glycolysis in the myocardium. We have demonstrated in a previous study (Ichihara and Abiko, 1975) that coronary artery ligation produces acceleration of glycogenolysis and elevation of phosphorylase activity in the region of myocardium that has been perfused by the ligated artery. We also have shown that the metabolic response to coronary artery ligation of the endocardial layers is more marked than that of the epicardial layers.

In the present study, we investigated the effect of pretreatment with nitroglycerin, dipyridamole, or propranolol on the acceleration of anaerobic metabolism being caused by coronary artery ligation. Because the endocardial layers are vulnerable to ischemia (Moir, 1972) and tend to proceed to glycogenolysis in response to ischemia more rapidly than the epicardial layers (Ichihara and Abiko, 1975), the effect of pretreatment with the drugs on endocardial metabolism was compared with that on epicardial metabolism.

531

MATERIALS AND METHODS

Mongrel dogs of either sex were anesthetized with pentobarbital sodium (30 mg/kg, I.V.). Under artificial respiration, the chest was opened to permit free access to the left ventricular wall. One of the small branches of the left anterior descending coronary artery was isolated and ligated with a silk thread 5 min after an intravenous injection of saline, nitroglycerin (20 μg/kg), dipyridamole (250 μg/kg), or propranolol (1 mg/kg). Immediately before, or 1.5, 3, 7, or 30 min after, coronary artery ligation, the ischemic region that had been perfused by the ligated artery was rapidly removed with scissors and immediately pressed and frozen with freezing clamps chilled with liquid nitrogen. Thus prepared, the pressed and frozen myocardium was cracked into fragments with a chisel chilled with liquid nitrogen so that the fragments originating in the endocardial and epicardial layers could be collected separately. Each of the endo- and epicardial frozen tissue samples (fragments) was analyzed for determination of glycogen (Seifter *et al.*, 1950), lactate (Barker and Summerson, 1941), glucose-6-phosphate (G-6-P), adenosine triphosphate (ATP), and phosphocreatine (PCr) (Bergmeyer, 1974), and phosphorylase activity (Cornblath *et al.*, 1963). Details of the analytical methods have been described elsewhere (Ichihara and Abiko, 1975).

RESULTS

Dogs were divided into four groups: saline-pretreated (control), nitroglycerin-pretreated, dipyridamole-pretreated, and propranolol-pretreated. Each group was further divided into five subgroups according to the time when the heart was removed: 1) the subgroup in which the heart was removed immediately before coronary ligation, 2) the subgroup in which the heart was removed 1.5 min after coronary ligation, 3) the subgroup in which the heart was removed 3 min after coronary ligation, 4) the subgroup in which the heart was removed 7 min after coronary ligation, and 5) the subgroup in which the heart was removed 30 min after coronary ligation. Each of the five subgroups consisted of six to eight dogs.

Glycogen Content

The myocardial glycogen content decreased maximally 3 min after coronary artery ligation in control dogs. The endo- and epicardial glycogen contents in the myocardium removed before and 3 min after coronary artery ligation are illustrated in Figure 1.

In control dogs, the endocardial glycogen decreased from 11.04 ± 0.75 (mean ± S.E.M.) to 7.63 ± 0.46 mg/g wet tissue ($p < 0.01$), and the epicardial glycogen decreased from 9.24 ± 0.60 to 6.81 ± 0.48 mg/g wet tissue ($p < 0.01$) after 3 min of coronary artery ligation. In dogs pretreated with nitroglycerin or

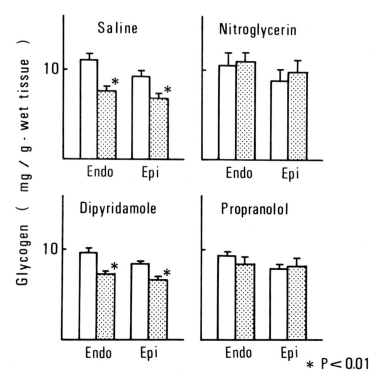

Figure 1. The endocardial (Endo) and epicardial (Epi) glycogen contents before (empty columns) and 3 min after (stippled columns) coronary artery ligation, in saline-pretreated (control), nitroglycerin-pretreated, dipyridamole-pretreated, and propranolol-pretreated dogs. Each column represents the mean ± S.E.M. (brackets).

propranolol, however, the endo- and epicardial glycogen did not change even after 3 min of coronary artery ligation. In dogs pretreated with dipyridamole, the endo- and epicardial glycogen decreased after coronary artery ligation as in control dogs.

Phosphorylase Activity

In control dogs, the activity of phosphorylase *a* increased markedly within 3 min after coronary artery ligation. Increase in the activity of phosphorylase *a* caused by coronary artery ligation corresponded closely to a decrease in myocardial glycogen. In dogs pretreated with nitroglycerin or propranolol, however, coronary artery ligation did not increase the activity of phosphorylase *a* within 30 min of coronary artery ligation. In dogs pretreated with dipyridamole, coronary artery ligation increased the activity of phosphorylase *a* to a small extent.

G-6-P and Lactate Content

Immediately after coronary artery ligation, both G-6-P and lactate contents increased markedly (especially in the endocardial layers) in control and dipyridamole-pretreated dogs. In dogs pretreated with nitroglycerin, however, both G-6-P and lactate contents did not increase markedly, even after coronary artery ligation. In dogs pretreated with propranolol, both G-6-P and lactate contents increased slightly after coronary artery ligation.

ATP and PCr Content

The content of ATP did not change appreciably in all the experiments, regardless of coronary artery ligation and/or pretreatment with nitroglycerin, dipyridamole, or propranolol, with the exception of a relatively low content of ATP in the myocardium removed 1.5 min after coronary artery ligation in dipyridamole-pretreated dogs. A marked decrease in the PCr content in the myocardium (especially in the endocardial layers) was observed after coronary artery ligation in control dogs and in dogs pretreated with dipyridamole. In dogs pretreated with nitroglycerin or propranolol, however, the PCr content did not change as markedly.

DISCUSSION

It was demonstrated in the present study that propranolol completely inhibited the decrease in myocardial glycogen and the increase in phosphorylase activity being caused by coronary artery ligation. The above results indicate that the breakdown of myocardial glycogen following coronary artery ligation is caused by stimulation of β-adrenergic receptors in the heart. According to Wollenberger, myocardial hypoxia or ischemia produces a release of catecholamines from the heart (Wollenberger and Shahab, 1965). Consequently, it is possible to assume that catecholamine release occurs following coronary artery ligation to activate phosphorylase and to accelerate the breakdown of glycogen.

The effect of pretreatment with nitroglycerin was very similar to that with propranolol in terms of the breakdown of glycogen and the activation of phosphorylase caused by coronary artery ligation. Because nitroglycerin is not considered to inhibit β-adrenergic receptors, the mechanism of action of nitroglycerin on the myocardial metabolism is probably different from that of propranolol.

Dipyridamole increases coronary blood flow markedly. Therefore, we assumed that dipyridamole could influence myocardial metabolism. However, it was not possible to demonstrate the action of dipyridamole on myocardial metabolism in terms of the breakdown of glycogen and the activation of phosphorylase following coronary artery ligation. The endocardial glycogenolysis after coronary artery ligation was more rapid and marked than the epicardial glycogenolysis, even in the presence of dipyridamole.

It is concluded that nitroglycerin, as well as propranolol, inhibits glycogenolysis and the activation of phosphorylase following coronary artery ligation, but that dipyridamole does not.

REFERENCES

BARKER, S. B., and SUMMERSON, W. H. 1941. The colorimetric determination of lactate acid in biological material. J. Biol. Chem. 138:535–554.

BERGMEYER, H. U. (ed.). 1974. Methods of Enzymatic Analysis, pp. 1238–1242 (G6P), pp. 1777–1781 (PCr), pp. 2101–2110 (ATP). Academic Press, New York.

CORNBLATH, M., RANDLE, P. J., PARMEGGIANI, A., and MORGAN, H. E. 1963. Regulation of glycogenolysis in muscle: Effects of glucagon and anoxia on lactic production, glycogen content, and phosphorylase activity in the perfused isolated rat hearts. J. Biol. Chem. 238:1592–1597.

ICHIHARA, K., and ABIKO, Y. 1975. Difference between endocardial and epicardial utilization of glycogen in the ischemic heart. Am. J. Physiol. 229:1585–1589.

MOIR, T. W. 1972. Subendocardial distribution of coronary blood flow and the effect of antianginal drugs. Circ. Res. 30:621–627.

SEIFTER, S., DAYTON, S., NOVIC, B., and MUNTWYLER, E. 1950. The estimation of glycogen with the anthrone reagent. Arch. Biochem. Biophys. 25:191–200.

WOLLENBERGER, A., and SHAHAB, L. 1965. Anoxia-induced release of noradrenaline from the isolated perfused heart. Nature 207:88–89.

Mailing address:
Kazuo Ichihara, Ph.D.,
Department of Pharmacology, Asahikawa Medical College,
Asahikawa 078-11 (Japan).

Recent Advances in Studies on
Cardiac Structure and Metabolism, Volume 12
Cardiac Adaptation
Edited by T. Kobayashi, Y. Ito, and G. Rona
Copyright 1978 University Park Press Baltimore

STUDIES ON EXPERIMENTAL CORONARY INSUFFICIENCY. I: EFFECTS OF A PHYSIOLOGICAL DOSE OF ADRENALINE AND NORADRENALINE ON MYOCARDIAL METABOLISM IN DOGS WITH GRADED CORONARY CONSTRICTION

O. IIMURA, C. WAKABAYASHI, T. KOBAYASHI, and M. MIYAHARA

Second Department of Internal Medicine,
Sapporo Medical College, Sapporo, Japan

SUMMARY

To investigate the mechanism by which catecholamines produce myocardial ischemia, the effect of intracoronary-administered adrenaline and noradrenaline was studied in dogs with graded coronary constriction. A physiological dose of catecholamines was favorable for augmentation or improvement of myocardial metabolism and cardiac function in dogs without or with slight coronary constriction. However, in dogs with moderate or severe coronary constriction, similar doses of catecholamines produced myocardial ischemia and cardiac dysfunction.

INTRODUCTION

In our previous studies (Miyahara, 1969; Iimura and Miyahara, 1971), it was revealed that intravenous infusion of catecholamines (CA), in doses corresponding to amounts of endogenous release during anginal attack or immediately after Master's exercise test, results in ischemic changes of ECG, in most cases, and in cardiac pain in about one-third of the patients with angina pectoris. In contrast no such changes occur in normal subjects. A significantly greater increase of cardiac effort index (Katz and Feinberg, 1958), calculated as an index of cardiac work, also was found in patients with angina pectoris as compared to that in normal subjects. On the other hand, following the administration of angiotensin-II, ischemic changes were seldom observed in patients with marked elevations of this index.

From these findings, it was suggested that a physiological dose of CA could be a trigger to the precipitation of anginal attack in patients, by way of more marked increase of cardiac work and, possibly, by augmentation of myocardial metabolism. Therefore, the present investigation was undertaken to elucidate the

effects of intracoronary-administered CA on cardiac hemodynamics and myocardial metabolism in dogs with graded constriction of the coronary artery.

MATERIALS AND METHODS

In anesthetized open-chest dogs, a Griggs type autoperfusing cannula (Griggs *et
al.,* 1968) was introduced into the left main coronary artery through the
brachiocephalic artery and aorta. The tip of the cannula was secured by ligation
around the orifice of the left main coronary artery. A polyethylene catheter was
placed from the coronary sinus to the left subclavian vein via the right atrium. A
short tube and another catheter were introduced into the left ventricle through
the apical ventricular wall and into the left femoral artery, respectively (Figure
1). Observations were begun 20 min after completion of the animal preparation,
and the extracorporeal loop of the autoperfused circuit was gradually tightened
to reduce the coronary blood flow (CBF) to a desired level.

The animals were divided into four groups according to the degree of CBF
reduction; that is, Grade 0, no reduction; Grade I, reduction less than 25%;
Grade II, between 26–49%; Grade III, more than 50% of the control value. The
hemodynamic and metabolic determinations were made before and after reduction of CBF and following the intracoronary administration of 0.2 μg/kg/min of
adrenaline (Ad) or 0.4 μg/kg/min of noradrenaline (NA) for 5 min by a constant
perfusion pump. These administration doses were twice as much as those used in
the clinical experiment mentioned above.

RESULTS

As shown in Figure 2, coronary constriction produced ST depression in the
electrocardiogram in Grades II and III. Following the intracoronary administration of Ad or NA, a moderate ST depression occurred in Grade II, and an
elevation of depressed ST occurred in Grade III. However, there were no clearly
notable changes in Grades 0 and I, except a slight ST depression following Ad in
Grade I.

Mean coronary blood pressure (m-CBP) was reduced proportionate to the
degree of coronary constriction, while both the intracoronary-administered Ad
and NA did not significantly affect m-CBP in any group. A reduction of
coronary vascular resistance (CVR) after Ad and NA was observed; the reduction
was particularly remarkable in Grades 0 and I after NA. CA produced an increase
of CBF in Grades 0 to II, where the effect of NA on CBF was more marked than
that of Ad, while no increase was observed after either Ad or NA in Grade III.

The first derivative of left ventricular pressure, dP/dt_{max}, was clearly increased by NA and moderately increased by Ad. However, in Grade III it was
moderately decreased by Ad and, on the average, not changed by NA. Left

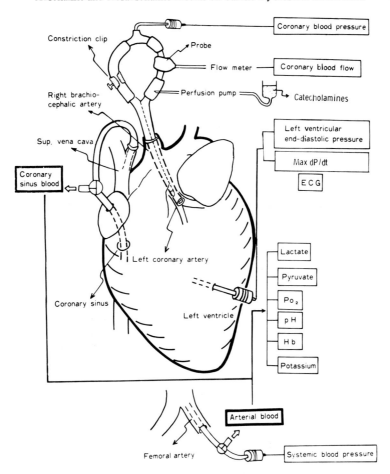

Figure 1. Schematic representation of the experimental preparation. Hemodynamic parameters and lead II of ECG were simultaneously and continuously recorded on a multichannel recorder (RM 85, Nihonkoden Co., Ltd., Tokyo, Japan). The oxygen saturation level and pH were determined by a gas electrode method (Radiometer Blood Gas Analyzer, BM 5-3-MK 2, Denmark Radiometer Co., Ltd., Denmark). Lactate and pyruvate concentration in arterial and coronary sinus blood were measured by the enzymatic method (Marbach and Weil, 1967.)

ventricular end-diastolic pressure (LVEDP) was slightly lowered by Ad in Grades 0 and I, and by NA in Grades 0 to II. In Grade III, constriction itself produced a moderate elevation of LVEDP, and both Ad and NA markedly elevated the end-diastolic pressure.

On the other hand, changes in myocardial oxygen consumption (MVO_2) by coronary constriction and following the administration of Ad and NA were quite similar to those in CBF. Both the arterio-coronary sinus difference of lactate (Δ

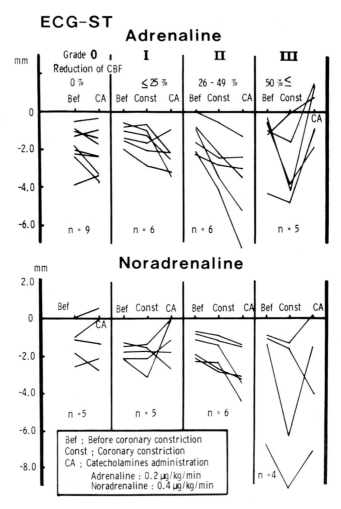

Figure 2. The effect of graded coronary blood flow reduction and the intracoronary infusion of adrenaline and noradrenaline on electrocardiographic ST segments in four groups. Changes of ST segment are measured in lead II of ECG.

lactate) and the myocardial extraction rate of lactate were decreased slightly in Grade II and moderately in Grade III after coronary constriction. They were slightly increased following Ad and NA in Grade 0, while slightly decreased in Grade II and markedly decreased in Grade III. Thus, in Grade III, lactate production was clearly found following the infusion of CA. The decreasing effects of Ad on Δlactate and on the extraction rate were significantly greater than those of NA. Lactate-pyruvate ratio in coronary sinus blood (L/P_{cs}) was not affected by coronary constriction and by CA in Grades 0 to II, while it was elevated significantly by both Ad and NA in Grade III. The arterio-coronary

Effect of Adrenaline and Noradrenaline (Summary— I)

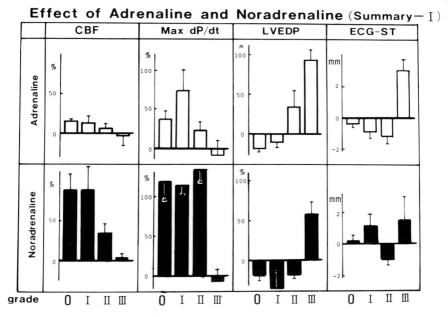

Figure 3. The effect of intracoronary-administered adrenaline (0.2 μg/kg/min) and nor-adrenaline (0.4 μg/kg/min) on coronary blood flow (CBF), dP/dt$_{max}$, and left ventricular end-diastolic pressure (LVEDP), expressed as the percent change of the value before the infusion, and on ECG-ST in mm.

sinus difference of potassium (ΔK) was increased by Ad and NA in Grades 0 to II. In Grade III, coronary constriction and CA produced a marked loss of potassium from the myocardium.

DISCUSSION

As shown in Figures 3 and 4, which summarize the effects of Ad and NA on the cardiac hemodynamics and the myocardial metabolism in dogs with graded coronary constriction, an augmentation of cardiac function and myocardial metabolism by Ad and NA in Grades 0 and I was observed. However, in Grade II, less of an increase of CBF by NA and a decrease of Δlactate and a slight elevation of L/P$_{cs}$ and of LVEDP by Ad, with moderate depression of ECG-ST, were noted. In Grade III, significant elevations of LVEDP and ST, remarkable lactate production, an increase of L/P$_{cs}$, potassium loss, and any significant changes in CBF and dP/dt$_{max}$ were observed following the administration of Ad and NA.

From these findings, it is suggested that, although a physiological dose of CA augments or improves the cardiac function and myocardial metabolism in dogs without or with slight coronary constriction, similar doses of CA produce myocardial ischemia with cardiac dysfunction in dogs with moderate or severe

Effect of Adrenaline and Noradrenaline (Summary — II)

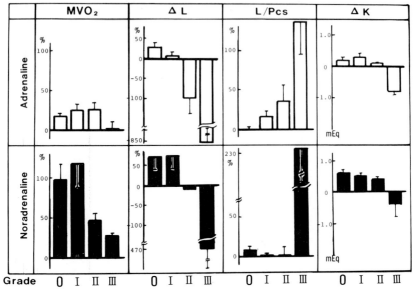

Figure 4. The effect of intracoronary-administered adrenaline and noradrenaline on myocardial oxygen consumption (MVO_2), arterio-coronary sinus difference of lactate (Δ lactate), and lactate-pyruvate ratio in coronary sinus blood (L/P_{cs}), expressed as the percent change of the value before the infusion, and on arterio-coronary sinus difference of potassium (Δ K) expressed as mEq/liter.

coronary constriction. This study supports the clinical findings reported previously and indicates the role of the activity of the sympathetic nervous system in the pathogenesis of angina pectoris.

REFERENCES

GRIGGS, D. M., JR., NAKAMURA, Y., LEUNISSEN, R. L. A., NAGANO, S., and LIPANA, J. G. 1968. Auto-perfused cannula to facilitate measurement of coronary flow. Med. Res. Eng. 7:30–33.

IIMURA, O., and MIYAHARA, M. 1971. Ischemic heart disease and catecholamines. Jpn. Circ. J. 35:973–978.

KATZ, L. N., and FEINBERG, H. 1958. The relation of cardiac effort to myocardial oxygen consumption and coronary flow. Circ. Res. 6:656–669.

MARBACH, E. P., and WEIL, M. H. 1967. Rapid enzymatic measurement of blood lactate and pyruvate. Use and significance of metaphosphoric acid as a common precipitant. Clin. Chem. 13:314–325.

MIYAHARA, M. 1969. A role of sympathoadrenal system in pathogenesis of ischemic heart disease. Acta Cardiol. 13(suppl.):174–184.

Mailing address:
O. Iimura, M.D.,
Second Department of Internal Medicine,
Sapporo Medical College, S-1, W-16, Sapporo (Japan).

Recent Advances in Studies on
Cardiac Structure and Metabolism, Volume 12
Cardiac Adaptation
Edited by T. Kobayashi, Y. Ito, and G. Rona
Copyright 1978 University Park Press Baltimore

STUDIES ON EXPERIMENTAL CORONARY INSUFFICIENCY. II: EFFECTS OF β-ADRENERGIC BLOCKING AGENT (PROPRANOLOL) ON METABOLIC RESPONSE TO ADRENALINE AND NORADRENALINE IN DOGS WITH CORONARY CONSTRICTION

O. IIMURA, C. WAKABAYASHI, T. KOBAYASHI,
T. SHOJI, S. YOSHIDA, and M. MIYAHARA

Second Department of Internal Medicine,
Sapporo Medical College, Sapporo, Japan

SUMMARY

To obtain further information on the mechanism by which catecholamines produce myocardial ischemia, the effects of propranolol on metabolic and mechanical responses to adrenaline or noradrenaline were investigated in coronary-constricted dogs. Propranolol suppressed the myocardial ischemia produced by noradrenaline and adrenaline in dogs with moderate coronary constriction.

INTRODUCTION

In the study reported in the preceding chapter, it was reported that the intracoronary administration of a small dose of catecholamines (CA) results in myocardial ischemia in dogs with moderate or severe coronary constriction (Iimura *et al.,* 1977). In this study, to gain a better understanding of the mechanism by which CA induces myocardial ischemia, the effect of β-adrenergic blocking agent on metabolic and mechanical responses to intracoronary administered CA was investigated in dogs with moderate coronary constriction.

MATERIALS AND METHODS

In anesthetized open-chest dogs, the left main coronary artery was cannulated with a Griggs type autoperfusing cannula (Griggs *et al.,* 1968). Propranolol, 0.2 mg/kg, was injected intravenously about 20 min after completion of the animal preparation, which has been described in detail in the preceding chapter. Beginning 10 min after the injection of propranolol, the extracorporeal loop of the autoperfused circuit was gradually tightened to reduce the coronary blood flow (CBF) to a desired level. Only dogs with CBF reduction between 26 and 49% of the control value before constriction, as moderately coronary-constricted animals, were used in this experiment. The intracoronary infusion of 0.2 μg/kg/min of adrenaline (Ad) or 0.4 μg/kg/min of noradrenaline (NA) was begun 10 min after coronary constriction. The infusion was continued for 5 min.

RESULTS

Effects of Propranolol on Cardiac Function and Myocardial Metabolism in Open-chest Dogs without Coronary Constriction (20 cases)

Ten minutes after propranolol, heart rate was significantly reduced from 133 ± 5 to 107 ± 3 beats/min, $p < 0.001$, and dP/dt_{max} was significantly reduced from 2587 ± 176 to 1938 ± 128 mm Hg/sec, $p < 0.01$, while other hemodynamic and metabolic parameters were not significantly changed.

Effects of Propranolol on Responses to CA in Dogs without Coronary Constriction

Propranolol significantly suppressed: 1) increases of CBF, $p < 0.05$, and myocardial oxygen consumption (MVO$_2$), $p < 0.05$, by NA, 2) decreases of coronary

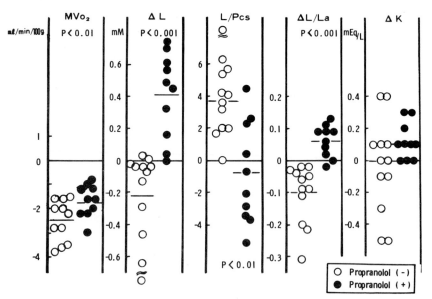

Figure 1. The individual changes in myocardial oxygen consumption (MVO$_2$), arterio-coronary sinus difference of lactate (ΔL), lactate-pyruvate ratio in coronary sinus blood (L/P$_{cs}$), lactate extraction rate (ΔL/La), and arterio-coronary difference of potassium (ΔK) by the coronary constriction which reduced coronary blood flow between 26 and 49% of the control value.

vascular resistance (CVR), $p < 0.01$, by both Ad (5 cases; control, 9 cases) and NA (5 cases; control, 5 cases), and left ventricular end-diastolic pressure (LVEDP), $p < 0.05$ in Ad and $p < 0.02$ in NA, and 3) an increase of dP/dt_{max}, $p < 0.05$ in Ad and $p < 0.02$ in NA, by both Ad and NA. Although there was no statistical difference, propranolol slightly augmented the increase of the arterio-coronary sinus difference of lactate (Δlactate) and the myocardial extraction rate of lactate by Ad.

Effects of Propranolol on Responses to Coronary Constriction

On the average, propranolol significantly contributed to a decrease of heart rate. A tendency was also observed to counteract the effect of coronary constriction that was manifested in the depression of ECG-ST and a slight elevation of LVEDP. As shown in Figure 1, propranolol partially inhibited a decrease of

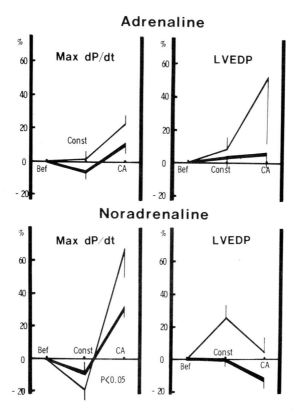

Figure 2. The effect of propranolol (0.2 mg/kg) on the changes of dP/dt_{max} and on left ventricular end-diastolic pressure (LVEDP) following intracoronary infusion of adrenaline and noradrenaline in coronary-constricted dogs. Bef = before coronary constriction; Const = coronary constriction; Ad = adrenaline (0.2 μg/kg/min); NA = noradrenaline (0.4 μg/kg/min); —— = propranolol pretreatment (–)); —— = propranolol pretreatment (+).

MVO$_2$ by coronary constriction. Furthermore, it was particularly interesting to note that increases of both Δlactate and the lactate extraction rate and a decrease of lactate-pyruvate ratio in coronary sinus blood (L/P$_{cs}$) were observed in dogs with propranolol pretreatment (10 cases), in contrast to decreases of the former and an increase of the latter in dogs without propranolol (12 cases).

Effects of Propranolol on Responses to CA in Dogs with Coronary Constriction

In dogs with coronary constriction, propranolol counteracted a decrease of CVR and depressions of ST by both Ad (5 cases; control, 6 cases) and NA (5 cases; control, 6 cases), and counteracted an increase of MVO$_2$, where $p < 0.05$, in all cases. The ST depression following Ad was almost completely inhibited by the pretreatment of propranolol.

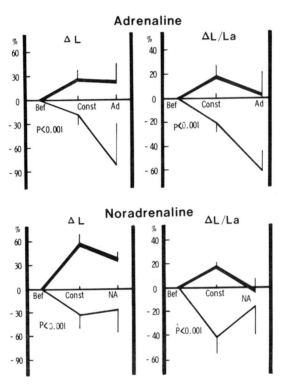

Figure 3. The effect of propranolol (0.2 mg/kg) on the changes of arterio-coronary sinus difference of lactate (ΔL) and on lactate extraction rate (ΔL/L$_a$) following intracoronary infusion of adrenaline and noradrenaline in coronary-constricted dogs. Bef = before coronary constriction; Const = coronary constriction; Ad = adrenaline (0.2 μg/kg/min); NA = noradrenaline (0.4 μg/kg/min); —— = propranolol pretreatment (–); —— ˈ= propranolol pretreatment (+).

Propranolol also suppressed an increase of dP/dt_{max} by NA, while it did not affect that by Ad. The values of LVEDP in the animals with propranolol were always lower than those in the dogs without this drug (Figure 2).

On the other hand, propranolol showed a tendency to suppress the decrease of both Δlactate and the lactate extraction rate by Ad, and to change both from a decrease to an increase by NA, on the average (Figure 3), while the drug did not clearly have an effect on L/P_{cs} and on arterio-coronary sinus difference of potassium in these experimental animals.

DISCUSSION

Initially in this investigation, clearly suppressing effects of propranolol on decreases of Δlactate, the lactate extraction rate, and MVO_2, and on an increase of L/P_{cs} by the coronary constriction were observed. These results might support the use of propranolol for the pretreatment of acute coronary insufficiency.

On the other hand, this drug inhibited decreases of Δlactate and the lactate extraction rate, an increase of L/P_{cs}, a depression of ECG-ST following Ad, and increases of dP/dt_{max} and MVO_2 following NA in the coronary-constricted animals.

Thus, it is suggested that propranolol mainly suppressed each augmentation of myocardial metabolism by Ad and of cardiac function by NA, indicating that propranolol can protect or improve the ischemic changes produced by CA, at least, in dogs with moderate coronary constriction.

REFERENCES

GRIGGS, D. M., JR., NAKAMURA, Y., LEUNISSEN, R. L. A., NAGANO, S., and LIPANA, J. G. 1968. Auto-perfused cannula to facilitate measurement of coronary flow. Med. Res. Eng. 7:30–33.

IIMURA, O., WAKABAYASHI, T., KOBAYASHI, T., and MIYAHARA, M. 1977. Studies on experimental coronary insufficiency. I: Effect of a physiological dose of adrenaline and noradrenaline on myocardial metabolism in dogs with graded coronary constriction. Preceding chapter in this volume.

Mailing address:
O. Iimura, M.D.,
Second Department of Internal Medicine,
Sapporo Medical College, S-1, W-16, Sapporo (Japan).

Recent Advances in Studies on
Cardiac Structure and Metabolism, Volume 12
Cardiac Adaptation
Edited by T. Kobayashi, Y. Ito, and G. Rona
Copyright 1978 University Park Press Baltimore

VIABILITY AND HISTOPATHOLOGY OF ELEVEN FRESH, ANTIBIOTIC-TREATED ALLOGRAFTS REMOVED THREE WEEKS TO THREE YEARS AFTER IMPLANTATION

N. AL-JANABI,[1] H. E. OLSON,[2] T. AMMERANTE,[2] and D. N. ROSS[2]

[1] School of Medicine,
Al-Mustansiriyah University,
Baghdad, Iraq
[2] The National Heart Hospital and
Cardiothoracic Institute,
University of London,
London, England

SUMMARY

Changes in metabolic activity of removed heart valve allografts have been measured. The fresh heart valves were sterilized and stored in antibiotic solution before implantation in patients. Viability was determined before insertion and after removal from patients by two methods: 1) tissue culture, and 2) autoradiography, using tritiated thymidine. The length of storage in the Hank's antibiotic or nutrient-antibiotic medium before insertion did not seem to influence the final metabolic activity nor the structural integrity of the allografts when they were removed.

Results from the present study show that the most severe degenerative changes occur in valves stored in Hank's solution and then implanted in the mitral position. The viability percentage declined progressively during the time that a valve treated in this manner was functioning in a patient.

INTRODUCTION

There has been a steady utilization of aortic valve homografts (allografts) over the past 12 years (Ross, 1962, 1964; Barratt-Boyes, 1964; Angell *et al.,* 1968).

Allograft valves have been collected during routine autopsies under clean but nonsterile conditions within 48 hours of the donor's death. They subsequently have been treated with Hank's antibiotic nutrient-antibiotic solution before implantation. These valves have been found to be satisfactory clinical substitutes (Karp and Kirklin, 1969; Barratt-Boyes, 1971). It is assumed that these valves retain donor-viable fibroblasts that are able to continue to function and service the collagen matrix after implantation in the recipient and that they can ensure long-term function.

By using an autoradiographic technique, it has been shown that valves sterilized in antibiotics remain viable for varying periods of time, that is, their living (metabolically active) fibroblasts are capable of synthesizing both deoxyribonucleic acid (Al-Janabi *et al.*, 1972) and protein (Al-Janabi *et al.*, 1973). Preservation of these two metabolic systems provides a possible means of self-repair of the valve structure and offers the prospect of a permanent replacement. The viability of the fibroblasts has been further enhanced by storing the valves in a nutrient-antibiotic solution instead of Hank's balanced salt-antibiotics solution (Al-Janabi and Ross, 1973).

The purpose of this study was to compare the viability and the structural integrity of the allograft valves at the time of implantation and after removal from the recipient, at intervals ranging from 23 to 1,001 days.

MATERIALS AND METHODS

From 1970 to 1975, approximately 500 fresh, human, aortic valve allografts treated with antibiotic solution were studied. Each had been removed under clean but nonsterile conditions during routine autopsies performed within 48 hours of a donor's death. The allografts were dissected and histologically investigated, and the percentage of viable cells was determined. They were then sterilized by storage in either Hank's antibiotic solution (1970–1971) or nutrient-antibiotic solution (1972–1975) (Table 1); the storage temperature for both methods was 4°C. Eleven of these grafts subsequently were removed at a second operation at intervals ranging from 23 to 1,001 days after the day that they had been implanted in a recipient.

Table 1. The antibiotic formula

Gentamycin	4mg/ml	1. In Hank's solution[a] (1970–1971)
Methicillin	10mg/ml	
Erythromycin		
Lactobionate	6mg/ml	2. In nutrient medium 199 + 10% calf serum[a]
Nystatin	2,500U/ml	(1972– present time)

[a]Purchased from Wellcome Reagent Ltd., Beckenham, Kentucky.

The excised material from these 11 allograft valves was divided into two groups:

1. Group 1 consisted of seven aortic valves that had been stored in Hank's antibiotic solution ($4°C$) before insertion for periods varying from 10 to 40 days. Five had been inserted in the mitral position and the remaining two in the aortic site.
2. Group 2 consisted of four valves stored in nutrient-antibiotic solution for 10 to 37 days before insertion. All four valves were placed in the aortic position.

The 11 valves were examined macroscopically, and viability studies using tritiated thymidine were carried out before fixing them in 10% formal saline for histological investigation.

RESULTS

Histological and Pathological Data

Group 1 (stored in Hank's antibiotic solution)   The five aortic valves in the mitral position were grouped according to the length of survival in the patient. (See Table 2.) The allografts had been in patients for 93, 272, 553, 658 and 1,001 days, respectively. Histological examination showed preservation of the normal architecture of the valve leaflets (Figure 1) with occasional foci of degeneration of collagen tissue, which were particularly prominent in the valve leaflet that had survived for 685 days. This section also showed a thin covering of fibroblasts on both surfaces of the leaflets (Figure 2). The extent of this covering, however, could not be related to the length of survival in the body. The leaflets that had survived 553 days were thickened and showed partial destruction of normal architecture with foci of calcification.

Group 2 (stored in nutrient-antibiotic solution)   These four valves had remained in the body for 23, 27, 81, and 151 days, respectively. The specimen with the shortest duration showed normal architecture, but with foci of inflammatory cells, including neutrophils at the base. The next two valves showed perforation of one valve leaflet each and vegetations consisting predominantly of fibrin and inflammatory cells, including neutrophils and plasma cells. The appearances were suggestive of infective endocarditis, although no etiological agent could be found. The architecture was preserved in the former but destroyed in the latter.

Viability

Viability of the allografts in Group 1 declined at a faster rate during their time in patients than those of Group 2. However, the decline did not appear to coincide with the time that the valve was functioning in a recipient, except in the case of

Table 2. Details of antibiotic-treated aortic valve allografts

Case no.	Donor Age	Donor Sex	Recipient Age	Recipient Sex	Ster. & pres. storage time days in antibiotic Hank's	Nutrient	Position of homograft Valve	Viability percentage Before insertion	After removal	Days in patient	Cause of removal
1	–	–	38	M	–	12	Ao.	–	35%	23	Dehiscence of valve which had become loose along the whole of the right coronary sinus
2	–	–	41	F	–	10	Ao.	–	–	151	Notes not available
3	29	M	14	M	–	37	Ao.	55	40	27	Perf. 1.5cm in diameter at the base of the right coronary sinus
4	41	M	62	M	–	32	Ao.	60	45	81	Dehiscence of part of right and noncoronary cusps
5	73	F	13	M	35	–	Mit.	60	35	553	Valve prolapse and calcium with three cusps thickened
6	15	M	13	M	40	–	Mit.	60	40	93	Gross mitral regurgitation and dehiscence around valve attachment
7	66	F	27	M	20	–	Ao.	53	46	195	Separation at two sites along the upper suture line of the left coronary sinus
8	–	–	62	F	20	–	Mit.	42	20	272	? Prolapse
9	–	–	62	M	–	–	Ao.	35	20	606	Some prolapse of the noncoronary cusp allowing moderate regurgitation
10	52	M	52	F	10	–	Mit.	45	35	685	Peripheral dehiscence of valve
11	–	–	41	M	–	–	Mit.	Cusp is acellular	35	1001	Homograft was reported competent

Ao = aortic; Mit = mitral.

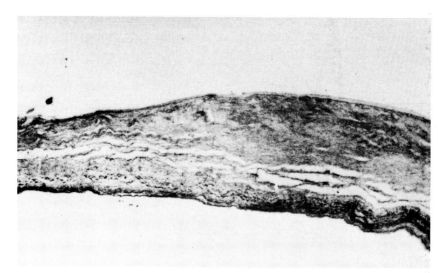

Figure 1. Photomicrograph of part of an aortic valve allograft (homograft; HRI) showing preservation of normal architecture. The elastic component is seen in the lower part of the valve cusp. Elastic van Gieson, × 180.

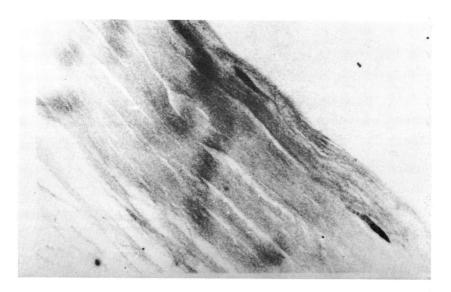

Figure 2. High power view of an aortic valve allograft (homograft), showing a layer of fibroblasts and collagen covering part of the surface of the homograph (HR2). Hematoxylin and eosin, × 580.

the fresh valve implanted for the longest time, which was acellular after 1,001 days. The viability percentage of Group 2 valves declined by 15% in only the two cases for which full information was available; whereas, the decline in viability of those valves in Group 1 varied between 7% and 25%. The allografts placed in the mitral position showed a greater loss of viability than those placed in the aortic position.

DISCUSSION

From the present study of 11 fresh aortic allograft valves (sterilized and stored in antibiotic solution) that had been removed from recipients, much information has been gained about the behavior of donor fibroblasts from the time of collection to the time of implantation and until their subsequent removal. Although tissue culture has been employed in our research laboratory and by other researchers (Mohri *et al.*, 1962; Barratt-Boyes, 1971; Angell, Desaneralle, and Shumway, 1972; Gavin, Herdson, and Barratt-Boyes, 1972) to investigate the presence of living cells in the fresh, antibiotic-treated valves, this method alone cannot determine the percentage of cells remaining viable.

We thus attempted to measure the mitotic index of the donor fibroblast before insertion. This was accomplished by autoradiography with the use of tritiated thymidine. Thymidine is a precursor, or building block, of deoxyribonucleic acid. When labeled with tritium, a radioisotope giving the best autoradiographic resolution, the utilization of thymidine by the viable (mitotically active) cells can be traced (Fitzgerald *et al.*, 1953; Taylor, 1960, 1965). This pyrimidine base is incorporated into the DNA of chromosomes during their replication. This method can be regarded as superior to tissue culture because it quantitatively determines the number of mitotically active nuclei at the time of assessment.

From the study reported here, as well as a previous one (Al-Janabi *et al.*, 1972), it has been shown quantitatively (by autoradiography) and qualitatively (by tissue culture) that valves freshly procured and treated with antibiotics are viable and can be implanted in a viable state, i.e., they have been implanted with metabolically active fibroblasts capable of synthesizing both DNA and protein. The influence of viability on long-term function of the valve is more difficult to establish, although short-term function does not appear to be affected.

The viability and histological changes found in fresh allografts in the present study are somewhat different quantitatively from those changes found in allografts that were chemically sterilized (Hudson, 1966; Smith, 1967; Gavin *et al.*, 1972). In these antibiotic-treated grafts, the number of viable fibroblasts declined progressively during the time that the valve was functioning in the recipient but did not fall to zero. The viability percentage at the time of implantation was approximately 20–30% greater than at the time of removal.

When the allograft was removed, the length of storage before insertion did not seem to influence the final structure of the allograft. Results show that the most severe degenerative changes were noted in valves stored in Hank's solution and then implanted in the mitral position. From the present study it can be concluded that some donor fibroblasts still are present in a normal viable state, as determined by autoradiography at the time of insertion, even after 40 days of storage in the antibiotic solution. The percentage of viability declined progressively during the time the valve was functioning in the patient. The only acellular cusp was found in the case of allograft No. 11, which was removed 1,001 days after insertion. Our findings also suggested that there is less destrruction of the collagen and elastic fibers in fresh, antibiotic-treated allografts than in chemically sterilized ones.

Acknowledgments The authors are grateful to Mr. Ramzi Jasim and R. Parker for their valuable practical assistance. We also wish to thank Miss C. Grimes, F. Kuthair, and N. Abdul Zahra for technical assistance in the preparation of this chapter.

REFERENCES

AL-JANABI, N., GIBSON, K., ROSE, J., and ROSS, D. N. 1973. Protein synthesis in fresh aortic and pulmonary valve allografts as an additional test viability. Cardiovasc. Res. 8:247–250.

AL-JANABI, N., GONZALEZ-LAVIN, L., NEIROTTI, R., and ROSS, D. N. 1972. Viability of fresh aortic valve homografts: A quantitative assessment. Thorax 27:83–86.

AL-JANABI, N., and ROSS, D. N. 1973. Enhanced viability of fresh aortic homografts stored in nutrient medium. Cardiovasc. Res. 8:817–822.

ANGELL, W. W., DESANERALLE, P., and SHUMWAY, N. E. 1972. Progress in cardiovascular diseases.

ANGELL, W. W., STINSON, E. B., IBEN, A. B., and SHUMWAY, N. E. 1968. Multiple valve replacement with fresh aortic homograft. J. Thorac. Cardiovasc. Surg. 56:323–332.

BARRATT-BOYES, B. G. 1964. Homograft aortic valve replacement in aortic incompetence and stenosis. Thorax 19:131–150.

BARRATT-BOYES, B. G. 1971. Long-term follow up of aortic valve grafts. Br. Heart J. 33:60.

FITZGERALD, P. J., SIMMEL, E., WEINSTEIN, J., and MATI, C. 1953. Radiography theory, technique and application. Lab. Invest. 2:181–222.

GAVIN, J. B., HERDSON, P. B., and BARRATT-BOYES, B. G. 1972. The pathology of chemically sterilized human heart valve allografts. Pathology 4:175.

HUDSON, R. E. B. 1966. Pathology of the human aortic valve homografts. Br. Heart J. 28:291.

KARP, R. B., and KIRKLIN, J. W. 1969. Replacement of diseased aortic valve with homografts. Ann. Surg. 169:921–926.

MOHRI, H., REICHENBACH, D. B., BARRES, R. W., and MERENDINO, K. A. 1969. Homologous aortic valve transplantation alterations in viable and nonviable valves. J. Thorac. Cardiovasc. Surg. 56:767.

ROSS, D. N. 1962. Homograft replacement with aortic valve. Lancet 2:487–489.

ROSS, D. N. 1964. Homotransplantation of the aortic valve in subcoronary position. J. Thorac. Cardiovasc. Surg. 47:413.

SMITH, X. 1967. Pathology of human aortic valve homografts. Thorax 22:114–138.

TAYLOR, J. H. 1960. Nucleic acid synthesis in relation to the cell division cycle. Ann. N.Y. Acad. Sci. 90:409–421.

TAYLOR, J. H. 1965. Distribution of tritium labeled DNA among chromosomes during meiosis. J. Cell Biol. 25(Suppl.):57–67.

Mailing address:
Dr. N. Al-Janabi,
School of Medicine, Al-Mustansiriya University
Baghdad—F.O. Box 14132 (Iraq).

REPERFUSION
OF
ISCHEMIC MYOCARDIUM

Recent Advances in Studies on
Cardiac Structure and Metabolism, Volume 12
Cardiac Adaptation
Edited by T. Kobayashi, Y. Ito, and G. Rona
Copyright 1978 University Park Press Baltimore

CORONARY MICROCIRCULATORY FACTORS CARDIAC MUSCLE CELL INJURY

G. RONA, I. HÜTTNER, M. BOUTET, M.-C. BADONNEL

Department of Pathology, McGill University,
Montreal, Quebec, Canada

SUMMARY

Coronary artery ligation with or without reperfusion was carried out in Wistar rats to study the role of coronary microcirculatory factors and membrane permeability alteration of cardiac muscle cell in the evolution of cardiac muscle cell injury by using the fine structural extracellular protein tracer, horseradish peroxidase (HRP). The findings were compared with those obtained in noncoronarogenic myocardial injury models following administration of norepinephrine, a pressor, and isoproterenol, a depressor catecholamine.

Following left coronary artery ligation lasting for 10 and 20 minutes, some of the collaterals in the ischemic zone were perfused by the tracer, but the number of patent capillaries decreased during 60-min ligation. The inhomogeneous involvement of cardiac muscle cells in ischemic injury correlated well with these microcirculatory findings. In comparison to permanent ischemia, an abrupt deterioration of the cardiac muscle cell alteration occurred after reperfusion with influx of HRP into the damaged cells. The binding of tracer to myofilaments was, however, a later event as compared to that seen in the catecholamine models. The latter observation implies that, in addition to microcirculatory factors, direct cardiac muscle cell stimulation should also be considered in the evolution of noncoronarogenic myocardial injury.

INTRODUCTION

Advances in technique for morphological investigations such as electron microscopic histochemistry and autoradiography and, more recently, utilization of fine structural diffusion tracers and freeze-fractured cardiac muscle cell preparations have made possible the acquisition of new information on the underlying biochemical changes and functional correlates of cardiac muscle cell injury. Recently, in addition to *in vivo* models, various *in vitro* preparations such as Langendorff isolated perfused heart and tissue slicing techniques and isolated cell systems have been used. While the latter methods offer advantages over intact heart for studies of cardiac muscle cell reaction to injury, they have, in our view, quite limited scope with respect to allowing inferential deductions for

This work was supported by Canadian Medical Research Council Grant No. MA-3635.

the human condition in which coronary circulatory factors also play a prominent role.

During the past two decades, our research group has investigated myocardial reaction and adaptation to insult by applying various experimental procedures such as catecholamine administration, coronary artery ligation, and hypertensive and toxic injuries. The relevant findings of these studies have been reviewed elsewhere (Rona, 1971). Insults applied in these procedures by interrupting the generation of energy or by depleting metabolic substrates may produce cardiac muscle cell lesion of a biochemical nature and adaptive or reversible retrogressive changes. At some point, which has been termed tentatively "the point of no return," and is regarded as a bioenergetic failure, the ability of the cardiac muscle cell to react to a disequilibrium is exceeded, and the process continues through complex biochemical and subsequent structural changes from degeneration on to necrosis. The biochemical defect responsible for the irreversible loss of cardiac muscle cell function is not clear (Williamson *et al.*, 1976), but certain ultrastructural changes such as peripheral clumping of the nuclear chromatin, myofilament disintegration, loss of sarcoplasmic tubules and peripheral couplings, mitochondrial granular densities, plasma membrane discontinuity, and intrasarcoplasmic fibrin deposition represent some of the signs of irreversible cardiac muscle cell lesion (Rona, 1971). The evolution of cardiac muscle cell injury and the repair processes also are influenced by other variables, in addition to the intensity of the stimulus applied. Furthermore, the chances of recovery of the injured cell depend on the varied participation of the intrasarcoplasmic components in the early stages of cellular alteration observed in various experimental models.

Some of the pertinent ultrastructural changes of cardiac muscle cell following injury have been reviewed in previous meetings of the Study Group (Rona *et al.*, 1970, 1973, and 1975a; Dusek, Boutet, and Rona, 1973). Consequently, we have chosen in this chapter to report our findings concerning the role of coronary microcirculatory factors and membrane permeability alterations of cardiac muscle cell injury produced by coronary artery ligation with or without subsequent myocardial reperfusion. A comparison is made to our previous observations of a noncoronarogenic model, the catecholamine-induced myocardial injury.

MATERIALS AND METHODS

Left coronary artery ligation was carried out by the simplified method of Selye *et al.* (Selye *et al.*, 1960) in male Wistar rats weighing 200–300 g. The effect of reperfusion was studied following ligature lasting for 10, 20, and 60 min with subsequent 10- and 60-min release. Samples taken from the center, the periphery of left ventricular infarct, and from the remote right ventricular myocardium

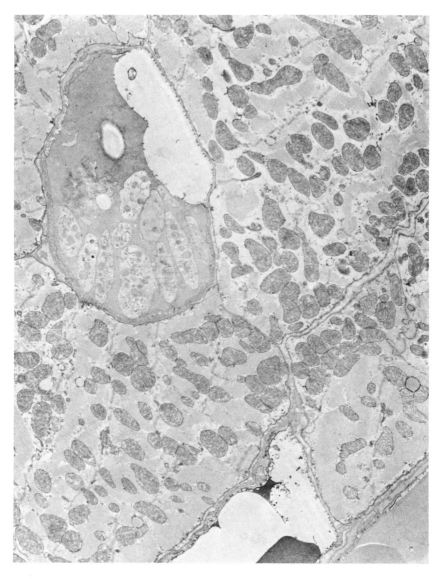

Figure 1. Left ventricular myocardium 20 min after permanent ischemia including the 10-min HRP circulation time. One capillary (left upper corner) is partly occluded by aggregated platelets and bleb-like swelling of an endothelial cell. Another capillary with ballooned endothelium (lower middle) contains electron dense HRP reaction product. A third capillary (right lower corner) appears structurally intact but not perfused by HRP. Cardiac muscle cells apart from some intracellular edema are structurally normal. Lead staining. X 6,600.

were processed for electron microscopy, as described previously (Boutet, Hüttner, and Rona, 1976). Sham-operated animals were used for control. Horseradish
peroxidase (HRP), Sigma type II, was injected under ether anesthesia through a
femoral vein in a dose of 10 mg/100 g body weight, dissolved in 0.5 ml of saline.
Rats were sacrificed following 10-min HRP circulation time by perfusion of
aldehyde fixative through a canula introduced into the right carotid artery.
Tissue blocks from rats not injected with HRP were examined for endogenous
peroxidase reaction.

OBSERVATIONS

Permanent Ischemia

The center of the ischemic area following 10- and 20-min ligation showed
inhomogeneous involvement of the coronary capillaries and cardiac muscle cells.
The lumen of some capillaries was compromised by the ballooning of endothelial
cells, while, in others, platelet aggregations were noted (Figure 1). Focally,
cardiac muscle cells showed relaxed sarcomeres. HRP was localized in the lumen

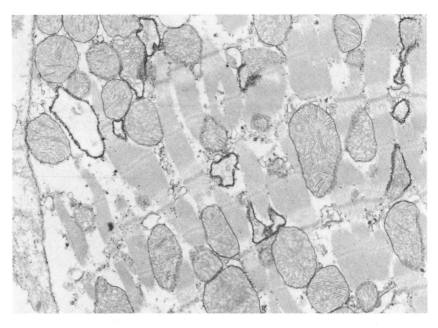

Figure 2. Cardiac muscle cell from left ventricular myocardium following 60-min permanent ischemia and 10 min after HRP injection. Sarcomeres are in extreme relaxation. While
the sarcolemmal membrane appears to be continuous, HRP reaction product binds to
ribosomes free in sarcoplasm and aggregated on intrasarcoplasmic membranes. Lead staining.
× 14,300.

of some capillaries, indicating some open circulation, at this stage, in the ischemic area. While the interstitium adjacent to perfused capillaries was positive for HRP, only low density reaction product was detected focally elsewhere. Cardiac muscle cells were free of reaction product.

The center of infarct following 60 min of ligature showed a greater proportion of nonperfused capillaries as compared to that observed following 10- and 20-min ligation. Many cardiac muscle cells showed extremely relaxed sarcomeres and mitochondria with polygonal configuration. Some vesicular structures were observed, a few of which could be identified as representing dilated profiles of sarcoplasmic reticulum. Ribosomes were prominent as free aggregates in the sarcoplasm and also in a linear arrangement on the external surface of some mitochondria. HRP reaction product was identified on these ribosomes (Figure 2). Reaction product also appeared to bind directly to the external mitochondrial membranes (Figure 3). In contrast to our experience with the catecholamine-induced myocardial injuries, in the model with permanent ischemia the relaxed myofilaments were free of reaction product. The periphery of the ischemic area contained more perfused capillaries than the center, and the interstitium was positive for HRP. Cell damage was less prevalent.

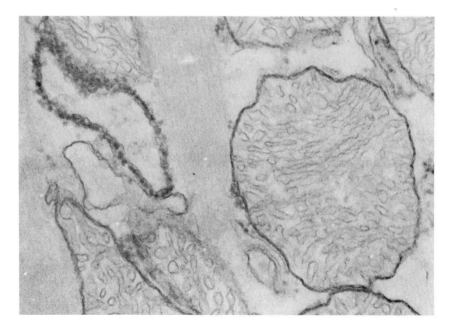

Figure 3. Detail of cardiac muscle cell prepared from unstained section of myocardial tissue presented in Figure 2. HRP reaction product labels ribosomes aggregated on intrasarcoplasmic membrane profile and also binds to external mitochondrial membranes. × 66,000.

Ischemia with Reperfusion

Ten-minute reperfusion following 10-min ischemia resulted in the reopening of many capillaries, as evidenced by HRP reaction product in the lumen.

In myocardium ischemic for 10 min followed by 60-min reperfusion, cardiac muscle cells with otherwise normal ultrastructure contained abundant lipid droplets (Figure 4). Other cells showed damage with contraction bands and edema (Figure 5). The contracted myofilaments at this stage were free of reaction product, while ribosomes and intracellular membrane structures again were labeled.

Reperfusion following 60 min of ischemia led to a dramatic deterioration of the cardiac muscle cell lesion as compared to the picture observed in the myocardium permanently ischemic for the same length of time. The cardiac muscle cells showed marked mitochondrial changes characterized by their irregular shape as well as by the presence of linear densities and electron dense granular deposits. Myofilament changes consisted of hypercontraction and irregular contraction-band formation. HRP reaction product was found in ribosomes and intracellular membranes as well as in the interior of altered mito-

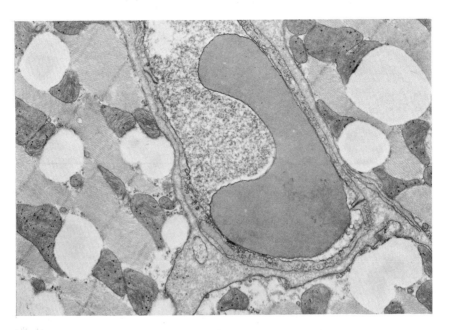

Figure 4. Sixty-minute reperfusion following 10-min ischemia. Injection of HRP started simultaneously with release. Lumen of a structurally intact capillary contains HRP reaction product, and the tracer also is noted in the interstitium. Cardiac muscle cells with normal ultrastructure contain many lipid droplets. Lead staining. × 14,300.

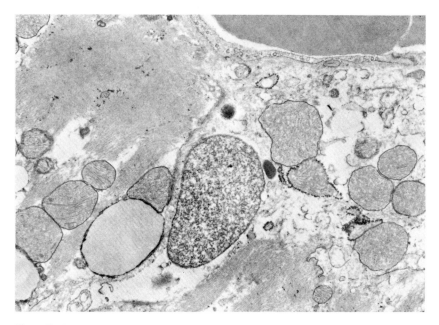

Figure 5. Another area of left ventricular myocardium reperfused following 10-min ischemia. Two cardiac muscle cells contain contraction bands. HRP reaction product is noted on some aggregated ribosomes and intrasarcoplasmic membranes. HRP-filled oval structure in the center probably is derived from a destroyed capillary. Lead staining. × 14,300.

chondria and also was deposited heavily on hypercontracted myofilaments (Figures 6 and 7).

DISCUSSION

Our observations obtained in ischemic rat myocardium with or without reperfusion indicated that, following 10- and 20-min ligation of left coronary artery, some of the collaterals remain patent as reflected by the presence of HRP in the lumen of some capillaries. However, the number of perfused capillaries decreased with time. While this microcirculatory observation may explain the inhomogeneous nature of subsequent cardiac muscle cell injury, progressive occlusion of capillaries by endothelial cell swelling and aggregated platelets excludes further microcirculatory adjustment.

Reperfusion modified the picture of ischemic myocardium. Even after 10-min ischemia, reperfusion resulted in pronounced contraction-band formation and edema in some cardiac muscle cells. A dramatic acceleration of the ultrastructural changes occurred by reperfusion following 60-min ligation. Further-

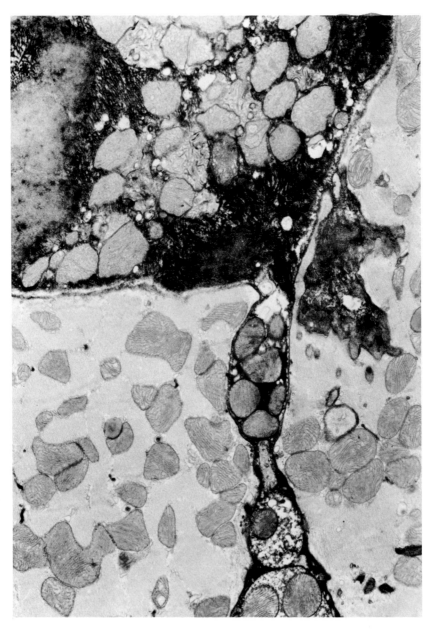

Figure 6. Ten-minute reperfusion following 60-min ischemia. Heavy deposit of HRP reaction product is evident on contracted myofilaments in one of the cardiac muscle cells. Also the external membranes and cristae of mitochondria are labeled with peroxidase. Lead staining. × 14,300.

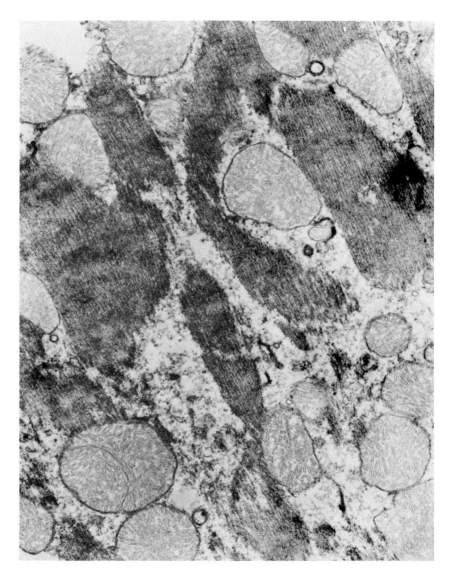

Figure 7. Ten-minute reperfusion following 60-min ischemia. HRP deposit on myofilaments and external mitochondrial membranes. Lead staining. × 22,400.

more, applying the extracellular diffusion tracer, HRP, furnished evidence that influx of plasmatic substances into cardiac muscle cells with altered sarcolemmal membrane may be one of the mechanisms whereby perfusion aggravates ischemic injury. While this deleterious effect of reperfusion has been discussed widely in systemic morphological studies by Jennings and associates (Kloner, Ganote, and Jennings, 1974; Jennings, Ganote, and Reimer, 1975; Jennings, 1976) our recent investigation furnished comparative rheological evidence with the fine structural diffusion tracer, HRP, on the underlying microcirculatory mechanism. The frustrating dilemma is that, while prolongation of ischemia increases the size of irreversibly damaged myocardium in the peripheral twilight zone (Braunwald, 1976), reperfusion apparently produces even more cardiac muscle cell damage.

The effect of reperfusion in the ischemic model can be correlated with observations obtained in the noncoronarogenic cardiac muscle cell injury induced by catecholamines. The sarcolemmal permeability alteration has been shown to be an early event following norepinephrine infusion (Boutet, Hüttner, and Rona, 1974; Rona, Boutet, and Hüttner, 1975b) in which overstimulated cardiac muscle cells are permanently exposed to circulatory plasma constituents. However, in the isoproterenol-induced cardiac muscle injury, tracer studies disclosed permeability alteration of the cardiac muscle cell membranes only following the return of blood pressure toward normal levels and the resumption of coronary microcirculatory transport (Boutet, Hüttner, and Rona, 1973). This reperfusion of the ischemic myocardium, in addition to unmasking membrane damage, may contribute to the cardiac muscle cell injury by the overflow of plasmatic substances not only into the interstitium but also into the cell interior.

The clarification of some interesting observations on the ischemic model requires further study. We have no explanation for the affinity of ribosomes to the external membranes of altered mitochondria nor for their endogenous peroxidase activity. It is worthwhile to correlate these findings with the similar affinity of lanthanum to the periphery of damaged mitochondria (Hoffstein *et al.,* 1975), implying the possible accumulation of negatively charged sites at this location.

Another observation that remains to be elucidated is the early binding of HRP to contracted myofilaments in the norepinephrine model (Boutet, Hüttner, and Rona, 1974; Rona, Boutet, and Hüttner, 1975a) as constrasted with the late appearance of this phenomenon in the reperfused ischemic model. The clarification of this problem is important because HRP deposition may be considered as a marker for plasma constituents.

Whereas some of the peroxidase positive cells may eventually recover, loss of barrier function of the sarcolemmal membrane may lead to further events detrimental to the cardiac muscle cell. These include transmembrane influx of

Ca^{2+} that, according to Fleckenstein's theory, produces myofilament overstimulation, excessive breakdown of ATP by the Ca^{2+}-activated myofibrillar ATP-ase, high energy phosphate deficiency, and Ca^{2+} overload of mitochondria (Fleckenstein et al., 1969, 1974). Sarcolemmal alteration also may allow leaking of intracellular constituents, including enzymes necessary for cellular reconstitution; and intrasarcoplasmic deposition and binding of macromolecules to contractile proteins could impede myofilament reassembly, all of which would contribute to irreversible cardiac muscle cell damage (Rona, Hüttner, and Boutet, in press). It is also logical to suggest that cardiac muscle cells with sarcolemmal membrane permeable to macromolecules, such as HRP, are reversibly, or even irreversibly, nonfunctional. Intracellular channels that exist at the gap junctions between adjacent cardiac muscle cells (Revel and Karnovsky, 1967; McNutt and Weinstein, 1970) could be blocked promptly by the raised Ca^{2+} concentration within the sarcoplasm (Loewenstein, Nakas, and Socolar, 1967).

The observations presented in this experimental study may be relevant to the assessment of the role of coronary perfusion in the evolution of myocardial changes in man with patent coronary arteries as well as in myocardium of patients following coronary thrombosis and reperfusion. Acceleration of cardiac muscle cell alteration following reperfusion as compared to permanent ischemia may have important significance for assessing infarct size from accompanying serum enzyme changes and may bring into question the rationale of therapy designed for reperfusion of the acutely infarcted myocardium.

REFERENCES

BING, R. J., CASTELLANOS, A., GRADEL, E., LUPTON, C., and SIEGEL, A. 1956. Experimental myocardial infarction: Circulatory, biochemical and pathological changes. Am. J. Med. Sci. 232:533–534.

BOUTET, M., HÜTTNER, I., and RONA, G. 1973. Aspect microcirculatoire des lésions myocardiques provoquées par l'infusion de catécholamines. Etude ultrastructurale à l'aide de traceurs de diffusion. 1. Isoproterenol. Pathol. Biol. (Paris) 8:811–825.

BOUTET, M., HÜTTNER, I., and RONA, G. 1974. Aspect microcirculatoire des lésions myocardiques provoquées par l'infusion de catécholamines. Etude ultrastructurale à l'aide de traceurs de diffusion. 2. Norépinephrine. Pathol. Biol. (Paris) 5:377–387.

BOUTET, M., HÜTTNER, I., and RONA, G. 1976. Permeability alteration of sarcolemmal membrane in catecholamine-induced cardiac muscle cell injury. Lab. Invest. 34:482–488.

BRAUNWALD, E. 1976. Introductory Remarks. Circulation 53(Suppl. I):1–2.

DUSEK, J., BOUTET, M., and RONA, G. 1973. Ultrastructural changes in isoproterenol - induced experimental atrial necrosis. In E. Bajusz and G. Rona (eds.), Recent Advances in Studies on Cardiac Structure and Metabolism. Vol. 2: Cardiomyopathies, pp. 423–432. University Park Press, Baltimore.

FLECKENSTEIN, A., DORING, A. H., and LEDER, O. 1969. The significance of high energy phosphate exhaustion in the etiology of isoproterenol-induced cardiac necrosis and its prevention by iproveratril, compound D 600 or prenylamine. *In* M. Lamarche and R. Royer (eds.), Symposium International on Drugs and Metabolism of Myocardium and Striated Muscle, pp. 11–22. Nancy, France.

FLECKENSTEIN, A., JANKE, J., DORING, H. J., and LEDER, O. 1974. Myocardial fiber necrosis due to intracellular Ca overload—a new principle in cardiac pathophysiology. *In* N. S. Dhalla (ed.), Recent Advances in Studies on Cardiac Structure and Metabolism Vol. 4: Myocardial Biology, pp. 563–580. University Park Press, Baltimore.

HOFFSTEIN, S., GENNARO, D. E., FOX, A. C., HIRSCH, J., STREULI, F., and WEISS-MANN, G. 1975. Colloidal lanthanum as a marker for impaired plasma membrane permeability in ischemic dog myocardium. Am. J. Pathol. 79:207–218.

JENNINGS, R., GANOTE, C. E., and REIMER, K. A. 1975. Ischemic tissue injury. Am. J. Pathol. 81:179–195.

JENNINGS, R. B. 1976. Relationship of acute ischemia to functional defects and irreversibility. Circulation 53(Suppl. I):26–29.

KLONER, R. A., GANOTE, C. E., and JENNINGS, R. B. 1974. The "no-reflow" phenomenon after temporary coronary occlusion in the dog. J. Clin. Invest. 54:1496–1508.

LEE, S. H., DUSEK, J., and RONA, G. 1971. Electron microscopic cytochemical study of glutamic oxalacetic transamenase activity in ischemic myocardium. J. Mol. Cell. Cardiol. 3:103–109.

LOEWENSTEIN, W. R., NAKAS, M., SOCOLAR, S. J. 1967. Junctional membrane uncoupling: permeability transformation at a cell membrane junction. J. Gen. Physiol. 50:1865–1891.

McNUTT, N. S., and WEINSTEIN, R. S. 1970. The ultrastructure of the nexus: A correlated thin section and freeze-cleave study. J. Cell Biol. 47:666–688.

REVEL, J. P., and KARNOVSKY, M. J. 1967. Hexagonal array of subunits in intercellular junctions of the mouse heart and liver. J. Cell Biol. 33:C7–C12.

ROBERTS, R., AMBOS, H. D., CARLSON, E. M., and SOBEL, B. E. 1975. Improved quantification of myocardial infarction based on analysis of serum CPK isoenzymes. Am. J. Cardiol. 35:166a.

RONA, G. 1971. Cardiac adaptation to insult. Symposium on Metabolism and Disease. Health and Welfare Canada. pp. 50–59.

RONA, G., DUSEK, J., HÜTTNER, I., and KAHN, D. S. 1970. Studies on myocardial resistance. *In* V. Zambotti and M. G. Arrigoni (eds.), Institute Lombardo—Accademia di Scienze e Lettere, pp. 173–204. Succ. Fusi-Pavia.

RONA, G., BOUTET, M., HÜTTNER, I., and PETERS, H. 1973. Pathogenesis of isoproterenol-induced myocardial alterations. Functional and morphological correlates. *In* N. S. Dhalla (ed.), Recent Advances in Studies on Cardiac Structure and Metabolism. Vol. 3: Myocardial Metabolism, pp. 507–525. University Park Press, Baltimore.

RONA, G., BOUTET, M., and HÜTTNER, I. 1975a. Membrane permeability alterations as manifestation of early cardiac muscle cell injury. *In* A. Fleckenstein and G. Rona (eds.), Recent Advances in Studies on Cardiac Muscle Structure and Metabolism. Vol. 6: Pathophysiology and Morphology of Myocardial Cell Alteration, pp. 439–451. University Park Press, Baltimore.

RONA, G., BOUTET, M., and HÜTTNER, I. 1975b. New approach in studying cardiac muscle cell injury. Postgrad. Med. J. 51:334–339.

RONA, G., HÜTTNER, I., and BOUTET, M. 1977. Microcirculatory changes in myocardium with particular reference to catecholamine-induced cardiac muscle cell injury. *In* H. Meessen (ed.), Handbuch der Allgemeinen Pathologie. Vol. III/7: Allgemeine Pathologie der Mikrozirkulation, pp. 791–888. Springer-Verlag, New York.

SELYE, H., BAJUSZ, E., GRASSO, S., and MENDELL, P. 1960. Simple techniques for the surgical occlusion of coronary vessels in the rat. Angiology 11:398–407.

SOBEL, B. E. 1976. Infarct size, prognosis, and causal contiguity. Circulation 53(Suppl. I):146–148.

WILLIAMSON, J. R., SCHAFFER, S. W., FORD, C., and SAFER, B. 1976. Contribution of tissue acidosis to ischemic injury in the perfused rat heart. Circulation 53(Suppl. I):3–14.

Mailing address:
G. Rona, M.D., Ph.D.,
Department of Pathology, McGill University,
3775 University Street, Montreal 112, Quebec (Canada).

Recent Advances in Studies on
Cardiac Structure and Metabolism, Volume 12
Cardiac Adaptation
Edited by T. Kobayashi, Y. Ito, and G. Rona
Copyright 1978 University Park Press Baltimore

THE EFFECTS OF CORONARY ARTERY LIGATION ON TRANSMURAL HIGH-ENERGY PHOSPHATES FOLLOWING 20 MINUTES OF BLOOD REFLOW

C. A. RAMEY and J. W. HOLSINGER, JR.

Research Service, U. S. Veterans Administration Hospital,
Newington, Connecticut,
and
Departments of Pediatrics and Medicine, University of Connecticut Health Center,
Farmington, Connecticut, USA

SUMMARY

Normal or elevated levels of ATP and phosphocreatine (PCr) were observed from the subepicardium to the subendocardium of the canine left ventricle after five and 20 minutes of left circumflex artery occlusion followed by 20 minutes of blood reflow. However, after two or four hours of occlusion, followed by reflow, ATP and PCr levels were markedly depressed, and a significant decreasing subepicardial to subendocardial gradient appeared, suggestive of inhibition of oxidative metabolism during extended periods of ischemia but not during short periods of ischemia.

INTRODUCTION

Historically, the investigation of the phenomenon of myocardial infarction generally has been approached through the study of the pathogenesis of atherosclerosis. The role of the myocardium has received much less attention, although many facets of ischemic change have been delineated using selective artery ligation.

Jennings, Whartman, and Zudyk (1957) have standardized a canine model for producing experimental ischemia. Utilizing ligation of the left circumflex artery (LCA), they have produced a readily definable area of predictable ischemia in the posterolateral wall of the left ventricle (LV).

Of the three layers of the LV, the subendocardial region has been known to have a particular susceptibility to hypoxic damage and may be the first to suffer from inadequate tissue perfusion (Kirk and Honig, 1964). Although regional ventricular blood flow has been studied extensively, less is known about the transmural metabolism of normal and ischemic tissue. Significant transmural gradients have not been reported in normal tissue by Dunn and Griggs (1975) for phosphocreatine (PCr), adenosine triphosphate (ATP), and lactate, but have been by Crass et al. (1976) for triglycerides and glycogen, and by Lundsgaard-Hansen (1967) for glycolytic enzyme activities. In the present study, the effects of restoration of blood flow after varying periods of ischemia were examined in terms of transmural ATP and PCr levels in the left ventricle.

MATERIALS AND METHODS

Forty adult mongrel dogs (weighing 20–25 kg) were randomly divided into control and experimental groups. The dogs were anesthetized (Nembutal, 30 mg/kg, i.v.) and then immediately intubated, using a balloon-cuffed endotracheal tube, and ventilated with a mixture of 100% oxygen and room air, using a positive pressure respirator. Arterial pH, pO_2, and pCO_2 were monitored and maintained within physiological range. The ECG was monitored through lead II.

The heart was exposed through a sternotomy and suspended in the pericardial sac. The LCA was dissected free from the great cardiac vein under the left atrium at a point approximately 5 mm from the origin of the LCA. A suture snare was positioned around the isolated artery and the vessel was occluded in experimental animals for 5, 20, 120, or 240 min, followed by 20 min of blood reflow, or it was left patent in control animals.

Following occlusion, animals that did not develop cyanosis of the posterolateral wall and/or elevation of the ST segment were not utilized. After the specified time interval had elapsed, transmural biopsies were taken through the posterolateral wall of the LV in the region of the posterior papillary muscle. Tissue samples were immediately frozen intact in liquid nitrogen. For all analyses, the frozen transmural samples were divided into three portions as follows: 1) the epicardial fat and blood vessels were trimmed away and the next 2–3 mm were retained as the subepicardial (s-epi) specimen; 2) the middle 2 mm of tissue were used for midventricular (mid) analyses, and 3) the inner 2 mm, including the endocardium with any residual papillary muscle removed, were used for the subendocardial (s-endo) region.

Tissue metabolites were extracted as described by Lamprecht and Stein (1965). ATP and PCr were assayed spectrophotometrically at 340 nm in the same reaction mixture (Lamprecht and Stein, 1965; Lamprecht and Traushold, 1965).

All meristic data were statistically analyzed with values expressed as the mean ± S.E.M. Statistical significance of each parameter was tested using standardized techniques (Snedecor and Cochran, 1967), which included the one-way analysis of variance and the F-test followed by contrasts and comparisons.

RESULTS

Figure 1 shows transmural ATP content in experimental animals after either 5, 20, 120, or 240 min of LCA occlusion with 20 min of reflow, or the content in

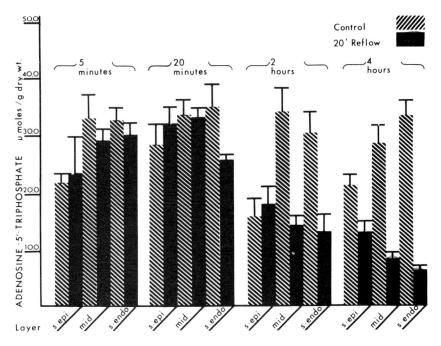

Figure 1. Transmural adenosine triphosphate (ATP) content after varying durations of ischemia followed by 20 min of blood reflow. Control and ischemic time intervals are indicated at the top of the figure. Transmural layers include: subepicardium (s-epi), midventricular (mid), and subendocardium (s-endo). Values are expressed as mean ± S.E.M. for control hearts (solid bars) and ischemic hearts (hatched bars).

control animals paired in time with the experimentals. Occlusion followed by reflow significantly ($p < 0.01$) affected ATP levels but was dependent on layer ($p < 0.01$) and time ($p < 0.01$) effects. Reflow stores of ATP were maintained in all layers after 5 min of occlusion. After 20 min of occlusion, reflow ATP levels were maintained in all layers except the subendocardium which showed a 26% decrease. Following 120 min of occlusion, the decrease in reflow levels of ATP had expanded to include both the subendocardium, down 58% (30.6 ± 3.2 to 12.8 ± 3.3, μmol/g dry weight), and the midventricular layer, down 60% (34.3 ± 4.3 to 13.8 ± 3.5, μmol/g dry weight). By 240 min of occlusion, ATP levels had decreased in all three layers significantly ($p < 0.01$) in comparison to controls with a subepicardial depression of 41%, midventricular depression of 73%, and subendocardial depression of 81%. In addition, reflow levels of ATP at 120 and 240 min of occlusion demonstrated a decreasing gradient from the subepicardium to the subendocardium.

Signficant ($p < 0.02$) changes in PCr reflow levels were observed under these conditions (Figure 2), which were also time-dependent ($p < 0.01$). A significant ($p < 0.01$) increasing outer-to-inner gradient occurred after 5 and 20 min, and,

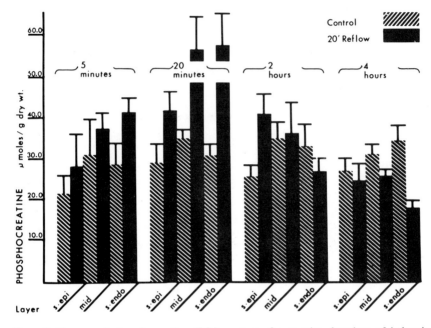

Figure 2. Transmural phosphocreatine (PCr) content after varying durations of ischemia followed by 20 min of blood reflow. Control and ischemic time intervals are indicated at the top of the figure. Transmural layers include: subepicardium (s-epi), midventricular (mid), and subendocardium (s-endo). Values are expressed as mean ± S.E.M. for control hearts (black bars) and ischemic hearts (hatched bars).

after 20 min of occlusion, PCr levels were significantly ($p < 0.01$) above control levels in all layers. After 120 min, reflow levels of PCr were maintained near control levels, but the transmural gradient was reversed. Subepicardial PCr increased 60.4% (25.5 ± 3.4 to 40.9 ± 6.8, µmol/g dry weight, $p < 0.01$), midventricular stores were maintained, and subendocardial levels were reduced 19%, although not significantly (32.6 ± 5.3 to 26.4 ± 3.9, µmol/g dry weight). After 4 hr of LCA occlusion and 20 min of blood reflow, PCr levels were maximally depressed in all layers, the subendocardial stores being most reduced (34.2 ± 3.7 to 17.2 ± 2.1, µmol/g dry weight). Transmural layer differences in reflow levels of PCr were significant ($p < 0.01$), with subendocardial PCr demonstrating the greatest increase after 5 and 20 min of occlusion and demonstrating the greatest decrease at 120 and 240 min.

DISCUSSION

Kloner, Ganote, and Jennings (1974) have suggested that a "no-reflow" phenomenon occurs in the left ventricle after 20–40 min of LCA occlusion. Extension of ischemia beyond 40 min should be identified by a significant decrease in mitochondrial oxidative metabolism, with a concomitant reduction in ATP and PCr.

Our data support this hypothesis. In the first 20 min of occlusion, reflow appears to have produced a metabolically reactive, hyperemic response for PCr, particularly in the subendocardium. However, after 2 and 4 hr of occlusion, restoration of the blood flow was incapable of returning either ATP or PCr to control levels, the subendocardium being most severely affected. During the first 20 min of occlusion, acceleration of glycolysis may result in accumulation of substrates of oxidative metabolism. With restoration of blood flow, the mitochondria then could respond in a metabolically hyperemic fashion, accounting for normalization of ATP and the "overshoot" in PCr. Eventual necrosis and rupture of mitochondria during the 2- and 4-hr occlusions prevent any significant oxidative metabolism from occurring following restoration of blood flow.

Although peripheral regions of the infarct have not been examined, these studies suggest that normal metabolism can be restored to the center of the ischemic zone by restoration of blood flow within 20 min, but not if the ischemic insult is prolonged for 2 or 4 hr.

REFERENCES

CRASS, M. F., III, HOLSINGER, J. W., JR., SHIPP, J. C., ELIOT, R. S., and PIEPER, G. M. 1976. Transmural gradients in the ischemic dog left ventricle: Metabolism of endogenous triglycerides and glycogen. In P. Harris, R. J. Bing, and A. Fleckenstein (eds.), Recent Advances in Studies on Cardiac Structure and Metabolism. Vol. 7: Biochemistry and Pharmacology of Myocardial Hypertrophy, Hypoxia, and Infarction, pp. 225–230. University Park Press, Baltimore.

DUNN, R. B., and GRIGGS, D. M., JR. 1975. Transmural gradients in ventricular tissue metabolites produced by stopping blood flow in the dog. Circ. Res. 37:438–445.

JENNINGS, R. B., WHARTMAN, W. B., and ZUDYK, Z. 1957. Production of an area of homogeneous myocardial infarction in the dog. Arch. Pathol. 63:580–585.

KIRK, E. S., and HONIG, C. R. 1964. Nonuniform distribution of blood flow and gradients of oxygen tension within the heart. Am. J. Physiol. 207:661–668.

KLONER, R. A., GANOTE, C. E., and JENNINGS, R. B. 1974. The "no-reflow" phenomenon after temporary coronary occlusion in the dog. J. Clin. Invest. 54:1496–1508.

LAMPRECHT, W., and STEIN, P. 1965. Creatine phosphate. In H. U. Bergmeyer (ed.), Methods of Enzymatic Analysis, pp. 610–616. 2nd Ed. Academic Press, New York.

LAMPRECHT, W., and TRAUSHOLD, I. 1965. ATP: Determination with hexokinase and glucose-6-phosphate dehydrogenase. In H. U. Bergmeyer (ed.), Methods of Enzymatic Analysis, pp. 543–551. 2nd Ed. Academic Press, New York.

LUNDSGAARD-HANSEN, P., MEYER, C., and RIEDWYL, H. 1967. Transmural gradients of glycolytic enzyme activities in left ventricular myocardium. I. The normal state. Pfluegers Arch. 297:89–106.

SNEDECOR, G. W., and COCHRAN, W. 1967. Statistical Methods, p. 593. Iowa State University Press, Ames, Iowa.

Mailing address:
Craig A. Ramey, Ph.D.,
U.S. Veterans Administration Hospital,
555 Willard Avenue, Newington, Connecticut 06111 (USA).

Recent Advances in Studies on
Cardiac Structure and Metabolism, Volume 12
Cardiac Adaptation
Edited by T. Kobayashi, Y. Ito, and G. Rona
Copyright 1978 University Park Press Baltimore

TRANSMURAL GRADIENTS IN ISCHEMIC CANINE LEFT VENTRICLE: EFFECTS OF BLOOD REFLOW ON GLYCOLYTIC INTERMEDIATES

J. W. HOLSINGER, JR., C. A. RAMEY, and T. B. ALLISON

Veterans Administration, Hospital Newington, Connecticut,
and Departments of Medicine, Pediatrics, and Pharmacology,
University of Connecticut School of Medicine,
Farmington, Connecticut, USA

SUMMARY

Following two and four hours of left ventricular ischemia, 20 minutes of blood reflow cannot produce a complete return to normal oxidative metabolism in ischemic canine myocardium. Glycolysis remains increased and aerobic metabolism is most extensively depressed in the subendocardium.

INTRODUCTION

For a number of years, the subendocardial region of the left ventricular wall has been known to have a particular susceptibility to hypoxic damage, and it may be the first to suffer from inadequate tissue perfusion. Even in the normal heart, several factors support this vulnerability to ischemic damage. For example, the subendocardium has the lowest tissue partial pressure of oxygen (Kirk and Honig, 1964b), despite higher stress factors (Kirk and Honig, 1964a), and, therefore, a higher metabolic oxygen demand. A subendocardial to subepicardial gradient in the severity of ischemia following acute coronary occlusion has been described previously (Jennings, Ganote, and Reimer, 1975). Regional differences in glycogen and triglyceride metabolism have been found in ischemic canine left ventricle (LV) (Crass *et al.*, 1976). Under the conditions studied, the subendocardium was characterized by a faster rate of glycogenolysis and demonstrated the least ability to mobilize tissue triglycerides relative to the subepicardial and midmyocardial zones. The glycolytic intermediate, glucose-6-phosphate, has been found to accumulate to a much greater extent over a four-hour period of ischemia in the subendocardium as compared to the subepicardium (Allison *et al.*, in press). Lactate also accumulates during ischemia to a greater degree in the subendocardium compared to the subepicardium. This increase in lactate suggests that pyruvate entry into the Kreb's cycle is inhibited, with a resulting shift in equilibrium favoring lactate production. With the data provided by these experiments, the effects of blood reflow on the transmural metabolism of the acutely ischemic myocardium were examined.

MATERIALS AND METHODS

Mongrel dogs weighing 20–25 kg were anesthetized with intravenous sodium pentobarbital and ventilated with a mixture of room air and 100% oxygen using a positive pressure respirator. Arterial pO_2, pCO_2, and pH were monitored and maintained within physiological range. The heart was exposed through a midline sternotomy, and the left circumflex coronary artery (LCA) was isolated. In groups of five dogs, the LCA was occluded for either 5, 20, 120, or 240 min, after which blood reflow was instituted for 20 min. Each group of animals was accompanied by a paired, time-equivalent control group, in which all experimental procedures were carried out, except actual occlusion of the circumflex coronary artery. After the stated time intervals, a transmural biopsy was obtained through the posterolateral wall of the LV and placed in liquid nitrogen

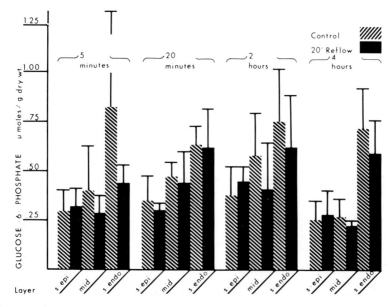

Figure 1. Glucose-6-phosphate content after varying durations of ischemia and 20 min of blood reflow. Control and ischemic time intervals are indicated at the top of the figure. An additional 20 min of blood reflow occurred in ischemic animals and an additional 20 min were added to the control period for each group; s-epi = subepicardium; mid = midventricular; s-endo = subendocardium. Values for control hearts are indicated by hatched bars, those for ischemic hearts by solid bars.

within seconds. Transmural sections were cut with an electrically powered circular saw. For the subepicardium (s-epi), the outer 1 mm was removed and discarded and the next inner 2 mm were taken for analyses. For the midventricular (mid) area, the middle 2 mm of the plug were taken. For the subendocardium (s-endo), the inner 2 mm of the left ventricular wall, including endocardium, were used. Extractions and analyses of glucose-6-phosphate, lactate, pyruvate, and lactate/pyruvate ratio in the transmural sections were performed as described previously (Allison *et al.*, in press).

RESULTS

Glucose-6-phosphate (Figure 1) demonstrated a significant ($p < 0.01$) layer effect with a gradient from subepicardium to subendocardium, with the latter demonstrating the greatest accumulation. There was no significant difference between control and experimental groups, and the layer effect was independent of time. Glucose-6-phosphate returned to normal in all four time groups following 20 min of blood reflow. In general, subepicardial levels appeared to be somewhat higher than controls, while subendocardial levels tended to be somewhat lower.

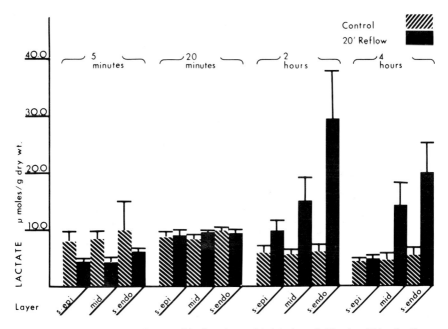

Figure 2. Lactate content after varying durations of ischemia and 20 min of blood reflow. Conditions are identical to those for Figure 1.

Lactate (Figure 2) demonstrated a significant ($p < 0.01$) treatment effect that was dependent on layer ($p = 0.01$) and time ($p < 0.01$). After 5 min of ligation followed by 20 min of reflow, lactate levels, when expressed as a percentage of controls, were significantly diminished in all three layers (s-epi, 41%; mid, 48%; s-endo, 38%). After 20 min of ligation followed by 20 min of reflow, there was no change in lactate levels in any layer of the heart. However, in the 120 min time group, lactate levels increased from 32% in the subepicardium to 349% in the subendocardium. In the 240 min group, lactate increased by 43% in the subepicardium, by 263% in the midmyocardium, and by 281% in the subendocardium.

DISCUSSION

Glucose-6-phosphate is a key intermediate in the initial portion of the glycolytic pathway, while lactate is a key intermediate in the final portion. During periods of ischemia, accumulation of glucose-6-phosphate indicates inhibition of glycolysis at the phosphofructokinase step, while accumulation of lactate represents a decreased entry of pyruvate into the Kreb's cycle in the mitochondria. Increased levels of lactate reflect a decreased oxidative metabolic state and are greater when blood reflow is restricted (Rovetto, Whitmer, and Neely, 1973).

As suggested by Jennings and Ganote (1974), 40 min of ischemia produces irreversible damage to the mitochondria; therefore, during ischemic insult of greater than 40 min, significant mitochondrial metabolism would not be expected to occur following restoration of blood flow. Our data indicate that, during the first 20 min of ischemia, reflow results in a return to normal of both glycolytic and mitochondrial metabolism. However, following 2 and 4 hr of ischemia, only glycolysis has responded to restoration of blood flow, in that glucose-6-phosphate levels have returned to control levels while subendocardial lactate levels remain significantly elevated. This implies that the entry of pyruvate into the mitochondria remains inhibited and that inhibition of phosphofructokinase has been removed allowing glycolysis to proceed. Thus, these data lend metabolic support to the concept that a "no-reflow" phenomenon (Kloner, Ganote, and Jennings, 1974) exists after extended periods of ischemia and that aerobic metabolism is most extensively depressed in the subendocardium.

REFERENCES

ALLISON, T. B., RAMEY, C. A., and HOLSINGER, J. W., JR. Transmural gradients of left ventricular tissue metabolites after circumflex artery ligation in dogs. J. Mol. Cell. Cardiol. In press.

CRASS, M. F., III, HOLSINGER, J. W., JR., SHIPP, J. C., ELIOT, R. S., and PIEPER, G. M. 1976. Transmural gradients in ischemic dog left ventricle: Metabolism of endogenous triglycerides and glycogen. In P. Harris, R. J. Bing, and A. Fleckenstein (eds.),

Recent Advances in Studies on Cardiac Structure and Function. Vol. 7: Biochemistry and Pharmacology of Myocardial Hypertrophy, Hypoxia, and Infarction, pp. 225–230. University Park Press, Baltimore.

JENNINGS, R. B., and GANOTE, C. E. 1974. Structural changes in myocardium during acute ischemia. Circ. Res. 34 and 35(suppl. III):156–168.

JENNINGS, R. B., GANOTE, C. E., and REIMER, K. A. 1975. Ischemic tissue injury. Am. J. Pathol. 81:179–198.

KIRK, E. S., and HONIG, C. R. 1964a. An experimental and theoretical analysis of myocardial tissue pressure. Am. J. Physiol. 207:361–367.

KIRK, E. S., and HONIG, C. R. 1964b. Nonuniform distribution of blood flow and gradients of oxygen tension within the heart. Am. J. Physiol. 207:661–668.

KLONER, R. A., GANOTE, C. E., and JENNINGS, R. B. 1974. The "no-reflow" phenomenon after temporary coronary occlusion in the dog. J. Clin. Invest. 54:1496–1508.

ROVETTO, M. J., WHITMER, J. T., and NEELY, J. R. 1973. Comparison of the effects of anoxia and whole heart ischemia on carbohydrate utilization in isolated working rat hearts. Circ. Res. 32:699–711.

Mailing address:
J. W. Holsinger, Jr. M.D.,
Chief of Staff, Veterans Administration Hospital,
555 Willard Avenue, Newington, Connecticut 06111 (USA).

Recent Advances in Studies on
Cardiac Structure and Metabolism, Volume 12
Cardiac Adaptation
Edited by T. Kobayashi, Y. Ito, and G. Rona
Copyright 1978 University Park Press Baltimore

FUNCTION OF CARDIAC SARCOPLASMIC RETICULUM FOLLOWING CARDIOPULMONARY BYPASS IN HUMAN SUBJECTS

R. W. LENTZ, D. A. BARNHORST, G. K. DANIELSON,
J. D. DEWEY, and C. E. HARRISON, JR.

Mayo Clinic and Mayo Foundation,
Rochester, Minnesota, USA

SUMMARY

The function of the cardiac sarcoplasmic reticulum (SR) was evaluated in 44 patients with nonischemic mitral valve disease and chronic heart failure (Group I) and in 28 patients with congenital subvalvular pulmonic obstruction and right ventricular hypertrophy (Group II). Heart muscle was removed approximately 15 min after the establishment of cardiopulmonary bypass and about 4 min after first aortal cross-clamping. Cats served as an additional experimental control. The SR was isolated by the method of Harigaya and Schwartz (1969). ^{45}Ca uptake (5 mM sodium oxalate) and binding were quantitated by Swinny Millipore filtration. Free calcium ion concentrations ranging from 1×10^{-7} M to 8×10^{-6} M were obtained by glycoletherdiaminetetraacetic acid (EGTA) buffering. Control studies in cats did not reveal a significant difference between left and right heart calcium uptake or binding. Compared with the nonfailing group (II), the SR of the failing group (I) showed a significant depression of calcium uptake ($p < 0.0001$) and binding ($p < 0.01$) at various ATP concentrations. The SR of both human groups revealed a high calcium affinity characterized by low, not significantly different, dissociation constants of about 1.8×10^{-7} M. There was no significant difference in the Ca^{2+}-sensitive SR ATPase activities of Groups I and II. The impaired SR calcium transport in the chronically failing human heart is interpreted as representing a true biochemical lesion of the myocardium, probably forming part of a more complex intracellular dysfunction. No direct correlation with any clinical parameter in the patients with failing hearts was found.

INTRODUCTION

Over recent years, many investigators have described a depressed function of the sarcoplasmic reticulum (SR) isolated from failing cardiac muscle. In the experimental animal, this has been documented in acute heart failure (Gertz *et al.*, 1967) and in various models of chronic heart failure (Harigaya and Schwartz, 1969; Gertz, Stam, and Sonnenblick, 1970; McCollum *et al.*, 1970; Muir *et al.*,

This investigation was supported in part by Research Grant HL-12997 from the National Institute of Health, Public Health Service, and by a grant from Smith, Kline Co., Inc.

1970; Suko, Vogel, and Chidsey, 1970; Sulakhe and Dhalla, 1971, 1973; Sordahl *et al.*, 1973; Ito, Suko, and Chidsey, 1974). It also has been demonstrated in the terminally failing and ischemic human myocardium (Harigaya and Schwartz, 1969; Lindenmayer *et al.*, 1971; Schwartz *et al.*, 1973). The purpose of the present investigation was to evaluate the cardiac SR function in patients with nonischemic mitral valve disease and chronic congestive heart failure.

MATERIALS AND METHODS

During corrective cardiac surgery, myocardial tissue, such as left ventricular papillary muscle or right ventricular bands of the crista supraventricularis, was removed from two groups of patients. Group I was comprised of 44 patients (28 females, 16 males, mean age 56 years) with nonischemic mitral valve disease and historical or clinical evidence for chronic congestive heart failure. Group II consisted of 28 patients (11 females, 17 males, mean age 15 years) with congenital cardiac abnormalities that all included subvalvular pulmonary stenosis. Patients in Group II had right ventricular hypertrophy without evidence for cardiac failure and served as the best available form of control. The tissue samples were removed approximately 15 min after establishment of cardiopulmonary bypass and about 4 min after aortal cross-clamping. Adult cats served as an additional experimental control.

The SR was isolated by the slightly modified method of Harigaya and Schwartz (1969). SR ^{45}Ca uptake (oxalate present), or binding (oxalate absent), or both were determined by using either glycoletherdiaminetetraacetic acid (EGTA)-free assays as outlined by Harigaya and Schwartz (1969) or media containing EGTA in various concentrations (Ogawa, 1968; Ogawa *et al.*, 1971) and 100 mM KCl, 20 mM imidazole (pH 6.8, 30°C), 5 mM $MgCl_2$, 10 μM ^{45}Ca-$CaCl_2$, 1 or 5 mM Tris-ATP, and about 0.1 mg/ml of SR protein. The SR calcium accumulation was measured by Millipore filtration and liquid scintillation counting. The SR ATPase activities were quantitated by the release of inorganic phosphate (Pi) to the EGTA-free reaction medium. The inorganic phosphate was measured by the method of Marsh (1959). The SR-specific, Ca^{2+}-sensitive ATPase activity was defined by the difference between the total SR ATPase activity (10 μM $CaCl_2$ in the reaction assay) and that of the basic and nonspecific SR ATPase (no calcium present).

RESULTS

Calcium Uptake

The ability of the SR to accumulate calcium in the presence of 5 mM sodium oxalate was significantly decreased in the failing group (I) as compared to the

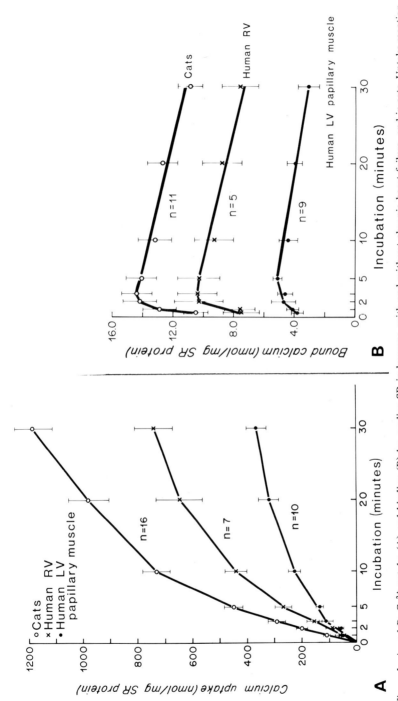

Figure 1. A and B. Ca²⁺ uptake (A) and binding (B) by cardiac SR in humans, with and without chronic heart failure, and in cats. Uptake reaction media: 100 mM KCl, 20 mM Tris-HCl (pH 7.0), 10 mM MgCl₂, 2 mM tris-ATP, 100 μM ⁴⁵Ca-CCl, 5 mM Na oxalate, 0.3 mg/ml of SR protein. Temperature, 30°C; 5 mM Na azide present during tissue homogenization; Millipore filtration. Binding reaction media: 10 μM ⁴⁵Ca-CaCl₂, no oxalate, 0.1 mg/ml of SR protein; otherwise as above.

587

nonfailing group (II) ($p < 0.0001$) or to the cats. The time course of the uptake reaction is shown in Figure 1A.

Calcium Binding

Both human and cat SR vesicles reached their points of apparent peak calcium binding after about 3 min (Figure 1B), the half-maximal time being less than 30 sec. The SR of Group I, again, bound significantly less calcium than that of Group II ($p < 0.01$) or of the cats. This significant difference in peak binding between the failing and nonfailing hearts also could be seen when varying ATP concentrations (1, 2, and 5 mM) were used to start calcium binding by the same SR sample. Figure 2 illustrates this for two different SR incubation assays, the one containing a total calcium concentration of 1×10^{-5} M $CaCl_2$ and no EGTA, the other containing additionally 2.6 μM EGTA to establish a free calcium concentration of 8×10^{-6} M. Control studies in cats did not reveal significant differences between left and right heart calcium uptake or binding.

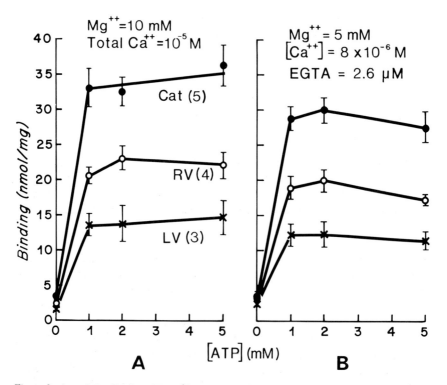

Figure 2. A and B. Cardiac SR Ca^{2+} binding with varying [ATP] in humans with and without chronic heart failure and in cats. Reaction media in A as described for Figure 1B. Reaction media in B as described in text.

Table 1. Dissociation constants (K_D) for cardiac SR Ca^{2+} binding

	K_D ([Ca^{2+}] for 1/2 B_{max})		
	Humans		
[ATP]	Failing left ventricle (Group I)	Nonfailing right ventricle (Group II)	Cats
	($\times$ 10^{-7} M)		
1 mM	2.2 ± 0.4 (7) $p = 0.04$	1.8 ± 0.5 (4) $p = 0.2$	3.1 ± 0.4 (5) $p < 0.01$
5 mM	1.2 ± 0.2 (8)	1.1 ± 0.3 (7)	1.4 ± 0.3 (7)

Human and cat microsomes showed very low calcium dissociation constants (K_D) of approximately 1.8×10^{-7} M (Table 1), a finding consistent with a high SR calcium affinity. This was observed during a series of experiments in which the 3-min SR peak binding was compared at various EGTA-stabilized calcium ion concentrations ranging from 1×10^{-7} M to 8×10^{-6} M. The reactions were started with 1 and 5 mM ATP. At neither ATP concentration did the dissociation constants differ significantly between Groups I and II or in the cats, but they diminished in part significantly with increasing ATP concentrations. They were not correlated with the degree of maximal SR calcium binding.

SR ATPase Activities

The difference between the two human groups in their Ca^{2+}-sensitive (azide-insensitive) SR ATPase activities did not reach significance. During active calcium binding, 15 ± 3 (mean ± S.E.) nmol of Pi/mg of SR per min were released in Group I ($n = 4$), 24 ± 5 in Group II ($n = 4$), and 14 ± 4 ($n = 6$) in the cat assays.

Purity of SR Preparations

The total protein yield of the SR preparations of both humans and cats did not differ significantly, thus excluding the likelihood of heterogeneously distributed "denaturated" protein. ^{45}Ca was added to the homogenates of cardiac muscle in each of the three groups (three experiments in each group). Its distribution in the pellets and supernatants of each of the three groups was similar, suggesting uniform concentrations of calcium-binding proteins among Group I, Group II, and cat cardiac muscle. No significant difference was demonstrated in SR cat calcium binding in the presence and absence of 5 mM sodium azide (three paired experiments). The (Na^+,K^+)-ATPase activity indicating sarcolemmal contaminants was similar in all groups: Group I (1.3 ± 0.4 μM Pi/mg per hr, $n = 5$), Group II (1.3 ± 0.6, $n = 3$), cats (2.6 ± 0.6, $n = 12$).

Clinical Parameters

No significant correlation could be established between the impaired SR calcium accumulation in Group I and clinical parameters, such as additional valve disease, etiology, New York Heart functional classification, abnormalities present in electrocardiographic tracings, size of cardiac silhouettes, hemodynamic findings, or anesthetics used during surgery. There was no significant relationship with the duration of preoperative cardiac symptoms. In neither human group was there a correlation between SR calcium binding and age or sex.

DISCUSSION

The data of this study on human and cat heart microsomes confirm the observations of others who reported a depressed SR function in chronically failing hearts. We found that this was also the case in patients who had chronic congestive heart failure but no evidence for clinically significant coronary disease. The impaired SR calcium transport in these failing hearts does not appear to represent methodological artifacts but rather a true biochemical disturbance in the course of excitation-contraction coupling. It cannot be explained by diminished ATP hydrolysis. Neither the Ca^{2+}-activated SR ATPase activities nor the microsomal calcium affinities changed significantly. Whether this lesion is a cause of or a sequel to heart failure is unknown.

REFERENCES

GERTZ, E. W., HESS, M. L., LAIN, R. F., and BRIGGS, F. N. 1967. Activity of the vesicular calcium pump in the spontaneously failing heart-lung preparation. Circ. Res. 20:477–484.

GERTZ, E. W., STAM, A. C., JR., and SONNENBLICK, E. H. 1970. A quantitative and qualitative defect in the sarcoplasmic reticulum in the hereditary cardiomyopathy of the Syrian hamster. Biochem. Biophys. Res. Commun. 40:746–753.

HARIGAYA, S., and SCHWARTZ, A. 1969. Rate of calcium binding and uptake in normal animal and failing human cardiac muscle: Membrane vesicles (relaxing system) and mitochondria. Circ. Res. 25:781–794.

ITO, Y., SUKO, J., and CHIDSEY, C. A. 1974. Intracellular calcium and myocardial contractility. V. Calcium uptake of sarcoplasmic reticulum fractions in hypertrophied and failing rabbit hearts. J. Mol. Cell Cardiol. 6:237–247.

LINDENMAYER, G. E., SORDAHL, L. A., HARIGAYA, S., ALLEN, J. C., BESCH, H. R., Jr., and SCHWARTZ, A. 1971. Some biochemical studies on subcellular systems isolated from fresh recipient human cardiac tissue obtained during transplantation. Am. J. Cardiol. 27:277–283.

McCOLLUM, W. B., CROW, C., HARIGAYA, S., BAJUSZ, E., and SCHWARTZ, A. 1970. Calcium binding by cardiac relaxing system isolated from myopathic Syrian hamsters (strains 14.6, 82.62, and 40.54). J. Mol. Cell. Cardiol. 1:445–457.

MARSH, B. B. 1959. The estimation of inorganic phosphate in the presence of adenosine triphosphate. Biochem. Biophys. Res. Commun. 32:357–361.

MUIR, J. R., DHALLA, N. S., ORTEZA, J. M., and OLSON, R. E. 1970. Energy-linked calcium transport in subcellular fractions of the failing rat heart. Circ. Res. 26:429–438.

OGAWA, Y. 1968. The apparent binding constant of glycoletherdiaminetetraacetic acid for calcium at neutral pH. J. Biochem. (Tokyo) 64:255–257.

OGAWA, Y., HARIGAYA, S., EBASHI, S., and LEE, K. S. 1971. Sarcoplasmic reticulum: Calcium uptake and release systems in muscle. Methods Pharmacol. 1:327–346.

SCHWARTZ, A., SORDAHL, L. A., ENTMAN, M. L., ALLEN, J. C., REDDY, Y. S., GOLDSTEIN, M. A., LUCHI, R. J., and WYBORNY, L. E. 1973. Abnormal biochemistry in myocardial failure. Am. J. Cardiol. 32:407–422.

SORDAHL, L. A., McCOLLUM, W. B., WOOD, W. G., and SCHWARTZ, A. 1973. Mitochondria and sarcoplasmic reticulum function in cardiac hypertrophy and failure. Am. J. Physiol. 224:497–502.

SUKO, J., VOGEL, J. H. K., and CHIDSEY, C. A. 1970. Intracellular calcium and myocardial contractility. III. Reduced calcium uptake and ATPase of the sarcoplasmic reticular fraction prepared from chronically failing calf hearts. Circ. Res. 27:235–247.

SULAKHE, P. V., and DHALLA, N. S. 1971. Excitation-contraction coupling in heart. VII. Calcium accumulation in subcellular particles in congestive heart failure. J. Clin. Invest. 50:1019–1027.

SULAKHE, P. V., and DHALLA, N. S. 1973. Excitation-contraction coupling in heart. X. Further studies on the energy-linked calcium transport by subcellular particles in the failing heart of myopathic hamster. Biochem. Med. 8:18–27.

Mailing address:
Carlos E. Harrison, Jr., M.D.,
Mayo Clinic and Mayo Foundation,
Rochester, Minnesota 55901 (USA).

Recent Advances in Studies on
Cardiac Structure and Metabolism, Volume 12
Cardiac Adaptation
Edited by T. Kobayashi, Y. Ito, and G. Rona
Copyright 1978 University Park Press Baltimore

EVALUATION OF PERFUSION CONDITIONS
IN CARDIOPULMONARY BYPASS

S. C̄ANKOVIĆ-DARRACOTT,[1] M. V. BRAIMBRIDGE,[1]
J. CHAYEN,[2] and L. BITENSKY[2]

[1] Department of Cardiothoracic Surgery, St. Thomas' Hospital,
London, England
[2] Division of Cellular Biology, Kennedy Institute of Rheumatology,
London, England

SUMMARY

Fresh sections of left ventricular drill biopsies, taken at the beginning and end of cardio-pulmonary bypass in 164 patients undergoing aortic valve replacement, have been analyzed for myocardial function. This has been assessed by changes in biochemical function, measured by semi-quantitative histochemical methods, and by changes in birefringence, measured quantitatively by polarization microscopy. It has been shown that continuous perfusion at 32°C with the heart beating provided better preservation than did the other three perfusion procedures, in all of which the heart was fibrillating. More recently, in a small number of cases, cardioplegic arrest has been found to give even better preservation.

INTRODUCTION

Over the past 12 years, the value of histochemical and birefringence analysis of myocardial function has been established in studies on 1,575 left ventricular biopsies from patients undergoing open-heart surgery for various conditions (Niles *et al.,* 1964; Braimbridge *et al.,* 1973a; Braimbridge *et al.,* 1973b). For the present study on the effect of various conditions of perfusion, attention has been confined to hearts subjected to a single defect.

MATERIALS AND METHODS

This study was made on full thickness left ventricular biopsies taken with an air-powered drill (Braimbridge and Niles, 1964) from 164 patients undergoing aortic valve replacement. The first biopsy was taken immediately before the insertion of the left ventricular vent, and the second was taken when the vent was removed at the end of bypass.

This work was supported by a grant from the British Heart Foundation.

The biopsies were chilled, sectioned, and reacted histochemically. The results were graded semi-quantitatively as described by Braimbridge *et al.* (1973b) and were assessed by nonparametric statistics (Siegel, 1956).

To measure the changes in birefringence, the selected myocardial fibers were placed at the 45° position in a quantitative polarizing microscope (Zeiss), and the optical path difference (in nm) was measured by means of a Brace-Kohler $\lambda/30$ compensator. A solution of ATP (2 mM) was then added, and the new optical path difference (OPD) measured.

RESULTS AND DISCUSSION

The changes in OPD measure the change in birefringence induced by ATP. The value of such measurements in detecting deteriorating myocardial function has been established in other studies using dogs (Darracott *et al.*, 1973). An example in the human heart is shown in Table 1. In this patient undergoing aortic valve replacement, perfusion of the left coronary artery proved to be very difficult. After 165 minutes, when the valve had been inserted, the heart was unable to function normally without supportive bypass. After a further 90 minutes of supportive bypass, the birefringence change in the affected epimyocardium had fallen to a disastrously low value and that of the endomyocardium was moderately altered. At postmortem the muscle produced virtually no change in birefringence, which is consistent with the view that this parameter reflects living function.

For assessment of the effects of bypass, an increase in the histochemical gradings of two units was defined as a moderate deterioration, while an increase of four or more units was taken to indicate severe deterioration (Braimbridge *et al.*, 1973b). With regard to the change in birefringence, a decrease of 0.7–1.48 nm was graded as moderate deterioration, and a decrease of greater than 1.48 nm (as in Table 1) was indicative of severe deterioration in function.

In the present study, five bypass procedures have been used: three groups involving fibrillating hearts, one group of beating hearts perfused continuously at 32°C, and one group treated by cardioplegic arrest. In this series of 164 patients, the histochemical results (Table 2) show that the best preservation was achieved

Table 1. Change in birefringence in a deteriorating heart caused by severe atheroma of the left coronary artery

Time on bypass	Epimyocardial (nm)	Endomyocardial (nm)
Beginning	3.22	4.62
165 min	3.21	4.01
255 min (DOT)	1.40	3.54
Post-mortem	0.00	0.42

Table 2. Histochemical and birefringence assessment of the preservation of the myocardium in patients during aortic valve replacement[a]

	Perfusion system				
	Intermittent		Continuous		Cardioplegia
	10–15°C (n = 26)	30°C (n = 12)	30°C (n = 50)	32°C (n = 66)	16°C (n = 10)
Average period of aortic occlusion	104 min	69 min	98 min	96 min	85 min
Average % time left coronary artery perfused	21	34	73	70	0
Average % time right coronary artery perfused	18	20	47	61	0
HISTOCHEMISTRY					
Good preservation	73	67	90	92	100
Moderate deterioration	19	33	10	8	0
Severe deterioration	8	0	0	0	0
BIREFRINGENCE					
Good preservation	84	67	72	85	100
Moderate deterioration	10.5	33	14	15	0
Severe deterioration	5.5	0	14	0	0

[a]Results given as percentage of each group showing any particular classification.

with either continuous perfusion at 32°C or at 30°C. The birefringence measurements were in agreement in that they showed best preservation with the perfusion at 32°C. However, they also demonstrated that more severe deterioration of this function occurred during continuous perfusion at 30°C when the heart was fibrillating. Intermittent perfusion of fibrillating hearts at 30°C appeared to give less satisfactory preservation than did continuous perfusion at this temperature, although the numbers studied were too few for definite conclusions. Lowering the temperature to 10–15°C did not improve the situation, i.e., by both forms of assessment, more patients showed severe deterioration.

Among the, at present, small number of hearts subjected to cardioplegic arrest, all showed good preservation with no deterioration.

The potential value of the birefringence measurements as an immediate prognostic guide is shown in a study on 27 patients undergoing aortic valve replacement. In 21 of these patients, the birefringence values at the end of bypass were equal to, or greater than, those at the beginning. In six, however, the second value was markedly lower than the first. Of this series, only those six patients caused clinical concern in that they showed low cardiac output and severe dysrhythmias post-operatively.

REFERENCES

BRAIMBRIDGE, M. V., DARRACOTT, S., BITENSKY, L., and CHAYEN, J. 1973a. Cytochemical analysis of left ventricular biopsies in open-heart surgery: A pilot study. Beitr. Pathol. 148:255–264.
BRAIMBRIDGE, M. V., DARRACOTT, S., CLEMENT, A. J., BITENSKY, L., and CHAYEN, J. 1973b. Myocardial deterioration during aortic valve replacement assessed by cellular biological tests. J. Thorac. Cardiovasc. Surg. 66:241–246.
BRAIMBRIDGE, M. V., and NILES, N. R. 1964. Left ventricular drill biopsy. J. Thorac. Cardiovasc. Surg. 47:685–686.
DARRACOTT, S., BRAIMBRIDGE, M. V., BITENSKY, L., and CHAYEN, J. 1973. Myocardial deterioration during perfusion of isolated dog heart assessed by cellular biological tests. J. Thorac. Cardiovasc. Surg. 66:247–254.
NILES, N. R., CHAYEN, J., CUNNINGHAM, G. J., and BITENSKY, L. 1964. The histochemical demonstration of adenosine triphosphatase activity in the myocardium. J. Histochem. Cytochem. 12:740–743.
SIEGEL, S. 1956. Non-parametric Statistics. McGraw-Hill Book Co., New York.

Mailing address:
Sally C̄anković-Darracott, B.Sc.,
Department of Cardiothoracic Surgery, St. Thomas' Hospital,
London, SE1 (England).

Recent Advances in Studies on
Cardiac Structure and Metabolism, Volume 12
Cardiac Adaptation
Edited by T. Kobayashi, Y. Ito, and G. Rona
Copyright 1978 University Park Press Baltimore

ULTRASTRUCTURAL CHANGE IN MYOCARDIUM SUBSEQUENT TO ISCHEMIC CARDIOPLEGIA "NO-REFLOW PHENOMENON"

M. SUNAMORI,[1] R. HATANO,[1] T. SUZUKI,[1]
N. YAMAMOTO,[1] T. TSUKUURA,[1] T. YAMADA,[1]
T. KUMAZAWA,[2] M. NAKAGAWA,[2] and T. SUNAGA[3]

[1] Department of Surgery, Tokyo Medical and Dental
University, Yushima, Bunkyo-ku, Tokyo, Japan
[2] Department of Anesthesia, Tokyo Medical and Dental
University, Yushima, Bunkyo-ku, Tokyo, Japan
[3] Department of Internal Medicine, Tokyo Medical and
Dental University, Yushima, Bunkyo-ku, Tokyo, Japan

SUMMARY

Mongrel dogs were subjected to cardiopulmonary bypass with hemodilution and to normo-thermic anoxic arrest for 30 minutes, to study the subepicardial and the subendocardial myocardial ultrastructure and the DPTI/TTI ratio. "No-reflow phenomenon" was demon-strated in the myocardium after cardiopulmonary bypass, associated with normothermic anoxic arrest. No-reflow phenomenon was a contributing factor to subendocardial ischemia in the normotrophied ventricle after open-heart surgery. Severe hemodilution with hemo-globin less than 5.0 g% resulted in irreversible damage in both myocardial layers.

INTRODUCTION

It has been known since the 1930s that the subendocardium is more easily injured than the subepicardium, although the pathogenesis of subendocardial vulnerability is not clarified yet. Subendocardial ischemia after open-heart sur-gery is a distinct complication that may become fatal.

The authors studied the morphological differences between the subepicardial and subendocardial myocardium of mongrel dogs subjected to cardiopulmonary bypass in an attempt to determine the pathogenesis of subendocardial vulner-ability to ischemia. In addition, the relationship between hemodilution and the fine structure of the subendocardium subjected to anoxic arrest, supported by cardiopulmonary bypass, was studied.

MATERIALS AND METHODS

Thirteen mongrel dogs were anesthetized with GOF (0.7%) or GO-Morphine (3 mg/kg) and left thoracotomy was performed. Cardiopulmonary bypass was instituted with the prime of Ringer-lactate solution, with no hyperosmolar solution, such as mannitol, added. The dogs were divided into two groups according to the degree of hemodilution; in Group 1, hemoglobin was diluted to less than 5.0 g%, and, in Group 2, hemoglobin concentration was between 5 and 10 g%.

After total cardiopulmonary bypass was obtained, the ascending aorta was cross-clamped for 30 min to produce anoxic arrest of the myocardium.

Transmural myocardial biopsy was performed, and specimens were divided into subepicardial and the subendocardial layers, which were fixed in 1% of glutaraldehyde solution (pH 7.20, 0°–4°C), and washed out with phosphate-buffered sucrose solution and stained with 2% osmium tetroxide solution (pH 7.20, 0°–4°C). Then, specimens were embedded in Epon-812. Ultrathin sections were obtained by Porter-Blum MT-II microtome. Sections were stained with lead acetate and uranyl acetate. Electron microscopic examination was made with the Hitachi HT-12S.

The supply-demand relationship of the subendocardium was studied by DPTI/TTI ratio, which was measured by the pressure curves of the left ventricular and arterial pressures by using planimetry.

A catheter was inserted into the coronary sinus to obtain coronary sinus venous blood for studying the oxygen content and the metabolites, such as glucose, lactate, pyruvate, glutamic oxalo-acetic transaminase (GOT), glutamic pyruvic transaminase (GPT), lactate dehydrogenase (LDH), and creatine phosphokinase (CPK).

Transmural biopsy was carried out before cardiopulmonary bypass, after the cessation of anoxic arrest, and during recovery at 120 min after the unclamping of the aorta.

RESULTS

Results on the metabolic changes were similar to the previous reports.

With regard to ultrastructural changes of the myocardium, there were no differences between the ultrastructural changes of the subepicardial and the subendocardial myocardium before cardiopulmonary bypass. The ultrastructural changes after anoxic arrest included changes in the mitochondria, such as swelling, vacuolation, disarray of the cristae, and lysis, as well as formation of contraction bands, widening of the intercalated discs, interstitial edema, and narrowing of capillary lumen associated with endothelial cell swelling (Figures 1 and 2). These findings were observed in both layers of the myocardium after anoxic arrest and in the recovery period following the restoration of coronary circulation. However, the subendocardial layer was injured more markedly than the subepicardial layer.

The dogs in Group 1, except for two, were unable to survive more than 45 min after restoration of coronary circulation, and fine structure of the myo-

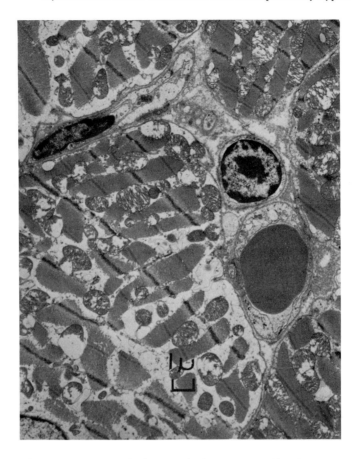

Figure 1. The ultrastructure of the left ventricular subendocardium immediately after 30 min of anoxic arrest with moderate hemodilution: loss of glycogen granules, interstitial edema, swelling of capillary endothelial cells, narrowing of capillary lumen, and degeneration of the mitochondria. Original magnification: ✕ 6,000.

cardium in both myocardial layers was severely damaged, with interstitial edema and more marked mitochondrial changes in the subendocardial than in the subepicardial layer.

Changes in the supply-demand relationship (DPTI/TTI ratio) were as follows:

In Group 1, the ratio was 0.85 ± 0.34 at 30 min after restoration of coronary circulation and 0.80 ± 0.37 at 60 min, after which it returned to the normal level.

In Group 2, the ratio was 0.74 ± 0.19 at 30 min and 0.85 ± 0.13 at 60 min after restoration of coronary circulation, after which it returned to the normal level.

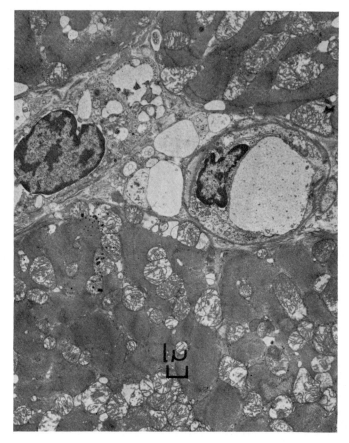

Figure 2. Ultrastructure of the left ventricular subepicardial layer, immediately after 30 min of anoxic arrest with moderate hemodilution (compare to Figure 1). Original magnification: × 6,000.

DISCUSSION

Myocardial ultrastructural changes after open-heart surgery were reported to include depletion of glycogen, interstitial edema, degenerative changes of the mitochondria, contraction bands, and swelling of capillary endothelial cells.

The no-reflow phenomenon has been reported in the brain (Ames *et al.,* 1968), in the kidney (Sommers and Jamison, 1971), and in the ischemic myocardium after the ligation of the coronary artery (Kloner, Ganote, and Jennings, 1974; Willerson *et al.,* 1975).

It appears that the no-reflow phenomenon also is responsible for the subendocardial myocardial vulnerability observed in this study after cardiopulmonary bypass. Ultrastructural damages were more marked in the subendocardium after anoxic arrest; the subendocardial ischemia was assessed by DPTI/TTI ratio (Buckberg *et al.,* 1972) during the recovery period after restoration of coronary circulation.

Severe hemodilution with hemoglobin concentration less than 5 g% has a deleterious effect on the myocardium.

Acknowledgments   The authors extend their appreciation to Mr. H. Miyamoto for his excellent assistance in the use of the electron microscope.

REFERENCES

AMES, A., III, WRIGHT, R. L., KOWADA, M., THURSTON, J. M., and MAJNO, G. 1968. Cerebral ischemia. II: The no-reflow phenomenon. Am. J. Pathol. 52:437–453.

BUCKBERG, G. D., FIXLER, D. E., ARCHIE, J. P., and HOFFMAN, J. I. E. 1972. Experimental subendocardial ischemia in dogs with normal coronary arteries. Circ. Res. 30:67–81.

KLONER, R. A., GANOTE, C. E., and JENNINGS, R. B. 1974. The no-reflow phenomenon after temporary coronary occlusion in the dog. J. Clin. Invest. 54:1496–1508.

SOMMERS, W. K., and JAMISON, R. L. 1971. The no-reflow phenomenon in renal ischemia. Lab. Invest. 25:635–643.

WILLERSON, J. T., WATSON, J. T., HUTTON, I., *et al.* 1975. Reduced myocardial reflow and increased vascular resistance following prolonged myocardial ischemia in the dog. Circ. Res. 36:771–781.

Mailing address:
Makoto Sunamori, M.D.
First Department of Surgery, Tokyo Medical and Dental University,
1-5-45, Yushima, Bunkyo-ku, Tokyo (Japan)

TISSUE CULTURE
OF
CARDIAC MUSCLE CELLS

Recent Advances in Studies on
Cardiac Structure and Metabolism, Volume 12
Cardiac Adaptation
Edited by T. Kobayashi, Y. Ito, and G. Rona
Copyright 1978 University Park Press Baltimore

TISSUE CULTURE OF MYOCARDIAL CELLS:
INTRODUCTORY REMARKS

A. WOLLENBERGER

Division of Cellular and Molecular Cardiology, Central
Institute of Heart and Circulatory Regulation Research,
Academy of Sciences of the DDR, Berlin, German Democratic Republic

As can be seen from Figure 1, tissue culture of beating myocardial cells had its beginnings about 65 years ago. The figure is a reproduction of part of the first page of a paper by Burrows (1912) entitled, "Rhythmische Kontraktionen der isolierten Hermuskelzelle außerhalb des Organismus." Burrows was a student of Ross Harrison who, only five years earlier in 1907 (Harrison, 1907), had inaugurated the area of modern tissue culture with his work on the cultivation of nerve tissue. In his paper, Burrows described that, several days after small pieces of embryonic chick heart were placed in medium consisting essentially of blood plasma and embryo extract, a few spontaneously contracting cells were seen growing out of the explant. These cells sometimes became isolated from neighboring cells and each would beat at its own intrinsic rate. This observation was in harmony with the old view that the cell was the elementary structural and functional unit of heart muscle, a view which, at the beginning of this century, was superseded temporarily by the belief, or rather the misbelief, of histologists that cardiac tissue was a syncytium. The observation also provided support for the myogenic, as opposed to the neurogenic, theory of the heart beat.

Without underrating the fundamental importance of Burrows' findings, there are certain disadvantages inherent in the method of explant culture. Thus, the number of pulsating cells is very low compared to the number of quiescent ones. Cultivation is possible only in natural nutrient media that contain a host of undefined components. Autolysis in hypoxic necrotizing regions in the interior of the explants can release additional, undefined, biologically active substances capable of affecting the living cells. Furthermore, it can be argued that the spontaneous rhythmic activity of cells in the outer growth zone of the explanted cardiac muscle fragments may have originated in the body of the explant, which might still harbor functionally intact nerve elements. These drawbacks were largely overcome when Rinaldini (1954) and Cavanough (1955) succeeded, by the use of trypsin (Moscona 1952), in dissociating embryonic avian heart muscle

605

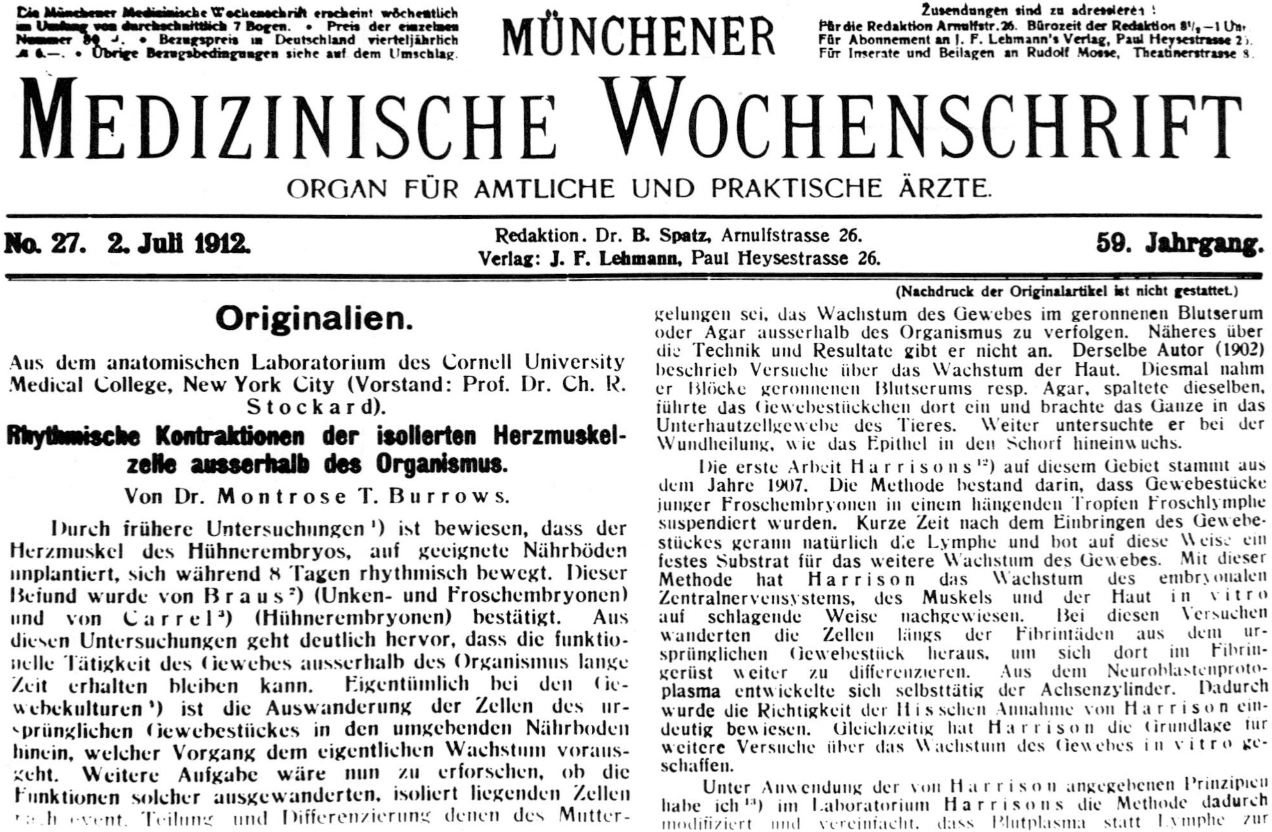

Die Münchener Medizinische Wochenschrift erscheint wöchentlich im Umfang von durchschnittlich 7 Bogen. • Preis der einzelnen Nummer 34 J. • Bezugspreis in Deutschland vierteljährlich 4 L—. • Übrige Bezugsbedingungen siehe auf dem Umschlag.

Zusendungen sind zu adressieren:
Für die Redaktion Arnulfstr. 26. Bürozeit der Redaktion 8½—1 Uhr.
Für Abonnement an I. F. Lehmann's Verlag, Paul Heysestrasse 26.
Für Inserate und Beilagen an Rudolf Mosse, Theaterstrasse 8.

MÜNCHENER MEDIZINISCHE WOCHENSCHRIFT

ORGAN FÜR AMTLICHE UND PRAKTISCHE ÄRZTE.

No. 27. 2. Juli 1912.

Redaktion. Dr. B. Spatz, Arnulfstrasse 26.
Verlag: J. F. Lehmann, Paul Heysestrasse 26.

59. Jahrgang.

Originalien.

(Nachdruck der Originalartikel ist nicht gestattet.)

Aus dem anatomischen Laboratorium des Cornell University Medical College, New York City (Vorstand: Prof. Dr. Ch. R. Stockard).

Rhythmische Kontraktionen der isolierten Herzmuskelzelle ausserhalb des Organismus.

Von Dr. Montrose T. Burrows.

Durch frühere Untersuchungen[1] ist bewiesen, dass der Herzmuskel des Hühnerembryos, auf geeignete Nährböden implantiert, sich während 8 Tagen rhythmisch bewegt. Dieser Befund wurde von Braus[2] (Unken- und Froschembryonen) und von Carrel[3] (Hühnerembryonen) bestätigt. Aus diesen Untersuchungen geht deutlich hervor, dass die funktionelle Tätigkeit des Gewebes ausserhalb des Organismus lange Zeit erhalten bleiben kann. Eigentümlich bei den Gewebekulturen[4] ist die Auswanderung der Zellen des ursprünglichen Gewebestückes in den umgebenden Nährboden hinein, welcher Vorgang dem eigentlichen Wachstum vorausgeht. Weitere Aufgabe wäre nun zu erforschen, ob die Funktionen solcher ausgewanderten, isoliert liegenden Zellen noch existent, Teilung und Differenzierung denen des Mutter-

gelungen sei, das Wachstum des Gewebes im geronnenen Blutserum oder Agar ausserhalb des Organismus zu verfolgen. Näheres über die Technik und Resultate gibt er nicht an. Derselbe Autor (1902) beschrieb Versuche über das Wachstum der Haut. Diesmal nahm er Blöcke geronnenen Blutserums resp. Agar, spaltete dieselben, führte das Gewebestückchen dort ein und brachte das Ganze in das Unterhautzellgewebe des Tieres. Weiter untersuchte er bei der Wundheilung, wie das Epithel in den Schorf hineinwuchs.

Die erste Arbeit Harrisons[12] auf diesem Gebiet stammt aus dem Jahre 1907. Die Methode bestand darin, dass Gewebestücke junger Froschembryonen in einem hängenden Tropfen Froschlymphe suspendiert wurden. Kurze Zeit nach dem Einbringen des Gewebestückes geriet natürlich die Lymphe und bot auf diese Weise ein festes Substrat für das weitere Wachstum des Gewebes. Mit dieser Methode hat Harrison das Wachstum des embryonalen Zentralnervensystems, des Muskels und der Haut in vitro auf schlagende Weise nachgewiesen. Bei diesen Versuchen wanderten die Zellen längs der Fibrinfäden aus dem ursprünglichen Gewebestück heraus, um sich dort im Fibringerüst weiter zu differenzieren. Aus dem Neuroblastenprotoplasma entwickelte sich selbsttätig der Achsenzylinder. Dadurch wurde die Richtigkeit der Hisschen Annahme von Harrison eindeutig bewiesen. Gleichzeitig hat Harrison die Grundlage für weitere Versuche über das Wachstum des Gewebes in vitro geschaffen.

Unter Anwendung der von Harrison angegebenen Prinzipien habe ich[14] im Laboratorium Harrisons die Methode dadurch modifiziert und vereinfacht, dass Blutplasma statt Lymphe zur

606

Figure 1. Reproduction of part of the first page of Burrows' 1912 paper on rhythmic contractions of heart cells in tissue culture.

into discrete single cells, a large fraction of which exhibited spontaneous rhythmic contractile activity when explanted and cultured *in vitro*. Dr. Harary (Harary and Farley, 1963) applied this technique to post-natal mammalian heart muscle. It also has become possible to keep cultures of beating myocardial cells alive for several weeks in chemically defined media (Halle and Wollenberger, 1970).

When dissociated single heart cells that are suspended in culture media are allowed to settle on a glass or plastic substrate, they spread out and form connections with each other if the cell density is sufficiently high; they may aggregate to a pulsating solid monolayer, or they may even grow to multilayers. Such aggregates could be considered to be tissues. The same applies to the multicellular, spherical bodies formed from suspensions of single heart cells by gyrorotary motion (Fishman and Moscona, 1971). It is only in this sense that we can speak of "tissue culture" of heart cells when dealing with aggregates of cells that at the outset of cultivation existed as single isolated individuals. Such cultures are more correctly classified as "cell cultures"; the term tissue culture is reserved for those situations in which compact tissue is the starting material for cultivation.

In keeping with the introductory nature of these remarks, suffice it to state without further comment that, as models for the study of problems of cardiac cellular structuration, metabolism, and function, cultures of dispersed beating cardiac cells have their limitations which must be recognized. However, they offer unique possibilities for an experimental attack on a variety of problems of myocardial biology that are not, or are much less, amenable to solution by work with intact heart muscle. Significant advances in this direction are presented in this volume.

At a time when the cost of laboratory animals and materials is steadily rising, it seems appropriate to note that cell culture is a relatively inexpensive technique. It enables the experimenter to reduce the number of test animals and to work with minute amounts of drugs and other substances that may be scarce and expensive. In measuring frequency and other parameters of contraction, an individual, isolated heart cell—a microheart, so to speak—of which there may be thousands or more in a culture dish, carries the same statistical weight as a whole organ. If a line of beating myocardial cells were available, the economical advantage of working with heart cell cultures would be utilized to the fullest. This would provide us with a continuous supply of a population of such cells more homogeneous than the primary cultures hitherto in use. Professor Paul (1970) from Glasgow stated some time ago that one of his graduate students had succeeded in subculturing beating cells from the heart of two-day-old rabbit embryos; but, to this author's knowledge, no report from his or any other laboratory has appeared in the literature concerning the continuous cultivation of beating heart cells. The idea does not seem to be entirely utopian, particularly because it has been reported that myocardial cells possessing well differentiated myofibrils can pass through periods of rapid DNA synthesis and can undergo mitosis, both *in vivo* (Goldstein, Claycomb, and Schwartz, 1974) and *in vitro* (Kasten, 1972).

REFERENCES

BURROWS, M. T. 1912. Rhythmische Kontraktionen der isolierten herzmuskelzelle außerhalb des organismus. Munch. Med. Wochenschr. 59:1473–1475.

CAVANOUGH, M. W. 1955. Pulsation, migration and division in dissociated chick embryo heart cells *in vitro*. J. Exp. Zool. 128:573–589.

FISHMAN, D. A., and MOSCONA, A. A. 1971. Reconstruction of heart tissue from suspensions of embryonic myocardial cells: Ultrastructural studies on dispersed and reaggregated cells. *In* N. Alpert (ed.), Cardiac Hypertrophy, pp. 125–139. Academic Press, New York.

GOLDSTEIN, M. A., CLAYCOMB, W. C., and SCHWARTZ, A. 1974. DNA synthesis and mitosis in well-differentiated mammalian cardiocytes. Science 183:212–213.

HALLE, W., and WOLLENBERGER, A. 1970. Differentiation and behavior of isolated embryonic and neonatal heart cells in a chemically defined medium. Am. J. Cardiol. 25:292–299.

HARARY, I., and FARLEY, B. 1963. *In vitro* studies on single beating rat heart cells. I. Growth and organization. Exp. Cell Res. 29:466–474.

HARRISON, R. G. 1907. Observations on the living developing nerve fiber. Proc. Soc. Exp. Biol. Med. 4:140–145.

KASTEN, F. H. 1972. Rat myocardial cells *in vitro:* Mitosis and differentiated properties. *In Vitro* 8:128–149.

MOSCONA, A. 1952. Cell suspensions from organ rudiments of the early chick embryo. Exp. Cell Res. 3:535–539.

PAUL, J. 1970. Personal communication.

RINALDINI, L. M. 1954. A quantitative method for growing animal cells. Nature 173:1134–1135.

Mailing address:
A. Wollenberger, Ph.D.,
Division of Cellular and Molecular Cardiology,
Central Institute of Heart and Circulatory Research,
Academy of Sciences of the DDR, 1115 Berlin-Buch (German Democratic Republic).

Recent Advances in Studies on
Cardiac Structure and Metabolism, Volume 12
Cardiac Adaptation
Edited by T. Kobayashi, Y. Ito, and G. Rona
Copyright 1978 University Park Press Baltimore

EFFECT OF ENVIRONMENTAL FACTORS AND TISSUE CULTURE METHODOLOGY IN PRODUCING AND STUDYING CULTURED CARDIAC CELLS

P. PADIEU,[1] C. FRELIN,[1] A. PINSON,[2] F. CHARBONNÉ,[3] and P. ATHIAS[1]

[1] School of Medicine, University of Dijon, Dijon, France
[2] Hadassah Medical School, Hebrew University, Jerusalem, Israel
[3] School of Medicine, University of Clermont-Ferrand, France

SUMMARY

Improvement in the method of heart cell cultures is described and justified in relation to environmental factors. The validity of such cardiac cell culture for cardiac research is discussed in light of particular cellular activities: differentiation of lipoprotein lipase, myoglobin biosynthesis, glucose and fatty acid metabolism, pleiotypic responses (protein, RNA, and DNA biosyntheses, substrates transports) to serum stimulation, and the architectonic growth of muscle and nonmuscle cells.

INTRODUCTION

In a living economy, the understanding of the differentiation of specific functions in a tissue during its development or maintenance is often hampered by multiple interactions between tissues, organs, and the numerous compounds carried by body fluids.

At the same time as other *in vitro* methods, tissue culture was developed as a tool for cellular biology. The culture of pieces of tissue, or organotypic cultures, was done for the first time by Harrison in 1907 when he followed the growth of neuronal axons. Strangeways and Fell (1927) successfully extended the method, while Wolff and Haffen (1952) simplified it. The culture of isolated cells, or histiotypic cultures, was first proposed in 1903 by Jolly, who grew blood cells, and, in 1912, Burrows first observed the divisions and association of myoblasts in a beating structure from fragments of chick heart, demonstrating the myogenetic origin of heart contraction.

These investigations were supported by contracts from : INSERM (ATP 6, ATP 21, CRL 6), DGRST (ACC BFM), CNRS (ERA 267), and NATO, and fellowships from INSERM, CNRS, and DGRST for one of the authors (A.P.).

Both then and now, dissociating tissue into isolated cells is a major difficulty in cardiac cell culture, as well as selecting a cell population from an organ. Although trypsin dissociation was first used in 1916 by Rous and Jones, this technique was forgotten until Moscona revived it in 1952. In 1955, Cavanaugh isolated and grew cells from the hearts of chick embryos, and a few years later Harary and Farley (1960) succeeded in growing cardiac cells from postnatal rats.

The main advantages of heart cell cultures are: 1) the reproducible production of relatively large amounts of biological material into many experimental units, i.e., culture dishes, from a single initial inoculum; 2) *in vitro* production of a rhythmic automatic neomyocardium; 3) ability to control the extracellular space; 4) facility of medium modification for time-course analyses; 5) simplicity of quantitative $^{14}CO_2$ production *in situ* in incubation chambers (Pinson and Padieu, 1974a).

In spite of these advantages, one could ask whether such cultured cells really reproduce genuine cardiac tissue or whether they represent an artificial living system. Cells adapt themselves to culture conditions, and, moreover, certain types of cells grow preferentially. But such cultures *in vitro* have the ability to acquire and maintain rhythmic and automatic contraction; therefore, they are ideally suited for cardiac research. Our intention in this chapter is to examine and define the validity of this biological system. It is therefore necessary to gain an understanding of the response of the cell to its differentiating program in relation to extracellular influences that act through the culture medium.

METHODS AND DISCUSSION

Culture of Cardiac Cells

Culture method remains essentially the same as described initially by Harary and Farley (1960) or by Harary, Hoover, and Farley (1974). Minced hearts from one- to five-day-old rats are dissociated by agitation by a magnetic stirring in a trypsin solution. After a certain period of agitation, the isolated cells in suspension are decanted into a centrifuge tube while stopping the trypsin activity. The cells are pelleted by centrifugation and then resuspended in culture medium. Before seeding, cells are counted so that they can be inoculated as desired, between 5.10^5 and 2.10^6 per 20-cm^2 dish.

Several improvements have been introduced in this laboratory in order to protect the cells from the many aggressions caused by changes from their normal environment (Chessebeuf *et al.*, 1974). Particularly, modifications have been made to provide protection from three major cellular aggressions that arise from the actions of trypsin, media, and water during explantation and recovery until the onset of growth. Cells are dissociated in 0.1 g/100 ml of trypsin (Calbiochem, grade B) at 35–36°C in a reconstituted Ham F10 medium minus Ca^{2+} and Mg^{2+} at pH 7.4 in a flask (25- or 50-ml) for suspension culture (Wheaton 35 66 75).

The magnetic stirrer is suspended vertically, thereby preventing shearing of the cells. The initial trypsinization occurs in 10 min with a stirrer speed of 150 rpm; the supernatant is decanted off, fresh trypsin is added, and the process is repeated two more times, but at 400 rpm the third time. Then, the fourth, fifth, and sixth trypsinizations, necessary to disintegrate all the tissues, last 25 min each at 400 rpm. At each trypsinization the cell suspension is decanted into a 16-ml culture tube containing 6 ml of fetal calf serum (FCS) (Gibco). The tube is then centrifuged for 10 min, without exceeding 100 g, thus avoiding cell damage. The FCS stops the action of trypsin, but, more importantly, it protects the cells and their membranes altered by trypsin. The plating efficiency is far better after this serum treatment than with other sera.

The third most important modification is the use of very pure water. Spring water (100 liters), bottled in glass, is passed downward (20 ml/min) through tandem containers (35-liters) filled with charcoal that has not been pretreated in any way. The purified water is then led directly to an all glass, refluxing, continuous flow still. The once run water is then batch-distilled three times (eliminating heads and tails) in a specially designed Vigreux column 3.5 m high with improved adiabatic characteristics and a timed reflux head (20 sec reflux, 6 sec flush) at a flow of 0.8 liter/hr. The water is used as soon as possible for culture medium preparation or stored at $4°$ C.

Observing the original method of Harary and Farley (1960), the culture medium is supplemented with FCS and human serum (HS), 10% each, and 13 mg/100 ml of $CaCl_2$. It has been verified that serum of the adult human best promotes growth, particularly of the AB group, but, because of its scarcity, we use serum from a pooled A and O group (1:1).

In conclusion, five factors seem to be of major significance in the successful growth of heart cells (or any others): 1) the purity of water, 2) the trypsinization medium, 3) the trypsin inhibition by FCS, 4) the joint use of HS and FCS, and 5) the elimination of all physical stress that may alter cell integrity. Pure mechanical dissociation is more deleterious than the use of trypsin, which is, at present, the least cell damaging proteolytic enzyme when compared to pronase, collagenase, hyaluronidase, etc. As a result of trypsin activity variations, it is necessary to adjust the concentration of trypsin by comparing the yield in viable, isolated cells. Grade B trypsin contains $MgSO_4$, which has a beneficial effect on cell dissociation. Therefore, this amount of added Mg^{2+} is maintained for other trypsins.

The culture unit, including a sterile room, is protected under a positive pressure by air-conditioned air sterilized through absolute filters.

Cellular Activities of Cultured Heart Cells and Interactions with Culture Medium

The cellular activities of the culture are regulated by trophic factors, i.e., nutrients and hormones, as far as specific enzymes and hormone targets are present in the cells; therefore, two kinds of factors may act within such cultures:

1. Extracellular factors: energetic nutrients, plastic nutrients for macromolecular syntheses, among which vitamins, hormones, and some nutrients are essential. Most of them are supplied by the synthetic medium except for lipids; hormones and more or less known factors are supplemented by the sera.
2. Intracellular factors, restricted to gene action because their relations to extracellular factors are frequently ill-defined.

Two sets of events observed in cardiac cell cultures are described below. First, the specific metabolism of cardiac origin is discussed, and, second, the growth events that are the response of "normal" cultured cells to serum stimulation and that can be partly related to cardiac cell lineage are considered.

Specific metabolisms of cultured cardiac cells: Activities of specific proteins

Lipoprotein lipase as a marker of lipid metabolism differentiation Harary, McCarl, and Farley (1966) have shown that cardiac cells were unable to grow and to beat in a synthetic culture medium. Its supplementation with fatty acids (FA) restored beating but not growth. Conversely, upon supplementation with delipidated serum, the culture resumed growth but not contractions. As in the heart (Bing *et al.,* 1954), the cultured cells must contain the necessary enzymes to metabolize lipids providing most of the energetic needs. Therefore, the assay of membrane lipoprotein lipase (LPL) has been chosen as a marker of this lipid metabolism in the culture because triglycerides (TG) cannot be taken up by the heart cell without prior hydrolysis to FA by LPL. There is a correlation between LPL activity and the ability of heart to assimilate TG; moreover, this enzyme is highly adaptative (for references see Pinson, Frelin, and Padieu, 1973). In cell cultures (Pinson, Frelin, and Padieu, 1973), after days 4–6, there is a sharp fourfold increase of activity of LPL with a plateau at about day 12 (Figure 1). In the presence of puromycin, there is a small increase of LPL activity. Comparing LPL to the curve for $[^3H]$ thymidine uptake, the LPL activity begins to increase after the period of exponential growth of the culture. Therefore, the development of LPL activity marks the myoblast maturation to a true myocyte for mechanical work sustained by the differentiation of lipid metabolism enzymes.

Myoglobin Myoglobin levels in the normal heart have been quantified (Nahani, 1973) by chromatography. Myoglobin increases slowly from the birth level of 200 μg/g of fresh tissue, until it sharply increases to 400 μg/g between days 6–8, and stays at this plateau until day 21. Then, myoglobin increases strongly to 800 μg/g between days 21–26 and then slowly increases again to reach a value of 1.25 mg/g at 3 months. In culture the biosynthesis of myoglobin was followed by the measurement of $[\Delta^{-14}C]$ aminolevulinate incorporation (Figure 1), despite the small amount of 5–15 μg/g fresh cells. This showed that in heart cells in culture there is a significant biosynthesis of

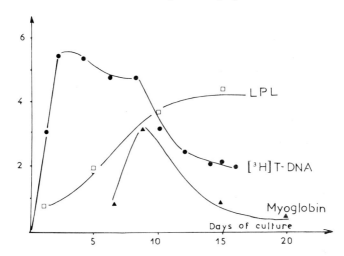

Figure 1. Cellular activities of cultured rat cardiac cells as a function of culture age. LPL: progression of lipoprotein lipase activity (1 unit = 100 μEq/protein/hr). Myoglobin: cpm of [Δ-^{14}C]aminolevulinate (1 unit = 1,000 cpm) incorporated per g of fresh cells. [^{3}H]T-DNA : cpm of [^{3}H]thymidine incorporated into DNA/20 cm^2 dish (1 unit - 2.10^3 cpm).

myoglobin; but, as shown by the label incorporation decrease after day 12, the biosynthesis stays repressed at a basal level. Nevertheless, it must be emphasized that the maximal label incorporation in myoglobin in culture is coincident with the maximal LPL biosynthesis.

Specific metabolisms of cultured cardiac cells: Energetic process

Glucose metabolism (Frelin *et al.*, 1974) Glucose metabolism was studied with [U-^{14}C]glucose in confluent cultures 4–8 days old. In Figure 2 the solid line represents the decrease of extracellular glucose from an initial concentration of 1 mg/ml to 0 mg/ml at 30 hr. The heavily dashed line gives the decrease of total radioactivity, the dotted line shows the radioactivity attributable to compounds other than glucose, and the lightly dashed line represents the lactate concentration. The uptake of glucose is 10–20 times higher than in the heart *in vivo.*

Therefore, the cardiac cells in culture must face this important uptake of glucose either by storing it as glycogen or by excreting it as catabolites. The glycogen maximum label occurs 2–4 hr after change of medium and then decreases exponentially with a half-life of less than 10 hr. After 15 hr the labeling decrease follows another exponential curve, with a half-life of about 100 hr. Key enzymes of glycolysis and of the Krebs cycle have been assayed. Their activities increased three to five times and plateaued at day 8, except for hexokinase, which did not change, and for lactate dehydrogenase, which in-

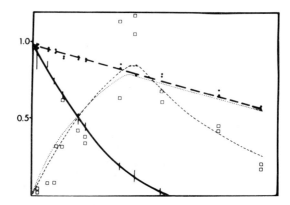

Figure 2. Metabolism of glucose during one medium change of 60 hr. Solid line (——) = decrease of glucose (1 unit = 1 mg/ml) for two determinations. Heavy dashes with filled circles (–•–•–•) = radioactivity of the medium (1 unit = 4.10^4 cpm). Dotted line (.....) = evolution of the concentration of radioactive compounds of the medium other than glucose (1 unit = 4.10^4 cpm). Light dashes with open square (–□–□–) = lactate concentration in the medium (1 unit = 20 μmol/dish).

creased by a factor of 20 and exhibited a shift to muscular isoenzymes. Therefore, glucose cannot be stored at as great an extent as glycogen in cultured cardiac cells, as *in vivo*. Excess cellular glucose excreted as lactate appears as a cellular adaptation and as the only route for the cell to eliminate such an enormous excess, suggesting that the uptake of glucose has lost control in culture and that glycogen metabolism is impaired (Anastasia and McCarl, 1973).

Lipids Because LPL developed in culture cells, study has been done in the laboratory on the utilization of normal (palmitate) and abnormal (erucate) FA (Pinson and Padieu, 1974b, 1976; Pinson, 1975). Palmitate oxidation reaches a maximum of 14 nmol/h/mg of protein at day 5 and then decreases to a still important basal level of 2.5 nmol/h/mg of protein at day 10. The maximal palmitate utilization at day 5 seems to be related to the need of energy for macromolecular biosyntheses in addition to cellular maintenance.

Specific metabolisms of cultured cardiac cells: Effects of serum on cellular activities (Frelin and Padieu, 1976) The pleiotypic effects of medium replacement were studied in 4–6-day-old cultures because confluency was reached in two days as a result of high seeding density. Immediately after each medium change, α-aminoisobutyrate and glucose transports increase, and RNA and protein syntheses are doubled. DNA biosynthesis (very low in absence of serum) begins after 12 hr but is preceded by a parallel sixfold increase of the activity of the phosphopentose pathway beginning with the medium change (Frelin *et al.*, 1974). The DNA biosynthesis is followed by a wave of mitoses. This sequence

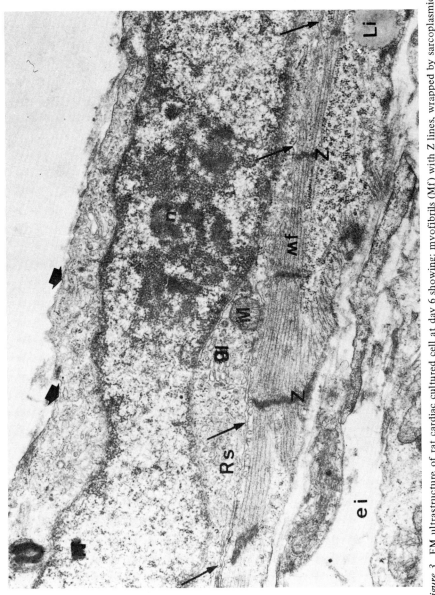

Figure 3. EM ultrastructure of rat cardiac cultured cell at day 6 showing: myofibrils (Mf) with Z lines, wrapped by sarcoplasmic reticulum (Rs), and with mitochondria (M); Golgi apparatus (gl); sarcoplasmic reticulum under the sarcolemma (thin arrows); lipid vacuoles (li); nucleus (N) and nucleolus (n). Between the Z lines, high class polysomes are evident. Some myofilaments are seen in an oblique section (bottom right). The bottom part shows parts of fibroblasts that have excreted some fibrillar material in the extracellular space (ei). × 20,000.

615

of events suggests that the stimulated cells were in early G1 phase at the time of medium change, and that for a cell cycle of 30 hr the exit time of the G1 phase is around 12–15 hr. DNA biosynthesis following the shift to a fresh medium is linearly related to the amount of serum up to 30%. It is also the case for protein biosynthesis; however, above 20% there is no increase, thus suggesting the existence of another limiting factor, which is the isoleucine content of the medium. In comparison to fibroblast cultures (see references in Frelin and Padieu, 1976), stimulation by serum of RNA and protein synthesis is less serum-dependent, while DNA biosynthesis is very much dependent. Serum growth factors are thermostable and dialysable in contrast to fibroblast serum growth factors. Catecholamines and prostaglandin E1 appear, at present, to be the most potent activators of DNA biosynthesis. We may conclude that cardiac cells in culture, more differentiated than fibroblasts, have acquired a certain independence toward serum for the expression of their genetic characteristics. However, they remain strongly serum-dependent for DNA replication until this cellular activity is, as *in vivo*, progressively lost as the culture ages.

Cell Types and Architectonic Development of the Culture

Heart cell cultures are generally composed of a mixture of muscle and nonmuscle cells that may be recognized in young sparse culture by PAS staining of glycogen (Polinger, 1973). However, as the culture ages, myoblasts become progressively insensitive to staining, probably because of defects in glucose and glycogen metabolisms (Anastasia and McCarl, 1973; Ferlin *et al.*, 1974). Searching for new histochemical criteria, Azan staining revealed a striking architectural organization. Muscle cells appear in a layer of cells on the substratum. Cells overlapping by their ends may be seen as several layers by electron microscopic (EM) observation. Although the intensity of staining decreases as the culture ages, muscle cells still remain conspicuous after 10 days in culture. Such cells exhibit in EM (Cedergren and Harary, 1964) a muscular structure, highly developed (Figure 3) (Charbonné, 1976). Electrophysiological study by single cell impalement allows the recording, for over 20 min, of typical 80 mV overshooting (+ 15 mV) action potentials of a following cell or of a pacemaker cell with slow diastolic depolarization (Athias *et al.*, 1977).

Nonmuscle cells start forming several layers on top of the myoblastic cells and appear after staining from yellow to blue color. At days 4–6 (Figure 4), condensed extracellular material is strongly stained in blue and observed in older culture (Figure 5) as long, fibrous, blue, extracellular material interwoven between the cells with a denser staining in the vicinity of the myoblast layer. An array of histochemical methods led to the presumptive identification of collagen. Gas chromatographic assays of proline and hydroxyproline in the total cellular proteins (free hydroxyproline was always absent in the medium) showed that hydroxyproline ranged from 20 nmol/dish at day 2 to 60 nmol/dish at day 8 and

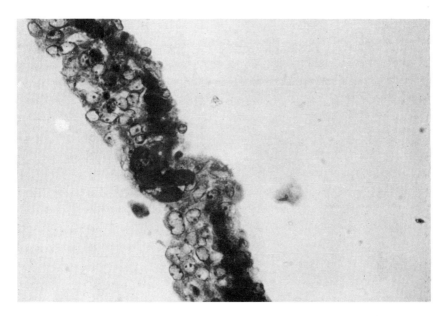

Figure 4. Six-day-old rat cardiac cell culture stained with Azan: darkly stained area represents the substratum layer of muscle cells and condensed collagenic material. Nonmuscle cells are on the top of muscle cells. × 400.

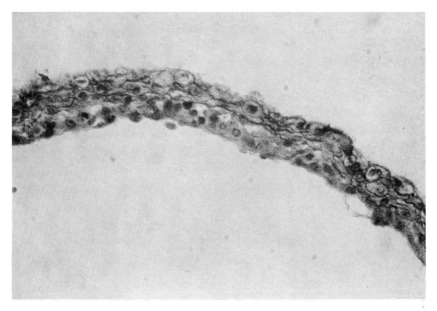

Figure 5. Fourteen-day-old culture (as in Figure 4) stained with Azan. In the muscle layer stain is weak. Fibrous extracellular material is clearly outlined around nonmuscle cells. × 400.

390 nmol/dish at day 14. Moreover, the hydroxyproline/proline ratio gave the relative importance of the amount of collagen in the culture. This ratio was 0.07 ± 0.02 at day 2 and averaged 0.155 ± 0.025 at days 12–14. Therefore, in the case of the exclusive presence of collagen (hydroxyproline/proline = 1) 15% of total polypeptidic proline may be engaged in collagen. Such a ratio would have never been reached in the case of the sole biosynthesis of elastin. This collagenic material is revealed on EM preparations as a dense padded fibrous material but with no cross-striations. This collagen and associated extracellular proteins are very likely synthesized by fibroblasts that exhibit a highly developed granular reticulum.

CONCLUSIONS

The practical consequences of these investigations on the growth of cultured cardiac cells can be expressed in the following ways:

1. Growth of nonmuscle cells is reduced when seeding at high density and then is better controlled in confluent cultures.
2. Cardiac cell cultures contain both muscle cells and nonmuscle cells that behave as highly differentiated cells: myocytes synthesizing muscular enzymes and proteins, and fibroblasts synthesizing collagen.
3. Cellular responses to serum stimulation exhibit specific patterns that can be correlated, to some extent, to cardiac development in the organism.

Therefore, such a culture, which is composed of cells and medium, needs to be considered as a whole and requires a complete and thorough investigation so that its biochemical, physiological, and pharmacological properties may be understood in order to use it as a tool for research in cardiology.

Acknowledgments We thank Mrs. A. Athias, O. Bonnard, and N. Pitoizet for their excellent technical assistance.

REFERENCES

ANASTASIA, J. V., and McCARL, R. L. 1973. Effects of cortisol on cultured rat heart cells. Lipase activity, fatty acid oxidation, glycogen metabolism and ATP levels as related to the beating phenomenon. J. Cell Biol. 57:109–117.
ATHIAS, P., MOALIC, J. M., FRELIN, C., KLEPPING, J., and PADIEU, P. 1977. Potentials de repos et d'activité de cellules cardiaques de rat dissociées en culture. C. R. Soc. Biol. 171:86–90.

BING, R. J., SIEGEL, A., UNGAR, I., and GILBERT, M. 1954. Metabolism of the human heart. II. Studies in fat, ketone and aminoacid metabolism. Am. J. Med. 16:504–515.

BURROWS, M. T. 1912. Rhythmical activity of isolated heart muscle cell *in vitro.* Science 36:90.

CAVANAUGH, M. W. 1955. Pulsation, migration and division in dissociated chick heart cells *in vitro.* J. Exp. Zool. 128:573.

CEDERGREN, B. and HARARY, I. 1964. *In vitro* studies on single beating rat heart cells. VI. Electron microscope studies of single cells. J. Ultrastruct. Res. 11:428–442.

CHARBONNÉ, F. 1976. Culture primaire de cellules myocardiques ventriculaires de coeurs de rat nouveau-né. Etude ultrastructurale. Action des acides érucique et palmitique. Thèse Doctorat Pharmacie, Université de Clermont-Ferrand, Clermont-Ferrand.

CHESSEBEUF, M., OLSSON, A., BOURNOT, P., DESGRÈS, J., GUIGUET, M., MAUME, G., MAUME, B. F., PÉRISSEL, B., and PADIEU, P. 1974. Long term cell culture of rat liver epithelial cells retaining some hepatic functions. Biochimie 56:1365–1379.

FRELIN, C. 1974. Croissance et modifications métaboliques des myoblastes cardiaques de rat en culture. Thèse Doctorat 3ème cycle Sciences, Université de Dijon, Dijon.

FRELIN, C., PINSON, A., MOALIC, J. M., and PADIEU, P. 1974. Energy metabolism of beating rat heart cell cultures. II. Glucose metabolism. Biochimie 56:1597–1602.

FRELIN, C., and PADIEU, P. 1976. Pleiotypic response of rat heart cell in culture to serum stimulation. Biochimie 58:953–959.

HARARY, I., and FARLEY, B. 1960. *In vitro* studies of single isolated beating heart cells. Science 131:1674–1675.

HARARY, I., McCARL, R. L., and FARLEY, B. 1966. Studies *in vitro* on single beating heart cells. IX. The restoration of beating by serum lipids and fatty acids. Biochem. Biophys. Acta 115:15–22.

HARARY, I., HOOVER, F., and FARLEY, B. 1974. The isolation and cultivation of rat heart cells. *In* S. P. Colowick and N. O. Kaplan (eds.), Methods in Enzymology. Vol. 32: S. Flescher and L. Packer (eds.), Biomembranes, Part B, pp. 740–745. Academic Press, New York.

HARRISON, R. G. 1907. Observation on the living developing nerve fiber. Proc. Soc. Exp. Biol. Med. 4:140.

JOLLY, J. 1903. Sur la durée de vie et de la multiplication des cellules animales en dehors de l'organisme. C. R. Soc. Biol. (Paris) 55:1266.

MOSCONA, A. 1952. Cell suspensions from organ rudiments and aggregation of cells from organ rudiments of the early chick embryo. J. Anat. 86:287–294.

NAHANI, J. 1973. Biosynthèse de la myoglobine par des cellules cardiaques postnatales en culture tissulaire. Thèse Doctorat 3ème cycle Sciences. Université de Dijon, Dijon.

PINSON, A. 1975. Métabolisme de l'acide palmitique et de l'acide érucique par les cellules cardiaques bathmotropes de rat en culture. Thèse Doctorat en Sciences, Université de Dijon, Dijon.

PINSON, A., FRELIN, C., and PADIEU, P. 1973. The lipoprotein lipase activity in cultured beating heart cells of the postnatal rat. Biochimie 55:1261–1264.

PINSON, A., and PADIEU, P. 1974a. Quelques aspects du métabolisme des acides gras à longue chaîne par les cellules bathmotropes de coeur de rat en culture. Biochimie 56:1587–1596.

PINSON, A., and PADIEU, P. 1974b. Erucic acid oxidation by beating heart cells in culture. FEBS Lett. 39:88–90.

PINSON, A., and PADIEU, P. 1976. Erucic acid metabolism by cultured beating heart cells of the postnatal rat. *In* P. Harris, R. S. Bing, and A. Fleckenstein (eds.), Recent Advances in Studies on Cardiac Structure and Metabolism. Vol. 7: Biochemistry and Pharmacology of Myocardial Hypertrophy, Hypoxia, and Infarction, pp. 29–40. University Park Press, Baltimore.

POLINGER, I. 1973. Identification of cardiac myocytes *in vivo* and *in vitro* by the presence of glycogen and myofibrils. Exp. Cell Res. 76:243–252.

ROUS, P., and JONES, F. S. 1916. A method for obtaining suspension of living cells from the fixed tissues and for the plating of individual cells. J. Exp. Med. 23:549–555.

STRANGEWAYS, T. S. P., and FELL, H. B. 1926. Experimental studies on the differentiation of embryonic tissues growing *in vivo* and *in vitro*. In the development of the undifferentiated limb. Proc. R. Soc. Lon. (Biol.) 99:340–366.

WOLFF, E., and HAFFEN, K. 1952. Sur une étude de cultures d'organes embryonnaires *in vitro*. Texas Rep. Biol. Med. 10:463–472.

Mailing address:
Dr. Prudent Padieu,
Laboratoire de Biochimie Médicale, Faculté de Médecine,
7, bd Jeanne d'Arc, 21033 Dijon (France).

Recent Advances in Studies on
Cardiac Structure and Metabolism, Volume 12
Cardiac Adaptation
Edited by T. Kobayashi, Y. Ito, and G. Rona
Copyright 1978 University Park Press Baltimore

FETAL MOUSE HEARTS IN ORGAN CULTURE STUDIES IN CARDIAC METABOLISM

J. S. INGWALL[1] and K. WILDENTHAL[2]

[1] Department of Medicine, University of California,
San Diego, California, USA
[2] Departments of Physiology and Internal Medicine,
University of Texas Health Science Center at Dallas,
Southwestern Medical School, Dallas, Texas, USA

SUMMARY

The fetal mouse heart in organ culture is an experimental model that combines the advantages of long-term cell culture models with those of conventional short-term models employing intact tissue. We have used this model to probe several control mechanisms that are important in myocardial metabolism. Intact cultured hearts maintain characteristics of the differentiated state for many days in culture: spontaneously rhythmic contractions, appropriate responsiveness to neurotransmitters, and synthesis of organ-specific substances. However, a slow, progressive loss of some characteristics of differentiation (e.g., maintenance of normal levels of myofibrillar proteins) occurs, and catabolic processes become dominant. Stability is greater in younger, smaller hearts. Deterioration *in vitro* can be slowed by supplying hearts with creatine or insulin. These substances, which probably act through different mechanisms, stimulate certain synthetic processes and/or retard degradative processes.

When cultured hearts are deprived of oxygen and glucose, many changes similar to those that accompany myocardial ischemia and infarction *in vivo* are produced: depletion of ATP, loss of tissue enzymes, development of ultrastructural abnormalities, and stimulation of intracellular repair processes. These results suggest that this system may provide a useful model for studying responses of intact hearts to anoxia and to anoxia coupled with substrate deprivation.

As with all *in vitro* systems, cultured hearts are maintained under relatively unphysiological conditions; accordingly, it is essential to exercise caution in extrapolating results to the adult myocardium. Nevertheless, our experience with cultured fetal mouse hearts suggests to us that use of this model has wide potential for elucidating many characteristics of myocardial metabolism. It is an especially valuable technique for exploring problems in which the effects of long-term interventions on intact myocardial tissue must be studied under precisely controlled conditions.

Work described in this chapter has been supported by grants from the National Heart and Lung Institute (HL 17682) and the San Diego County Heart Association to Dr. Ingwall and by grants from the National Heart and Lung Institute (HL 14706, HL 17669, HL 18087, HL 06298), the American Heart Association and the Moss Heart Fund to Dr. Wildenthal.

Dr. Wildenthal is the recipient of a USPHS Research Cancer Development Award (HL 70125).

INTRODUCTION

Myocardial metabolism has been studied in many models, including such diverse models as intact animals, isolated perfused hearts and muscle strips, and isolated heart cells in monolayer culture. Conventional preparations for studying intact myocardial tissue *in vivo* or *in vitro* suffer from the disadvantages of being stable for only brief periods of time and/or of being rather poorly controlled. In contrast, models using spontaneously beating myocardial cells in monolayer culture offer the advantages of ease and reproducibility of obtaining many replicate heart preparations, the ability to manipulate experimental conditions, and long-term stability; but extrapolation of the responses of isolated cells to the intact heart is often limited. One culture model combines the advantages of working with a spontaneously beating intact heart with the advantages of a culture model: the intact beating fetal mouse heart in organ culture. In this chapter we discuss how the cultured fetal mouse heart model can be used to study changes in myocardial metabolism: 1) during development, 2) as a result of supplying hearts specific metabolites and hormones, and 3) in response to stress, namely, oxygen and substrate deprivation.

RESULTS AND DISCUSSION

Characterization of Fetal Mouse Hearts in Organ Culture: Influence of Fetal Age and Time in Culture

Pregnant mice usually have 8–14 fetuses. To prepare organ cultures, hearts are isolated aseptically from 14–21-day fetal mice (term ~21–22 days) and placed on stainless steel grids at a gas-medium interface in organ culture dishes (Wildenthal, 1971a). Culture dishes are placed in sealed chambers gassed with 95% O_2 and 5% CO_2 at 37°C. Supplied a chemically defined medium such as medium 199, minimum essential medium (MEM), or Earle's salt solution (Grand Island Biological Co.), these hearts will beat in culture for four to eight days before dying (Wildenthal, 1971a; Wildenthal, 1973a), slowly losing myocardial mass throughout the culture period (50 ± 6% after three days). The rate of loss of cardiac mass can be reduced and viability extended to two to four weeks if hearts are supplied with insulin, serum, and hydrocortisone (Wildenthal, 1970; Wildenthal, 1971a; Wildenthal, 1972a; Griffin and Wildenthal, 1974; Wildenthal, Griffin, and Ingwall, 1976a). Cultured mouse hearts beat spontaneously and rhythmically and respond to most cardioactive drugs in a manner similar to the adult myocardium. For example, they develop bradycardia when supplied acetylcholine or propranolol and tachycardia when supplied with catecholamines, glucagon, or triiodothyronine or when made hyperthermic (Wildenthal, 1971b; Wildenthal, 1972b; Wildenthal *et al.,* 1973; Wildenthal, 1973d; Wildenthal, 1974; Wildenthal *et al.,* 1976).

Hearts obtained from 14–21-day-old fetuses are progressively more differentiated. Substrate utilization assumes a more adult-like pattern with increasing age (Wildenthal, 1973a; Wildenthal, 1973b), and responsiveness to cardioactive drugs becomes more mature (Wildenthal, 1973d; Wildenthal *et al.,* 1976). Increasing differentiation with age also is reflected in changes in the specific activities of cardiac enzymes. The activity of the muscle-specific protein creatine kinase (CPK) monotonically increases from 50 ± 5 mIU/mg wet weight in 0.5-mg hearts isolated from 14-day fetuses to 450 ± 20 mIU/mg wet weight in 8-mg hearts from 21-day fetuses (Figure 1). The increase in accumulation of CPK is primarily because of increased accumulation of the muscle-specific isoenzyme, MM-CPK. In hearts from 14-day fetuses, the specific activity of MM-CPK is barely measurable (~1 mIU/mg wet weight); whereas in hearts isolated from fetuses at term the specific activity of MM-CPK is 325 ± 20 mIU/mg wet weight. In contrast to these impressive changes in accumulation of CPK, the specific activity of the glycolytic enzyme lactic dehydrogenase (LDH) does not change during this time of development (Figure 1).

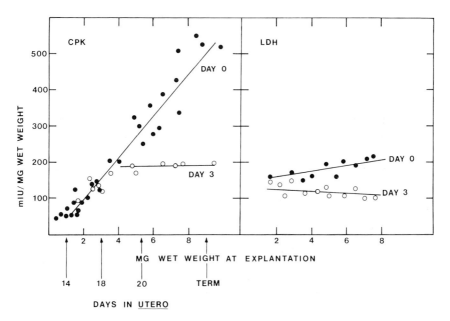

Figure 1. The specific activities of CPK (left panel) and of LDH (right panel) in freshly explanted fetal mouse hearts (day 0, filled circles) and after three days in culture (day 3, open circles). CPK activity was measured using the coupled enzyme method of Rosalki (1967); LDH activity, using the method of Bernstein and Everse (1975). Each entry represents the mean of enzyme activities obtained from 2–20 hearts and is accurate within 10%.

The differentiated state is maintained in culture, but catabolism exceeds anabolism (Wildenthal, 1972a; Wildenthal, Griffin, and Ingwall, 1976; Wildenthal and Griffin, 1976). The specific activities of both CPK and LDH progressively decrease with time in culture, and the effect on CPK is greater than on LDH. As shown in Figure 1, after day 3 in culture, the specific activity of CPK has decreased to ~200 mIU/mg wet weight for hearts weighing $\geq$ 4 mg, an average decrease in specific activity of ~50%. After day 3 in culture, the average decrease in specific activity of LDH is ~30%. Changes in the specific activity of MM-CPK with time in culture and with increasing size of the hearts are similar to the changes observed for total CPK activity (Table 1). In cultured hearts the distribution of the three isoenzymes (BB-, MB-, and MM-CPK) is not the same as in freshly explanted hearts. The BB-isoenzyme is preferentially lost, presumably because of oxidation. As a result, cultured hearts contain proportionately more MM-CPK activity than freshly explanted hearts. These results show that the amount of CPK and LDH per unit cardiac mass decreases with time in culture.

Other experiments also suggest increased catabolism with time in culture. Measurements of the rate of synthesis of total proteins and of the contractile protein myosin heavy chain suggest that muscle-specific protein synthesis becomes preferentially depressed during the culture period. The rate of myosin heavy-chain synthesis in 19–21-day-old hearts cultured for three days is approximately two-thirds of the rate observed in littermate hearts cultured for one day, while the rate of total protein synthesis is approximately the same. In addition, the specific activities of several lysosomal hydrolytic enzymes were greater in hearts cultured for three days compared to values obtained for freshly explanted hearts: acid phosphatase (150 ± 6%, $n = 4$), cathepsin D (206 ± 15%, $n = 4$), and β-acetylglucosaminidase (280 ± 28%, $n = 4$) (Wildenthal, Griffin, and Ingwall, 1976; Wildenthal and Griffin, 1976; Wildenthal et al., 1976).

These results show that the accumulation and synthesis of muscle-specific proteins such as CPK and myosin decrease with time in culture while lysosomal enzymes increase. They also show that the loss is progressively greater as the age and size of the heart increase. Hearts obtained from fetuses near term are too large to be perfused adequately, contain hypoxic cores, and are least suitable for long-term culturing (Wildenthal, 1971a).

Effects of Metabolites and Hormones
on the Accumulation and Synthesis of Muscle Proteins

During the last trimester of development, fetal mouse hearts become increasingly more differentiated, as evidenced by the appearance and rapid accumulation of the muscle-specific isoenzyme of CPK. During this time in development, the accumulation of total creatine (free creatine plus creatine phosphate) in the heart also increases (from ~0.5 nmol/mg wet weight in 1-mg hearts to 3.8 nmol/mg wet weight in 8-mg hearts). As described above, culturing hearts in the absence of creatine for

Table 1. Effect of time in culture and of creatine (5 mM) on the specific activities of CPK and MM-CPK in mouse hearts

mg wet weight/heart	CPK (mIU/mg wet weight)			MM-CPK (mIU/mg wet weight)		
	freshly explanted	cultured two days	cultured two days with creatine	freshly explanted	cultured two days	cultured two days with creatine
2.4	130	110 (85%)	145 (122%)	66	68 (103%)	107 (162%)
3.0	170	150 (88%)	175 (103%)	114	90 (79%)	120 (104%)
3.6	210	150 (72%)	175 (83%)	140	104 (74%)	130 (92%)
4.8	290	160 (55%)	200 (69%)	195	132 (68%)	200 (103%)
5.8	350	160 (46%)	225 (64%)	235	145 (62%)	210 (90%)
6.4	380	195 (51%)	220 (58%)	255	155 (60%)	170 (67%)
7.2	435	185 (42%)	210 (48%)	290	150 (52%)	185 (64%)

Total CPK activity was determined using the coupled enzyme reaction of Rosalki (1967). Isoenzyme composition was determined by measuring the fluorescence of NADPH generated by the isoenzymes separated by cellulose acetate strip electrophoresis (Klein, Shell, and Sobel, 1973; Ingwall, 1976). Data are presented as the specific activities (mIU/mg wet weight) and were obtained using two to six hearts for each analysis. The values in parentheses represent the percentage of corresponding values of freshly explanted hearts. Values for heart weight refer to freshly explanted hearts.

three days leads to an ~50% depletion in the specific activity of CPK; at the same time the intracellular creatine concentration falls ~50% (Ingwall, 1976). In order to test whether the increases in both creatine content and CPK activity in the developing heart and the loss of both creatine content and CPK activity in cultured hearts may be causally related, cultured hearts were supplied with creatine and the accumulation and rates of synthesis of several muscle-specific and nonspecific proteins were measured. The intracellular creatine concentration in hearts supplied with 5 mM creatine for two days was 7.5 ± 0.8 nmol/mg wet weight compared to only 1.3 ± 0.1 nmol/mg wet weight (n = 8) in hearts supplied control medium (Ingwall, 1976). The results shown in Table 2 suggest that muscle-specific protein synthesis in cardiac muscle is selectively enhanced by creatine. The relatively small, but significant, increases in the rate of uptake of labeled amino acid and in total protein content compared to the larger increases in the rate of myosin heavy-chain synthesis and in CPK activity reflect a selective increase in one subgroup of cellular proteins, namely, the muscle-specific proteins, with little or no change in the nonspecific proteins (Ingwall *et al.,* 1975b; Ingwall and Wildenthal, 1976). A comparison of the specific activities of total CPK and of MM-CPK in freshly explanted hearts and in creatine-supplied and control-cultured hearts is shown in Table 1. Although enzyme levels in creatine-supplied hearts are significantly greater than in littermate hearts cultured in the absence of creatine (137 ± 5.5%, n = 7 for MM-CPK), enzyme levels do not exceed those found in freshly explanted hearts (97 ± 12.3%, n = 7 for MM-CPK). These results suggest that in hearts depleted of creatine the accumulation and rate of synthesis of muscle-specific proteins are depressed and that high levels of intracellular creatine maintain the differentiated state.

It is well known that the rate of protein synthesis is dependent on the energy state of the cell. To test whether or not creatine alters the adenylate and guanylate energy charges in cultured hearts, the relative proportions of the purine ribonucleotides were measured in littermate hearts cultured for two days with or without creatine, using high-pressure liquid chromatography (Ingwall, Kaufman, and Mayer, 1976). It was found that the adenylate energy charge (ATP + ½ADP/ATP + ADP + AMP) was the same in freshly explanted hearts (0.89 ± 0.02, n = 5), in hearts cultured in the absence of creatine (0.88 ± 0.02, n = 4), and in hearts cultured in the presence of 5 mM creatine (0.88 ± 0.02, n = 4). However, compared to the guanylate energy charge (GTP + ½GDP/ GTP + GDP + GMP) in freshly explanted fetal hearts (0.88 ± 0.01, n = 6), the guanylate energy charge in hearts cultured in the absence of creatine was depressed (0.78 ± 0.04, n = 4), while the guanylate energy charge in creatine-supplied hearts was not (0.87 ± 0.01, n = 4). That is, in hearts demonstrating reduced muscle-specific protein synthesis, the guanylate energy charge is depressed, and, in hearts in which catabolism is retarded (creatine-supplied hearts), the guanylate energy charge is the same as in freshly explanted hearts. The

Table 2. Summary of the effects of creatine and insulin on protein content of fetal mouse hearts cultured for two days

	Percentage of matched control cultures	
	+ creatine (5 mM)	+ insulin (50 μg/ml)
Cardiac mass		
mg wet weight/heart	102 ± 2.4 (22)	115 ± 2.0 (20)*
mg protein/heart	106 ± 1.9 (32)*	116 ± 2.5 (20)*
Muscle-specific proteins		
Rate of myosin heavy-chain synthesis[a]	130 ± 6.5 (22)*	134 ± 7.4 (18)*[d]
CPK activity[b]	123 ± 5.6 (21)*	118 ± 2.7 (12)*
MM-CPK isoenzyme activity[b]	140 ± 9.0 (13)*	
Nonspecific proteins		
Uptake of radiolabeled amino acid	106 ± 2.7 (22)*	122 ± 4.0 (18)*
Rate of total protein synthesis		113 ± 3.7 (18)*[d]
Rate of total protein degradation		78 ± 4.1 (15)*[d]
LDH activity[b]	104 ± 3.2 (18)	101 ± 3.8 (12)
LDH isoenzyme composition[b]	same as control (27)	same as control (12)
Lysosomal enzymes		
Acid phosphatase activity[c]	101 ± 1.3 (8)	94 ± 1.2 (6)*
Cathepsin D activity[c]	97 ± 3.0 (7)	85 ± 2.8 (6)*

Each experiment compared 4–12 littermate hearts cultured under identical conditions except for the addition of creatine or insulin. The values in parentheses refer to the number of litters tested. An asterisk denotes values $p < 0.05$ that the experimental group is the same as control using Student's t-test for paired data.
[a]Measured using the method of Paterson and Strohman (1972) as described by Ingwall and Wildenthal (1976).
[b]Measured as described in the legends to Table 1 and Figure 1.
[c]Measured as described by Ingwall and Wildenthal (1976).
[d]Corrected for changes in the specific activity of intracellular amino acid pools (Wildenthal, Griffin, and Ingwall, 1976).

627

guanylate energy charge appears to reflect the ability of myocardial cells to synthesize muscle-specific proteins. These results suggest a possible mechanism for creatine-stimulated muscle protein synthesis: high creatine phosphate contents may maintain the relatively high guanosine triphosphate (GTP) concentration required for polypeptide chain initiation and elongation.

Supplying cultured fetal mouse hearts with insulin also tends to maintain enzyme levels found in freshly explanted hearts. Compared to littermate hearts cultured in the absence of insulin, insulin-supplied hearts have greater protein content, higher CPK activity, increased incorporation of labeled amino acids into myosin heavy chain, and increased rate of total protein synthesis (Table 2; Wildenthal, 1972a; Wildenthal, 1973c; Wildenthal, Griffin, and Ingwall, 1976; Wildenthal, 1976). Insulin also has a marked effect on degradative processes in the cultured heart: insulin decreases the rate of protein degradation and the total activity of several lysosomal hydrolyases including acid phosphatase, β-acetyl-glucosaminidase, and cathepsin D (Wildenthal, 1973c; Wildenthal, 1975; Wildenthal, Griffin, and Ingwall, 1976; Wildenthal, 1976). It also reduces the proportion of lysosomal enzymes present in the nonsedimentable fraction of the tissue homogenate (Wildenthal, Griffin, and Ingwall, 1976; Wildenthal, 1976). These results suggest the possibility that insulin may function in part by altering lysosomal enzyme activity and/or availability. The mechanisms by which creatine and insulin act are probably different. In some experiments, we have supplied fetal mouse hearts with both creatine and insulin and found the effects on protein synthesis to be additive.

The results described here show that both creatine and insulin function to maintain relatively high levels of muscle-specific proteins in cultured hearts and that control mechanisms operating at the levels of protein synthesis, protein degradation, and maintenance of high energy stores are involved. If the control mechanisms operating in the fetal heart also function in the adult heart, these results define new regulatory mechanisms important in cardiac metabolism.

Alterations in Cardiac Metabolism in
Response to Oyxgen and Substrate Deprivation

In an attempt to define the determinants of cell viability, we have examined the temporal relationships between changes in mechanical performance, in high-energy phosphate stores and in cytoplasmic enzyme release in fetal mouse hearts both during transient oxygen and substrate deprivation and during subsequent resupply of oxygen and substrate (DeLuca, Ingwall, and Bittl, 1974; Ingwall et al., 1975a; Roeske, Ingwall, and DeLuca, 1975). The ATP content of hearts at the end of 1, 3, 4, 5, or 8 hr of oxygen and glucose deprivation and after 1 or 4 hr of resupply of oxygen and glucose has been compared with the ATP content of continuously oxygenated hearts (Figure 2). Deprivation leads to cessation of beating and ATP depletion. If oxygen and glucose are resupplied after 1 hr of

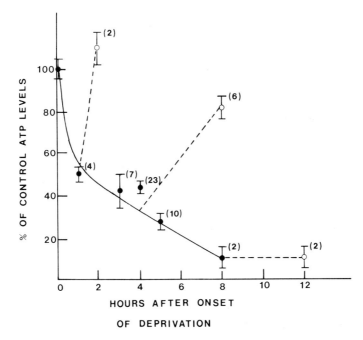

Figure 2. Percentage change in ATP levels at the end of 1, 3, 4, 5, or 8 hr of oxygen and glucose deprivation (filled circles) and 1 or 4 hr after resupply of oxygen and glucose (open circles) from ATP levels in continuously oxygenated hearts. ATP levels after 24 hr of recovery were the same as values found at the end of 4 hr of recovery (not shown). ATP content was assayed using firefly luciferase; control values were ~35 nmol/mg of protein (Ingwall *et al.,* 1975a; Roeske, Ingwall, and DeLuca, 1975). The numbers in parentheses represent the number of litters tested. Data are taken from DeLuca, Ingwall, and Bittl (1974), Ingwall *et al.* (1975a), and Roeske, Ingwall, and DeLuca (1975).

deprivation, beating resumes within minutes, ATP levels return to or exceed control values and no enzyme depletion is observed during the following 24 hr of recovery (DeLuca, Ingwall, and Bittl, 1974). If the insult is extended to 4 hr, ATP levels are depressed to 20–40% of control values; upon resupply of oxygen and glucose, beating resumes slowly, ATP levels return to 60–80% of control values, and 4–16 hr after resupply of oxygen and substrate as much as 30–40% of CPK and LDH contents are depleted from the heart (Ingwall *et al.,* 1975a; Roeske, Ingwall, and DeLuca, 1975). If the insult is extended to 8 hr, no recovery is observed.

The changes in ATP levels in deprived mouse hearts correlate well with changes in mitochondrial integrity (Sybers *et al.,* 1974; Ingwall *et al.,* 1975a). Mitochondrial swelling and decreased matrix density are observed in deprived hearts within 1 hr after the onset of deprivation. After 4 hr of insult, most of the cells in the hearts show these changes as well as glycogen depletion and some disorientation of the myofibrils. Upon resupply of oxygen and glucose, however, mitochondria resume normal appearance. The rapid return of the swollen mitochondria to normal appearance, coupled with the rapid resynthesis of ATP, indicates that 4 hr of deprivation does not irreversibly damage most mitochondria. This may not be surprising because the mitochondrial membranes appear to be intact in many of the cells. Extending the period of deprivation to longer times and/or insulting the hearts at elevated temperatures leads to irreversible cell injury, and recovery is no longer possible (Roeske, Ingwall, and DeLuca, 1975).

While maintaining high ATP levels in myocardial tissue is obviously important, beating and extent of recovery in this model do not appear to be tightly coupled to the absolute ATP content. The average time to asystole during deprivation is 8 min, a time before significant depression in ATP content or in the adenylate energy charge occurs (Roeske et al., 1976; Kaufman et al., in press). Resumption of beating, although often with depressed force of contraction and slower rates, occurs within minutes after restoration of oxygen and glucose, i.e., before ATP levels and the adenylate energy charge are significantly returned toward control (Ingwall et al., 1975a; Roeske et al., 1976; Kaufman et al., in press).

What may be more important than the extent of ATP depression is the duration of the insult. ATP catabolism has been shown to occur by the following pathway: ATP → ADP → AMP → adenosine → inosine → hypoxanthine. It has not been possible to demonstrate de novo ATP synthesis in mouse hearts cultured for 24–48 hr; rather, ATP synthesis occurs via salvage pathways through inosine and hypoxanthine (Kaufman et al., in press). Hence, if inosine and hypoxanthine are lost from the hearts during insult, return to control ATP levels during resupply of oxygen and glucose is not possible.

Figure 3 shows the results of an experiment in which loss of radiolabeled purine bases and nucleosides from the hearts to the medium was measured in littermate hearts continuously oxygenated and hearts deprived of oxygen and glucose for 2, 4, 6, or 8 hr. The results show that a significant proportion of the radiolabeled bases and nucleosides (identified as being exclusively hypoxanthine and inosine by two-dimensional, thin-layer chromatography (Kaufman et al., in press)), which would otherwise be available for conversion to ATP via salvage pathways, has been lost from the heart during insult. It is tempting to speculate that interventions designed to maintain mitochondrial membrane integrity, coupled with a supply of the deprived myocardium with nontoxic nucleosides or bases, would prevent irreversible damage to the jeopardized myocardium.

The loss of nucleosides and bases from fetal mouse hearts during the period of insult is in contrast to the loss of macromolecules that occurs during the recovery period (Ingwall et al., 1975a; Roeske, Ingwall, and DeLuca, 1975).

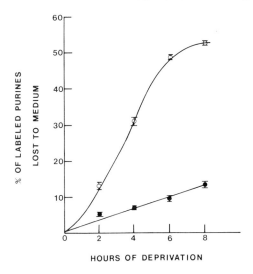

Figure 3. Percentage of radioactive purines lost to the culture medium from continuously oxygenated hearts (filled circles) and from littermate hearts deprived of oxygen and glucose for 2, 4, 6, or 8 hr (open circles). Hearts were prelabeled for 18 hr with [^{14}C] adenine (0.5 μCi/ml, Schwartz/Mann, specific activity 53 mCi/mol). Radiolabeled medium was removed and hearts were washed five times using unlabeled medium; the cpm/ml of the final two washes was < 0.3% of the labeling medium (178,000 ± 2000 cpm/ml). 2, 4, 6, or 8 hr later, radioactivity (cpm) of hearts and of media was determined for hearts deprived of oxygen and glucose and for littermate hearts continuously oxygenated. Total cpm for each dish (i.e., heart plus medium) averaged 39,300 ± 800 (n = 16). Data represent the mean of values obtained using two litters.

After 4 hr of deprivation, loss of enzymes such as LDH and CPK does not occur to any significant extent until 4–6 hr after resupply of oxygen and glucose. All of the LDH activity depleted from insulted hearts is found in the culture medium; CPK activity is not (Ingwall and DeLuca, in preparation). These results suggest that enzyme depletion may be energy dependent. In addition to passive "leakage" of macromolecules from damaged or dying cells to the medium, release via lysosomes also may occur. Ultrastructural analyses of hearts that were deprived and then resupplied with oxygen and glucose show the appearance of autophagic vacuoles containing damaged mitochondria and myofibrils in an otherwise normal-appearing cell (Ingwall *et al.,* 1975a; Sybers *et al.,* 1974). It seems likely that these vacuoles, presumably lysosomes, represent a repair mechanism whereby focally damaged areas in a cell are sequestered. It is not known whether this repair mechanism functions in the adult myocardium.

Acknowledgments We would like to acknowledge our many collaborators in these studies: J. W. Covell, M. DeLuca, E. E. Griffin, N. F. Hall, I. A. Kaufman, S. E. Mayer, W. R. Roeske, and H. D. Sybers. We also acknowledge the excellent assistance of D. Buccigrossi, S. C. Jascinski, M. Kennedy, P. Kolb, P. C. Morton, L. Nimmo, J. R. Wakeland, and R. Watson.

REFERENCES

BERNSTEIN, L. H., and EVERSE, J. 1975. Determination of isoenzymes of lactic dehydrogenase. Methods Enzymol. 41:47–52.

DeLUCA, M. A., INGWALL, J. S., and BITTL, J. A. 1974. Biochemical responses of myocardial cells in culture to oxygen and glucose deprivation. Biochem. Biophys. Res. Comm. 59:749–756.

GRIFFIN, E. E., and WILDENTHAL, K. 1974. Control of cardiac protein balance by hydrocortisone. Circulation 50(suppl. III):12.

INGWALL, J. S. Creatine and the control of muscle-specific protein synthesis in cardiac and skeletal muscle. Circ. Res. 38(suppl. I):115–123.

INGWALL, J. S., DeLUCA, M., SYBERS, H. D., and WILDENTHAL, K. 1975a. Fetal mouse hearts: A model for studying ischemia. Proc. Natl. Acad. Sci. USA 72: 2809–2813.

INGWALL, J. S., KAUFMAN, I. A., and MAYER, S. E. Purine nucleotide and creatine contents in differentiating cardiac muscle. J. Cell Biol. 70(part 2):239a.

INGWALL, J. S., MORALES, M. F., STOCKDALE, F. E., and WILDENTHAL, K. 1975b. Creatine: A possible stimulus for skeletal and cardiac muscle hypertrophy. In P. E. Roy and P. Harris (eds.), Recent Advances in Cardiac Structure and Metabolism. Vol. 8: The Cardiac Sarcoplasm, pp. 467–486. University Park Press, Baltimore.

INGWALL, J. S., and WILDENTHAL, K. 1976. Role of creatine in the regulation of cardiac protein synthesis. J. Cell Biol. 68:159–163.

KAUFMAN, I. A., HALL, N. F., DeLUCA, M. A., INGWALL, J. S., and MAYER, S. E. Metabolism of adenine nucleotides in the cultured fetal mouse heart. Am. J. Physiol. In press.

KLEIN, M. S., SHELL, W. E., and SOBEL, B. E. 1973. CPK isoenzymes after intramuscular injections, surgery and myocardial infarction. Cardiovasc. Res. 7:412–418.

PATERSON, B., and STROHMAN, R. C. 1972. Myosin synthesis in cultures of differentiating chicken embryo skeletal muscle. Dev. Biol. 29:113–138.

ROESKE, W. R., INGWALL, J. S., and DeLUCA, M. A. 1975. Biochemical responses of the ischemic fetal mouse heart to temperature. Clin. Res. 23(2):83A.

ROESKE, W. R., INGWALL, J. S., KRAMER, M., and COVELL, J. W. 1976. The relationship of control and ischemic myocardial function to mechanical recovery in cultured fetal mouse hearts. Clin. Res. 24:88A.

ROSALKI, S. B. 1967. An improved procedure for serum creatine phosphokinase determination. J. Lab. Clin. Med. 69:696–705.

SYBERS, H. D., INGWALL, J. S., DeLUCA, M. A., and ROSS, J., JR. 1974. Ultrastructure of fetal mouse hearts in organ culture: Effects of anoxia. In C. J. Arceneaux (ed.), Proceedings, 32nd Annual Meeting, Electron Microscopy Society of America, pp. 30–31. Claitors Publishing Division, Baton Rouge.

WILDENTHAL, K. 1970. Factors promoting the survival and beating of intact fetal mouse hearts in organ culture. J. Mol. Cell. Cardiol. 1:101–104.

WILDENTHAL, K. 1971a. Long-term maintenance of spontaneously beating mouse hearts in organ culture. J. Appl. Physiol. 30:153–157.

WILDENTHAL, K. 1971b. Responses to cardioactive drugs of fetal mouse hearts maintained in organ culture. Am. J. Physiol. 221:238–241.

WILDENTHAL, K. 1972a. Protein breakdown inhibited by insulin to improve heart culture. Nature 239:101–102.

WILDENTHAL, K. 1972b. Studies of fetal mouse hearts in organ culture: Evidence for a direct effect of triiodothyronine in enhancing cardiac responsiveness to norepinephrine. J. Clin. Invest. 51:2702–2709.

WILDENTHAL, K. 1973a. Studies of fetal mouse hearts in organ culture: Metabolic requirements for prolonged function *in vitro* and the influence of cardiac maturation on substrate utilization. J. Mol. Cell. Cardiol. 5:87–99.

WILDENTHAL, K. 1973b. Fetal maturation of cardiac metabolism. *In* R. S. Comline *et al.* (eds.), Fetal and Neonatal Physiology, pp. 181–185. Cambridge University Press, Cambridge.

WILDENTHAL, K. 1973c. Inhibition by insulin of cardiac cathepsin D activity. Nature 243:226–227.

WILDENTHAL, K. 1973d. Maturation of responsiveness to cardioactive drugs: Differential effects of acetylcholine, norepinephrine, theophylline, tyramine, glucagon, and dibutyryl cyclic AMP on atrial rate in hearts of fetal mice. J. Clin. Invest. 52:2250–2258.

WILDENTHAL, K. 1974. Studies of mouse hearts in organ culture: The influence of prolonged exposure to triiodothyronine on cardiac responsiveness to acetylcholine, isoproterenol, glucagon, theophylline, and dibutyryl cyclic AMP. J. Pharm. Exp. Ther. 190:272–279.

WILDENTHAL, K. 1975. Lysosomes and lysosomal enzymes in the heart. *In* J. T. Dingle and R. Dean (eds.), Lysosomes in Biology and Pathology. Vol. 4, pp. 167–190. London, North-Holland.

WILDENTHAL, K. 1976. Hormonal and nutritional substrate control of cardiac lysosomal enzyme activities. Circ. Res. 39:441–446.

WILDENTHAL, K., ALLEN, D. O., KARLSSON, J., WAKELAND, J. R., and CLARK, J. M., JR. 1976. Responsiveness to glucagon in fetal hearts: Species variability and apparent disparities between changes in beating, adenylate cyclase activation, and cyclic AMP content. J. Clin. Invest. 57:551–559.

WILDENTHAL, K., GRIFFIN, E. E., and INGWALL, J. S. 1976. Hormonal control of cardiac protein and amino acid balance. Circ. Res. 38(suppl. I):138–144.

WILDENTHAL, K., and GRIFFIN, E. E. 1976. Reduction by cycloheximide of lysosomal proteolytic enzyme activity and rate of protein degradation in organ-cultured hearts. Biochim. Biophys. Acta 444:519–524.

WILDENTHAL, K., HARRISON, D. R., TEMPLETON, G. H., and REARDON, W. C. 1973. A method for measuring the contractions of small hearts in organ culture. Cardiovasc. Res. 7:140–144.

WILDENTHAL, K., WAKELAND, J. R., MORTON, P. C., and GRIFFIN, E. E. Inhibition of cardiac protein degradation by agents that cause lysosomal dysfunction. Circulation. In press.

Mailing address:
Joanne S. Ingwall, Ph.D.,
Department of Medicine, Harvard Medical School, and Peter Bent Brigham Hospital,
721 Huntington Ave., Boston, Massachusetts 02115 (USA).

Recent Advances in Studies on
Cardiac Structure and Metabolism, Volume 12
Cardiac Adaptation
Edited by T. Kobayashi, Y. Ito, and G. Rona
Copyright 1978 University Park Press Baltimore

THE EFFECT OF
THE RECIPROCAL RELATIONSHIP OF Ca^{2+}
AND cAMP ON THE CONTROL OF BEATING
IN CULTURED RAT HEART CELLS

I. HARARY and G. A. WALLACE

Laboratory of Nuclear Medicine and Radiation Biology,
University of California at Los Angeles,
Los Angeles, California, USA

SUMMARY

The demonstration of Ca^{2+} control of the cAMP level in heart cells and the localization of the Ca^{2+} activator protein of cAMP phosphodiesterase on the sarcoplasmic reticulum (SR) have led us to postulate a model whereby the Ca^{2+} flux is related to the cAMP flux. The model suggests that the increase in cytosol Ca^{2+} automatically results in an increase in SR Ca^{2+} and a subsequent decrease in cAMP to allow for the periodic flux of Ca^{2+} and cAMP in the contraction cycle.

INTRODUCTION

Ca^{2+} has long been known to be intimately involved in the contraction cycle of the heart by its direct participation in both excitation-contraction coupling and myofibril contraction (Katz, 1970). In this capacity, the Ca^{2+} concentration is required to fluctuate with the cycle. cAMP has also been shown to be related to heart contraction through its effect on cellular uptake and sequestering of Ca^{2+}. The expected variation of cAMP concentration with contraction resulting from this relation has been demonstrated (Brooker, 1975). It therefore would also be expected, if contraction Ca^{2+} and cAMP are linked, that the cyclic changes in their concentrations would be coordinated with each other and the contraction cycle. It is the purpose of this chapter to provide an observation that will serve as a link between cAMP and Ca^{2+} and the contraction cycle, and to present a model whereby the increase in Ca^{2+} in systole automatically leads to a reduction of Ca^{2+} and subsequently restores the initial condition.

Supported in part by ERDA Contract EY–87–C–03–0012 with the University of California at Los Angeles.

Evidence has been accumulating the cAMP potentiates that entry of external Ca^{2+} into the heart cell (Reuter, 1974), perhaps through phosphorylation of the plasma membrane (Hui, Drummond, and Drummond, 1976). In addition, it is generally agreed that the sarcoplasmic reticulum (SR) is phosphorylated by cAMP-dependent protein kinases and that the phosphorylated membranes facilitate Ca^{2+} entry into the SR (Kirchberger *et al.,* 1972). This suggests that cAMP stimulates accumulation of Ca^{2+} by the cell and also causes a subsequent decrease in the cytosol by the uptake of Ca^{2+} by the SR. The last step leads to a decrease in Ca^{2+} below the level needed for myofibril contraction, but, in itself, would only lead to a one-cycle contraction. A necessary further step is a mechanism for recycling that includes a decrease in Ca^{2+} uptake, a decrease in Ca^{2+} in the SR, a decrease in cytosol cAMP, and a subsequent increase in the cAMP to allow the cycle to start again. In this chapter evidence is presented for a hypothesis that the feedback effect of Ca^{2+} on the cAMP level provides a closing link in the circle, such that the cycle may continue.

DISCUSSION

Ca^{2+}, cAMP, and Beating

Our experiments with cultured heart cells (Harary, Hoover, and Farley, 1974) demonstrated that both noradrenaline and Ca^{2+} control the concentration of

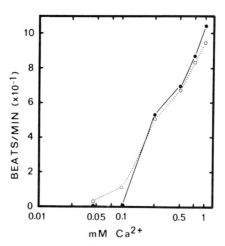

Figure 1. Beating of heart cells conditioned in high or low Ca^{2+} medium. Two-day-old cultures were incubated in fresh medium for 2 hr before the addition of experimental medium (●); beating rates in duplicate were measured 10 min after treatment. ○ = beating rates of heart cells treated as above but with an additional incubation in $4.5 \times 10^{-5} M\, Ca^{2+}$ for 2 hr before the addition of experimental medium. The solid symbol at $4.5 \times 10^{-5} M\, Ca^{2+}$ indicates the beating rate 10 min after the cells were placed on this medium. The open symbol at $4.5 \times 10^{-5} M\, Ca^{2+}$ indicates the beating rate 2 hr after the cells were placed on this medium.

cAMP, which in turn regulates the utilization of Ca^{2+} (Harary *et al.,* 1976). Addition of noradrenaline or depletion of Ca^{2+} in the external medium resulted in cells that could beat at a lower concentration of external Ca^{2+} compared to the controls. In a preliminary experiment, it was shown that noradrenaline increased the cAMP concentration and also increased the rate of beating at external Ca^{2+} concentrations (3×10^{-5} M) which normally would not support beating. Through its action on cAMP, noradrenaline appeared to increase the ability of heart cells to utilize Ca^{2+} for beating.

A decrease of Ca^{2+} in the cells, caused by incubating the cells in a Ca^{2+}-depleted medium, also led to an increased utilization of Ca^{2+} for beating. Heart cells containing a normal Ca^{2+} concentration ceased beating at an external Ca^{2+} concentration below 10^{-4} M. In cultures preincubated for 2 hr in 3×10^{-6} M Ca^{2+} medium, beating was restored by 4.5×10^{-5} M Ca^{2+}. In another experiment, cells incubated in 4.5×10^{-5} M Ca^{2+} stopped beating, as expected, but, within 2 hr, they resumed beating spontaneously (Figure 1). Cells incubated in a medium with high Ca^{2+} had a greater minimum external Ca^{2+} requirement to maintain beating than did cells incubated in a low Ca^{2+} medium. This indicated that the external Ca^{2+} concentration was involved in controlling the effect of Ca^{2+} on beating, perhaps indirectly controlling the intracellular level of Ca^{2+} through an effect on cAMP.

If cAMP is related to the sensitivity of heart cells to Ca^{2+}, then its concentration should respond directly to changes in external Ca^{2+}. When cells were incubated for 2 hr in various concentrations of Ca^{2+}, their content of cAMP increased from 3 pmol to 6 pmol per mg of protein as the concentration of Ca^{2+} decreased from 10^{-3} M to 10^{-4} M (Figure 2). Thus, a decrease in cellular Ca^{2+} increased the cAMP and decreased the external Ca^{2+} requirement for beating,

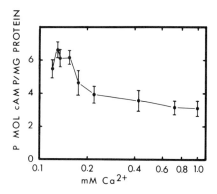

Figure 2. Effect of external Ca^{2+} on cellular concentration of cAMP. Two-day-old cultures were incubated for 2 hr in growth medium with different Ca^{2+} concentrations, and cAMP was determined. Each point represents an average of four plates. The vertical bars represent standard error of mean. A *t*-test was performed on grouped cAMP values between 10^{-4} M and 2×10^{-4} M and between 2×10^{-4} M and 10^{-3} M. Level of significance was $p < 0.001$.

perhaps through the concomitant increase in cAMP. In this way, Ca^{2+} may regulate its own effect on contractility.

Ca^{2+} may affect the concentration of cAMP by an effect on cAMP phosphodiesterase (PDE). This enzyme is stimulated by an "activator" protein, which is activated by Ca^{2+} (Kakiuchi and Yamazaki, 1970). Thus, a decrease in Ca^{2+} would cause a decrease in cAMP phosphodiesterase activity and a resultant increase in cAMP.

Localization of cAMP Phosphodiesterase Activator

In order to study the regulation of cAMP degradation, the protein activator and PDE were purified from the rat heart, and the Ca^{2+} requirement for activity was measured (Wallace and Harary, 1975). In order to produce a soluble preparation of activator, we found it necessary to freeze and thaw the homogenate prepared from the rat heart. The necessity for freezing and thawing the ventricles in order to solubilize the activator protein suggested that the activator might be associated with a membrane in the intact cell. Therefore, membrane fractions were prepared from fresh heart (Kidwai et al., 1971) to determine whether or not the activator protein was associated with any of the cellular membranes. Plasma membranes and mitochondrial membranes showed no activity. Activator activity was found in the sarcoplasmic membranes but only if fresh ventricles were used in the membrane preparations; no particulate activator was found in a frozen-thawed ventricle preparation. The activator was solubilized from the sarcoplasmic reticulum.

The PDE activator protein also was partially purified by a procedure involving ammonium sulfate fractionation and affinity column chromatography with cAMP PDE bound to Sepharose 4B.

Model for Beating, Ca^{2+} and cAMP Interactions

The localization of the Ca^{2+} activator protein of PDE in the SR system provides a logical link in the Ca^{2+} and cAMP cycle. cAMP regulates the Ca^{2+} level by affecting Ca^{2+} uptake and sequestering; Ca^{2+}, in turn, affects the cAMP level. The Ca^{2+} activator localization in the SR has led us to postulate a model that provides an automatic mechanism for the subsequent decrease in cytosol Ca^{2+} following the increase of Ca^{2+} present during systole. The model further suggests that Ca^{2+} sequestered in the SR plays a major role in controlling the cAMP level.

The steps for the model are outlined in Figure 3, beginning with the depolarization of the sarcolemma:

Step 1. Cellular Ca^{2+} level is low. Ca^{2+} enters the cell. The cAMP level is high and is consistent with the uptake of Ca^{2+} (Reuter, 1974; Hui, Drummond, and Drummond, 1976).

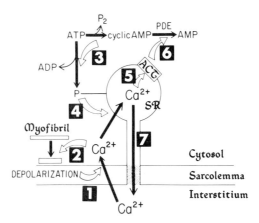

Figure 3. Steps in the variation of Ca^{2+} and cAMP in the heart. ACT = PDE activator; SR = sarcoplasmic reticulum.

Step 2. Cytosol Ca^{2+} increases. Myofibrils shorten. Ca^{2+} influx stops.

Step 3. The high cAMP also has caused a phosphorylation of the SR (Kirchberger *et al.*, 1972).

Step 4. Phosphorylation leads to an increased uptake of Ca^{2+} by the SR (Kirchberger *et al.*, 1972). Ca^{2+} moves from the myofilament falling below the activation threshold for contraction (10^{-7} M).

Step 5. Higher level of Ca^{2+} near the SR, on the membrane and in the SR stimulates PDE activity, through the PDE activator associated with the SR, and causes a decrease in the cAMP.

Step 6. The decrease in cAMP, in turn, leads to a decrease in phosphorylation, continued or increased dephosphorylation of the phosphorylated SR (Tada, Kirchberger, and Li, 1975) and, consequently, less uptake of Ca^{2+}.

Step 7. Ca^{2+} passes through the SR and the T system to the external medium. Both Steps 6 and 7 lead to a decrease in Ca^{2+} in the SR.

Step 8. The decrease in SR Ca^{2+} results in an increase in cAMP by the continued action of adenyl cyclase and the decreased action of PDE.

We are thus returned to Step 1 in which we have a low level of cytosol Ca^{2+} and a high level of cAMP, thereby priming the pump for the next round.

The contraction cycle is represented in Figure 4. Stages A → B: the Ca^{2+} rises in the cytoplasm with no change in the SR Ca^{2+} or in cAMP. Stages B → C: the cytosol Ca^{2+} falls and SR Ca^{2+} rises. cAMP falls with the rise in SR Ca^{2+}. Stages C → D: the SR Ca^{2+} falls and cAMP rises with no change in the cytosol Ca^{2+}. The unique features of this model are the variation of cAMP only with the SR Ca^{2+}

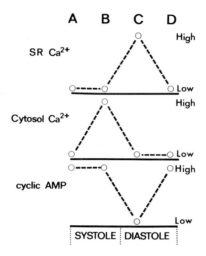

Figure 4. The variation in SR Ca²⁺, cytosol Ca²⁺, and cAMP with the stages of the contraction cycle of the heart.

and the emptying of the SR and the T system to the outside medium, allowing both the cytosol and SR to be low in Ca^{2+}.

A possible variant of this model, which differs only in the source of contractile Ca^{2+}, is still a matter of some dispute. In the variant model, the flux of cytosol Ca^{2+} into and out of the SR is the mechanism by which the cytosol Ca^{2+} is altered. The steps of Ca^{2+} and cAMP flux during the contraction cycle are represented in Figure 5.

In diastole we have a low level of cAMP and cytosol Ca^{2+} and a high level of SR Ca^{2+}.

1. Ca^{2+} flows from the SR to the cytosol. The SR is dephosphorylated. The drop in SR Ca^{2+} leads to an increase in cAMP and cytosol consistent with the levels in systole.
2. High Ca^{2+} causes contraction. High cAMP results in phosphorylation of the SR.
3. The more active, phosphorylated SR takes up cytosol Ca^{2+} leading to a decrease in cytosol Ca^{2+} and an increase in SR Ca^{2+}.
4. High SR Ca^{2+} leads to activation of the Ca^{2+} activator of PDE and a decrease in cAMP.
5. We are returned to the diastolic phase with low cytosol Ca^{2+}, high SR Ca^{2+}, and low cAMP.

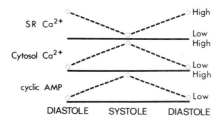

Figure 5. Steps of the variation of Ca^{2+} and cAMP in the heart when the direct source of contractile Ca^{2+} is from the SR.

Support for the model and its variant is derived from the following observations:

1. The systolic phase of contraction occurs when the Ca^{2+} and the cAMP levels are high. Diastole corresponds to a lower level of cAMP (Brooker, 1975). These observations are consistent with the timing suggested by the models.
2. The cAMP-stimulated protein kinase phosphorylation of the SR results in an enhanced uptake of Ca^{2+} (Kirchberger *et al.*, 1972).
3. The Ca^{2+} activator protein (Kakiuchi and Yamazaki, 1970) has been shown to be localized in the SR of the rat heart (Wallace and Harary, 1975).
4. The cAMP of Ca^{2+} depleted rat heart cells in culture was shown to increase, indicating a general reciprocal relation of Ca^{2+} and cAMP (Harary *et al.*, 1976).
5. Consistent with the SR control of the cAMP level is the recent observation that adenyl cyclase also is localized on the SR and the sarcolemma (Katz *et al.*, 1974).

The adenyl cyclase of the sarcolemma has been reported to be inhibited by Ca^{2+} (Kirchberger, Iorio, and Katz, 1974). Although it has not yet been shown if the SR adenyl cyclase is also inhibited by Ca^{2+}, this would be consistent with the direction of the control of cAMP by the SR activator of PDE. A decrease in cAMP therefore could be caused by the decreased activity of adenyl cyclase and increased activation of PDE caused by SR Ca^{2+}.

The choice of models largely depends upon the choice of the mechanism of Ca^{2+} flux. In the first model (Figures 3 and 4), the contractile Ca^{2+} enters the cell from the extracellular space and leaves the SR directly to the outside. In the variant model (Figure 5), the Ca^{2+} level adjacent to the myofilament is controlled by the flux in and out of the SR directly into the cytosol.

The arguments for external Ca^{2+} as a source of contractile Ca^{2+} are reviewed by Langer (1974). Studies of the contraction force decay in Ca^{2+}-free solution correlate the decay rate with kinetics of the exchange rate of Ca^{2+} in the interstitial space. There is a loss of contraction despite the presence of more than enough cellular Ca^{2+} to saturate the myofilaments. The importance of external Ca^{2+} also is shown by the inhibitory effect of La^{3+} which acts by replacing the membrane Ca^{2+} located externally. This results in an inhibition of Ca^{2+} influx in the heart and inhibits contraction only in the heart and not in skeletal muscle, which is thought to contain an internal source of contractile Ca^{2+}. The dependence of heart muscle upon an immediate source of extracellular Ca^{2+} is in marked contrast to skeletal muscle which is primarily dependent upon stores localized in the sarcotubular system (Winegrad, 1968). Finally, the positive inotropic effect of solutions low in Na^+ is consistent with the abrupt increase of Ca^{2+} uptake and transport to the myofilaments (Langer, 1974).

In support of the variant model (Figure 3), it has been shown that the cAMP increase in the heart occurs after membrane depolarization in synchrony with the contraction (Wollenberger et al., 1973). However, the data are not precise enough to rule out an increase in cAMP just before depolarization, depicted in Figure 4. In addition, high cAMP in the cytosol is consistent with the binding of Ca^{2+} to the external membrane and the cellular uptake of Ca^{2+}. The inward Ca^{2+} current across the sarcolemma, as studied by the voltage clamp technique, is increased by noradrenaline and dibutyryl cAMP (Reuter, 1974). The low Ca^{2+} in the cytosol during diastole would also be consistent with a high level of cAMP because low Ca^{2+} allows higher activity of sarcolemmal adenyl cyclase (Kirchberger et al., 1974). A suggested mechanism, relating the roles of both internal and external Ca^{2+} for the heart, is that the entry of a small amount of Ca^{2+} is necessary to trigger the release of Ca^{2+} from the SR or other stores of Ca^{2+}, such as the mitochondria (Ebashi, 1969). Whatever mechanism proves to be correct, the crucial point of each model is the demonstration of how the flow of Ca^{2+} into the SR stimulated by cAMP and the control of cAMP by the SR Ca^{2+} synchronizes the SR activity with the contraction cycle.

CONCLUSIONS

We are suggesting that the increase in Ca^{2+} must, of itself, automatically result in the subsequent decrease of cAMP to allow for the periodic flux of Ca^{2+} and cAMP in a contraction cycle. A mechanism for this resides in the effect of the increased Ca^{2+} content of the SR which activates the activator protein of cAMP phosphodiesterase and results in a decrease in cAMP. High SR Ca^{2+} leads to decreased cAMP, and low SR Ca^{2+} results in an increase in cAMP. The levels vary cyclically, one step out of synchrony with each other. Thus, the depolarization of the sarcolemma and the entry of Ca^{2+} into the cells cause contraction and a series of events leading to the restoration of the state necessary for the repetition of the cycle. These events serve as the periodic priming of the SR pump, consistent with the contraction cycle.

REFERENCES

BROOKER, G. 1975. Implications of cyclic nucleotide oscillations during the myocardial contraction cycle. Adv. Cycl. Nucl. Res. 5:435–452.

EBASHI, S. 1969. Ca ion as a basis of pharmacological actions. Proc. Fourth Intl. Congr. Pharm. (Basel) 1:32–54.

HARARY, I., HOOVER, F., and FARLEY, B. 1974. The isolation and cultivation of rat heart cells. In S. Fleischer and L. Packer (eds.), Methods of Enzymology, pp. 740–745. Academic Press, New York.

HARARY, I., RENAUD, J. F., SATO, E., and WALLACE, G. A., 1976. Calcium ions regulate cAMP and beating in cultured heart cells. Nature 261:60–61.

HUI, C.-H., DRUMMOND, M., and DRUMMOND, G. I. 1976. Calcium accumulation and cyclic AMP-stimulated phosphorylation in plasma membrane-enriched preparation of myocardium. Arch. Biochem. Biophys. 173:415–427.

KAKIUCHI, S., and YAMAZAKI, R. 1970. Calcium dependent phosphodiesterase activity and its activating factor from brain. Biochem. Biophys. Res. Commun. 41:1104–1110.

KATZ, A. M. 1970. Contractile proteins of the heart. Physiol. Rev. 50:63–158.

KATZ, A. M., TADA, M., REPKE, D. I., IORIO, J. M., and KIRCHBERGER, M. A., 1974. Adenylate cyclase: Its probable localization in sarcoplasmic reticulum as well as sarcolemma of the canine heart. J. Mol. Cell. Cardiol. 6:73–78.

KIDWAI, A. M., RADCLIFFE, M. A., DUCHON, G., and DANIEL, E. E. 1971. Isolation of plasma membrane from cardiac muscle. Biochem. Biophys. Res. Commun. 45:901–910.

KIRCHBERGER, M. A., IORIO, J. M., and KATZ, A. M. 1974. Control of cardiac sarcolemmal adenylate cyclase by calcium ions. J. Clin. Invest. 53:80A.

KIRCHBERGER, M. A., TADA, M., REPKE, D. I., and KATZ, A. M. 1972. Cyclic adenosine 3′,5′-monophosphate-dependent protein kinase stimulation of calcium uptake by canine cardiac microsomes. J. Mol. Cell. Cardiol. 4:673–680.

LANGER, G. A. 1974. Ionic movements and the control of contraction. In G. A. Langer and A. J. Brady (eds.), The Mammalian Myocardium, pp. 193–217. John Wiley & Sons Inc., New York.

REUTER, H. 1974. Localization of beta-adrenergic receptors, and cyclic nucleotides on action potentials, ionic currents and tension in mammalian cardiac muscle. J. Physiol. 242:429–451.

TADA, M., KIRCHBERGER, M. A., and LI, H.-C. 1975. Phosphoprotein phosphatase-catalyzed dephosphorylation of the 22,000 dalton phosphoprotein of cardiac sarcoplasmic reticulum. J. Cycl. Nucl. Res. 1:329–338.

WALLACE, G. A., and HARARY, I. 1975. Localization of the cyclic adenosine 3′:5′-monophosphate phosphodiesterase activator protein in rat heart. Biochem. Biophys. Res. Commun. 67:810–817.

WINEGRAD, S. 1968. Intracellular calcium movements of frog skeletal muscle during recovery from tetanus. J. Gen. Physiol. 56:191–217.

WOLLENBERGER, A., BABSKII, E. B., KRAUSE, E. B., GERZ, S., BLOOM, D., and BOGDANOVA, E. V. 1973. Cyclic changes in levels of cyclic AMP and cyclic GMP in frog myocardium during the cardiac cycle. Biochem. Biophys. Res. Commun. 55:446–452.

Mailing address:
Dr. Isaac Harary,
Laboratory of Nuclear Medicine and Radiation Biology,
University of California at Los Angeles,
900 Veteran Avenue, Los Angeles, California 90024 (USA).

Recent Advances in Studies on
Cardiac Structure and Metabolism, Volume 12
Cardiac Adaptation
Edited by T. Kobayashi, Y. Ito, and G. Rona
Copyright 1978 University Park Press Baltimore

ELECTRICAL PROPERTIES OF CULTURED HEART CELLS

N. SPERELAKIS and M. J. McLEAN

Department of Physiology,
University of Virginia School of Medicine,
Charlottesville, Virginia, USA

SUMMARY

The findings reported in this chapter indicate the wide variety of electrophysiological properties that can be achieved in cultured heart cells isolated from old embryonic chick hearts (ventricles). Some cells have reverted (partially dedifferentiated) properties resembling the young embryonic state, namely, no fast Na^+ channels, a low P_K, and high automaticity. Other cells have only partly reverted properties, and still other cells retain or regain their highly differentiated electrical properties, including a large number of fast Na^+ channels, a low number of slow Na^+ channels, a high P_K, and no automaticity. Many factors, some unknown, seem to influence the degree of differentiation observed in culture, including the following: reaggregation, aging in culture, and low serum media (possibly via inhibition of cell division). Culturing in media containing elevated K^+ plus ATP seems to improve the incidence of highly differentiated cells. The trypsin-dispersed cultured cells retain their pharmacological receptors; this is particularly clear for the highly differentiated cells. It would appear that a highly differentiated morphology is accompanied by highly differentiated membrane properties, whereas the reverse is not necessarily true, i.e., some cells have highly differentiated electrical properties with a reverted ultrastructure. Immature myocardial cells do not continue to differentiate, either electrically or morphologically, *in vitro*. This is true of reaggregate cell cultures prepared from young embryonic hearts and of organ-cultured intact young hearts. However, addition of a RNA-enriched fraction obtained from adult chicken hearts does allow electrical differentiation to proceed after a lag period of several days. Hence, the cultured cells can be used to study and answer a wide variety of multidisciplinary questions that are difficult or impossible to answer in intact cardiac muscle.

INTRODUCTION

The use of cultured heart cells in various multicellular organizations affords unique advantages over intact myocardium for answering certain types of questions. For example, the following types of studies can be performed on monolayer networks of interconnected cells: 1) Simultaneous recording of transmembrane potentials and contractions can be made on single cells using photoelectric

The work of the authors summarized and reviewed in this article was supported by grants from the U.S. Public Health Service (HL-11155, HL-18711, and 5SO1RR05431-13).

techniques. 2) Because cardiac muscle is a one- or two-dimensional system, studies of electrotonic spread of current and cell-to-cell interactions are facilitated. 3) The electrogenesis of various components of the action potential and the electrogenesis of pacemaker potentials can be studied in isolated single cells in which propagation from, or interaction with, contiguous cells is eliminated. 4) Voltage clamp experiments can be done on isolated single cells in which there can be no question as to adequate voltage control over the entire cell membrane, and in which the membrane current densities can be measured. 5) Because the cells are denervated, the direct effect of various chemicals and pharmacological agents on the myocardial cells can be determined without complications caused by neural and systemic influences. 6) The problem of diffusion lag in the interstitial fluid space is reduced or eliminated, thus facilitating ion-flux studies in a simple two-compartment system. 7) Microelectrophoretic injection of various substances can be done while observing electrical and mechanical effects on the injected cell. 8) The cultured cells can be maintained in various experimental media to attempt to change the composition of the cell membranes and to ascertain the concomitant changes in membrane transport and electrical properties. Cultured heart cells can be grown in chemically defined media (Halle and Wollenberger, 1971), and antibiotics may be omitted from the culture medium if sterile procedures are followed carefully. 9) Finally, by using hearts of various embryonic ages, some fundamental questions of development can be answered.

The first account of cultured heart cells was given by Burrows (1912), who observed the independent pulsatory activity of single cells and foresaw its significance as a direct confirmation of the myogenic theory of heart muscle. Although cardiac muscle was traditionally regarded as a branching syncytium, Lewis (1928) rejected this concept in favor of cellular independence, on the basis of studies of cultured heart cells. Monophasic action potentials were recorded using relatively large-tipped electrodes (Hogg, Goss, and Cole, 1934), and larger potentials were obtained by impalement of cultured heart cells with finer microelectrodes (Mettler *et al.*, 1952; Fänge, Persson, and Thesleff, 1952; Crill, Rumery, and Woodbury, 1959; Sperelakis and Lehmkuhl, 1965). Details of the methodology for satisfactory intracellular recordings have been given by Sperelakis (1967, 1972b).

MATERIALS AND METHODS: CULTURED HEART CELL PREPARATIONS

Many tissues can be grown in culture as explants of small minced pieces from which some cell types grow out and form monolayer sheets. However, the cells emigrating from the explant, e.g., fibroblasts, may or may not include the cell type that one is interested in studying (myocardial cell, in this instance). Therefore, discussion in this chapter deals only with cases in which the myocardial cells are dissociated from the ventricle and/or atrium by use of proteolytic enzymes to loosen the intercellular matrix plus some sort of mechanical shearing force. Trypsin is generally used for heart cell dispersal, and it can be shown that the reaggregated cells have electrophysiological and pharmacological properties identical to those of cells in the original myocardium from which they were derived. That is, exposure to the trypsin, at the concentrations and times necessary for cell dispersal, does not permanently damage the cell membrane or its receptors. Embryonic or early postnatal tissue is generally used because the myocardial cells are more easily freed from the tissue. Various procedures are available for increasing the proportion of myocytes to nonmyocytes, e.g., fibroblasts or endothelioid cells, in the culture, such as differential stickiness (Hyde *et al.,* 1969); but, even without using these, the percentage of beating myocardial cells may be 50–90%.

Although cultured heart cells do undergo mitosis (Mark and Strasser, 1966; DeHaan, 1967; Kasten, 1972; Kelly and Chacko, 1976), there is no general agreement as to whether or not the mitotic state affects the state of differentiation. Some investigators suggest that dividing cells are not in a highly differentiated state. However, mitosis apparently proceeds without loss, or with only transient loss, of myofibrils. Mitosis and organogenetic movements continue when the cells are depolarized in high K^+ (Pappano and Sperelakis, 1969; Manasek and Monroe, 1972). It is not clear whether contact inhibition of cell division occurs among heart cells *in vitro.* Multilayer regions can be found in cultures produced at high-plating density, and cells do overgrow one another. The density of cells plated may influence their viability and function through secretion of factors into the medium ("conditioned medium") (see, for example, Gordon and Brice, 1974).

Cultured heart cells can be studied as various types of preparations. First, they can be kept as suspensions of cells for some types of experiments. Second, they can be plated on glass or plastic at a low density ($<10^5$ cells/ml) so that, in many instances, isolated single cells can be found stuck to the substrate. Third, the cells can be plated at a higher density (e.g., 0.5×10^6 cells/ml) so that loose monolayer networks of cells and rosette patterns are formed. Cells within such groups usually contract synchronously. Cells plated at a still higher density ($>10^6$ cells/ml) and for longer periods will form confluent sheets. In some regions, the sheets are one cell thick, i.e., monolayers; whereas, in other regions, some cells overlap and form multilayers two or more cells thick. Large areas of the sheets contract synchronously.

In addition to these types of cell formations, special reaggregations of cells can be prepared. For example, the cells can be grown as long, thin strands, either by using a fiberglass filament as the substrate (Sperelakis and McLean, unpublished observation) or by making a fine scratch on a coating on which the cells will not stick (Lieberman *et al.,* 1972). The cells can be reaggregated into small spheres of about 100–500 μm in diameter by either plating onto cellophane (to which they do not adhere very well and therefore pull free and form small spherical reaggregates (McLean and Sperelakis, 1976)), or gyrotation according to the Moscona method (1961) for about 48 hr.

The strand and spherical reaggregate preparations are useful because they are easier to impale with one or two microelectrodes and because the cells tend to retain their highly differentiated electrical properties (see book edited by Lieberman and Sano, 1976, for results from several laboratories). In contrast, the cells in monolayer networks and sheets revert back to the young embryonic state. Such reverted cells are also useful for studying certain properties, such as the mechanism of changes in cation channels and K^+ permeability and the electrogenesis of pacemaker potentials. In fact, reverted ventricular myocardial cells make a good model for study of the properties of cardiac nodal cells. The discussion which follows of the electrical properties of cultured heart cells is divided into two major categories: 1) reverted monolayers, and 2) highly differentiated reaggregates. We have presented here principally the results from our own laboratory, but the reader is referred to the book edited by Lieberman and Sano (1976) for reviews by numerous experts.

RESULTS AND DISCUSSION

Changing Electrical Properties During Intact Heart Development *in Situ*

Absence of fast Na$^+$ channels in young hearts   In order to determine the state of membrane differentiation of the cultured cells, comparison has been made with the properties of intact chick hearts at different stages of development *in situ.* The electrical properties of the cells undergo sequential changes during development, as shown in Figure 1. Young (2–4 days *in ovo*) myocardial cells possess slowly-rising (10–20 V/sec) action potentials preceded by pacemaker potentials. Hyperpolarizing current pulses do not greatly increase the rate of rise of the action potential, and excitability is not lost until the membrane is depolarized to less than −25 mV. The upstroke is generated by Na$^+$ influx through tetrodotoxin (TTX)-insensitive, slow Na$^+$ channels. Kinetically fast Na$^+$ channels that are sensitive to TTX make their initial appearance on about day 5, and the maximal rate of rise of the action potential ($+\dot{V}_{max}$) suddenly jumps to about 50–70 V/sec. The fast Na$^+$ channels increase in density thereafter, until about day 18, when the adult maximal rate of rise of about 150 V/sec is achieved. During an intermediate stage of development (from about day 5 to day 8), both slow and fast Na$^+$ channels coexist in the membrane. TTX causes a reduction in $+\dot{V}_{max}$ to about the rate observed in young cells, i.e., 10–20 V/sec, but the action potentials and accompanying contractions persist. After about day 8, the action potentials are completely abolished by TTX, despite increased stimulus intensity, and depolarization to less than −50 mV now abolishes excitability. This indicates that the battery of action potential-generat-

INTACT HEARTS

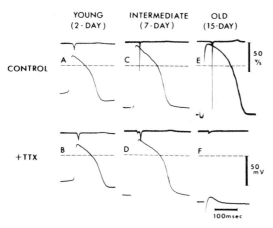

Figure 1. Development of sensitivity to TTX of intact embryonic chick hearts with increasing embryonic age. A–B: Intracellular recordings from a two-day-old heart before (A) and 20 min after (B) the addition of TTX (20 μg/ml). C–D: Recordings from a seven-day-old heart before (C) and 2 min after (D) the addition of TTX (2 μg/ml). Note depression of the rate of rise in D. E–F: Recordings from a 15-day-old heart before (E) and 2 min after (F) the addition of TTX (1 μg/ml). The action potentials were abolished, and excitability was not restored by strong field stimulation in F. The upper traces give dV/dt; this trace has been shifted relative to the V-t trace to prevent obscuring dV/dt. The horizontal broken line in each panel represents zero potential. dV/dt calibration (in E) and voltage and time calibrations (in F) pertain to all panels. (Modified from Sperelakis and Shigenobu, 1972.)

ing Na^+ channels consists predominantly of fast Na^+ channels; most of the slow Na^+ channels have been inactivated (either by removal from the membrane, or by masking), and insufficient numbers remain to support regenerative excitation. Addition of some positive inotropic agents increases the number of slow Ca^{2+}-Na^+ channels in the membrane and leads to regaining of excitability in cells whose fast Na^+ channels have been inactivated.

Low K^+ permeability in young hearts   The young chick hearts have a low K^+ permeability (P_K). This accounts for the low resting potentials of about −40 mV and for the high incidence of automaticity in the ventricular area of the tubular heart. As shown by resting potential versus log $[K^+]_o$ curves for hearts of different ages (Figure 2), the low resting potentials in young hearts are caused by a high P_{Na}/P_K ratio of about 0.2, attributable to a low P_K rather than to an internal $[K^+]_i$ substantially lower than that of old hearts. The $[K^+]_i$ level is about 130 mM in three-day-old hearts compared to 150 mM in 15-day hearts; hence, the K^+ diffusion potential (E_K) is not greatly different (about −91 mV at a $[K^+]_o$ of 4 mM for three-day hearts). As development proceeds, P_K increases rapidly so that the P_{Na}/P_K ratio is about 0.1 by day 5 and is between 0.05 and

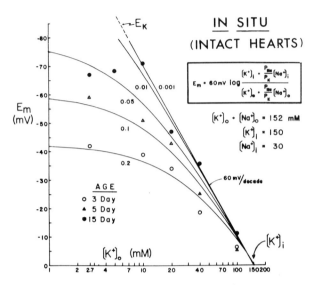

Figure 2. Resting potential (E_m) plotted as a function of $[K^+]_0$ on a logarithmic scale for three representative hearts of different ages. $[K^+]_0$ was elevated by substitution of K^+ for equimolar amounts of Na^+. Continuous lines give theoretical calculations from the constant-field equation (inset) for P_{Na}/P_K ratios of 0.001, 0.01, 0.05, 0.1, and 0.2. Calculations were made assuming $[K^+]_i$ and $[Na^+]_i$ values shown. For a P_{Na}/P_K ratio of 0.001, the curve is linear over the entire range with a slope of 60 mV/decade, i.e., it closely follows E_K. Symbols give representative data obtained from embryonic chick hearts at days 3 (○), 5 (△), and 15 (●). The data for the three-day heart follow the curve for a P_{Na}/P_K ratio of 0.2, those for five-day heart follow the theoretical curve for 0.1, and those for the 15-day heart follow the curves for 0.01 to 0.05. The estimated intracellular K^+ activities ($[K^+]_i$) obtained by extrapolation to zero potential are nearly the same for all ages. (Modified from Sperelakis and Shigenobu, 1972.)

0.01 by day 15. The increase in resting potential parallels the increase in P_K. The input resistance of the cells is high in young hearts (about 13 MΩ), and it declines in parallel with the increase in P_K (to a final value of about 4.5 MΩ). As predicted from Figure 2, young hearts are less sensitive to elevation of $[K^+]_0$. Carmeliet *et al.* (1976) also have shown from ^{42}K flux measurements that P_K is several-fold lower in six-day hearts than in 19-day hearts.

The presence of pacemaker potentials is determined by P_K in cells that have a low P_{Cl}, as do myocardial cells. The low P_K in young cells makes for automaticity as well as low resting potentials. The incidence of pacemaker potentials in cells in young hearts is very high, and this incidence decreases during development, roughly in parallel with the increase in P_K. Automaticity is absent in the ventricular cells of the older hearts.

Low (Na^+,K^+)-ATPase activity and high cAMP level in young hearts The (Na^+,K^+)-ATPase specific activity is low in the young hearts and increases progressively during development, reaching the final adult value by about day 18

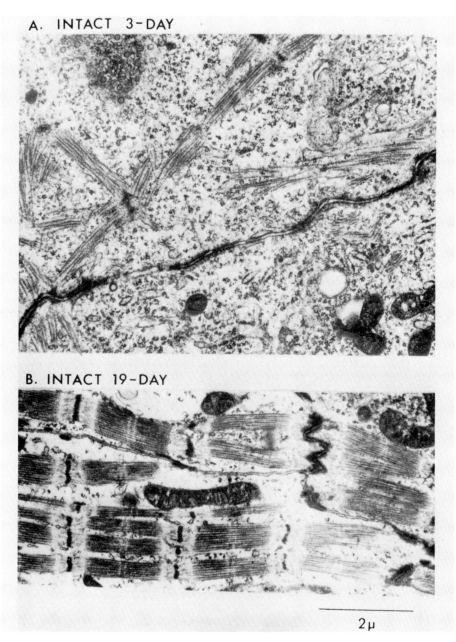

A. INTACT 3-DAY

B. INTACT 19-DAY

2 μ

Figure 3. Cell ultrastructure of young (three days *in ovo*) and old (19 days *in ovo*) intact embryonic chick hearts *in situ*. A: three-day ventricular cells demonstrating paucity and nonalignment of myofibrils. Ribosomes are abundant in the cytoplasm. The contiguous cells are held in close apposition by desmosomes. B: 19-day ventricular cells with abundant and aligned myofibrils. A convoluted intercalated disc appears between contiguous cells. Calibration given in B also applies to A.

(Sperelakis, 1972). Although the Na^+-K^+ pump capability is thus low in young hearts, it must be sufficient to maintain a relatively high $[K^+]_i$, possibly because of the low P_K. That is, in young hearts the pump capability is low, but the ion leak is correspondingly low.

The cAMP level is very high in young hearts, and it decreases during development, first rapidly and then more slowly, reaching the final adult level by about day 16 (McLean et al., 1975). Because elevation of cAMP leads to an increase in the number of available slow Ca^{2+}-Na^+ channels (Shigenobu and Sperelakis, 1972), the decrease in cAMP level during development could be related to the decrease in density of slow channels.

Few and nonaligned myofibrils in young hearts   Electron microscopy of young hearts shows that there are only few and short myofibrils (Figure 3A). The sarcomeres are not complete, and the myofibrils run in all directions, i.e., they often run perpendicular to one another. There is an abundance of ribosomes and rough endoplasmic reticulum, and large pools of glycogen are found in certain regions of the cells. As development progresses, the number of myofibrils increases, and they become aligned, as illustrated in Figure 3B. By day 18 the ultrastructure of the myocardial cells is indistinguishable from the adult morphology.

Cultured Myocardial Cells Dispersed from Old Embryonic Hearts

Reversion to the young embryonic state in standard monolayer culture

Loss of myofibrils   When ventricular myocardial cells are trypsin-dispersed from 16–20-day-old embryonic chick hearts and placed into a standard monolayer cell culture, the cells lose many of their myofibrils within a short time. Cells in a monolayer culture are illustrated with light microscopy in Figure 4A and with electron microscopy in Figure 4B. As shown, after several days in culture there are only few and incomplete myofibrils. Thus, the ultrastructure rapidly reverts to that characteristic of the young embryonic state (compare Figure 4B with Figure 3A). However, the cells tend to regain more myofibrils after long periods in culture (Mark and Strasser, 1966) and closely resemble the adult ultrastructure if placed into media containing low serum concentrations (which presumably inhibit cell division and favor differentiation) (Jones et al., personal communication).

Loss of fast Na^+ channels and gain of slow Na^+ channels   When the monolayer cells, cultured for 3–14 days, are impaled with microelectrodes, it is found that the resting potentials are low, the action potentials are slowly-rising ($+\dot{V}_{max}$ of 3–15 V/sec), and the overshoot is small (see Figure 5C). Hyperpolarizing current pulses increase action potential amplitude (see Figure 7B), but $+\dot{V}_{max}$ is increased only a relatively small amount. With depolarizing pulses, $+\dot{V}_{max}$ decreases and goes to zero at an E_m of about −20 mV; spontaneous contractions cease at a $[K^+]_o$ of about 50 mм, corresponding to a resting potential of about

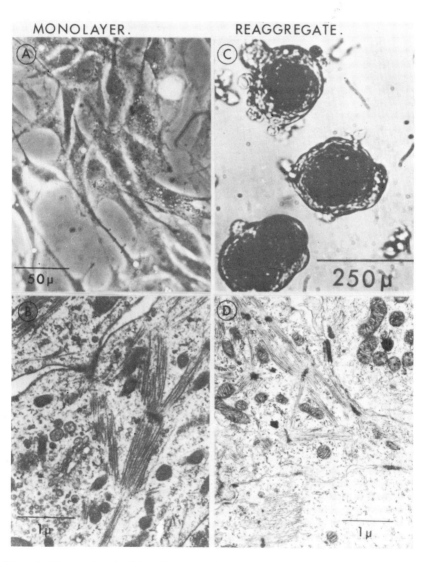

Figure 4. Micrographs of 19-day-old embryonic chick ventricular cells cultured as mono-layers (A–B) and in spherical reaggregates (C–D). A: Low power phase contrast micrograph showing cell arrangement. B: Electron micrograph showing paucity and nonalignment of myofibrils in cells. C: Low power light micrograph showing several spherical reaggregates. D: Electron micrograph of several cells showing sparse, incomplete, and nonaligned myofibrils.

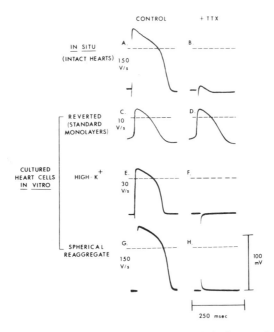

Figure 5. Comparison of electrophysiological properties of the intact, old (16-day) embryonic chick heart *in situ* (A–B) with those of trypsin-dispersed, old ventricular myocardial cells in cultures prepared by three different methods (C–H). A–B: Intact heart; control action potential (A) was rapidly-rising (150 V/sec), had a high stable resting potential (about −80 mV), and was completely abolished by tetrodotoxin (TTX; 0.1 µg/ml) (B). C–D: Standard reverted monolayers; control action potential was slowly-rising (10 V/sec) and was preceded by a pacemaker potential, the resting potential was low (about −50 mV) (C), and TTX did not alter the action potential (D). E–F: Partially reverted cells cultured as monolayers in media containing elevated K⁺ concentration (25 mM); control action potential had a rate of rise of 30 V/sec (E), lacked a pacemaker potential, had a moderately high resting potential (−60 mV), and was completely abolished by TTX (F). G–H: Highly differentiated cells in spherical reaggregate culture; control action potentials were rapidly-rising (150 V/sec), the resting potentials were high (−80 mV)(G), and TTX abolished the action potentials (H).

−15 mV (see Figure 6). TTX has no effect on the rate of rise or overshoot of the action potential (Sperelakis and Lehmkuhl, 1965) (Figure 5D). The loss of TTX sensitivity in monolayer culture has been confirmed (Roseen and Fuhrman, 1971; McDonald, Sachs, and DeHaan, 1972; Renaud, 1973). The action potentials closely resemble those found in young embryonic hearts (compare Figure 5C with Figure 1A), not those found in old embryonic hearts from which the cells were derived (compare Figure 5C–D with Figure 5A–B or with Figure 1E–F). Thus, the ventricular cells taken from 16–20-day embryonic hearts revert back to the early embryonic state (or partially dedifferentiate) with respect to the action potential-generating mechanism, namely, fast Na⁺ channels are lost and slow Na^+ channels are gained. This reversion occurs rapidly, being complete within 24 hr (McLean and Sperelakis, 1974).

The inward current during the action potential is carried mainly by the Na^+ ion because the overshoot is a function of log $[Na^+]_o$, the slope approaching the theoretical 60 mV/decade; $+\dot{V}_{max}$ is also dependent on $[Na^+]_o$, and excitability is abolished at 28 mM Na^+ and below. Li^+ cannot substitute for Na^+ for carrying current through the slow Na^+ channels during the action potentials. However, a small inward Ca^{2+} current undoubtedly normally participates in the electro-genesis of the rising phase and overshoot of the action potential. In fact, in cells whose excitability is abolished in zero Na^+ (Li^+, choline$^+$, or sucrose replace-ment), the elevation of $[Ca^{2+}]_o$ to 10 mM or more, or the addition of Sr^{2+}(5–10 mM) or Ba^{2+} (2–10 mM), leads to rapid reappearance of action potentials. Thus, purely divalent cation spikes can be produced in cultured heart cells, as has been done recently for Purkinje fibers (Vereecke and Carmeliet, 1971). The divalent cations presumably pass through either slow Ca^{2+} channels or the slow Na^+ channels.

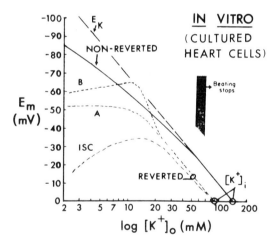

Figure 6. Resting potential (E_m) as a function of the external K^+ concentration for chick embryonic heart cells in monolayer culture (reverted) and in cultured spherical reaggregates (nonreverted). The line labeled E_K has a slope of 60 mV per tenfold change in $[K^+]_o$. Reverted cells: With elevation of $[K^+]_o$ from 2.7 to 10–15 mM, the resting potentials of some cells are almost unaffected (curve A), whereas those of other cells become slightly hyperpolarized (curve B). Isolated single cells (ISC) that are not beating spontaneously usually have a much lower resting potential, but they become markedly hyperpolarized at 10–15 mM $[K^+]_o$ (curve labeled ISC). All cells depolarize as $[K^+]_o$ is elevated above 20 mM, and extrapolation of linear region of curve to zero potential gives $[K^+]_i$ of 90–100 mM. Spontaneous synchronous beating of cell groups ceases at 50–60 mM $[K^+]_o$. Non-reverted cells: The curve for cells in cultured spherical reaggregates fits a theoretical plot of values calculated from the constant-field equation for P_{Na}/P_K ratio of 0.02. The plot extrapolates to a $[K^+]_i$ of about 130 mM.

Decrease in P_K *and gain of automaticity* Shortly after separation from the ventricle, many of the myocardial cells in suspension will beat spontaneously at independent rhythms. This indicates that the normally nonpacemaker ventricular cells of old embryonic hearts rapidly gain automaticity upon cell separation. This suggests that a marked decrease in P_K occurs. When the cells are allowed to adhere to the glass for a few days and are subsequently impaled, the resting potentials are low and many cells exhibit pacemaker potentials (Figure 5C). The input resistance increases, the average value being close to double (10 MΩ) that of cells in intact hearts. These facts are consistent with a low P_K. A plot of resting potential versus log $[K^+]_o$ suggests that the extrapolated $[K^+]_i$ is 90–100 mM in the reverted cells (Figure 6), corresponding to an E_K (at a $[K^+]_o$ of 4 mM) of −82 mV. This value is considerably higher (numerically) than the measured average resting potential of about −55 mV, hence suggesting that P_K is low (high P_{Na}/P_K ratio). Thus, P_K also tends to revert back toward the young embryonic state in cultured monolayers. In fact, in some isolated single cells in culture, P_K is so low that the cells are depolarized beyond the level that action potentials can be produced (beyond the inactivation potential for the slow channels); therefore, these cells are not spontaneously contracting. However, if impaled with one or two microelectrodes, it is seen that the membrane resistance is very high and that spontaneous action potentials and contractions appear upon application of hyperpolarizing current pulses (see Figure 8 J–L). As shown

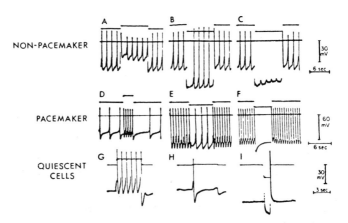

Figure 7. Effect of polarizing current on nonpacemaker and pacemaker reverted heart cells in monolayer culture. A–C: Nonpacemaker cell; frequency of firing unaltered by current pulses of 0.6 (A) and 1.4 nA (B); at 1.5 nA, action potentials prevented, but driving junctional potentials remain at unaltered frequency (C). D–F: Three pacemaker cells; depolarizing current pulse of 1.2 nA markedly increases rate of firing (D), whereas hyperpolarizing pulses slow the frequency (E, 0.6 nA) or cause cessation of firing (F, 1.2 nA). G–I: Quiescent cells can be induced to fire during depolarizing current pulses (1.4 nA in G and 0.2 nA in H), or at the termination of hyperpolarizing current pulses (I, 2 nA).

in Figure 6, these cells exhibit a prominent hyperpolarization when $[K^+]_o$ is raised to 10–15 mM.

Some of the monolayer cells behave as nonpacemaker cells. As illustrated in Figure 7A–B, application of depolarizing or hyperpolarizing current pulses does not alter the frequency of firing in these cells. Sufficient hyperpolarization causes failure of the action potentials, but, unlike the true pacemaker cells, small driving junctional potentials continue at unaltered frequency during the pulse (Figure 7C); the junctional potentials probably represent the interaction with contiguous firing cells. In contrast, true pacemaker cells respond to small depolarizing current pulses by an increase in firing rate, and to small hyperpolarizing pulses by a decrease in firing frequency (Figure 7D–F); note the absence of

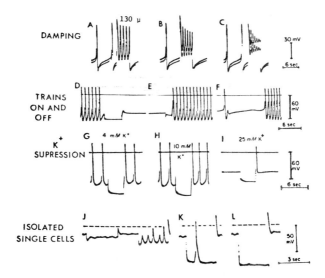

Figure 8. A–C: Impalement of one cell in a monolayer culture with two microelectrodes (130 μm apart) showing nearly identical potential changes in both electrodes when current is passed through one electrode. Depolarizing pulses of 9 (A), 10.2 (B), and 11.6 (C) nA were applied; note damping of responses. Bridge imbalance in C because of high current. D–E: Trains of spontaneous action potentials turned off (D) and on (E) by small hyperpolarizing pulses. Automatic firing was stopped by a 1.2 nA pulse too small to cause anodal-break excitation; firing reinstated by a larger pulse (1.8 nA) which produced anodal-break excitation (E). F: Spontaneous arrest of firing and resumption of firing in a cell; note depolarizing afterpotential following the hyperpolarizing afterpotential. G–I: Recordings from one true pacemaker cell illustrating suppression of automaticity by elevation of extracellular K^+. In 4 mM (G) and 10 mM (H) K^+, automaticity was not suppressed, whereas elevation of K^+ to 25 mM caused depolarization and cessation of spontaneous action potential generation; but anodal-break excitation elicited an action potential (I). Hyperpolarizing current pulses of 4.8 nA applied in each panel. J–L: Recordings from an isolated single cell in culture that was quiescent and had a very low resting potential. Hyperpolarizing current pulses of 0.2 and 0.4 nA (J), 0.8 nA (K), and 0.9 nA (L) elicited anodal-break responses as well as spontaneous firing during the pulse (J–K); the frequency of firing during the pulse was a function of the degree of hyperpolarization, indicating true pacemaker behavior.

junctional potentials in F when firing is abolished. The slope of the pacemaker potential is an exquisite function of E_m. Quiescent cells can be induced to exhibit trains of action potentials during application of long-duration depolarizing pulses (Figure 7G–H), and anodal-break excitation can be elicited by brief hyperpolarizing pulses (Figure 7I). Large depolarizing pulses result in the occurrence of damped oscillations during the pulse (Figure 8A–C). Some cells exhibiting pacemaker potentials function as latent pacemakers in that they are driven by true pacemaker cells which possess greater intrinsic firing rates. In some true pacemaker cells, application of a hyperpolarizing current pulse, large enough to shut off the train but too small to elicit anodal-break excitation, will "permanently" turn off the train (Figure 8D); subsequent application of a hyperpolarizing pulse sufficiently large to elicit anodal-break excitation (or of a brief depolarizing pulse just sufficient to trigger a single action potential) turns the train back on (Figure 8E). This suggests that each action potential is responsible for triggering the next one. In some cases, the train turns off and on paroxysmally (Figure 8F), and, in such cases, it can be seen that a depolarizing afterpotential follows the hyperpolarizing afterpotential.

Automaticity is suppressed by elevation of $[K^+]_o$ above 15 mM (Figure 8G–I), as expected by the increase in K^+ conductance (g_K). The g_K is a function of both P_K and $[K^+]_o$, and P_K also is increased in elevated $[K^+]_o$. Distinction between suppression of automaticity and depolarization block of excitability is demonstrated clearly in Figure 8I, in which automaticity of the same cell penetrated in G–H is completely suppressed, yet the cell is capable of producing anodal-break excitation. In addition, spontaneous firing did not occur during the hyperpolarizing pulse itself.

Automaticity is rapidly induced by 2–5 mM Ba^{2+} (Figure 9A–C), presumably because of its effect of decreasing P_K and of increasing the inward background depolarizing current. Partial depolarization is produced, and membrane resistivity is increased greatly. If the depolarization produced is too great (beyond the inactivation potential for the slow channels), the cell becomes quiescent but will fire spontaneous action potentials and contract concomitantly during the application of hyperpolarizing current pulses (Figure 9D–F). The frequency of firing produced is a function of the intensity of the hyperpolarizing current pulse. Sr^{2+} (5–10 mM) also has the ability to induce automaticity in quiescent cells concomitant with hyperpolarization (Figure 9G–I). At the higher Sr^{2+} concentrations, prominent depolarizing after-potentials are produced, and the action potentials ride on top of large sinusoidal-like oscillations. The effect of Sr^{2+} could be attributable to stimulation of an electrogenic Na^+ pump potential contribution to E_m. Both Sr^{2+} and Ba^{2+} hyperpolarize cells partially depolarized by ouabain or local anesthetic inhibition of the (Na^+, K^+)-ATPase, but the hyperpolarizing action of Ba^{2+} usually is masked by its prominent depolarizing action because of decreasing P_K.

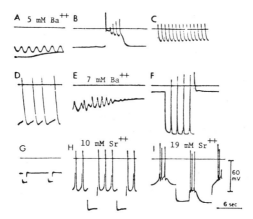

Figure 9. Effects of Ba²⁺ and Sr²⁺ on reverted cells in monolayer culture. A–C: In a quiescent cell, Ba²⁺ (5 mM) depolarized and induced spontaneous firing. A: Two successive sweeps superimposed at 20 sec after addition of Ba²⁺ showing onset of depolarization and oscillations. B: After 3 min, the action potentials acquired prolonged plateaus with repetitive discharges on the plateau. C: At 5 min, sustained depolarization occurred with repetitive action potentials. D–F: In a firing cell (D), Ba²⁺ (7 mM) rapidly depolarized and increased membrane resistance (E); repolarizing current pulse (1.2 nA), applied during the sustained depolarization, initiated action potentials during the pulse (F). G–I: In a quiescent cell (G), 10 mM Sr²⁺ produced hyperpolarization and converted the cell to a true pacemaker (H), as evidenced by cessation of firing during applied hyperpolarizing pulses of 4.8 nA. Elevation of Sr²⁺ to 19 mM (I) induced sinusoidal-like oscillations with several action potentials superimposed and produced prominent depolarizing afterpotentials; current pulse of 6.0 nA applied.

Decrease in (Na⁺,K⁺)-ATPase and increase in cAMP   The cultured monolayer cells have a lowered (Na⁺,K⁺)-ATPase specific activity (Sperelakis and Lee, 1971) and an elevated cAMP level (McLean *et al.*, 1975). In these respects, also, there seems to be some reversion toward an earlier embryonic state.

Partial reversion in elevated K⁺   It was found that separating the cells and culturing them in media containing elevated K⁺ (12–60 mM) helped the cells to retain more highly differentiated electrical properties (McLean and Sperelakis, 1974). (The cells were tested in normal K⁺ solutions.) The resting potentials were higher (about −60 mV), and automaticity was absent in most cells, indicating that P_K was not as greatly reverted. Although the action potentials were only slightly faster-rising ($+\dot{V}_{max}$ of about 30 V/sec), they were completely abolished by TTX (Figure 5E–F). Thus, it appears that some fast Na⁺ channels are retained and the number of slow Na⁺ channels is not greatly increased. Hyperpolarization by current injection did not greatly increase $+\dot{V}_{max}$, indicating that another population of fast Na⁺ channels, which were voltage inactivated, was not present. Therefore, culture in high K⁺ media acted to prevent complete reversion to the young embryonic state. Addition of ATP (5 mM) to the medium had a slightly beneficial effect, especially in combination with elevated K^+, for the retention or the regaining of differentiated membrane properties.

Retention of highly differentiated membrane electrical properties in cultured spherical reaggregates

Fast-rising TTX-sensitive action potentials and high-resting potentials Many cells in spherical reaggregates (see Figure 4C) (and in cylindrical strands) retain fully differentiated electrophysiological properties identical to those of the intact old embryonic hearts *in situ* (compare Figure 5G–H with Figure 5A–B). These cells had high-resting potentials of about −80 mV, and pacemaker potentials were absent; this indicates that P_K remained high. The plot of E_m versus log $[K^+]_o$ indicated a P_{Na}/P_K ratio of about 0.02, and a $[K^+]_i$ of about 130 mM (Figure 6). The input resistance averaged ∼5 MΩ. The action potentials had fast rates of rise (100–200 V/sec), and they were completely blocked by low concentrations of TTX (3 × 10^{-7} M). $+\dot{V}_{max}$ diminished as the cells were progressively depolarized by elevation of $[K^+]_o$, and all excitability was abolished at an E_m of about −50 mV. In addition, the chronaxie is brief (about 0.5 msec), indicative of high excitability comparable to that of adult cardiac muscle. Thus, these cells retained their full complement of fast Na^+ channels as well as a high P_K. Therefore, reversion to any significant extent did not occur in these cells. By a number of criteria, many cells in cultured spherical reaggregates are adult-like in electrical properties.

On the other hand, not all cells were of this type. Some cells in the same reaggregate, or cells in another reaggregate in the same culture vessel, had partially reverted. That is, there was a wide spectrum of degrees of reversion. In general, aging the cultures for several weeks greatly improved the incidence of highly differentiated cells. After a month in culture, many reaggregates exclusively contained electrically mature cells. (Aging was also a significant factor in achieving a more differentiated morphology and electrical properties in the monolayer cells.)

Pharmacological receptors To test for the retention of some pharmacological receptors in the reaggregates, experiments were done using the induction of slow Ca^{2+}–Na^+ channels in the sarcolemma as an assay. To facilitate the detection of induction of slow channels, the fast Na^+ channels and excitability were blocked using TTX (Figure 10 A–B). Then, the addition of agents, such as catecholamines, which rapidly increase the number of slow channels available for activation upon stimulation, caused the appearance of slow-rising overshooting action potentials (the "slow responses") which resemble the plateau component of the normal action potential (Figure 10C). The slow responses are accompanied by contractions, and it has been shown that both Ca^{2+} and Na^+ inward currents participate in the slow response (Schneider and Sperelakis, 1975). The slow responses are blocked by agents that block inward slow Ca^{2+} current,

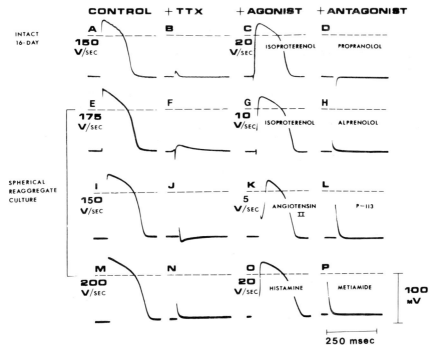

Figure 10. Demonstration of functional receptors for positive inotropic agents in intact old (16-day) embryonic chick hearts (A–D) and in cultured spherical reaggregates of trypsin-dispersed ventricular cells (E–P). Following blockade of the fast Na^+ channels by tetrodotoxin, positive inotropic agents induce slow responses that are blocked by specific antagonists. A–D: Recordings from a ventricular cell in an intact 16-day-old heart. The control rapidly-rising (150 V/sec) action potential (A) was abolished by tetrodotoxin (TTX: 0.1 μg/ml) (B). Addition of isoproterenol (10^{-6} M) induced a slowly-rising (20 V/sec) overshooting electrical response (C) that was blocked by propranolol (10^{-5} M) (D). E–H: Recordings from one cell in a cultured spherical reaggregate showing control action potential (E) abolished by TTX (0.1 μg/ml) (F); isoproterenol (3 × 10^{-5} M) induced a slow response (G) that was blocked by the specific β-adrenergic receptor antagonist, alprenolol (10^{-7} M). I–L: Recordings from one cell in another reaggregate showing control action potential (I) and its blockade by TTX (J); a slow response was induced by angiotensin II (10^{-6} M) (K) and was blocked by its competitive antagonist, P–113 (10^{-5} M) (L). M–P: Recordings from one cell in another reaggregate showing control action potential (M) and its blockade by TTX (N); histamine (10^{-5} M) induced a slow response (O) which was abolished by the H_2 antagonist, metiamide (10^{-5} M) (P).

including Mn^{2+}, La^{3+}, verapamil, and D-600. The effect of isoproterenol is blocked by β-adrenergic blocking agents (Figure 10 D,H), thereby indicating the presence of functional β-adrenergic receptors. Angiotensin II also induces the slow response, and its action is blocked by specific angiotensin-receptor blocking agents (Figure 10 I–L) (Freer *et al.*, 1976). Finally, the histamine induction of the slow response is blocked by histamine H_2-receptor blocking agents (but not by β-adrenergic antagonists or by H_1-receptor antagonists) (Figure 10 M–P) (Josephson *et al.*, 1976). Thus, the cells possess functional receptors for positive inotropic agents.

Reverted morphology Although the sarcolemmal electrical properties of most cells in a given reaggregate were highly differentiated, the ultrastructure of the cells in that same reaggregate exhibited the characteristic appearance of an immature cardiomyoblast (Figure 4D). There were only few and incomplete myofibrils, and there was a paucity of sarcoplasmic reticulum. The morphology was similar to that of reverted monolayer cells (compare Figure 4D with B) as well as to that of the three-day-old intact hearts (compare Figure 4D to Figure 3A). The cell borders had numerous desmosomes, but no gap-like junctions could be found. Cultured strand reaggregates described by Lieberman's group demonstrate a more highly differentiated morphology, including aligned myofibrils and well developed intercalated discs. Furthermore, Jones *et al.* (personal communication) have achieved highly differentiated morphology (and electrophysiology) in multilayer-cultured chick cells incubated in media with reduced serum concentrations.

Lack of low-resistance connections Evidence was obtained from double microelectrode impalements that cell-to-cell propagation occurs through the spheres. However, no evidence of low-resistance connections between cells impaled at various interelectrode distances (50–200 μm) could be obtained using applied currents of up to 40 nA. This was especially true of aggregates containing the most highly differentiated cells. In aggregates containing less differentiated cells with pacemaker potentials, moderate to strong electrotonic interaction between the two microelectrodes was obtained in about 50% of the cases. In contrast, DeHaan and Fozzard (1975) have reported strong electrotonic interactions between cells in their spherical reaggregates, and Lieberman (1973) has reported strong interaction in his strand preparations. Jongsma and van Rijn (1972) have reported strong electrotonic interaction in monolayers of rat heart cells, whereas Lehmkuhl and Sperelakis (1965) have reported weak or absent electrotonic interaction in monolayers of chick heart cells, except in the case where exceptionally long and thick fibers were impaled. Thus, it appears that cultured heart cells can be made to exhibit different degrees of electrotonic coupling.

Cultured Myoblastic Cells from
Young Embryonic Hearts Arrested in Development

Spherical reaggregate cultures When spherical reaggregate cultures were prepared from three-day-old embryonic hearts and cultured for 10 days, no evidence for differentiation was obtained. The impaled cells had low-resting potentials, pacemaker potentials, and slowly-rising (about 10 V/sec) action potentials that were not sensitive to TTX (Figure 11 A–B). In contrast, DeHaan

YOUNG (3 d.) MYOCARDIAL CELLS
(10 d. in vitro)

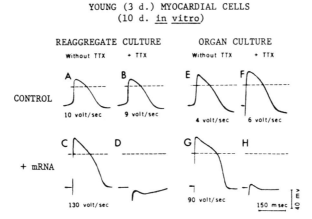

Figure 11. Arrest of development of young (3 days) embryonic myocardial cells in cultured reaggregates (A–B) and in organ-cultured intact hearts (E–F), and induction of further differentiation by culturing with RNA-enriched extracts from adult hearts (C–D, G–H). A–B: Recordings from one cell in a spherical reaggregate before (A) and after (B) TTX (1 μ g/ml), illustrating the failure of membrane differentiation, including lack of fast Na$^+$ channels. C–D: Recordings from one cell in a spherical reaggregate culture treated with RNA showing a fast rate of rise (130 V/sec) and a high resting potential (−75 mV) (C); TTX (0.1 μg/ml) rapidly abolished the action potential (D). E–F: Recordings from one cell in a three-day-old intact heart organ cultured for 10 days before (E) and after (F) addition of TTX (1 μg/ml), and showing the arrest of development. G–H: Recordings from one cell in an organ-cultured three-day-old heart treated with RNA showing a fast rate of rise (90 V/sec) (G) and complete blockade by TTX (H). Electric field stimulation applied in C, D, F, G, H.

and coworkers (1976) reported that reaggregates of four-day-old cells exhibited increasing rates of rise of the action potentials over several days in culture; because day 4 is on the edge of the intermediate period, it is possible that genes coding for the production of protein for fast Na$^+$ channels had been activated prior to culturing.

Organ-cultured intact young hearts When three-day-old chick embryonic hearts are placed intact into organ culture for 10–14 days, these muscle cells also do not continue to differentiate electrically or morphologically (Sperelakis and Shigenobu, 1974; Sperelakis *et al.,* 1974; Renaud and Sperelakis, 1976). The impaled cells have resting potentials and action potentials with properties identical to fresh three-day-old hearts (Figure 11 E–F). They do not gain TTX-sensitive fast Na$^+$ channels. In effect, the cells are arrested in the stage of differentiation attained at the time of explantation. The same was true for young hearts grafted onto the chorio-allantoic membrane of a host chick for purposes of blood perfusion. Therefore, something in the *in situ* environment of the heart in the developing embryo must control the appearance of the fast Na$^+$ channels.

Since the innervation reaches the heart on about day 5, a trophic influence of the neurons could trigger the next step in differentiation.

Induction of further differentiation in **vitro** *by RNA*   When reaggregates or organ-cultured hearts containing young cells whose development was arrested are incubated with RNA-enriched extracts from adult chicken hearts fast Na^+ channels appear *de novo,* resting potentials increase, automaticity ceases, and the rapidly rising action potentials are completely TTX-sensitive (McLean *et al.,* 1976) (Figure 11 C–D, G–H). These findings indicate that further differentiation can be induced *in vitro.* The inducing potency is unique to RNA-containing extracts from hearts, and is destroyed by pretreatment of the RNA with ribonuclease. Blockade of the induction by cycloheximide suggests that new protein synthesis results in the appearance of the fast Na^+ channel activity. Thus, the cultured young myocardial cells provide a model for studying genetic regulation of cell membrane properties.

REFERENCES

BURROWS, M. T. 1912. Rhythmische kontractionen der isolierten herzmuskelzelle ausserhalb des organismus. Münch. Med. Wochenschr. 59:1473–1475.

CARMELIET, E., HORRES, C. R., LIEBERMAN, M., and VEREECKE, J. S. 1976. Developmental aspects of potassium flux and permeability of the embryonic chick heart. J. Physiol. (Lond.) 254:673–692.

CRILL, W. E., RUMERY, R. E., and WOODBURY, J. W. 1959. Effects of membrane current on transmembrane potentials of cultured chick embryo heart cells. Am. J. Physiol. 197:733–735.

DeHAAN, R. L. 1967. Spontaneous activity of cultured heart cells. *In* R. D. Tanz, F. Kavaler, and J. Roberts (eds.), Factors Influencing Myocardial Contractility, pp. 217–230. Academic Press, New York.

DeHAAN, R. L., and FOZZARD, H. A. 1975. Membrane responses to current pulses in spheroidal aggregates of embryonic heart cells. J. Gen. Physiol. 65:207–222.

DeHAAN, R. L., McDONALD, T. F., and SACHS, H. G. 1976. Development of tetrodotoxin sensitivity of enbryonic chick hearts *in vitro. In* M. Lieberman and T. Sano (eds.), Developmental and Physiological Correlates of Cardiac Muscle, pp. 155–168. Raven Press, New York.

FÄNGE, R., PERSSON, H., and THESLEFF, S. 1952. Electrophysiologic and pharmacological observations on trypsin-disintegrated embryonic chick hearts cultured *in vitro.* Acta Physiol. Scand. 38:173–183.

FREER, R. J., PAPPANO, A. J., PEACH, M. J., BING, K. T., McLEAN, M. J., VOGEL, S. J., and SPERELAKIS, N. 1976. Mechanism of the positive inotropic action of angiotensin II on isolated cardiac muscle. Circ. Res. 39:178–183.

GORDON, H. P., and BRICE, M. C. 1974. Intrinsic factors influencing the maintenance of contractile embryonic heart cells *in vitro.* II. Biochemical analysis of heart muscle conditioned medium. Exp. Cell Res. 85:311–318.

HALLE, W., and WOLLENBERGER, A. 1971. Myocardial and other muscle cell cultures. *In* A. Schwartz (ed.), Methods in Pharmacology, Vol. 1, pp. 191–246. Appleton-Century-Crofts, New York.

HOGG, B. M., GOSS, C. M., and COLE, K. S. 1934. Potentials in embryo rat heart muscle cultures. Proc. Soc. Exp. Biol. Med. 32:304–307.

HYDE, A., BLONDEL, B., MATTER, A., CHENEVAL, J. P., FILLOUX, B., and GIRARDIER, L. 1969. Homo- and heterocellular junctions in cell cultures: An electrophysiological and morphological study. Prog. Brain Res. 31:283–311.

JONGSMA, H. J., and VAN RIJN, H. E. 1972. Electrotonic spread of current in monolayer cultures of neonatal rat heart cells. J. Membr. Biol. 9:341–360.

JOSEPHSON, I., RENAUD, J. -F., VOGEL, S., McLEAN, M., and SPERELAKIS, N. 1976. Mechanism of the histamine-induced positive inotropic action in cardiac muscle. Eur. J. Pharmacol. 35:393–398.

KASTEN, F. H. 1972. Rat myocardial cells *in vitro:* Mitosis and differentiated properties. *In Vitro* 8:128–150.

KELLY, A. M., and CHACKO, S. 1976. Myofibril organization and mitosis in cultured cardiac muscle cells. Develop. Biol. 48:421–430.

LEHMKUHL, D., and SPERELAKIS, N. 1965. Electrotonic spread of current in cultured chick heart cells. J. Comp. Cell. Physiol. 66:119–133.

LEWIS, W. H. 1928. Cultivation of embryonic heart muscle. Carnegie Inst. of Wash. Contrib. Embryol. No. 90 18:1–21.

LIEBERMAN, M. 1973. Electrophysiological studies of a synthetic strand of cardiac muscle. Physiologist 16:551–563.

LIEBERMAN, M., ROGGEVEEN, M. A., PURDY, J. E., and JOHNSON, E. A. 1972. Synthetic strands of cardiac muscle: Growth and physiological implications. Science 175:909–911.

LIEBERMAN, M., and SANO, T. 1976 (eds.). Developmental and Physiological Correlates of Cardiac Muscle. Raven Press, New York.

McDONALD, T. F., SACHS, H. G., and DeHAAN, R. L. 1972. Development of sensitivity to tetrodotoxin in beating chick embryo hearts, single cells, and aggregates. Science 176:1248–1250.

McLEAN, M. J., LAPSLEY, R. A., SHIGENOBU, K., MURAD, F., and SPERELAKIS, N. 1975. High cyclic AMP levels in young chick embryonic hearts. Dev. Biol. 42:196–201.

McLEAN, M. J., RENAUD, J. -F., SPERELAKIS, N., and NIU, M. C. 1976. mRNA induction of fast Na^+ channels in cultured cardiac myoblasts. Science 191:297–299.

McLEAN, M. J., and SPERELAKIS, N. 1974. Rapid loss of sensitivity to tetrodotoxin by chick ventricular myocardial cells after separation from the heart. Exp. Cell Res. 86:351–364.

McLEAN, M. J., and SPERELAKIS, N. 1976. Retention of fully differentiated electrophysiological properties of chick embryonic heart cells *in vitro.* Dev. Biol. 50:134–142.

MANASEK, F. J., and MONROE, R. G. 1972. Early cardiac morphogenesis is independent of function. Dev. Biol. 27:584–588.

MARK, G. E., and STRASSER, F. F. 1966. Pacemaker activity and mitosis in cultures of newborn rat heart ventricle cells. Exp. Cell Res. 44:217–233.

METTLER, F. A., GRUNDFEST, H., CRAIN, S. M., and MURRAY, M. R. 1952. Spontaneous electrical activity from tissue cultures. Trans. Am. Neurol. Assn. 77:52–53.

MOSCONA, A. 1961. Rotation mediated histogenetic aggregation of dissociated cells. Exp. Cell Res. 22:455–475.

PAPPANO, A. J., and SPERELAKIS, N. 1969. Low K^+ conductance and low resting potentials of isolated single heart cells. Am. J. Physiol. 217:1076–1082.

RENAUD, J. -F. 1973. Etude de l'évolution en culture primaire des cardiomyoblastes embryonnaires de poulet. Thesis. University of Nantes.

RENAUD, J. -F., and SPERELAKIS, N. 1976. Electrophysiological properties of chick embryonic hearts grafted and organ-cultured *in vitro.* J. Mol. Cell. Cardiol. 8:889–900.

ROSEEN, J. S., and FUHRMAN, F. A. 1971. Comparison of the effects of atelapidtoxin with those of tetrodotoxin, saxitoxin and batrachotoxin on beating of cultured heart cells. Toxicon 9:411–415.

SCHNEIDER, J. A., and SPERELAKIS, N. 1975. Slow Ca^{++} and Na^+ current channels induced by isoproterenol and methylxanthines in isolated perfused guinea pig hearts whose fast Na^+ channels are inactivated in elevated K^+. J. Mol. Cell. Cardiol. 7:249–273.

SHIGENOBU, K., and SPERELAKIS, N. 1972. Ca^{++} current channels induced by catecholamines in chick embryonic hearts whose fast Na^+ channels are blocked by tetrodotoxin. Circ. Res. 31:932–952.

SPERELAKIS, N. 1967. Electrophysiology of cultured heart cells. *In* T. Sano, V. Mizuhira, and K. Matsuda (eds.), Electrophysiology and Ultrastructure of the Heart, pp. 81–108. Bunkodo Company, Tokyo.

SPERELAKIS, N. 1972a. (Na⁺, K⁺)-ATPase activity of embryonic chick heart and skeletal muscles as a function of age. Biochim. Biophys. Acta 266:230–237.

SPERELAKIS, N. 1972b. Electrical properties of embryonic heart cells. *In* W. C. De Mello (ed.), Electrical Phenomena in the Heart, pp. 1–61. Academic Press, New York.

SPERELAKIS, N., FORBES, M. S., SHIGENOBU, K., and COBURN, S. 1974. Organ-cultured chick embryonic heart cells of various ages. Part II. Ultrastructure. J. Mol. Cell. Cardiol. 6:473–483.

SPERELAKIS, N., and LEE, E. C. 1971. Characterization of (Na⁺,K⁺)-ATPase isolated from embryonic chick hearts and cultured chick heart cells. Biochim. Biophys. Acta 233: 562–579.

SPERELAKIS, N., and LEHMKUHL, D. 1965. Insensitivity of cultured chick heart cells to autonomic agents and to tetrodotoxin. Am. J. Physiol. 209:693–698.

SPERELAKIS, N., and SHIGENOBU, K. 1972. Changes in membrane properties of chick embryonic hearts in development. J. Gen. Physiol. 60:430–453.

SPERELAKIS, N., and SHIGENOBU, K. 1974. Organ-cultured chick embryonic hearts cells of various ages. Part I. Electrophysiology. J. Mol. Cell. Cardiol. 6:449–471.

SPERELAKIS, N., SHIGENOBU, K., and McLEAN, M. J. 1976. Membrane cation channels—changes in developing hearts, in cell culture, and in organ culture. *In* M. Lieberman and T. Sano (eds.), Developmental and Physiological Correlates of Cardiac Muscle, pp. 209–234. Raven Press, New York.

VEREECKE, J., and CARMELIET, E. 1971. Sr action potentials in cardiac Purkyně fibers. Pfluegers Arch. 322:73–82.

Mailing address:
Nick Sperelakis, Ph.D.,
Department of Physiology, School of Medicine, University of Virginia,
Charlottesville, Virginia 22903 (USA).

Recent Advances in Studies on
Cardiac Structure and Metabolism, Volume 12
Cardiac Adaptation
Edited by T. Kobayashi, Y. Ito, and G. Rona
Copyright 1978 University Park Press Baltimore

PALMITATE OXIDATION BY
BEATING HEART CELLS IN CULTURE

A. PINSON,[1] C. FRELIN,[2] and P. PADIEU[2]

[1] Myocardial Research Group, Department of Biochemistry, The Hebrew University–
Hadassah Medical School, Jerusalem, Israel
[2] Laboratory of Medical Biochemistry, School of Medicine,
7 Blvd. Jeanne d'Arc, 21033 Dijon, Cedex, France

SUMMARY

Palmitic acid oxidation has been studied in cultures of beating heart cells. The data reported suggest:

1. The main source of fatty acids for oxidation in cell cultures is provided by lypolysis of preexisting intracellular fatty acids. Most fatty acids that have just entered the cell are not oxidized immediately. Thus, aged heart cells in culture seem to retain their ability to utilize fatty acids as their main energy source.
2. In cultured heart cells, the amount of CO_2 obtained from the carboxyl group was much higher than that obtained from the methyl group. On the other hand, β-hydroxybutyrate has been shown to be formed mainly from the methyl group. This may indicate that β-oxidation terminates at the β-hydroxybutyrate stage because of premature dissociation of this last intermediate from the enzyme complex.

INTRODUCTION

In 1954, Bing *et al.* showed that fatty acids serve as the main energy source for the heart. This finding and the fact that fatty acids have been much mentioned in the field of heart pathology have prompted numerous publications of studies concerned with cardiac fat metabolism, using perfused heart, tissue slices, and studies *in vivo* (for review, see Bing, 1965; Neely and Morgan, 1974).

Cardiac cells in culture readily lend themselves to metabolic studies. The cells appear to preserve their state of differentiation in culture as evidenced by their continuous beating and by their unchanged basic structure. The purpose of

This work was supported by research grants from the Institut National de la Santé et de la Recherche Médicale ATP No. 13.74–34 and the Délégation générale à la Recherche Scientifique et Technique: "Biologie et Fonction du Myocarde" No. 75–7–0320, and by a research grant obtained from the Chief Scientist, Ministry of Health, State of Israel.

667

the work discussed in this chapter was to study palmitic acid oxidation by beating heart cells in culture.

MATERIAL AND METHODS

Cultures from 3–4-day-old rats were obtained as described elsewhere (Pinson, Frelin, and Padieu, 1973). As far as possible, every series of experiments was carried out in cultures originating from the same seeded cell suspension.

Palmitic acid (purity grade 99%) was purchased from the Sigma Chemical Company. [16-^{14}C] Palmitic acid (specific activity 44.8 mCi/mmol) and [1-^{14}C] palmitic acid (specific activity 53 mCi/mmol) were purchased from the Commissariat à l'énergie atomique (CEA), Suclay (France).

Substrate preparation, 0.1 mmol potassium palmitate, containing about 2% of either [16-^{14}C] palmitate or [1-^{14}C] palmitate, was added to 100 ml of fetal bovine serum. Aliquots of the serum were stored at −20°C. For experimental work, the serum was diluted fourfold with Ham F10 culture medium (Ham, 1963). The final concentration of palmitate added to the incubation medium was 0.2 mM.

^{14}C-Carbon dioxide production was measured as described previously (Pinson and Padieu, 1974). β-Hydroxybutyrate was chromatographed on a Dowex 1 formate column (La Noue, Nicklas, and Williamson, 1970).

RESULTS

Palmitate Utilization as a Function of Culture Age

Figure 1 shows the oxidation of [1-^{14}C] palmitate as a function of the age of the culture. The maximal oxidative capacity occurred at the age of 4–5 days; the oxidation of palmitate then decreased and plateaued at a lower level after 10 days in culture.

Figure 2 shows the oxidation of [1-^{14}C] palmitate as a function of time by 7- and 14-day-old cultures.

Figure 3 shows $^{14}CO_2$ release as a function of time from [16-^{14}C] palmitate by 6-day-old cultures with or without preincubation with methyl-labeled palmitate.

Figure 4 shows the results using three different experimental systems: 6-day-old cultures were preincubated for 13 hr with [16-^{14}C] palmitate. After preincubation, the media were removed and CO_2 release was measured with one of the following: 1) no fatty acid, 2) unlabeled palmitate, or 3) labeled palmitate added to the new medium. This was compared to the results from the two other experimental systems in which $^{14}CO_2$ release from labeled palmitate was measured, with or without preincubation, with unlabeled palmitate. There was no significant difference in CO_2 release in the first three experimental systems,

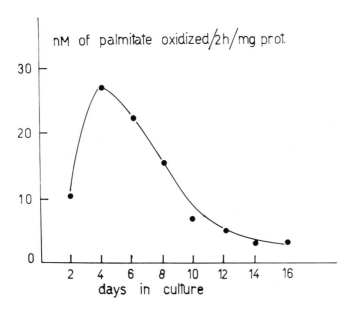

Figure 1. Oxidation of [1-^{14}C] palmitate as a function of culture age.

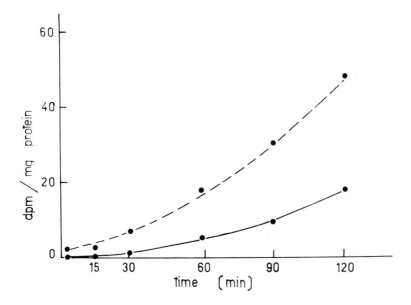

Figure 2. Oxidation of [1-^{14}C] palmitate as a function of incubation time. − − − − =
7-day-old cultures; ——— = 14-day-old cultures.

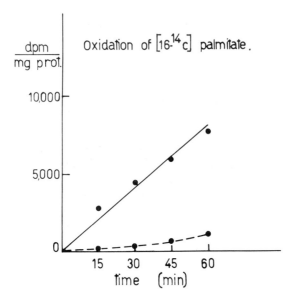

Figure 3. Release of $^{14}CO_2$ by 6-day-old cultured heart cells from [16-^{14}C]palmitate as a function of time. ———— = 18 hr of preincubation with [16-^{14}C]palmitate; – – – – = without preincubation.

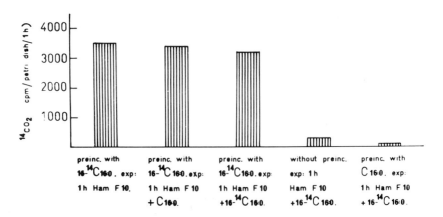

Figure 4. Experiments in which the release of $^{14}CO_2$ from [16-^{14}C]palmitate was measured in 6-day-old cultures. 1–3: The cultures have been preincubated with [16-^{14}C]palmitate for 13 hr; 4: without preincubation with palmitate; 5: after preincubation with unlabeled palmitate.

while CO_2 release without prelabeling was only about 8% of the total amount of CO_2 released with prelabeling and only 3% of the total release when cells were first preincubated with unlabeled palmitate.

Palmitate Oxidation

The difference in the amount of CO_2 released from the carboxyl group of palmitate and the amount released from the methyl group, shown in Figure 5, suggests that the carboxyl terminal of the molecule may have a different fate from that of the methyl terminal. Therefore we measured the radioactivity released into the trichloroacetic acid (TCA)-soluble fractions 1) of the cells and 2) of the extracellular medium, starting with $[1\text{-}^{14}C]$ palmitate and $[16\text{-}^{14}C]$ palmitate, respectively. As shown in Figure 6, the amount of label originating from the methyl-labeled palmitate was higher than that from the carboxyl-labeled palmitate. Also, it appears that there was a continuous release of label into the extracellular medium.

Data reported in Table 1 show that radioactivity released into the TCA-soluble fraction of the extracellular medium from methyl-labeled palmitate was much higher than that released from carboxyl-labeled palmitate. In both cases (with carboxyl- or with methyl-labeled palmitate), most of the water-soluble radioactivity was found to be β-hydroxybutyrate, as was further confirmed by thin layer chromatography (TLC) data.

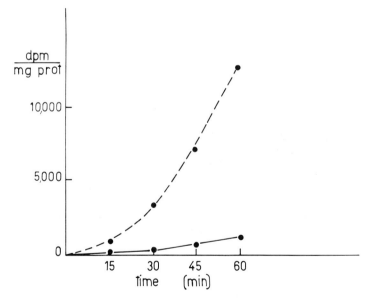

Figure 5. Oxidation of $[1\text{-}^{14}C]$ palmitate (– – –) and $[16\text{-}^{14}C]$ palmitate (———) as a function of time.

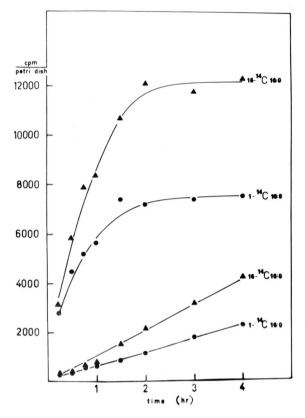

Figure 6. The TCA-soluble radioactivity measured as a function of time of incubation. Radioactivity from either [16-^{16}C]palmitate (▲——▲) or [1-^{14}C]palmitate (●——●) was measured in the intracellular fraction (the two upper curves) and in the extracellular fraction (the two lower curves).

Fatty acid analysis by gas-liquid chromatography (GLC) (Bézard, Boucrot, and Clément, 1964) failed to demonstrate the existence of appreciable amounts of the lower homologs of palmitate, which might explain this difference in radioactivity release. On the contrary, most of the radioactivity other than that occurring in palmitate was found in the higher homolog, oleate.

DISCUSSION

Palmitate Utilization as a Function of Culture Age

The rate of CO_2 production from [1-^{14}C]palmitate (Figure 1) reached its maximal level on the fourth to fifth day in culture and then decreased with aging. Similarly, $^{14}CO_2$ production from [1-^{14}C]palmitate by 14-day-old cells

Table 1. Radioactivity of the water-soluble fraction in the extracellular medium

	16-^{14}C 16:0	1-^{14}C 16:0
Total radioactivity of the water soluble fraction (cpm/petri dish)	279,000	104,600
Radioactivity of the β-hydroxybutyric acid fraction (cpm/petri dish)	229,800	70,700

Six-day-old cultures were incubated for 18 hr with either [1-^{14}C] palmitate or with [16-^{14}C] palmitate. β-Hydroxybutyrate was separated by a Dowex 1-formate column.

(Figure 2) occurred at a lower level and was delayed by about 20–30 min when compared to $^{14}CO_2$ production in 7-day-old cells.

This observation is in agreement with the findings of other researchers. Thus, it has been concluded previously that the decrease in palmitate oxidation is attributable to the lower energy requirements of aged cells in culture and that such cells lose their ability to utilize fatty acids as the principal energy source (Fujimoto and Harary, 1964; Anastasia and McCarl, 1973).

An alternative explanation for the decreased oxidation of fatty acids in aged cultures may be based on the results shown in Figures 3 and 4. These results suggest that the pool of oxidized free fatty acids (FFA) is derived mainly from lipolysis of intracellular esters already present in the cell and not from fatty acids that have just entered. It has been demonstrated that almost all fatty acids entering the cell are esterified within one minute of uptake (Stein and Stein, 1968). Therefore, the FFA taken up by the cells will be more diluted with unlabeled fatty acids derived by lipolysis in aged cells, which are richer in neutral lipids, than in younger cultures.

The decrease of fatty acid oxidation as a function of culture age (Figure 1) is apparent because it only reflects the oxidation of fatty acids that have entered the cell during the course of the experiment as a function of age of the culture. Preliminary data indicate that, if the same experiment (Figure 1) is performed when cultures are preincubated with labeled palmitate, the decrease in CO_2 released as a function of culture age is much reduced. This would indicate that cultured cardiac myocytes maintain their ability to utilize fatty acids as their main energy source.

Palmitate Oxidation

For almost three decades, it has been accepted that β-oxidation of fatty acids does not yield intermediates of the overall process as studied either *in vivo* or in the perfused heart by using [1-^{14}C], [6-^{14}C], or [11-^{14}C] palmitate (Weinman *et al.*, 1950; Evans, Opie, and Shipp, 1963). Minute amounts of the intermediates of β-oxidation have been detected in rat liver mitochondria (Stanley and Tubbs, 1975).

Also, lower homologs have been found in cultured heart cells that have been incubated with erucic acid (Pinson and Padieu, 1974a). The data reported in Figure 5 suggest, however, that in cardiac cell cultures the two terminals of the fatty acid molecule have different fates. Figure 6 demonstrates that, whereas the formation of labeled water-soluble molecules occurs from both ends of palmitate, it is much more significant from the ω end. It also shows that there is a continuous release of these water-soluble molecules into the extracellular medium.

Table 1 shows that after 18 hr of incubation with labeled palmitate, the major part of label in the extracellular medium was attributable to water-soluble molecules that were found to be mainly β-hydroxybutyrate. The labeled β-hydroxybutyrate derived from the carboxyl terminal of the fatty acid molecule is probably formed by condensation of two molecules of acetyl-CoA by the known pathway. However, if this were the only pathway of β-hydroxybutyrate formation, we would not expect to find any difference in the amounts of β-hydroxybutyrate formed from the carboxyl terminal or from the methyl terminal of palmitate. The differences that were observed may be attributable to the fact that β-hydroxybutyrate also is formed as an intermediate when β-oxidation of a fatty acid reaches the last four carbon atoms of the fatty acid chain. It may be speculated that the low amount of CO_2 and the high amount of β-hydroxybutyrate released from the methyl terminal are caused by a low affinity of β-hydroxybutyrate for the β-oxidation enzyme complex in certain metabolic states of the cell, which would result in its release from the enzyme surface.

It has been reported that, in perfused heart under anoxic conditions, lower homologs of palmitate are formed (Rabinowitz and Hercker, 1974). All our experiments were done under conditions of a constant rate of air flow. When either oxygen alone or oxygen/CO_2 flow was used, instead of a flow of air, the results reported in Figure 5 were unchanged.

CONCLUSIONS

Our data suggest that lypolysis and oxidation of preexisting intracellular fatty acids occur before the oxidation of fatty acids that have just entered the cell. Thus, the decrease in fatty acid oxidation as a function of culture age is apparent.

We have also suggested that under certain metabolic conditions β-oxidation of palmitate may terminate at the β-hydroxybutyrate stage because of premature dissociation of this last intermediate from the enzyme complex. This explanation is consistent with the differences noted in CO_2 production between [1-C^{14}]palmitate and [16-^{14}C]palmitate, as shown in this chapter.

REFERENCES

ANASTASIA, J. V., and McCARL, R. L. 1973. Effects of cortisol on cultured rat heart cells. Lipase activity, fatty acid oxidation, glycogen metabolism and ATP levels as related to the beating phenomenon. J. Cell Biol. 57:109–116.

BÉZARD, J., BOUCROT, P., and CLÉMENT, G. 1964. Cellecte d'esters d'acides gras marqués au tirtium et au carbone-14 élués par chromatographie gaz-liquide. J. Chromatogr. 14:368–377.

BING, R. J. 1965. Cardiac metabolism: A review. Physiol. Rev. 45:171–213.

BING, R. J., SIEGEL, A., UNGAR, I., and GILBERT, M. 1954. Metabolism of the human heart. II. Studies on fat, ketone and amino acid metabolism. Am. J. Med. 16:504–515.

EVANS, J. R., OPIE, L. H., and SHIPP, J. C. 1963. Metabolism of palmitic acid in perfused rat heart. Am. J. Physiol. 205:766–770.

FUJIMOTO, A., and HARARY, I. 1964. Studies *in vitro* on single beating heart cells. IV. The shift from fat to carbohydrate metabolism. Biochim. Biophys. Acta 86:74–80.

GREVILLE, G. D., and TUBBS, P. K. 1968. The catabolism of long chain fatty acids in mammalian tissues. Essays Biochem. 4:155–212.

HAM, R. G. 1963. An improved nutrient solution for diploid Chinese hamster and human cell lines. Exp. Cell Res. 19:515–526.

La NOUE, K. F., NICKLAS, W. J., and WILLIAMSON, J. R. 1970. Control of citric acid cycle activity in rat heart mitochondria. J. Biol. Chem. 245:102–111.

NEELY, J. R., and MORGAN, H. E. 1974. Relationship between carbohydrate and lipid metabolism and the energy balance of heart muscle: A Review. Ann. Rev. Physiol. 36:413–459.

PINSON, A., FRELIN, C., and PADIEU, P. 1973. The lipoprotein lipase activity in cultured beating heart cells of the post-natal rat. Biochimie 55:1261–1264.

PINSON, A., and PADIEU, P. 1974a. Erucic acid oxidation by beating heart cells in culture. FEBS Lett. 39:88–90.

PINSON, A., and PADIEU, P. 1974b. Quelques aspects du metabolisme des acides gras à longue chaine par les cellules bathmotropes de coeur de rat en culture. Biochimie 56:1587–1596.

RABINOWITZ, J. L., and HERCKER, E. S. 1974. Incomplete oxidation of palmitate and leakage of intermediary products during anoxia. Arch. Biochem. Biophys. 161:621–627.

STANLEY, K. K., and TUBBS, P. K. 1975. The role of intermediates in mitochondrial fatty acid oxidation. Biochem. J. 150:77–88.

STEIN, O., and STEIN, Y. 1968. Lipid synthesis, intracellular transport, and storage. III. Electron microscopic radiographic study of the rat heart perfused with tritiated oleic acid. J. Cell Biol. 36:63–77.

WEINMAN, E. O., CHAIKOFF, I. L., DAUBEN, W. G., GEE, M., and ENTENMAN, C. 1950. Relative rates of conversion of the various atoms of palmitic acid to carbon dioxide by the intact rat. J. Biol. Chem. 184:735–744.

Mailing address:
Arié Pinson, Ph.D.,
Myocardial Research Group, Department of Biochemistry,
The Hebrew University—Hadassah Medical School, Jerusalem (Israel).

Recent Advances in Studies on
Cardiac Structure and Metabolism, Volume 12
Cardiac Adaptation
Edited by T. Kobayashi, Y. Ito, and G. Rona
Copyright 1978 University Park Press Baltimore

SYNTHESIS AND PHOSPHORYLATION OF CANINE CARDIAC MYOSIN IN TISSUE-CULTURE ASSESSMENT OF HYPERTROPHYING FACTORS

J. WIKMAN-COFFELT, C. FENNER, and D. T. MASON

Section of Cardiovascular Medicine, Department of Medicine,
University of California, Davis, School of Medicine, Davis, California, USA

SUMMARY

Canine cardiac myosin, which was synthesized in a 14-day tissue culture, based on L-[^{3}H] leucine incorporation, was precipitated with goat γG antimyosin (cardiac-specific) and analyzed on dodecylsulfate gels. Incorporation of ^{32}PO$_4$ into myosin chains occurring in culture was the same as that obtained *in vivo* and appeared to be coupled with translation. Removal of ^{32}PO$_4$ from myosin heavy chains with base treatment indicated the presence of phosphoserine and phosphothreonine in canine cardiac myosin heavy chains. Further acid hydrolysis confirmed the data. The system described here, i.e., analyses of ^{32}PO$_4$ and L[^{3}H]leucine incorporation into myosin heavy chains, could be used as a system for assaying hypertrophying factors.

INTRODUCTION

Cardiac cells from chick embryos (Cavanaugh, 1955; DeHaan, 1967a) and neonatal rats (Harary and Farley, 1960, 1963) have been grown successfully *in vitro*. Recently, techniques were described for culturing fetal canine cardiac cells (Andreasen *et al.*, 1975). The techniques were similar to those described for growing chick embryo cardiac cells (DeHaan, 1967a, 1967b). The isolated cells grown in culture were characterized as principally myocytes by detecting glycogen granules histochemically and by the immunological precipitation of cardiac-specific myosin. Moreover, myosin is actively synthesized and phosphorylated in cultured canine cardiac cells to the same degree and specificity as *in vivo*. The phosphorylated peptide has been characterized (Fenner *et al.*, 1977). This

This work was supported in part by Research Program Project Grants HL 14780 and AMDD 16716 from the National Institutes of Health, Bethesda, Maryland, and by a research grant from the California Chapter of the American Heart Association.

system, as shown here, can be used to study the effects of hormones and cyclic nucleotides on myosin synthesis and phosphorylation.

MATERIAL AND METHODS

Canine and sheep cardiac cells were cultured as described earlier (Andreasen *et al.*, 1975), as were purification of myosin from cell cultures, assessment of myosin synthesis, and myosin phosphorylation (Andreasen *et al.*, 1975). Purification of the phosphorylated peptide of canine cardiac myosin heavy chains was described earlier (Andreasen *et al.*, 1975). Specific activity of the immunoprecipitated myosin was determined by elution of bound dye from polyacrylamide gels (Fenner *et al.*, 1975). The eluted dye and gel bands were dried, solubilized in H_2O_2, and analyzed in a scintillation counter after addition of 10 ml of scintillation fluor.

RESULTS AND DISCUSSION

When fetal canine cardiac cells were grown in culture, myocytes were the principal cells as distinguished by glycogen granules (Figure 1) and immuno-specific cardiac myosin (Andreasen *et al.*, 1975). When $^{32}PO_4$ was added to a

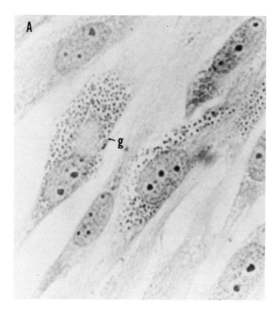

Figure 1. Fetal canine cardiac cells (A) after nine days of culture, stained for glycogen (g) granules. × 1,000.

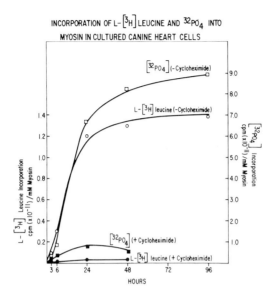

Figure 2. Effects of a protein synthesis inhibitor, cycloheximide, on myosin synthesis and phosphorylation. Six-week canine fetal hearts were cultured for nine days; cycloheximide (20 μg/ml) was added 1 hr before the isotope. Incubation was continued after addition fo the isotopes, L-[³H] leucine and ³²PO₄; cultures were terminated at the times indicated. In control samples no cycloheximide was added. Myosin was purified by immunoprecipitation, and specific activity was terminated as described in materials and methods.

12-day fetal canine cardiac tissue culture, myosin was increasingly labeled relative to time up to 48 hr; this was similar to L-[³H] leucine incorporation into myosin (Andreasen *et al.,* 1975). Incorporation of both L-[³H] leucine and ³²PO₄ were inhibited with cycloheximide (Figure 2), which has been shown to inhibit protein synthesis (Andreasen *et al.,* 1975).

When myosin was purified from cultured cardiac cells grown in the presence of ³²PO₄ for 30 min or 2 hr, there was neglible isotope incorporation. The limited isotope labeling time did not allow for characterization of the phosphorylated peptide. These results indicate that myosin phosphorylation did not occur during myosin isolation. A cell culture labeling time of 24–48 hr was used in the studies reported here.

For isolation and purification of the phosphorus-rich peptide of myosin heavy chains, the heavy chains of myosin labeled in tissue culture with ³²PO₄ were purified, subjected to partial acid hydrolysis, and applied to a Sephadex G-10 column. About 0.2% of myosin was recovered as the multiphosphorylated peptide. The phosphorus-rich peptide which eluted in the void volume for the Sephadex G-10 chromatograph was lyophilized, applied to a Dowex 1X8 chromatograph, and eluted with a gradient of 0–3 N formic acid from the ion-

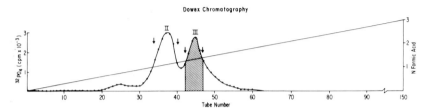

Figure 3. The void volume elute from the Sephadex G-19 column (Figure 2) was lyophilized and applied to a Dowex 1 × 8 column (0.9 × 30 cm) and eluted with 0–3 N formic acid.

exchange column (Figure 3). After lyophilization, Peak II from a Dowex chromatograph was applied to a high-voltage electrophoresis (Figure 4). This rechromatographed peptide coelectrophoresed with $^{32}PO_4$ (Peak II), while the other phosphorylated peptide (Peak III) from a Dowex chromatograph had a greater mobility than $^{32}PO_4$, migrating toward the anode at pH 1.9 (Figure 4).

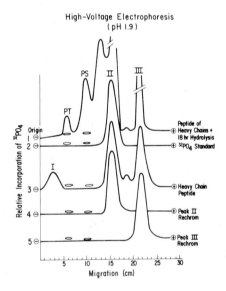

Figure 4. A radioscan of the multi-phosphorylated peptide subjected to high voltage electrophoresis as described in Materials and Methods. 1. Rechromatography of Peaks II and III from a Dowex 1 × 8 column after additional 18-hr acid hydrolyses (6 N HCl, 110°) of the purified peptide. PT = phosphothreonine standard stained with ninhydrin; PS = phosphoserine standard. 2. [^{32}P] orthophosphate standard. 3. Partial acid hydrolysis (6 N HCl, 2 hr, 110°) lyophilized and applied to Whatman 3 MM for electrophoresis). 4. Rechromatography on high voltage electrophoresis of Peak II obtained from Dowex 1 × 8 column and eluted with a 0–3 mN formic acid gradient as shown in Figure 3. 5. Same as 4 except rechromatography of Peak III from Dowex 1 × 8 column.

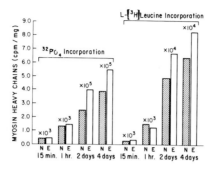

Figure 5. Effects of epinephrine on myosin heavy chain synthesis. Epinephrine (1 μg/ml) was added to culture media as described in Table 1. Incubation was continued for the time periods indicated, and synthesis of myosin heavy chains was analyzed as described in Table 1.

The covalently bound phosphate on the peptide could be removed with *E. coli* alkaline phosphomonoesterase or by alkaline treatment of the purified myosin or of the peptide (DeHaan, 1967a). Further treatment of the purified phosphorylated peptide from Peak III for 18 hr using acid conditions released phosphothreonine, phosphoserine, $^{32}PO_4$, and phosphorus-rich peptides (Figure 5, Peak I).

Table 1. Degree of myosin heavy chain synthesis in cell culture based on ^{32}P and L-[^3H]leucine incorporation

Control value	100%
Concentration of L-thyroxine	
0.1 μg/ml	110%
1.0 μg/ml	68%
10.0 μg/ml	74%
Concentration of norepinephrine	
0.1 μg/ml	88%
1.0 μg/ml	80%
10.0 μg/ml	71%

L-thyroxine or norepinephrine was added to a culture media containing ^{32}P (250 μCi/plate) and/or L-[^3H]-leucine (250 μCi/plate) of a 12-day cell culture of fetal canine cardiac cells. Incubation was continued for 18 hr, after which cells were harvested as described earlier (Andreasen *et al.,* 1975) and myosin heavy chains were purified.

Two agents that have been considered hypertrophying factors, L-thyroxine (Thyrum, Kritcher, and Luchi, 1970) and norepinephrine (Laks and Morady, in press), were added to the media in varying concentrations to determine how they would alter protein synthesis. Norepinephrine lowered protein synthesis at concentrations of 10 to 0.1 μg/ml. There was a minor elevation in protein synthesis with L-thyroxine at a low concentration (0.1 μg/ml) and inhibition at higher concentrations (1−10 μg/ml) (Table 1). The lack of a stronger response relative to elevations in protein synthesis with these hormones may be because of the lack of a direct effect on pure myocardial cells, posing the possibility that myocardial cell cultures may not be ideal for assessing hypertrophying factors. There also could be a lag before a surge in protein synthesis, necessitating longer labeling times. In the case of epinephrine, short labeling times gave little alteration in protein synthesis, whereas extended labeling times gave an elevation in protein synthesis (Figure 5).

REFERENCES

ANDREASEN, T., CASTLES, J. J., SAITO, Y. W., CHACKO, K., FENNER, C., MASON, D. T., and WIKMAN-COFFELT, J. 1975. The behavior of fetal canine cardiac cells in culture: Synthesis and phosphorylation of myosin. Dev. Biol. 47:366−375.

CAVANAUGH, M. W. 1955. Pulsation, migration and division in dissociated chick embryo heart cells *in vitro*. J. Exp. Zool. 128:573−589.

DeHAAN, R. L. 1967a. Introduction: Spontaneous activity of cultured heart cells. *In* R. L. DeHaan (ed.), Factors Influencing Myocardial Contractility, p. 217. Academic Press, New York.

DeHAAN, R. L. 1967b. Regulation of spontaneous activity and growth of embryonic chick hearts in tissue culture. Dev. Biol. 16:216−249.

FENNER, C., MASON, D. T., and WIKMAN-COFFELT, J. 1977. Purification of multiphosphorylated peptide from canine cardiac myosin heavy chains−Labeled in tissue culture. Anal. Biochem. 78:188−196.

FENNER, C., TRAUT, R. R., MASON, D. T., and WIKMAN-COFFELT, J. 1975. Quantification of coomassie blue stained proteins in polyacrylamide gels based on analyses of eluted dye. Anal. Biochem. 63:595−602.

HARARY, I., and FARLEY, B. 1960. *In vitro* studies of single isolated beating heart cells. Science 131:1674−1675.

HARARY, I., and FARLEY, B. 1963. *In vitro* studies of single beating heart cells. Growth and organization. Exp. Cell Res. 29:451−465.

LAKS, M., and MORADY, F. Norepinephrine the producer of myocardial, cellular hypertrophy, and/or necrosis, and/or fibrosis. Am. Heart J. In press.

THYRUM, P. T., KRITCHER, E. M., and LUCHI, R. J. 1970. Effect of L-thyroxine on the primary structure of cardiac myosin. Biochim. Biophys. Acta 197:335−336.

Mailing address:
Joan Wikman-Coffelt, Ph.D.,
Section of Cardiovascular Medicine,
Department of Medicine, University of California, Davis, School of Medicine,
Davis, California 95616 (USA).

Recent Advances in Studies on
Cardiac Structure and Metabolism, Volume 12
Cardiac Adaptation
Edited by T. Kobayashi, Y. Ito, and G. Rona
Copyright 1978 University Park Press Baltimore

PLEIOTROPIC EFFECT OF SERUM ON BEATING RAT HEART CELL CULTURES AND THEIR MODULATION BY HORMONES

C. FRELIN and P. PADIEU

Laboratory of Medical Biochemistry, School of Medicine,
7 Blvd. Jeanne d'Arc, 21033 Dijon, France

SUMMARY

The multiple effects of serum on metabolic activities and macromolecular syntheses of heart cell cultures are discussed in this chapter. This pleiotropic response, which is linearly related to the amount of serum used, allowed us to quantitatively test the growth-promoting activity of different hormones. In addition, the possible mediation of the serum effects by cyclic nucleotides is considered.

INTRODUCTION

Supplementation of synthetic culture media with serum is necessary to maintain rat heart cells in culture. Serum supplies free fatty acids that are essential for automatic rhythmic contractions (Harary, 1964) and for growth-promoting substances (Frelin and Padieu, 1976). Figure 1 shows that in confluent rat heart cell cultures each medium change is followed by a coordinated time-dependent response in cellular activities (pleiotropic response) that ultimately leads to mitoses. These results can be interpreted according to the following scheme: At the time of each medium change, cells are blocked in the early G_1 phase of the cell cycle, and, upon fresh, complete medium addition, part of the cell population is stimulated to divide. The precise timing of events thus reflects the synchronous progression of the stimulated cells through the entire cell cycle (phases G_1, S, G_2, and M). Then, cells are again synchronized in early G_1 by the combined effects of growth-promoting substance and isoleucine depletions (Frelin, Pinson, and Padieu, in preparation).

This investigation was supported by contracts from INSERM (ATP 21, CRL 6), DGRST (ACC BFM), and CNRS (ERA 267).

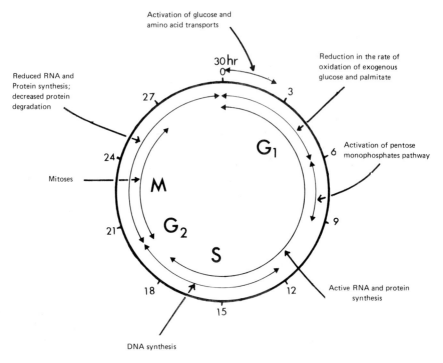

Figure 1. Timing of events induced by each medium change in heart cell cultures. After approximately 30 hr all stimulated cells are again blocked in the early G_1 phase of the cell cycle. The positions of the different phases of the cell cycle are indicated approximately.

The magnitude of the pleiotropic response, which indicates the number of stimulated cells, is linearly related to the concentration of serum.

MATERIALS AND METHODS

Primary cultures of heart cells derived from 3–4-day-old Wistar albino rats were prepared according to the method of Pinson, Frelin, and Padieu (1973). Ham F/10 medium supplemented with 10% pooled human serum, 10% fetal calf serum, and 13 mg% $CaCl_2$ was used to maintain the cells. The seeding density was approximately $1.7.10^6$ cells per 60-mm Petri dish, so that confluency was reached within one or two days. DNA and protein syntheses were measured as the incorporation of labeled precursors (tritiated thymidine and [^{14}C]leucine) into the cold 5% trichloracetic acid precipitable material, according to the procedure previously described (Frelin and Padieu, in press). Cultures used were generally four to six days old, a sufficient time period for cells to recover from the dissociation procedure. Moreover, at this age, cell sensitivity to serum stimulation is at its highest level (Frelin, Pinson, and Padieu, in preparation), and fibroblasts have not yet outnumbered myoblasts, which are still able to undergo mitoses (Masse and Harary, 1974). In such young cultures, the relationship between macromolecular synthesis and the concentration of serum is linear up to a serum concentration of 20%. From a series of Petri dishes prepared from the same cell suspension and seeded at identical cell densities, three groups of 3–5 plates each were used in *all experiments* to determine the relationship between the incorporation of tritiated thymidine or [^{14} C] leucine and the concentration of serum. These data provide a calibration curve for the culture used. All other plates were incubated simultaneously with 10% serum-supplemented medium, and the tested substance or hormone was added in small volume. An incubation time of 24 hr was chosen because this time period allowed all stimulated cells to synthesize DNA (Frelin and Padieu, 1976). Results are expressed in serum percent-equivalent as deduced from the calibration curves. By knowing the hormone concentration used and its normal range in the serum, it is possible to conclude whether or not the tested hormone or substance is the serum growth-promoting substance.

RESULTS

Table 1 summarizes the effects of various hormones on the serum-stimulated DNA and protein syntheses. Insulin activated both syntheses, but the concentration that produced a stimulation similar to 10% serum was nonphysiological as reported earlier for other cell cultures (Vaheri *et al.,* 1973). Cortisol slightly inhibited DNA synthesis but activated protein synthesis. This dual effect ruled out cortisol as the growth-promoting substance of serum, but might explain the variability in activity of different sera. Glucagon at nearly physiological concentrations slightly increased both DNA and protein syntheses as did isoproterenol and triiodothyroxine. It therefore seems that none of the hormones tested could alone account for the growth-promoting activity of serum. In all cell lines so far investigated in detail, growth is never regulated by a single hormone, but rather by a certain balance that differs with the cell type considered (Gospodarowicz and Moran, 1974; Mukherjee, Washburn, and Banerjee, 1973; Hayashi and Sato, 1976).

A decrease in the intracellular concentration of cAMP (Otten, Johnson, and Pastan, 1972) or an increase in the ratio of cGMP to cAMP (Rudland, Seeley, and Seifert, 1974) has been implicated as a primary event following serum stimulation of cells in culture.

In heart cell cultures, no significant variation in tritiated thymidine incorporation was detected when dibutyryl cAMP at concentrations ranging from 10^{-8} to 10^{-4} M was added to complete medium or serum-free medium. At 10^{-3} M, cAMP was found cytotoxic. Identical results were repeatedly obtained with 3-

Table 1. Influence of various treatments on DNA and protein syntheses

Treatment		DNA synthesis	Protein synthesis
Cortisol	10 ng/ml	4.50	19.70
	50 ng/ml	6.60	15.30
	100 ng/ml	11.90	18.30
Glucagon	30 pg/ml	12.0	11.0
	60 pg/ml	9.4	8.4
Insulin	44 nIU/ml	10.6	10.4
	0.11 mIU/ml	12.3	10.2
	18 mIU/ml	14.1	9.7
	0.8 IU/ml	18.3	18.7
Isoproterenol	5 μM	13.0	10.2
Triiodothyroxine (T_3)	1 μg/ml	11.5	10.5
Papaverine	1.5 mM	0	0
Theophylline	2 mM	1.5	0
Prostaglandin E_1	0.4 μg/ml	16.9	8.8

Results are expressed in serum percent-equivalent. Because all plates were incubated in the presence of 10% serum, all values lower than 10.0 mean an inhibiting effect of the substance while values higher than 10.0 mean a stimulating effect.

to 8-day-old cultures incubated either in low or high extracellular calcium concentration. Moreover, partial dialysis or heat treatment of serum did not affect these results. The more hydrophobic cAMP, tested over the same range of concentrations, was also without any effect. In contrast to these negative results, at 10^{-8} M, dibutyryl cAMP reduced glucose consumption by the cells and elicited a marked positive chronotropic effect at 10^{-4} M, as already noted by Krause *et al.* (1970). Papaverine and theophylline, two phosphodiesterase inhibitors, completely inhibited the effects of serum on both DNA and protein synthesis. Prostaglandin E_1, an activator of adenylate cyclase, stimulated DNA but not protein synthesis (Table 1). Dibutyryl cAMP did not affect total protein synthesis at concentrations lower than 10^{-5} M. At 10^{-4} M it produced a 40% stimulation, but only when 10% serum was present.

DISCUSSION

cGMP antagonizes the effects of cAMP in fibroblast cell lines (Kram and Tomkins, 1973; Rudland, Seeley, and Seifert, 1974). In heart cell cultures, the addition of cGMP (or dibutyryl cGMP) at concentrations ranging from 10^{-9} M to 10^{-4} M did not affect DNA synthesis at all serum and calcium concentrations. However, at 10^{-5} M, cGMP had a marked negative chronotropic effect, as already described (Krause, Halle, and Wollenberger, 1972). Thus, neither cAMP nor cGMP had any noticeable effect on serum stimulated macromolecular syntheses, although they did affect the beating activity.

Our data on effectors of enzymes regulating the intracellular level of cAMP also are puzzling. Two phosphodiesterase inhibitors, papaverine and theophylline, completely abolished the effects of serum on both DNA and protein synthesis. However, activators of adenylate cyclase, such as isoproterenol, glucagon, and prostaglandin E_1, are activators of DNA synthesis. This may indicate either a differential action of these compounds on beating cells and mitotic cells or, more probably, a compartmentalization of the intracellular cAMP pool.

The elucidation of the hormonal requirements for growth of heart cells in culture will be useful in advancing our understanding of cardiac muscle growth. Furthermore, the possibility of culturing heart cells in a fully chemically defined medium will enhance the importance of cell culture as an experimental tool.

Acknowledgment   Dr. Pike from the Upjohn Company is acknowledged for his generous gift of prostaglandin E_1.

REFERENCES

FRELIN, C., and PADIEU, P. 1976. Pleiotropic response of rat heart cells in culture to serum stimulation. Biochimie. 58:953–959.

FRELIN, C., PINSON, A., and PADIEU, P. Growth and energy metabolism in aging beating rat heart cell cultures. In preparation.

GOSPODAROWICZ, D., and MORAN, J. S. 1974. Stimulation of division of sparse and confluent 3T3 cell populations by a fibroblast growth factor, dexamethasone and insulin. Proc. Natl. Acad. Sci. USA 71:4584–4588.

HARARY, I. 1964. Studies on individual heart cells. Circ. Res. 15:120–127.

HAYASHI, I., and SATO, G. H. 1976. Replacement of serum by hormones permits growth of cells in a defined medium. Nature 259:132–134.

KRAM, R., and TOMKINS, G. M. 1973. Pleiotypic control by cyclic AMP: Interaction with cyclic GMP and possible role for microtubules. Proc. Nat. Acad. Sci. USA 70:1659–1663.

KRAUSE, E. G., HALLE, W., KALLABIS, E., and WOLLENBERGER, A. 1970. Positive chronotropic response of cultured isolated rat heart cells to N^6, 2'-0-dibutyryl-3':5'-adenosine monophosphate. J. Mol. Cell. Cardiol. 1:1–10.

KRAUSE, E. G., HALLE, W., and WOLLENBERGER, A. 1972. Effect of dibutyryl cyclic GMP on cultured beating rat heart cells. *In* P. Greengard, G. A. Robinson, and R. Paoletti (eds.), Advances in Cyclic Nucleotide Research. Vol. 1, pp. 301–306. Raven Press, Hewlet, N.Y.

MASSE, M. J., and HARARY, I. 1974. Role of cell division in the cytodifferentiation of rat heart cells in culture. Biochimie 56:1581–1585.

MUKHERJEE, A. S., WASHBURN, L. L., and BANERJEE, M. R. 1973. Role of insulin as a permissive hormone in mammary gland development. Nature 246:159–160.

OTTEN, J., JOHNSON, G. S., and PASTAN, I. 1972. Regulation of cell growth by cyclic adenosine 3',5'-monophosphate. J. Biol. Chem. 247:7082–7087.

PINSON, A., FRELIN, C., and PADIEU, P. 1973. The lipoprotein lipase activity in cultured beating heart cells of the post-natal rat. Biochimie 55:1261–1265.

RUDLAND, P. S., SEELEY, M., and SEIFERT, N. 1974. Cyclic GMP and cyclic AMP levels in normal and transformed fibroblasts. Nature 251:417–419.

VAHERI, A., RUOSLAHTI, E., HOUI, T., and NORDLING, S. 1973. Stimulation of density inhibited cell cultures by insulin. J. Cell. Physiol. 81:355–364.

Mailing address:
Christian Frelin,
Laboratoire de Biochemie Medicale, Faculte de Medecine,
7 Blvd. Jeanne d'Arc, 21003 Dijon (France).

Recent Advances in Studies on
Cardiac Structure and Metabolism, Volume 12
Cardiac Adaptation
Edited by T. Kobayashi, Y. Ito, and G. Rona
Copyright 1978 University Park Press Baltimore

EFFECTS OF ADRENALINE
AND METHYLISOBUTYLXANTHINE
ON ADENOSINE 3′:5′-MONOPHOSPHATE LEVELS
IN CULTURES OF BEATING HEART CELLS
OF THE NEWBORN RAT

A. WOLLENBERGER and R. IRMLER

Division of Cellular and Molecular Cardiology,
Central Institute of Heart and Circulatory Regulation Research,
Academy of Sciences of the DDR, Berlin German Democratic Republic

SUMMARY

(−)-Adrenaline caused concentration-dependent increases in cAMP levels and the rate of beating in eight-day-old heart cell cultures of newborn rats. Half-maximal increases in both parameters (5- and 0.2-fold, respectively) occurred at about 10^{-6} M. Following the addition of 3×10^{-7} M adrenaline, the cellular cAMP level rose to a maximum in 30 sec. The rise was abolished by 5×10^{-8} M (−)-propranolol and was greatly magnified by 10^{-4} M 1-methyl-3-isobutylxanthine. In the presence of the latter compound, the average rate of accumulation of cAMP in the cultures during the first 10 seconds of exposure to 3×10^{-7} M adrenaline was 8.78 pmol/mg of protein·sec, which is 230 times more rapid than the basal accumulation rate. These findings may be taken as evidence in support of the view that cAMP is involved in the positive chronotropic action of adrenaline on cardiac pacemaker cells.

INTRODUCTION

Whereas an association of the positive inotropic cardiac action of adrenergic catecholamines with increases in myocardial cyclic adenosine 3′:5′-monophosphate (cAMP) levels is amply documented (for literature references, see Osnes and Øye, 1975), no information exists about the relation of the positive chronotropic cardiac action of these agents to cAMP levels in the relevant tissues of the heart, which are the ones endowed with pacemaker properties. Examination of this relationship has apparently been hampered by difficulties in isolating the pacemaker regions of the heart for biochemical study without gross contamination by nonpacemaker tissue. This difficulty can be circumvented to a great extent by employing monolayer cultures of dissociated heart cells in which many, if not the majority of, myocardial cells can regain the facility of autorhythmicity that was lost early in embryogenesis (Wollengerger, 1964). In heart cell cultures enriched at the outset in myocardial cells, Moura and Simpkins (1975) found that positive chronotropic concentrations of adrenaline and noradrenaline as high as 10^{-6} M caused elevations in cAMP levels amounting to 50%, at the maximum. Since larger increases in cAMP content have been observed in isolated rat hearts following perfusion with solutions containing lower concentrations of adrenaline (Cheung and Williamson, 1965) and isoproterenol (Øye and Langslet, 1972), we decided to reinvestigate the problem and to try to obtain, at the same time, an estimate of the magnitude of stimulation by adrenaline of the cellular rate of synthesis of cAMP.

MATERIALS AND METHODS

Single cells were dissociated from the heart ventricles of newborn rats and were cultivated at 37°C as monolayers in Müller flasks (2.4×10^6 seeded cells in 3 ml) for eight days by procedures described in detail elsewhere (Halle and Wollenberger, 1971), using the chemically defined medium SM 20-I (Halle and Wollenberger, 1970) plus 10% calf serum and 2×10^{-6} M fluorodeoxyuridine (Kössler, 1972) as culture medium with a daily change of half of the medium for the first 7 days and changing to SM 20-I medium (without additions) for the eighth day. Toward the end of the eighth day, the medium was changed for the last time in the following way: After washing the cells with 1 ml of SM 20-I medium, 0.5 ml of this medium containing 30 mM Hepes buffer, pH 7.5, was added to the flasks, which then were gently shaken on a rocker apparatus for three hours. At the end of this period, the substances to be tested, dissolved in SM 20-I, were added to the flask in a volume of 10 μl with an Eppendorf micropipette. Addition of the same volume of pure SM 20-I had no effect on the beating rate of the cells and on the cAMP content. The cells were observed and prepared for assay of cAMP as indicated in the legends of Figures 1 and 2.

RESULTS AND DISCUSSION

Concentration-Response Relationship

Adrenaline produced a concentration-dependent increase in both cAMP levels and in the beating rate of the cultured heart cells (Figure 1). Maximal or near maximal effects were observed at concentrations of 3×10^{-5} and 3×10^{-4} M, which caused a tenfold increase in cAMP level, measured after two min, and a 40–45% increase in the rate of beating. According to Figure 1, a half-maximal (fivefold) increase in cAMP was produced by 1.02×10^{-6} M adrenaline. The concentration for producing a half-maximal rise in the rate of beating is very close to this value. At a concentration of 3×10^{-8} M, adrenaline did not accelerate beating, but elevated cAMP level by 40%. However, the statistical significance of this rise remains to be established. In any event, the present

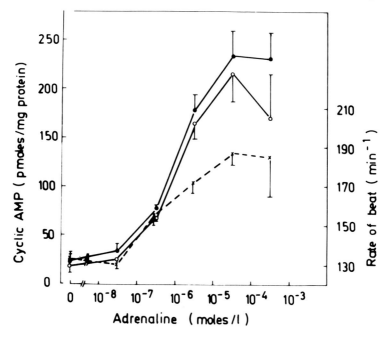

Figure 1. Log concentration-response curves for increases in the rat of beating and in cAMP levels of cultured rat heart cells in response to (–)-adrenaline. For observation of the cells, the culture flasks were placed on the warm stage of an inverted Zeiss-Jena phase contrast microscope, where the temperature of the medium was kept at $37 \pm 0.3°C$. The rates of beating of three or four selected groups of interconnected and usually synchronously beating cells were measured for 15 sec per group with a stop watch before and after addition of (–)-adrenaline-bi-(+)-tartrate, the total time taken for each series of counting being less than 2 min. The last counts following addition of adrenaline did not differ significantly from the first counts. For statistical evaluation of the results, the mean rate of beating of all observed groups of cells in a flask was taken as a single individual value. cAMP was determined separately in the cells and in the medium in reaction mixtures of 100 μl by the protein binding assay of Gilman (1970), using a crude cAMP-dependent protein kinase preparation from bovine adrenal cortex as the binding protein. Five to 10 sec before termination of a 120-sec exposure to adrenaline the medium was quickly removed by suction and 0.5 ml of an ice-cold 5% trichloroacetic acid (TCA) solution were quickly added at 120 sec to fix the cells. The cell monolayer grown on the glass surface was scraped off with a silicon rubber policeman. The cell suspensions from three flasks, corresponding to 0.7–1.0 mg of protein, were quantitatively transferred, with the help of washes with 0.2 ml each of 5% cold TCA, to one centrifuge tube for homogenization with a glass pestle. After a 10-min centrifugation at 4°C and 3,000 × g, the supernatant was shaken with 2–3 vol of water-saturated ether for four consecutive extractions of the TCA. Traces of ether were evaporated on an 80°C water bath. The residue was dissolved in 0.3 ml of 1 N NaOH for the determination of protein (Lowry *et al.,* 1951).

Inorganic salts and other substances in the TCA-free cell extract interfering with the cAMP assay were removed by successive passage of the extract through columns of the following materials (Mao and Guidotti, 1974; Salomon, Londos, and Rodbell, 1974): Dowex 50 WX8 (200–400 mesh, H^+ form, 0.4 × 5.5 cm), neutral alumina (Merck grade I, 0.4 × 4.6 cm), and Dowex 1 X2 (200–400 mesh, Cl^- form, 0.4 × 8 cm). The eluates from the Dowex 1 columns were lyophilized to dryness. The residues were dissolved in 150 μl of water and used for triplicate or quadruplicate determinations of cAMP. For the determination of the extent of recovery of cAMP, 0.1 pmol of [^{3}H]cAMP of specific activity 38.4 mCi/mmol was added to a 2.0–2.5-ml sample before chromatography. The recovery ranged from 79 to 100%. cAMP in TCA-treated incubation medium was determined in the same manner. The plotted values are the means and the vertical bars are the standard errors of the means from experiments with six culture flasks.

findings contrast with those of Birnbaum *et al.* (1975) and other researchers cited by them who reported that the dose-response curves for increases in rate and force of contraction of heart muscle preparations by catecholamines were two orders of magnitude to the left of those for increases in cAMP level. Our findings are compatible with, and may be taken as supporting evidence for, the view (see Wollenberger, 1975) that cAMP is involved in the positive chronotropic action of catecholamines on the heart.

Figure 1 also shows that efflux of cAMP from the cells during a two-minute exposure to adrenaline was of minor proportion, as long as the concentration of the amine did not exceed 3×10^{-5} M. When the concentration was raised to 3×10^{-4} M, a large fraction of the nucleotide that was formed (about 30%) was released into the medium.

Time Course of Response and Effect of 1-Methyl-3-Isobutylxanthine

The time course of the changes in cAMP levels in the heart cell cultures caused by adrenaline was studied at a concentration of the amine of 3×10^{-7} M. This

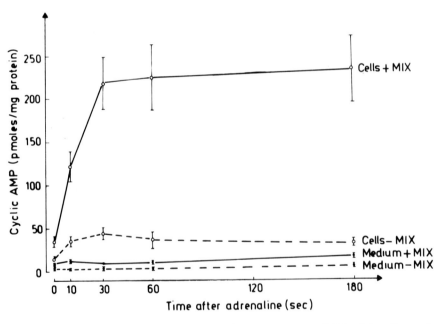

Figure 2. Time course of the effect of 3×10^{-7} M adrenaline on cAMP levels in cultures of neonatal rat heart cells in the absence and presence of 10^{-4} M of 1-methyl-3-isobutylxanthine (MIX). 1-Methyl-3-isobutylxanthine was added to the culture medium 10 min before the addition of adrenaline. For details of the experimental procedure see Materials and Methods and the legend of Figure 1. Each plotted point in the curves represents the mean of values from three experiments. The vertical bars represent ± standard errors of the means.

concentration causes, at two min, an increase in cellular cAMP amounting to 25% of the maximal increase obtainable by adrenaline under the same conditions (Figure 1). Figure 2 shows that 10 seconds after exposure to 3×10^{-7} M adrenaline, the level of cAMP in the cells had risen more than 2-fold. The maximal increase, amounting to a three-fold elevation of the basal level, was seen at 30 seconds. The cellular level of the nucleotide remained elevated for at least three minutes (Figure 2). Little change was seen in the cAMP concentration in the culture medium. The temporal pattern of the cellular change is very similar to that observed in response to adrenaline and other catecholamines by Moura and Simpkins (1975) in cultured dissociated rat heart cells and by Birnbaum *et al.* (1975) in intact heart muscle.

The cAMP phosphodiesterase inhibitor, 1-methyl-3-isobutylxanthine, 10^{-4} M, which produced a 2.5-fold increase in the basal cellular cAMP level and a 60% increase in the rate of beating, magnified manyfold the cAMP-raising action of 3×10^{-7} M adrenaline (Figure 2). Thirty seconds after addition of adrenaline the cellular cAMP level had risen to 218 pmol/mg of protein, which is a value 15 times higher than the basal cAMP level of the cells. Thereafter, cAMP continued to accumulate slowly in the cells and also in the medium (Figure 2). The effects of 10^{-4} M 1-methyl-3-isobutylxanthine and 3×10^{-7} M adrenaline on the rate of beating were at least additive, if not synergistic.

Effect of Adrenergic Blocking Agents

The β-adrenoreceptor blocker (−)-propranolol, at 5×10^{-8} M, completely blocked the rise in the cAMP level in the rat heart cell cultures in response to 3×10^{-7} M (−)-adrenaline. The adrenaline-induced acceleration of beating, on the other hand, was reduced only about 75% by propranolol. This could mean that the remaining 25% of this acceleration was caused by stimulation of α-adreno-receptors. However, the α-receptor blocker phentolamine, used in a concentration of 5×10^{-8} M, had no effect on the adrenaline-increased rate of beating. Higher concentrations were not tried.

Estimation of the Magnitude of Stimulation of cAMP Formation by Adrenaline

On the assumption that the destruction of cAMP in heart cell culture is completely inhibited by 10^{-4} M 1-methyl-3-isobutylxanthine, the rates of synthesis of cAMP before and at different times after the addition of 3×10^{-7} M adrenaline can be taken to equal the sums of the rates of cAMP accumulation in the cells and in the medium during the different time intervals marked in Figure 2 or indicated in its legend. A plot of these values (Figure 3) indicates that the rate of accumulation of cAMP in the culture increased 230-fold from a basal value of 0.038 pmol/mg of protein·sec to an average of 8.78 pmol/mg of protein·sec for the first 10 seconds of exposure to 3×10^{-7} M adrenaline. Thereafter, the accumulation rate declined rather rapidly. An explosive onset of the stimulatory effect of ad-

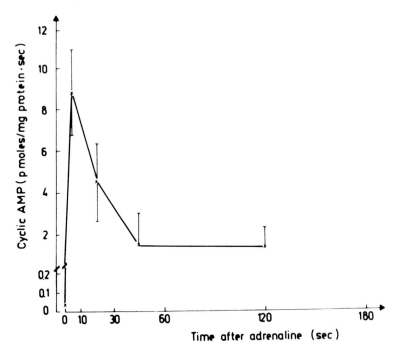

Figure 3. Rate of accumulation of cAMP in cultures of rat heart cells following exposure to 3×10^{-7} M adrenaline in the presence of 10^{-4} M methylisobutylxanthine. The curve is constructed from data presented in Figure 2. The plotted values following addition of adrenaline represent the average increment in cAMP levels per sec in the cultures (cells plus medium) during the successive time intervals marked by the points plotted in Figure 2. The value before addition of adrenaline (0 sec) represents the increment in cAMP level per sec in the cultures during a 10-min incubation in the presence of 10^{-4} M 1-methyl-3-isobutylxanthine. Means ± standard errors (vertical bars) of the results of three experiments for each point.

renaline on cAMP accumulation in heart muscle has been described before by Drummond and Hemmings (1973). The secondary decline in the velocity of cAMP formation might be attributed to one or more of the following factors: formation of an inhibitor of adenylate cyclase (Ho and Sutherland, 1971), inhibition of the enzyme by relatively high concentrations of cAMP (Lehotay and Murphy, 1975), depletion of a possibly very small cellular pool of ATP available for the cyclase reaction (McIlwain, 1972), and/or, possibly, desensitization of β-adrenoreceptors.

REFERENCES

BEAVO, J. A., ROGERS, N. L., CROFFORD, O. B., HARDMAN, J. G., SUTHERLAND, E. W., and NEWMAN, E. V. 1970. Effects of xanthine derivatives on lipolysis and on adenosine 3',5'-monophosphate phosphodiesterase activity. Mol. Pharmacol. 6:597–603.

BIRNBAUM, J. E., ABEL, P. W., AMIDON, G. L., and BUCKNER, C. K. 1975. Changes in mechanical events and adenosine 3',5'-monophosphate levels induced by enantiomers of isoproterenol in isolated rat atria and uteri. J. Pharmacol. Exp. Ther. 194:396–409.

CHEUNG, W. Y., and WILLIAMSON, J. R. 1965. Kinetics of cyclic adenosine monophosphate changes in rat heart following epinephrine administration. Nature 207:979–981.

DRUMMOND, G. I., and HEMMINGS, S. J. 1973. Role of adenylate cyclase-cyclic AMP in cardiac actions of adrenergic amines. In N. S. Dhalla and G. Rona (eds.), Recent Advances in Studies on Cardiac Structure and Metabolism. Vol. 3: Myocardial Metabolism, pp. 213–222. University Park Press, Baltimore.

GILMAN, A. G. 1970. A protein binding assay for adenosine 3':5'-cyclic monophosphate. Proc. Natl. Acad. Sci. USA 67:305–312.

HALLE, W., and WOLLENBERGER, A. 1970. Differentiation and behavior of isolated embryonic and neonatal heart cells in a chemically defined medium. Am. J. Cardiol. 25:292–299.

HALLE, W., and WOLLENBERGER, A. 1971. Myocardial and other muscle cell cultures. In A. Schwartz (ed.), Methods in Pharmacology, Vol. 1, pp. 191–246. Appleton-Century-Crofts, New York.

HO, R. J., and SUTHERLAND, E. W. 1971. Formation and release of a hormone antagonist by rat adipocytes. J. Biol. Chem. 246:6822–6827.

KÖSSLER, A. 1972. Myosingehalt und Aktivität der Kreatin-Phosphokinase in Rattenherz-Zellkulturen. Acta Biol. Med. Ger. 29:119–134.

LEHOTAY, D. C., and MURPHY, B. E. P. 1975. Inhibition of a parathyroid hormone-stimulated renal adenylate cyclase by cyclic AMP. Endocrine Res. Commun. 2:431–443.

LOWRY, O. H., ROSEBROUGH, N. J., FARR, A. L., and RANDALL, R. J. 1951. Protein measurement with the Folin phenol reagent. J. Biol. Chem. 193:265–275.

McILWAIN, H. 1972. Regulatory significance of the release and action of adenine derivatives in cerebral systems. Biochem. Soc. Symp. 36:69–85.

MAO, C. C., and GUIDOTTI, A. 1974. Simultaneous isolation of adenosine 3',5'-cyclic monophosphate (cAMP) and guanosine 3',5'-cyclic monophosphate (cGMP) in small tissue samples.

MOURA, A.-M., and SIMPKINS, H. 1975. Cyclic AMP in cultured myocardial cells under the influence of chronotropic and inotropic agents. J. Cell. Mol. Cardiol. 7:71–77.

OSNES, J.-B., and ØYE, I. 1975. Relationship between cyclic AMP metabolism and inotropic response of perfused rat hearts to phenylephrine and other adrenergic amines. Adv. Cyclic Nucleotide Res. 5:415–433.

ØYE, I., and LANGSLET, A. 1972. The role of cyclic AMP in the inotropic response to isoprenaline and glucagon. Adv. Cyclic Nucleotide Res. 1:291–300.

SALOMON, Y., LONDOS, C., and RODBELL, M. 1974. A highly sensitive adenylate cyclase assay method. Anal. Biochem. 58:541–548.

WOLLENBERGER, A. 1964. Rhythmic and arrhythmic contractile activity of single myocardial cells cultured in vitro. Circ. Res. Suppl. 14,15:184–201.

WOLLENBERGER, A. 1975. The role of cyclic AMP in the adrenergic control of the heart. In W. G. Nayler (ed.), Contraction and Relaxation in the Myocardium, pp. 113–190. Academic Press, New York.

Mailing address:
Albert Wollenberger, Ph.D.,
Division of Cellular and Molecular Cardiology,
Central Institute of Heart and Circulatory Regulation Research
Academy of Sciences of the DDR, 1115 Berlin-Buch (German Democratic Republic).

Recent Advances in Studies on
Cardiac Structure and Metabolism, Volume 12
Cardiac Adaptation
Edited by T. Kobayashi, Y. Ito, and G. Rona
Copyright 1978 University Park Press Baltimore

OUABAIN-INDUCED ARRHYTHMIAS
OF CULTURED MYOCARDIAL CELLS
AND THEIR IMPROVEMENT BY QUINIDINE

K. GOSHIMA

Institute of Molecular Biology, Faculty of Science,
Nagoya University, Chikusa-Ku, Nagoya, Japan

SUMMARY

Single-isolated myocardial cells obtained *in vitro* from fetal mouse heart developed various types of arrhythmic movements, such as fibrillatory and fluttering movements, in medium containing ouabain. The percentage of isolated myocardial cells that exhibited arrhythmic movements increased as ouabain concentration was increased. The arrhythmic movements induced by relatively low concentrations of ouabain were reduced by addition of quinidine. Cell clusters also developed various types of arrhythmic movements in medium containing ouabain. These arrhythmias became more severe when the ouabain concentration was increased. Under conditions such that approximately 43% of the single-isolated myocardial cells showed arrhythmias, many cells in cell clusters showed fibrillatory movements, but the cell clusters as a whole still maintained rhythmic beating. Under conditions in which about 65% of the single-isolated myocardial cells showed arrhythmias, cell clusters as a whole showed irregular beating. The cell clusters stopped beating under conditions in which about 79% of the single-isolated myocardial cells showed arrhythmias. Relatively mild types of arrhythmias of cell clusters were improved by addition of quinidine. From these observations, the genesis and improvement of arrhythmias of cell clusters were concluded to be essentially a result of the genesis and improvement of arrhythmic movements of the individual component cells in the clusters.

INTRODUCTION

There are two opposing concepts on the genesis of severe cardiac arrhythmias such as fibrillation and flutter in adult heart. One is the circus movement or reentry concept, which postulates disturbances of conduction of impulses between cells; the other is the ectopic focal stimulation concept, which postulates abnormal generation of impulses in pacemaker cells and/or nonpacemaker cells.

When heart tissue is dissociated into its component cells with the aid of trypsin and these cells are cultured *in vitro,* both single-isolated myocardial cells and cell clusters beat spontaneously (Harary and Farley, 1963; Wollenberger, 1964; Sperelakis and Lehmkuhl, 1964; DeHaan, 1967; Goshima, 1969). Single-isolated myocardial cells are completely separated from neighboring cells and no impulses are conducted between cells; thus, they beat independent of each other at widely varying rates of 10–230 beats/min at 36°C in standard medium. However, when the single-isolated myocardial cells come in contact forming cell clusters, all the myocardial cells in a given cell cluster beat synchronously at 100–180 beats/min at 36°C in standard medium. It is known that the synchronized beating is achieved by electrotonic spread of impulses between the cells (Goshima, 1969; Hyde et al., 1969). The beating rhythms of both single-isolated myocardial cells and cell clusters were regular and maintained stably in standard medium for at least five hours (Goshima, 1975).

It is known that cultured myocardial cells function in a manner basically similar to the adult heart in situ: the rates of spontaneous beating of both single-isolated myocardial cells and cell clusters change in response to changes of the external potassium and calcium concentrations and to changes of temperature of the medium in essentially the same way as does the beating of adult heart (Goshima, 1975); the acceleration of the beating rate by norepinephrine and dibutyryl cAMP was counteracted by dibutyryl cGMP (Goshima, 1976b). Cultured myocardial cells are separated anatomically and functionally from nerves, connective tissue and blood vessels; thus, they can be used to study the direct effects of ouabain, quinidine, and other cardioactive agents on myocardial cells.

It was reported previously that cultured myocardial cells showed arrhythmias under abnormal conditions (Wollenberger, 1964; Sano and Sawanobori, 1970; Goshima, 1975). Goshima (1976a) reported previously that single-isolated myocardial cells and cell clusters from fetal mouse heart showed various types of arrhythmias after incubation in medium containing ouabain or in medium with low potassium or high calcium concentration, and that the arrhythmias were improved by the addition of antiarrhythmic drugs, such as quinidine or procaine amide. This chapter describes studies on the relationship between the types of arrhythmias of cell clusters and the percentage of arrhythmic single-isolated cells.

MATERIALS AND METHODS

Mouse heart cells (13–17-day-old fetuses) were cultured as described previously (Goshima, 1976). After cultivation for one day, microscopic observations were performed at 36°C in the following medium: 116 mM NaCl, 1.0 or 5.4 mM KCl, 1.8 mM $CaCl_2$, 0.8 mM $MgSO_4$, 0.9 mM NaH_2PO_4, 5.5 mM glucose, amino acids, vitamins, 5% fetal bovine serum, and 10 mM BES (one of Good's buffers), pH 7.3.

RESULTS AND DISCUSSION

Single-Isolated Myocardial Cells

When single-isolated myocardial cells were incubated in medium containing ouabain, they developed the following three types of arrhythmic movements: 1) irregular, fibrillatory movement of comparatively high frequency (often more than 300/min) (called "fibrillatory movement" in this chapter); 2) irregular beating of comparatively low frequency, accompanied by continuous fibrillatory movement of comparatively high frequency (called "fluttering movement"); and 3) irregular, writhing movement of comparatively low frequency (called "writhing movement").

As shown in Figure 1, the percentage of single-isolated myocardial cells that exhibited arrhythmic movements increased as the ouabain concentration was increased. Figure 1 also shows that, on decreasing the potassium concentration of the medium, lower concentrations of ouabain could induce arrhythmias of single-isolated myocardial cells. The percentage of fibrillatory cells among total arrhythmic cells increased with an increase in the ouabain concentration.

After incubating cells in medium containing 10, 30, or 60 μM ouabain (1.0 mM KCl) for 20 to 30 min, quinidine was added stepwise in the presence of the ouabain. All three types of arrhythmias of single-isolated myocardial cells, induced by relatively low concentrations of ouabain, changed to normal, regular beating after the addition of quinidine (Table 1). However, arrhythmias induced by a high concentration of ouabain did not change to normal, regular beating following the addition of quinidine (Table 1).

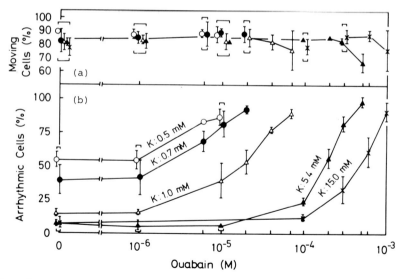

Figure 1. Influences of ouabain and potassium concentration on (a) moving cells (rhythmic plus arrhythmic) as a percentage of the total single-isolated myocardial cells and (b) arrhythmic cells as a percentage of the total beating cells. Points and bars show mean ± S.D. of values in three experiments. Totals of 150 to 300 cells were observed with each concentration of potassium.

Table 1. Improvement of ouabain-induced arrhythmias of single-isolated myocardial cells by
quinidine

Ouabain (μM)	Cells showing improvement by quinidine among total arrhythmic cells (%)
10	84
30	67
60	25

After incubating cells in medium containing 10, 30, or
60 μM ouabain (1.0 mM KCl) for 20 to 30 min, quinidine
sulfate was added. The concentration of quinidine was
increased stepwise every 5 to 20 min from 2.5 μM to 5,
7.5, 10, 15, 20, and finally 30 μM.

When single-isolated myocardial cells were incubated in medium with low
potassium or high calcium concentrations, they developed the same three types
of arrhythmias as those observed after the addition of ouabain. The percentage
of single-isolated myocardial cells that exhibited arrhythmias increased with a
decrease in the potassium concentration or an increase in calcium concentration.
These arrhythmias also were improved by addition of quinidine or procaine
amide.

Myocardial Cell Clusters

Cell clusters showed various types of arrhythmias after incubation for 10–30
min in medium containing various concentrations of ouabain (Table 2).

At low concentrations of ouabain, the beating of cell clusters as a whole was
synchronous and rhythmical, but many myocardial cells in the clusters showed
fibrillatory movements with a high frequency of approximately 300/min. The
fibrillatory movements disappeared following the addition of quinidine (Table 2).

At intermediary concentrations of ouabain, the beating of cell clusters as a
whole was synchronous but irregular, and many myocardial cells in the clusters
showed fibrillatory movements. The fibrillatory cells in the clusters contracted
synchronously with other beating cells in the clusters without cessation of their
fibrillatory movements. The time course of the genesis of irregular beating is
shown in Figure 2: the beating rate increased temporarily after the addition of
0.2 mM ouabain (5.4 mM KCl), and then rapidly decreased. The cell cluster
showed rhythmical beating for 2–5 min, but many myocardial cells in the cluster
showed fibrillatory movements. Then, the cell cluster showed irregular beating.
In this case, the cluster showed alternate strong and weak contractions at
irregular intervals. The irregular beating induced by intermediary concentrations

Table 2. Arrhythmias of cell clusters induced by ouabain in media of various potassium concentrations and their improvement by quinidine

Types of arrhythmias	Ouabain (μM)						Improvement by quinidine (5–50 μM)
	K⁺ (mM)	0.5 K⁺	0.7 K⁺	1.0 K⁺	5.4 K⁺	15 K⁺	
Normal beating				1–5	10–100	100–200	
Rhythmic beating with cellular fibrillation		0–1	0–5	10–25	100–200	200–300	+
Irregular beating with cellular fibrillation		4–8	5–15	15–40	150–350	350–570	+
No beating, only cellular fibrillation		8–15	10–20	30–50	250–450	450–600	± or –

After incubating cell clusters in various ouabain and potassium concentrations for 15 to 40 min, quinidine sulfate was added. Quinidine was added stepwise, because both rhythmic and arrhythmic beating of myocardial cells often stopped suddenly, but temporarily, after rapid increase in the quinidine concentration.

+ = improvement (normal, regular beating without significant cellular fibrillation was restored); ± = incomplete improvement (see text for detail); – = no improvement; ± or – = incomplete improvement was observed in 16 out of 35 clusters.

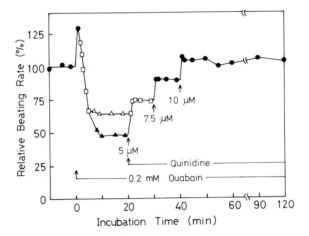

Figure 2. Genesis of irregular beating of a cell cluster in medium containing 0.2 mM ouabain (5.4 mM KCl) and its improvement by addition of quinidine. Final concentrations of 5, 7.5, and 10 μM quinidine sulfate were added at the times indicated by arrows. ● = normal, regular beating without significant cellular fibrillation; □ = rhythmic beating with continuous cellular fibrillation of many cells; △ ▲ = irregular strong and weak contractions with continuous cellular fibrillation of many cells (△ = strong and weak contractions counted, ▲ = only strong contractions counted).

of ouabain was improved by addition of quinidine (Table 2, Figure 2). Figure 3a shows the transmembrane potentials recorded from a cell cluster during irregular beating: irregular discharge of action potentials and small oscillatory potentials were recorded. After addition of quinidine, the oscillatory potentials disappeared and the rhythmic action potentials reappeared (Figure 3b).

At high concentrations of ouabain, the cell clusters stopped beating, but many myocardial cells in the clusters showed fibrillatory movements. The

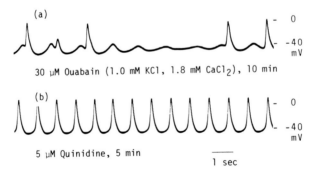

Figure 3. Transmembrane potentials recorded from a cell cluster: (a) after incubation in medium containing 30 μM ouabain (1.0 mM KCl) for 10 min, (b) 5 min after addition of 5 μM quinidine sulfate to (a).

beating cessation, induced by high concentrations of ouabain, was only incompletely improved by the addition of quinidine in 16 out of 35 clusters (Table 2). That is, fibrillatory movements slightly decreased, and irregular or regular beating was restored, although their contractions were weak.

As shown in Table 2, following a decrease of the potassium concentration in the medium, lower concentrations of ouabain could induce arrhythmias of cell clusters.

When cell clusters were incubated in medium with low potassium or high calcium concentrations, they developed the same types of arrhythmias as those observed when ouabain was added. These arrhythmias became more severe after a decrease in potassium concentration or an increase in calcium concentration. Relatively mild types of the arrhythmias also were improved by the addition of quinidine or procaine amide.

Relationship between Types of Arrhythmias of Cell Clusters and Percentage of Arrhythmic Single-Isolated Myocardial Cells

Table 3 gives the percentages of single-isolated myocardial cells showing arrhythmias at given concentrations of ouabain in media of various potassium concentrations in which cell clusters demonstrated rhythmic beating with cellular fibrillation, irregular beating, or stopped beating. Under conditions in which approximately 43% of the single-isolated myocardial cells demonstrated arrhythmias, many cells in cell clusters showed fibrillatory movements, but the cell clusters as a whole still maintained rhythmic beating. Under conditions in which about 65% of the single-isolated myocardial cells showed arrhythmias, many cells in cell clusters showed fibrillatory movements, and the cell clusters as a whole showed irregular beating. Under conditions in which about 79% of the single-isolated myocardial cells showed arrhythmias, the cell clusters as a whole stopped beating, but many myocardial cells in the clusters showed fibrillatory movements.

These observations show that the genesis and improvement of arrhythmias of cell clusters, induced by ouabain, are essentially caused by the genesis and

Table 3. Relationship between types of arrhythmias of cell clusters and percentage of arrhythmic single-isolated myocardial cells

Arrhythmic single-isolated cells (%)	Types of arrhythmias of cell clusters	Improvement by quinidine[a]
43	Rhythmic beating with cellular fibrillation	+
65	Irregular beating with cellular fibrillation	+
79	No beating, only cellular fibrillation	± or −

[a] +, ±, − = as in Table 2.

improvement of arrhythmias of individual component cells in the clusters (Goshima, 1976). These results suggest that severe cardiac arrhythmias, such as fibrillation and flutter in adult heart *in vivo,* may be, at least in part, the consequence of arrhythmias of individual component cells. Conduction of impulses between cells in clusters may contribute to prevention of severe arrhythmias of the cell clusters. Thus, under conditions in which less than 65% of the single-isolated myocardial cells developed arrhythmias, the cell clusters as a whole still maintained beating.

REFERENCES

DeHAAN, R. L. 1967. Regulation of spontaneous activity and growth of embryonic chick heart cells in tissue culture. Dev. Biol. 16:216–249.

GOSHIMA, K. 1969. Synchronized beating of and electrotonic transmission between myocardial cells mediated by heterotypic strain cells in monolayer culture. Exp. Cell Res. 58:420–426.

GOSHIMA, K. 1974. Initiation of beating in quiescent myocardial cells by norepinephrine, by contact with beating cells and by electrical stimulation of adjacent FL cells. Exp. Cell Res. 84:223–234.

GOSHIMA, K. 1975. Further studies on preservation of the beating rhythm of myocardial cells in culture. Exp. Cell Res. 92:339–349.

GOSHIMA, K. 1976a. Arrhythmic movements of myocardial cells in culture and their improvement with antiarrhythmic drugs. J. Mol. Cell. Cardiol. 8:217–238.

GOSHIMA, K. 1976b. Antagonistic influences of dibutyryl cyclic AMP and dibutyryl cyclic GMP on the beating rate of cultured mouse myocardial cells. J. Mol. Cell. Cardiol. 8:713–725.

GOSHIMA, K. 1977. Ouabain-induced arrhythmias of single isolated myocardial cells and cell clusters cultured *in vitro* and their improvement by quinidine. J. Mol. Cell. Cardiol. 9:7–23.

HARARY, I., and FARLEY, B. 1963. *In vitro* studies on single beating rat heart cells. I. Growth and organization. Exp. Cell Res. 29:451–465.

HYDE, A., BLONDEL, B., MATTER, A., CHENEVAL, J. P., FILLOUX, B., and GIRARDIER, L. 1969. Homo- and heterocellular junctions in cell cultures, an electrophysiological and morphological study. Prog. Brain Res. 31:283–311.

SANO, T., and SAWANOBORI, T. 1970. Mechanism initiating ventricular fibrillation demonstrated in cultured ventricular muscle tissue. Circ. Res. 26:201–210.

SPERELAKIS, N., and LEHMKUHL, D. 1964. Effects of current on transmembrane potentials in cultured chick heart cells. J. Gen. Physiol. 47:895–927.

WOLLENBERGER, A. 1964. Rhythmic and arrhythmic contractile activity of single myocardial cells cultured *in vitro.* Circ. Res. 14, 15 (suppl. II):184–201.

Mailing address:
Kiyota Goshima, Ph.D.,
Institute of Molecular Biology, Faculty of Science,
Nagoya University, Chikusa-ku, Nagoya 464 (Japan).

Recent Advances in Studies on
Cardiac Structure and Metabolism, Volume 12
Cardiac Adaptation
Edited by T. Kobayashi, Y. Ito, and G. Rona
Copyright 1978 University Park Press Baltimore

EXPERIMENTAL STUDIES ON CARDIAC ARRHYTHMIAS WITH SPECIAL REFERENCE TO FIBRILLATION IN HEART CELL CULTURE

S. YONEDA and S. TOYAMA

Department of Cardiology,
The Center for Adult Diseases, Osaka, Japan

SUMMARY

Fibrillation-like beating of cardiac muscle cells in culture was induced by altering the concentrations of various ions. Fine structural changes of cell membrane and intercellular alteration of cardiac muscle cells appeared to be more prominent in cells with fibrillation-like beating than in others. From the results of the present study, it may be concluded that fibrillation-like beating may occur in the presence of altered concentrations of certain ions, accompanied by fine structural changes in the cells.

INTRODUCTION

In order to clarify the mechanisms of cardiac arrhythmias and conduction disturbances, we studied the pathogenic mechanism in cardiac muscle cell culture. This method is a useful tool in the investigation of cardiac muscle cell behavior because the heart cells may be grown as monolayers and the movement of cells may be visualized. In addition, we undertook this study to investigate the possible relationship of subtle structural changes of the cells and their couplings in the genesis and progress of cardiac arrhythmias and fibrillation.

MATERIALS AND METHODS

Heart cells were isolated from the ventricles of ddY mouse embryos by slight modification of the method of Harary and Farley (1963) and were cultured with Eagle's minimum essential medium (MEM), containing 10% calf serum in 35-mm Petri dishes. Cardiac arrhythmias were induced by altered ionic concentrations of the medium, replaced by a proportional concentration of choline chloride. The investigation was observed visually by phase contrast microscopy at a temperature of 37°C. The structural changes of cultured cardiac muscle cells were studied by phase contrast technique and scanning electron microscopy (JSM–Sl).

RESULTS AND DISCUSSION

We observed by phase contrast microscopy that heart cells began to beat spontaneously and synchronously when in contact with one another. It has been well known that the mechanism of this synchronous beating is formed as a result of the intercellular connection (Halbert, Bruderer, and Lin, 1971; Yoneda *et al.,* 1975). By using scanning electron microscopy, we observed that numerous slender processes form bridges between adjacent cardiac muscle cells (Yoneda *et al.,* 1975). The cells thus draw closer to each other. These scanning electron microscopic findings in heart cell culture suggest that the slender processes and cell edge are the mode for intercellular contact. They also imply that subtle changes of intercommunication might be brought about at the ultrastructural level in association with arrhythmias, which frequently occur in various cardiac disorders.

In view of this, groups of approximately 10 cells, showing regular rhythmical beating at a rate of approximately 100 beats per min, were used in an attempt to determine whether or not fibrillation-like beating would be induced by changes in the concentration of the NaCl, KCl, or CaC_2 in the medium. Fibrillation-like beating occurred in certain conditions not only when the concentration of NaCl was reduced to 85%, 65%, 35%, or 10% in the medium, with concomitant changes in the concentrations of KCL and/or $CaCl_2$, but also when the concentration of NaCl was increased to 150%, with $CaCl_2$ reduced to 10% or KCl reduced to 10% or 35% in the medium. By scanning electron microscopy, we could detect various subtle changes in cell connections in the cells showing fibrillation-like beating as well as in those not showing fibrillation-like beating; a tendency was noted, however, for the cell membrane changes to be conspicuous in the cells showing fibrillation-like beating. Cell membrane changes were indicated by dissociation in cell-to-cell connection, crooking, irregularity, shortening, or disappearance of slender cell processes. Changes of cell body were detected only in cells with reduced potassium chloride in the medium.

REFERENCES

HALBERT, S. P., BRUDERER, R., and LIN, T. M. 1971. *In vitro* organization of dissociated rat cardiac cells into beating three dimensional structures. J. Exp. Med. 133:677–695.

HARARY, I., and FARLEY, B. 1963. *In vitro* studies on single beating rat heart cells: 1. Growth and organization. Exp. Cell Res. 29:451–465.

YONEDA, S., TANAKA, K., AKAGAMI, H., SHIBATA, N., and TOYAMA, S. 1975. Scanning electron microscopic studies on the formation of cardiac intercellular connection in culture. Jpn. Circ. J. 39:1321–1328.

Mailing address:
S. Yoneda, M.D.,
Department of Cardiology, The Center for Adult Diseases,
1-3-3 Nakamichi, Higashinari-ku, Osaka (Japan).

Recent Advances in Studies on
Cardiac Structure and Metabolism, Volume 12
Cardiac Adaptation
Edited by T. Kobayashi, Y. Ito, and G. Rona
Copyright 1978 University Park Press Baltimore

MYOCARDIAL DEPRESSANT FACTOR AND
RAT HEART MYOBLASTS IN TISSUE CULTURE

F. KÖLBEL,[1] P. VESELÝ,[2] F. FRANC,[2] and M. MALÝ[3]

[1] Third Medical Department, Faculty of General Medicine,
Charles University, Prague, Czechoslovakia
[2] Department of Experimental Biology and Genetics, and [3] Department of Physics,
Czechoslovak Academy of Sciences, Prague, Czechoslovakia

SUMMARY

Beating rat heart myoblasts in tissue culture are suitable for the demonstration of the effect of sera from patients with cardiogenic shock upon the contractility of heart muscle. Shock serum either promptly stops beating or causes discoordinated movements of the cultivated myoblasts (fibrillation). This effect of the shock serum is concentration-dependent. Hydrocortisone before and/or after treatment of the cultivated cells does not influence the effect of the shock serum. Calcium ions shorten the period of standstill of the muscle cells after washout of the shock serum.

INTRODUCTION

The presence of humoral factors depressing cardiac function in different types of shock was demonstrated first in 1943 and has been demonstrated repeatedly thereafter (Blalock, 1943; Lefer, 1973). The polypeptidic character of these substances was determined as well as their probable source in the splanchnic area, mainly in the lysosomes and zymogenic granules of pancreatic cells (Glenn and Lefer, 1970; Jones *et al.*, 1975). For the determination of these factors, preparations of cat papillary muscle were used (Lefer and Martin, 1970). This chapter demonstrates suitability of using beating embryonic rat heart muscle cells in tissue culture to study the effects of sera from patients with cardiogenic shock upon the patients' heart mechanical performance and properties.

MATERIALS AND METHODS

Preparation of Rat Heart Myoblasts

Rat heart myoblasts (RHM) were prepared from whole hearts of rat embryos 12–16 days old trypsinization. Dissociated cells were seeded into 60 X 15-mm Falcon polystyrene dishes in Eagle's minimum essential medium (MEM), supplemented with all the nonessential amino acids, sodium pyruvate, and 10% calf serum (Sevac, Prague), and incubated at 37°C in a humidified incubator for at least three days before the experiment. Cultures of myoblasts with good and regular frequency of contractions were selected for the examination of patients' sera. The medium was exchanged one day before the experiment, and 5 mM Hepes buffer and 5 mM Tes buffer (Calbiochem) were added to the medium in order to stabilize the pH around 7.4 during the experimental procedure which was carried out in the cinemicrographic apparatus MK-1, equipped for this purpose with a Videolux-1 CCTV Camera (HT, Hungary) and a CV-2100 ACE Videorecorder (Sony, Japan). The culture dish was placed in the MK-1 at 37°C and observed for 20 min until the frequency of pulsations became stabilized. Then, the lid of the culture dish was removed, and the contractility was checked again. If the pulsations were not disturbed by these manipulations, the treatment with different sera was started, and the behavior of myoblasts was recorded at TV speed (25 frames per sec) for further analysis.

Preparation of Sera

To obtain sera, blood samples were collected in polypropylene tubes and centrifuged immediately. The sera were frozen and stored at −20°C until their use. When used diluted, Eagle's MEM was added before testing, after thawing the sera.

Mathematical Operations

Changes in cell length were determined from the videorecording of the tissue culture at a speed of 25 frames per sec. The power spectra of the curves, depicted in Figure 1, were calculated on the Hewlett-Packard 9020 model calculator.

RESULTS AND DISCUSSION

In intact tissue cultures, three types of pulsations were observed: two-dimensional pulsations of isolated cells and/or of groups of cells and three-dimensional concentric pulsations of groups of cells (minihearts). The response of all of these types of pulsations to the different types of treatment was identical.

There was no significant difference in the frequency of pulsations of the cultures after the addition of the control (human as well as calf) sera and after the addition of the sera from patients who had recovered from cardiogenic shock (Table 1). All sera from patients with a developed clinical picture of cardiogenic shock either stopped the pulsations of the tissue culture immediately, or also caused a transitory period of discoordinated movements of the cells that could be called fibrillation (Table 1). The cessation of beating was sometimes ir-

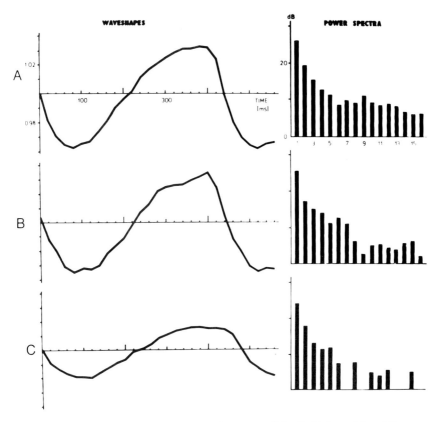

Figure 1. Changes in the dimensions of beating myocardial cells (left panels) and the power spectra calculated for each of the three curves (right panels). From top to bottom: A. findings in a control cell contracting in Eagle's MEM under conditions described in Materials and Methods; B. findings in a cell after spontaneous reappearance of rhythmic pulsations that followed the replacement of the 10% acute shock serum in Eagle's MEM by fresh Eagle's MEM; C. findings in a cell contracting in Eagle's MEM containing 1% of the serum used in Experiment B. For all three waveshapes, the descending segments of the curves correspond to contraction, and the ascending parts to relaxation of the cell.

reversible, irrespective of removal of the serum and/or of the treatment of the cells with hydrocortisone (1 µg/ml).

Sometimes the cellular standstill could be reverted by replacing the medium containing the shock serum with a fresh Eagle's MEM. The duration of the standstill was shortened by more than one-half by the admixture of $CaCl_2$ to the medium, replacing the shock serum (Table 2).

The slopes of the contraction, as well as of the relaxation, segments of the diagrammatic representation of movements of the cell recovering from the effect

Table 1. Influence of control sera, of sera from patients surviving cardiogenic shock, and of sera from patients in the acute phase of cardiogenic shock on the pulsations of rat heart myoblasts in tissue culture

Serum	Number of investigations	Standstill or fibrillation
Cardiogenic shock—Acute phase	15	15
Cardiogenic shock—Reconvalescence	2	0
Control—Human	1	0
Control—Calf	1	0

of the shock serum after its washout were almost identical to those of a control cell not exposed to any treatment (Figure 1, left middle and top panels). Similarly these characteristics were identical to the amplitudes of the pulsations, the duration of the diastolic plateau, and the length of the contractile cycle.

In a cell exposed to the influence of 1% shock serum causing a cellular standstill at higher concentrations, the amplitude of pulsations was markedly lower when compared to the previous two cells (Figure 1, bottom left panel). The contraction as well as the relaxation segments of the working cycle of this cell were markedly prolonged, as were the diastolic plateau and the whole contraction cycle.

A very sensitive indicator of the cell membrane tone was disclosed by the power spectra of the cardiac cell movements, mainly those with high harmonic levels (Figure 1, right panels). It is evident that in the cell recovering from the effect of the shock serum and with only minor changes in the characteristics of its contraction, the intensity of some oscillations with a high harmonic level is decreased. The slow movements of the cell exposed to the influence of the diluted shock serum are accompanied by a very pronounced defect of some types of the harmonic oscillations with high frequencies, which can be interpreted as physical sign of a decreased tone of the cellular membrane of the cell.

Table 2. Time necessary for spontaneous reappearance of rhythmic pulsations of rat heart myoblasts after replacement of the medium containing the shock serum by Eagle's MEM (HMEM) alone, and by Eagle's MEM supplemented with the addition of 9 mmol of calcium chloride

Shock serum replaced by	Standstill—duration (min)
HMEM	>20
HMEM + $CaCl_2$	10

REFERENCES

BLALOCK, A. 1943. Study of thoracic duct lymph in experimental crush injury and injury produced by gross trauma. Bull. Johns Hopkins Hosp. 72:54–61.

GLENN, T. M., and LEFER, A. M. 1970. Role of lysosomes in the pathogenesis of splanchnic ischemia shock in cats. Circ. Res. 27:783–797.

JONES, R. T., GARCIA, J. H., MERGNER, W. J., PENDERGRASS, R. E., VALIGORSKY, J. M., and TRUMP, B. F. 1975. Effect of shock on the pancreatic acinar cell. Arch. Pathol. 99:634–644.

LEFER, A. M. 1973. Blood-borne humoral factors in the pathophysiology of circulatory shock. Circ. Res. 32:129–139.

LEFER, A. M., and MARTIN, J. 1970. Relation of plasma peptides to the myocardial depressant factor in hemorrhagic shock in cats. Circ. Res. 26:59–69.

Mailing address:
F. Kölbel, M.D., Ph.D.,
Third Medical Department, Charles University Faculty of General Medicine,
U nemocnice 1, 128-21 Prague 2 (Czechoslovakia).

Recent Advances in Studies on
Cardiac Structure and Metabolism, Volume 12
Cardiac Adaptation
Edited by T. Kobayashi, Y. Ito, and G. Rona
Copyright 1978 University Park Press Baltimore

CARDIOTOXIC EFFECTS OF ADRIAMYCIN IN MAMMALIAN CARDIAC CELLS IN CULTURE

M. W. SERAYDARIAN and M. F. GOODMAN

Department of Biological Sciences, University of Southern California and
School of Nursing, University of California, Los Angeles, California, USA

SUMMARY

Cardiotoxicity of unknown etiology may preclude the use of adriamycin, a cancer chemo-
therapeutic agent. Mammalian cardiac cells in culture were used as a model system in the
study of the mechanisms involved. Adriamycin inhibited cell growth, particularly of the
fast-dividing nonmuscle cells. This inhibition might be a contributory factor to cardiomyopathy, but it does not explain the cessation of the rhythmic contractions characteristic
of myocardial cells in culture. The concentrations of ATP and phosphorylcreatine (PC) were
decreased in the adriamycin-treated cells, but the addition of creatine resulted in a several-
fold increase of PC. Therefore, the regulation of energy production and the potential to
maintain a high, steady-state concentration of PC were not impaired.

INTRODUCTION

The anthracycline antibiotic, adriamycin, is a promising new cancer chemothera-
peutic agent (Bonadonna *et al.*, 1970; Cortes, Ellison, and Yates, 1972). The
drug's action was attributed to the intercalation between base pairs of DNA
helices and the subsequent inhibition of DNA replication and/or RNA synthesis
(Pigram, Fuller, and Hamilton, 1972; Zunino *et al.*, 1972). Maintenance therapy
may be precluded, however, because of associated cardiotoxicity of unknown
etiology (Lefrak *et al.*, 1973). A possible involvement of mitochondria in the
cardiomyopathy has been suggested by several investigators (Buja *et al.*, 1973;
Jaenke, 1974). Furthermore, it has been suggested that, because of the quinone
structure, the activity of adriamycin could be attributable to the inhibition of
coenzyme Q_{10} -enzymes of the electron transfer processes of cell respiration in
addition to the intercalation within DNA helices (Henry, 1974; Iwamoto *et al.*,
1974). Gosalvez *et al.* (1974) indicated that the activity of adriamycin could not
be assigned to a specific site on the respiratory chain. Heart mitochondria

This investigation was supported by Research Grant HEW CA 17358 and by a grant
from the American Heart Association, Greater Los Angeles Affiliate.

isolated from adriamycin-treated rabbits showed a reduced respiratory control that disappeared within two weeks after interruption of the treatment. With intermittent treatment, State 4b respiration was affected, but continuous daily treatment led to the impairment of State 3 oxidations. The ADP/O ratio was not appreciably affected and the ATP levels were maintained (Ferrero *et al.*, 1976).

In the present study, mammalian cardiac cells in culture were used as a model system to investigate the mechanisms involved in the adriamycin cardiotoxicity. The preparation of mammalian cardiac cells in culture serves as a convenient cellular model independent of nervous, hormonal, and vascular controls, and the continuous rhythmic contractions are a good indication of physiological integrity. The cell population is heterogeneous, and the nonmyocardial cells divide faster than the myocardial cells, thus becoming more prevalent with culture age.

MATERIALS AND METHODS

Cardiac cells, derived from newborn rats, were cultured according to Harary and Farley (1963). The drug-treated cells were cultured in control medium for 24 hr, followed by a 3-hr treatment with 1.7 μM adriamycin (1 μg/ml), and then returned to control medium. Immediately following the 3-hr treatment with adriamycin, no difference could be observed between the control and experimental plates: beating rate ranged from 40 to 100 beats/min, depending on the batch, and the protein concentration was approximately 200 μg/plate (determined by the method of Lowry *et al.* (1951)).

RESULTS AND DISCUSSION

Adriamycin treatment inhibited growth of cells in culture (Figure 1). The cells continued to contract synchronously and rhythmically for 24–48 hr following adriamycin treatment, but then the beating ceased.

Cell Population

Cytological studies were undertaken in order to determine whether or not adriamycin treatment had a differential effect on the population of cells.

A distinction between the myocardial and the nonmyocardial cells in control cultures was made by demonstrating the presence of glycogen in the beating myocardial cells and its absence in the nonbeating cells, but the nuclei of all the cells were stained with hematoxylin (Clark, 1973). A similar correlation of glycogen and the myocardial cells was observed in embryonic chick heart cells in culture (Polinger, 1973).

Figure 2 shows that the relative proportion of myocardial to nonmyocardial cells in control culture was lower than in culture treated with adriamycin.

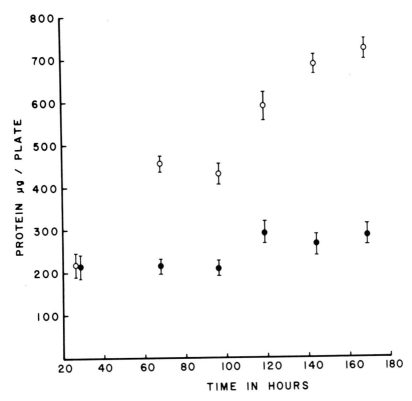

Figure 1. Growth curve of cardiac cells in culture. Control ○; adriamycin treated ●. Each value is an average of 10 determinations ± S.E.M.

Because nonmyocardial cells divide much faster than myocardial cells, the selectivity for myocardial cells was a result of susceptibility of the fast-proliferating nonmuscle cells to adriamycin. The inhibition of cell division of nonmuscle cells in the heart, e.g., capillary endothelial or fibroblasts, might be a contributory factor in the cardiomyopathy.

Energy Metabolism

The cessation of rhythmic contractions of cardiac cells in culture has been correlated in previous studies with an inhibition of energy metabolism; therefore, a possible effect of adriamycin on cell energetics was investigated. Cell extracts were analyzed for ATP and phosphorylcreatine (PC) as previously described (Seraydarian *et al.,* 1972). Table 1 demonstrates that the concentrations of ATP and PC were significantly lower in the adriamycin-treated cells. The low concentrations of ATP and PC could explain the failure of the cells to

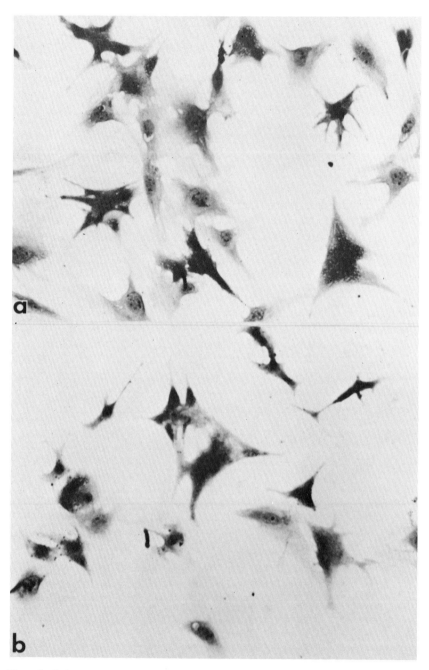

Figure 2. Cell population in culture. 1) Control culture, b) adriamycin-treated. Four-day-old cultures stained for glycogen (dark) and counterstained with hematoxylin (blue). The highly refractive myocardial cells are well differentiated from cells stained only with hematoxylin (only nuclei stained) and identified as nonmuscle. X 375.

Table 1. Effect of adriamycin on the concentration of ATP and PC

Conditions	Protein (µg/plate)	ATP (nmol/mg of protein)	PC (nmol/mg of protein)
Control (12)	564.8 ± 43.7	27.9 ± 0.8	26.4 ± 1.3
Adriamycin treated (12)	253 ± 19.4	16.1 ± 0.8	18.6 ± 1.7
5 mM creatine medium (12)	540 ± 42.2	26.7 ± 0.9	67.7 ± 3.3
Adriamycin treated; 5 mM creatine medium (12)	216 ± 11.3	17.1 ± 0.9	47.5 ± 2.2
50 mM creatine medium (15)	447.1 ± 34.2	20.2 ± 1.4	163 ± 7.8
Adriamycin treated; 50 mM creatine medium (13)	196.2 ± 23.2	13.0 ± 2.3	132 ± 11.6

All values are means ± S.E.M.; the number of experiments is given in parentheses.

maintain the rhythmic contractions in culture. Furthermore, if adriamycin cardiotoxicity were caused by a reduction of the maximal oxidative capacity of the mitochondria, as suggested by Ferrero *et al.* (1976), the heart would not be able to meet the demands of increased activity and the cells in culture would demonstrate a similar toxic effect.

When myocardial and skeletal muscle cells were grown in culture media enriched in creatine, the steady-state concentration of PC was greatly increased, but the concentration of ATP did not change (Seraydarian, Artaza, and Abbott, 1974). The new, high steady-state concentration depends on metabolism and was inhibited by metabolic inhibitors (Seraydarian, 1975). The only metabolic path known for the synthesis of PC is from ATP and creatine, catalyzed by creatine phosphokinase. Because the added creatine stimulates the rate of the transphosphorylation without depleting the ATP of the cell, the rate of oxidative phosphorylation must have been stimulated by the regeneration of mitochondrial ADP. Table 1 demonstrates an increase in the concentration of PC in the adriamycin-treated cells in the presence of 5 mM and 50 mM creatine. The new, high steady-state concentration of PC was comparable to that of control cells (Table 1). Unlike the metabolic inhibitors previously studied (Seraydarian, 1975), adriamycin did not impair the cells' potential to respond with an increase in energy production to the addition of creatine. This leaves unanswered the question of why the concentrations of ATP and PC were not maintained at control levels without the addition of creatine. Preliminary experiments indicate that the decrease in the concentration of ATP and PC in adriamycin-treated cultures might be related to the change in cell population, rather than to the effect of the drug on the mitochondria. Recent work by Bier and Jaenke (1976) also suggests that adriamycin does not alter mitochondrial function directly. The low energy charge remains a plausible, direct, underlying mechanism for the cessation of beating, and either the contractile machinery and/or the excitability could be affected.

Acknowledgment   The authors wish to thank Dr. N. R. Bachur for his generous gift of adriamycin.

REFERENCES

BIER, C. C., and JAENKE, R. S. 1976. Function of myocardial mitochondria in the adriamycin-induced cardiomyopathy of rabbits. J. Natl. Cancer Inst. 57:1091–1094.

BONADONNA, G., MONFARDINI, S., DELENA, M., FOSSATI-BELLANI, F., and BERETTA, G. 1970. Phase I and phase II evaluation of adriamycin. Cancer Res. 30:2572–2582.

BUJA, M., FERRANS, V. J., MAYER, R. J., ROBERTS, W. C., and HENDERSON, E. S. 1973. Cardiac ultrastructural changes induced by daunorubicin therapy. Cancer 32: 771–788.

CLARK, G. 1973. Staining Procedures. Williams and Wilkins Co., Baltimore.

CORTES, E. P., ELLISON, R. R., and YATES, J. W. 1972. Adriamycin in the treatment of acute myelocytic leukemia. Cancer Chemother. Rep. 56:237–243.

FERRERO, M. E., FERRERO, E., GAJA, G., and BERNELLI-ZAZZERA, A. 1976. Adriamycin: Energy metabolism and mitochondrial oxidations in the heart of treated rabbits. Biochem. Pharmacol. 25:125–130.

GOSALVEZ, M., BLANCO, M., HUNTER, J., et al.: 1974. Effects of anticancer agents on the respiration of isolated mitochondria and tumor cells. Eur. J. Cancer 10:567–574.

HARARY, I., and FARLEY, B. 1963. *In vitro* studies of beating heart cells in culture. I. Growth and organization. Exp. Cell Res. 29:451–465.

HENRY, D. W. 1974. Adriamycin (NSC-123127) and its analogs. Cancer Chemother. Rep. 4(Part 2):5–9.

IWAMOTO, Y., HANSEN, I. L., PORTER, T. H., and FOLKERS, K. 1974. Inhibition of coenzyme Q_{10}-enzyme, succinoxidase and NADH-oxidase, by adriamycin and other quinones having antitumor activity. Biochem. Biophys. Res. Commun. 58:633–638.

JAENKE, R. S. 1974. An anthracycline antibiotic-induced cardiomyopathy in rabbits. Lab. Invest. 30:292–304.

LEFRAK, E. A., PITHA, J., ROSENHEIM, S., and GOTTLIEB, J. A. 1973. A clinico-pathologic analysis of adriamycin cardiotoxicity. Cancer 32:302–314.

LOWRY, O. H., ROSEBROUGH, N. J., RAFF, A. L., and RANDALL, R. J. 1951. Protein measurement with Folin reagent. J. Biol. Chem. 193:265–275.

PIGRAM, W. J., FULLER, W., and HAMILTON, L. D. 1972. Stereochemistry of intercalation: Interaction of daunomycin with DNA. Nature (New Biol.) 235:17–19.

POLINGER, I. S. 1973. Identification of cardiac myocytes *in vivo* and *in vitro* by the presence of glycogen and myofibrils. Exp. Cell Res. 76:243–252.

SERAYDARIAN, M. W. 1975. Studies on the control of energy metabolism in mammalian cardiac muscle cells in culture. *In* P. E. Roy and P. Harris (eds.), Recent Advances in Studies on Cardiac Structure and Metabolism. Vol. 8: The Cardiac Sarcoplasm, pp. 181–190. University Park Press, Baltimore.

SERAYDARIAN, M. W., ARTAZA, L., and ABBOTT, B. C. 1974. Creatine and the control of energy metabolism in cardiac and skeletal muscle cells in culture. J. Mol. Cell. Cardiol. 6:405–413.

SERAYDARIAN, M. W., SATO, E., SAVAGEAU, M., and HARARY, I. 1972. *In vitro* studies of beating heart cells in culture. XII. The utilization of ATP and phosphocreatine in oligomycin and 2-deoxyglucose inhibited cells. J. Mol. Cell. Cardiol. 4:477–484.

ZUNINO, F., GAMBETTA, R., DIMARCO, A., and ZACCARO, A. 1972. Interaction of daunomycin and its derivatives with DNA. Biochim. Biophys. Acta 277:489–498.

Mailing address:
Maria W. Seraydarian, Ph.D.,
School of Nursing, The Center for the Health Sciences, University of California,
Los Angeles, California 90024 (USA).

Recent Advances in Studies on
Cardiac Structure and Metabolism, Volume 12
Cardiac Adaptation
Edited by T. Kobayashi, Y. Ito, and G. Rona
Copyright 1978 University Park Press Baltimore

CARDIOMYOPATHY *IN VITRO*

A. WADA,[1] Y. INUI,[1] H. FUSHIMI,[1] and S. ONISHI[2]

[1] The Center for Adult Diseases, Osaka, and
[2] College of Medical Technology, Osaka University, Japan

SUMMARY

Phase contrast microscopy of cultured embryonic heart cells showed the beating frequency decreased more rapidly and the regularity of the rhythm of the beating cells was lost sooner in heart cells from cardiomyopathic hamsters than from the control hamsters. Studies of cultured heart cells by differential interference contrast (with Nomarski's prism) and by electron microscopy revealed a significant impediment in the maturation of the sarcomeric units in the diseased animals compared to controls.

The incorporation of [^{14}C]leucine into acid-insoluble fractions was studied, and no significant difference in incorporation between the two groups was found. An analysis of polyacrylamide gel electrophoresis revealed the possible existence of a quantitative difference in one of the composing proteins of the erythrocyte membrane between the two groups.

The protein kinase activity of ghosts from the control group was more sensitive to cAMP than that from the diseased animals. In addition, the binding of [^{3}H]cAMP to the ghosts was almost identical between the two. The morphological and biochemical observations lead one to the plausible supposition that there are some differences in the interaction of the so-called catalytic and regulatory subunits between the two groups and that there is an impairment of the higher arrangement of myofibrils from their building blocks in the diseased hamster.

The significance of the existence of abundant corpuscles resembling neurosecretory granules was not established by this study. They may have an etiological significance or they may be related to a disturbed function in the cultured cells of the cardiomyopathic hamster.

INTRODUCTION

For more than 10 years, idiopathic cardiomyopathy in man has attracted much interest clinically, morphologically, and biochemically, but the pathogenesis of the disease is still not yet clear. Hence, experiments using animal models could be useful for studying of this disease. The authors were provided with an inbred strain of the Syrian hamster with a hereditary cardiomyopathy (BIO 14.6) from Bio-Research Institute, Boston, Massachusetts, and have used this animal for morphological and biochemical studies. Previous reports suggested that the delayed maturation of the sarcomeric units in this strain occurred in the neonatal heart cells (Bajusz *et al.,* 1969; Onishi *et al.,* 1970; Nadkarni, Hunt, and Heggtveit, 1972; Wada *et al.,* 1975). Therefore, it seemed important to investigate biochemical studies concerning pathomechanism of this disease and tissue cultures of heart cells from hamsters of this strain, because the beating cells provide a unique physical measurement of specific cellular function and metabolism. This chapter reports comparative observations made by phase contrast, differential interference contrast, and electron microscopy of the cultured heart cells of cardiomyopathic hamsters and healthy controls. In addition, the results of biochemical studies are presented.

MATERIALS AND METHODS

The experimental animals were obtained by brother-sister mating in our laboratory. They were kept in an air-conditioned room and were given Oriental CMF hamster chow and water *ad libitum.*

Culture of Beating Heart Cells

On the 16th day of gestation, the hearts were removed aseptically from the embryos of both cardiomyopathic and healthy hamsters and immediately immersed in a phosphate-buffered saline solution. Single heart cells were obtained as described previously (Wada *et al.,* 1976). The hearts were minced into small pieces and trypsinized three times for 15 min each. The last precipitate obtained was suspended in cold Eagle's minimum essential medium (MEM). After passing the suspension through gauze, the single cells, an average of 4.5×10^5 cells per dish in 2 ml of medium, were spread on a Falcon petri dish, 35 mm in diameter, coated with collagen. The culture medium was exchanged every three days and the cells were observed daily under an inverted phase contrast microscope with a temperature-regulated chamber.

Preparation Method for Differential Interference Contrast Microscope

The same number of heart cells was seeded on a cover glass in a petri dish. On the 1st, 2nd, 4th, and 7th days following incubation, the cultured monolayer cells on the cover glass were fixed with 2.5% glutaraldehyde made up in 0.1 M phosphate buffer for 30 min; then the cover glass was covered with another refined thin glass, 0.16 mm thick, and placed on a thin slide glass. The grown cells were observed with a differential interference contrast microscope with Nomarski's prism. Special care was taken to keep the cell moist during observations.

Preparation Method for Electron Microscope

The cultured cells were prepared in the following manner: After discarding the cultured medium, the petri dish containing adherent heart cells was washed several times with a phosphate-buffered saline solution. Then the cells were fixed with 2.5% glutaraldehyde, made up in 0.1 M phosphate buffer for 10 min, rinsed once in the buffer, and post-fixed with osmium tetroxide for 15 min. The cells were scraped off with a rubber policeman, dehydrated, and embedded in Epon. Ultrathin sections were stained with uranyl acetate and lead nitrate.

Preparation Method for Virological Study

To detect any viral infections related to this disease, hearts, kidneys, and livers of 120-, 50-, and 10-day-old cardiomyopathic hamsters, and embryo hearts at the 16th day of gestation were mashed in a mortar, 2 ml of MEM were added, and the preparation was centrifuged at 3,000 rpm for 10 min. The supernatants were placed over a monolayer of cultured kidney cells obtained from a green monkey and a human embryo. Degenerative changes of these cultured cells and the inhibitory effect of the supernatants on the cultured cells were checked under a microscope for 17 successive days following incubation.

Preparation Method of Erythrocyte Ghost

The heparinized blood was washed three times with a buffered saline solution containing 0.1 mM $MgSO_4$. Then, 40 vol of 5 mM phosphate buffer, pH 8.0, containing 0.1 mM $MgSO_4$ was added. The hemolyzed erythrocytes were washed by centrifugation three times at $10^4 \times$ g with the buffer used for hemolysis.

Polyacrylamide Gel Electrophoresis

The ghosts were dissolved with 1% sodium dodecylsulfate (SDS) and 10 mM 2-mercaptoethanol followed by heating for 5 min in boiling water. The gels (5% acrylamide) were subjected to electrophoresis for 15–20 min before sample application. The analysis on the gels, equilibrated with 0.03 M Tris-borate, pH 8.0, containing 0.1% SDS, was carried out with a current of 1 mA per tube for 1 hr. Gels were stained after electrophoresis with 0.1% Coomassie Blue in a mixture of ethanol, acetic acid, and water (50:10:40; v/v) overnight and destained with 25% ethanol in 5% acetic acid.

Assay of Protein Kinase Activity

The activity was measured in the reaction mixture consisting of 5 mM theophyllin, 30 mM $MgCl_2$, 0.1 mM NaF, 0.3 mM EDTA, 10 μM [γ-^{32}P] ATP, with or without 1 μM cAMP, and the ghost (ca. 300γ protein) in 20 mM imidazole buffer, pH 6.5. The reaction was started by the addition of [γ-^{32}P] ATP. After incubation for 10 min at 37°C, 1 mM 10% TCA was added, and the precipitate was washed three times by centrifugation with ice-cold 5% TCA. After washing with alcohol and ether, the precipitate was dissolved with Scentilamide OH and an aliquot was counted with a liquid scintillation counter, using Bray solution as a scintillator.

Autoradiography of ^{32}P Labeled Ghost
after SDS Polyacrylamide Gel Electrophoresis

The ghost was labeled with ^{32}P under the same conditions as that employed for the measurement of the enzymic activity. After incubation, the ghosts were washed with 5% TCA several times, followed by washing with ether. The material thus prepared was analyzed with SDS polyacrylamide gel electrophoresis in the same manner as the ghost. After electrophoresis, the gels were dried at room temperature, and radioactivity in the gel was detected by autoradiography using Kodak medical x-ray film.

Assay of cAMP Binding

The binding of cAMP to the ghost was measured by millipore filtration according to Gilman (1970). The total volume of the reaction mixture was 0.09 ml, consisting of 0.6 mM $MgCl_2$, 2 mM theophyllin, 0.3 μM $\sim$ 1.6 mM [^{3}H]cAMP, and the ghost (100γ protein) in 0.032 M acetate buffer, pH 4.5. The mixtures were kept in ice for 1 hr and applied to millipore filter paper (Type HA, 0.45μm) followed by buffer pH 4.5 with 6 mM $MgCl_2$ and 2 mM theophyllin. Measurements of the filter papers were made with a liquid scintillation counter using a toluene-based scintillator.

Thin-Layer Chromatography of Lipids Extracted from Lysosomal Fractions

The lysosome was prepared according to the method of Sawant *et al.* (1964). The lipid was extracted from the fraction by the method of Folch-Pi, Lees, and Sloane-Stanley (1957). After an application on silica gel G plate, the material was developed with petroleum ether, ether, and acetic acid (80:15:1; v/v) as a solvent system. After development, lipid fraction was visualized by iodine vapor; the fraction left at the origin was further chromatographed on silica gel G plate using chloroform, methanol, and water (80:15:4; v/v) as a solvent system. In addition, the lysosome prepared by the above mentioned method was analyzed with polyacrylamide gel electrophoresis in the same manner as the ghost.

Determination of Intracellular Concentration of Leucine

After being weighed, the excised heart was frozen and thawed several times and homogenized thoroughly with 4 vol of water. The homogenate was treated with trichloroacetic (TCA) acid at the final concentration of 8%. After centrifugation, TCA was removed with ether, and an aliquot was analyzed with an amino acid analyzer (Hitachi KLA-3B) to determine leucine content.

Determination of [^{14}C] Leucine Added
in the Grown Medium into the Acid-Insoluble Fraction

The primary culture prepared from heart tissue by trypsinization was treated with 2 mol of the radioactive growth medium consisting of leucine-free Eagle's

MEM containing 10% dialyzed calf serum and $[^{14}C]$ leucine (0.2 μCi) for 1 hr at 37°C. After incubation with the radioactive growth medium, cells were washed with ice-cold, buffered saline solution three times, and the washed cells were scraped off with a rubber policeman. After centrifugation, the cell pellet was frozen and thawed several times and homogenized with water, followed by an addition of TCA at the final concentration of 5%. The precipitate resulting from the TCA acidification was dissolved with NaOH, and an aliquot was used for counting the radioactivity incorporated and for protein determination by the method of Lowry *et al.* (1951).

RESULTS

Phase Contrast Microscopic Findings of Cultured Heart Cells

Within 20 hr of incubation, most of the dispersed cells from both cardiomyopathic and control hamsters began to beat at the bottom of the petri dish. As the incubation time progressed, the number of beating cells, singular or synchronous, increased. Counting technique of the beating frequency of the cultured cardiomyocytes from the diseased and control hamsters observed on the 2nd, 7th, and 10th days of incubation showed more rapid decline in the average beating frequency of the cells in the former than in the latter. The rhythm of the beating cells of the diseased hamsters tended to become irregular as the experimental period continued, while the regularity of the control cells was not changed significantly during the experiment. The results were compared under the same experimental conditions.

Differential Interference Contrast Microscopic Findings

The cells from the cardiomyopathic hamsters on the first day of cultivation were smaller than the cells from the control hamsters and were rather oval in shape, while the cells from the controls were mostly rectangular. Occasionally, two or more nuclei were observed in the diseased cells, and the nucleoli were usually more prominent than those in the controls. The arrangement of myofibrils in the diseased cells was comparatively more dissociated, and the mitochondria showed a greater variety in their size than in the controls (Figures 1 and 2). These findings of morphologically less developed organelles in the diseased cells continued to be found throughout the period of the observation.

Electron Microscopic Findings

The cultured cardiomyocytes of diseased hamsters were immature or primitive and showed generally less prominent formation of their myofibrils than the cardiomyocytes from control animals. In the cardiomyocytes of the diseased hamsters, the arrangement of the myofibrils was sparse and irregular, revealing a state of disarray. Z lines also were incompletely formed, and the cytoplasm was

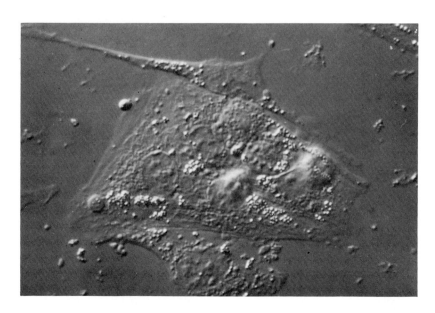

Figure 1. Differential interference contrast micrograph (Nomarski's prism) of cultured embryonic heart cells from a cardiomyopathic hamster on the first day of incubation. The cells are rather oval in shape with multiple nuclei. Mitochondria are more irregular in size, and myofibrils are less prominent than those in Figure 2. × 400.

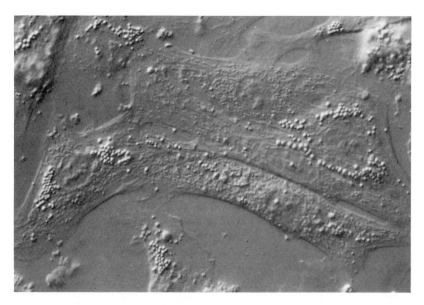

Figure 2. Differential interference contrast micrograph (Nomarski's prism) of cultured embryonic heart cells from a healthy control hamster on the first day of incubation. The cells are bigger than those in Figure 1 and are rectangular in shape. Myofibrils are well developed and more regularly arranged than those in Figure 1. × 400.

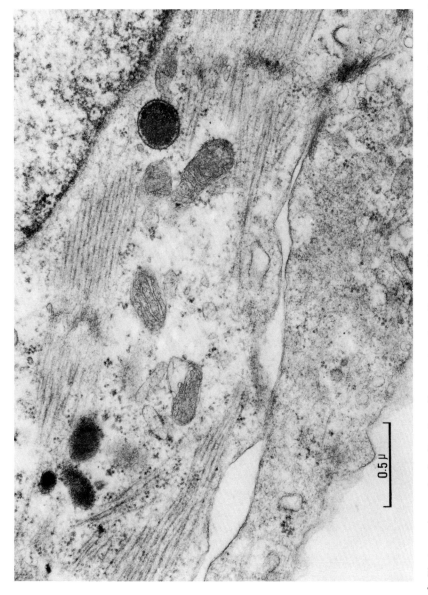

Figure 3. Electron micrograph of cultured cardiomyocytes of cardiomyopathic embryonic hamster on the fifth day of cultivation showing the sparse and intricate arrangement of the myofibrils, poorly formed Z lines, irregularly shaped mitochondria, relatively abundant polysomes, and the edematous matrix. Note the paranuclear corpuscle with its homogenously stained electron dense core with definite limiting membrane. × 20,000.

727

abundant with free ribosomes and polysomes. Mitochondria were irregular both in shape and size, and the matrix of the cytoplasm was edematous (Figure 3). In contrast, the cultured cardiomyocytes of the healthy hamsters, on the same day of cultivation, showed relatively well developed arrangements of myofibrils and Z lines. In addition, several densely stained corpuscles, similar to the neurosecretory granule, were characteristically observed in the paranuclear areas of the cultured cardiomyocytes in the diseased hamsters (Figure 3). Few such corpuscles were observed in the cultured heart cells of control hamsters.

Virological Findings

The incubated, cultured renal cells obtained from the green monkey and human embryo were completely unaffected by the addition of extracts from the hearts, kidneys, and livers of the cardiomyopathic hamsters that were checked. This finding demonstrated that no actual viral infections were involved in the development of the disease in this strain of hamster.

Biochemical Findings

The enzymatic activity of protein kinase in the absence of cAMP was higher in the diseased hamsters (166% compared to the control hamsters). When cAMP was presented at the concentration of 1 μM, the activity was stimulated by 116% in the diseased and by 209% in the control (Table 1). In this sense, the dependency on cAMP was higher in the control hamsters than in the diseased. The difference in the enzymatic activity in the presence or absence of cAMP between the two ghosts might be attributed to the difference in the acceptor protein of the ghost; therefore, autoradiography was carried out with the gels after electrophoresis of the labeled ghosts in the presence of 0.1% SDS. Although some undissolved proteins still remained at the origin, the major radioactivity among them was located in similar positions (Figure 4).

The binding of cAMP to ghosts was studied to determine whether or not the dependency of the activity on cAMP is related to its binding capacity to the ghost. The binding was measured by the method of Gilman (1970) using

Table 1. Protein kinase activity of the ghost

	BIO	RB
cAMP (−)	16,900	10,193
cAMP (+)	19,609	21,304

The concentration of cAMP was 1 μM. The figures indicate counts per min per mg of protein. BIO = the cardiomyopathic hamster; RB = the control.

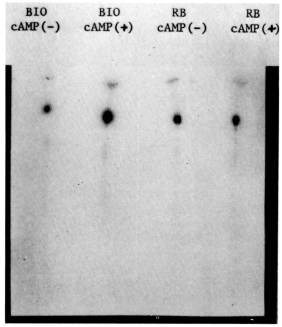

Figure 4. Autoradiography of ^{32}P labeled ghosts after SDS polyacrylamide gel electrophoresis. The electrophoresis was carried out from the top to the bottom as in the case of nonlabeled ghosts. The black portions correspond to those exposed to ^{32}P. The concentration of cAMP was 1 μM.

[^{3}H]cAMP. As shown in Table 2, the binding of cAMP was almost equal between the two in the concentration range of 0.3 μM to 1.6 mM cAMP. The same thing was true at 0.3 μM cAMP. A saturation phenomenon was observed in its kinetics when the concentration of cAMP increased more than 0.5 mM.

The incorporation of [^{14}C]leucine into acid-insoluble fraction from cultured heart cells of the cardiomyopathic hamsters and controls showed no significant difference (Table 3). Also, intracellular concentration of leucine in

Table 2. cAMP binding to the ghost cAMP

cAMP	BIO	RB
0.1 mM	874	728
0.5 mM	1,123	1,071
1.6 mM	1,086	1,216

The figures indicate counts per min bound per mg of protein. BIO = cardiomyopathic hamster; RB = control hamster.

Table 3. Incorporation of [^{14}C]leucine into acid insoluble fractions (cpm/mg of protein)

BIO	RB
118500	105035

The protein content was determined by Lowry's method with bovine serum albumin as the standard. The concentration of leucine in the growth medium was 16 μM. BIO = the cardiomyopathic hamster; RB = the control.

the cells from both groups was almost equal, 0.072 mM in the cardiomyopathic and 0.077 mM in the control, respectively.

Results of thin-layer chromatography of lipids and phospholipids showed no significant difference in their quality between diseased and control hamsters. Also, lysosomal fractions analyzed with polyacrylamide gel electrophoresis revealed similar patterns in both groups.

DISCUSSION

Few reports have been published on the tissue culture of heart cells of the cardiomyopathic hamster, and morphological studies of tissue cultures of this strain have not been reported previously. Our results indicate a tendency for the frequency of cultured cardiomyocytes from hamsters with a hereditary idiopathic cardiomyopathy to be lower and for the beating rate to decrease more rapidly than the rate in cells from healthy hamsters. Because the tissue cultures were carried out under the same conditions, the results are considered to be acceptable and appropriate, especially because the comparison of these findings to those of a differential interference contrast microscope and an electron microscope significantly showed insufficient formation of myofibrils in the cultured cells of the cardiomyopathic hamster.

The electron microscopic studies showed that the formation of myofibrils in the cultured heart cells was delayed more in the cardiomyopathic hamsters than in the normal animals, despite the presence of abundant-free ribosomes, or polysomes, and of well developed rough surfaced endoplasmic reticulum. Recently, Bester and Gevers (1973a, 1973b, 1975) demonstrated defective tRNA molecules in the cardiomyopathic hamster and their possible inhibiting effect on the biosynthesis of myofibrillar protein using ^{14}C labeled protein hydrolysate. Our results, on the contrary, showed that protein synthesis in the cardiomyopathic hamster was not impaired significantly. That is, protein synthesis in the diseased hamster appeared to be identical to that of the control, judging by the results of radioactive leucine incorporation into the acid-insoluble fraction. Although the significance of our results seems to be controversial, it may be speculated that the impaired assembly of myofilaments because of unknown factor(s) is a possible cause of underdeveloped ultrastructural features. An abundance of free ribosomes and polysomes in the cells from diseased hamsters was considered to be a reflection of attempted protein synthesis.

The results of our experiments using polyacrylamide gel electrophoresis revealed the existence of a quantitative difference in one of the composing proteins of the cell membrane, but not in lipids or in phospholipid, between the diseased and the control hamsters. The protein kinase activity enhanced by the addition of cAMP was somewhat higher in the controls than in the diseased hamsters. Namely, the enzyme from the control hamsters was more sensitive to cAMP addition than that from the diseased. On the other hand, cAMP, which had a different effect on the sensitivity to both enzyme preparations, bound to the enzymes in a similar fashion, as shown in Table 2. One possible explanation for the situation, at the present time, may be an assumption of a difference between the interaction of the catalytic and the regulatory subunits, if the existence of these units is valid in this system.

It is not known whether the membrane-bound corpuscles are neurosecretory or lysosomal granules. On a morphological basis, however, they appear to be neurosecretory, identical to the specific granules of type A reported by Berger *et al.* (1972). Early studies have suggested that specific granules may or may not contain amines (Bloom *et al.,* 1961; Nayler and Merrillees, 1964; Kuhn, Richards, and Tranzer, 1975), and in mammals these granules usually have been found in atrial myocardial cells (Bencosme and Berger, 1972). In our preliminary study, however, similar membrane-bound corpuscles were found in the vicinity of the Golgi apparatus in the right ventricular cardiomyocytes of the post-natal cardiomyopathic hamsters, but not in the control hamsters. Furthermore, these corpuscles showed a numerical increase roughly corresponding to the period of increasing hypertrophy of the right ventricular wall. The presence of the corpuscles in the cultured cardiomyocytes of the diseased hamsters seems to be quite interesting. Angelakos *et al.* (1972) reported a greater rate of norepinephrine formation in the heart during early life of the cardiomyopathic hamster as compared to a control group of the same age, and Bencosme and Berger (1972) stated that the corpuscles are related to a secretory function of myocardium. To determine whether the corpuscles might have been related to the etiology of the disease or might have acted to impede myocardial function, further studies are needed.

Throughout the experiments, no virus particles were noted during electron microscopic observations.

REFERENCES

ANGELAKOS, E. T., CARBALLO, L. C., DANIELS, J. B., KING, M. P., and BAJUSZ, E. 1972. Adrenergic neurohumors in the heart of hamsters with hereditary myopathy

732   Wada *et al.*

during cardiac hypertrophy and failure. *In* E. Bajusz and G. Rona (eds.), Recent Advances in Studies on Cardiac Structure and Metabolism. Vol. 1: Myocardiology, pp. 262–278. University Park Press, Baltimore.

BAJUSZ, E., BÜCHNER, F., ONISHI, S., and RICKERS, K. 1969. Hypertrophie des Herzmuskels bei erbbedingter Myopathie. Naturwissenschaften 56:568–569.

BENCOSME, S. A., and BERGER, J. M. 1972. Specific granules in human and non-human vertebrate cardiocytes. *In* E. Bajusz and G. Rona (eds.), Recent Advances in Studies on Cardiac Structure and Metabolism. Vol. 1: Myocardiology, pp. 327–339. University Park Press, Baltimore.

BERGER, J. M., SOSA-LUCERO, J. C., de la IGLESIA, F. A., LUMB, G., and BENCOSME, S. A. 1972. Relationship of atrial catecholamines to cytochemistry and fine structure of atrial specific granules. *In* E. Bajusz and G. Rona (eds.), Recent Advances in Studies on Cardiac Structure and Metabolism. Vol. 1: Myocardiology, pp. 340–350. University Park Press, Baltimore.

BESTER, A. J., and GEVERS, W. 1973a. Cell-free protein synthesis in heart and skeletal muscles from polymyopathic hamsters. Biochem. J. 132:193–201.

BESTER, A. J., and GEVERS, W. 1973b. Evidence for defective transfer ribonucleic acid in polymyopathic hamsters and its inhibitory effect on protein synthesis. Biochem. J. 132:202–214.

BESTER, A. J., and GEVERS, W. 1975. The synthesis of myofibrillar and soluble proteins in cell-free systems in intact cultured muscle cells from newborn polymyopathic hamster. J. Mol. Cell. Cardiol. 7:325–344.

BLOOM, G., ÖSTLUND, E., VON EULER, U. S., LISHAJKO, F., RITZÉN, M., and ADAMS-RAY, J. 1961. Studies on catecholamine containing granules of specific cells in cyclostome heart. Acta Physiol. Scand. 53(suppl. 185):1–34.

FOLCHI-PI, J., LEES, M., and SLOANE-STANLEY, G. H. 1957. A simple method for the isolation and purification of total lipids from animal tissue. J. Biochem. 226:495–509.

GILMAN, A. G. 1970. A protein binding assay for adenosine 3'-5'-cyclic monophosphate. Proc. Natl. Acad. Sci. 67:305–312.

KUHN, H., RICHARDS, G., and TRANZER, P. 1975. The nature of rat "specific heart granules" with regard to catecholamines: Investigation by ultrastructural cytochemistry. J. Ultrastruc. Res. 50:159–166.

LOWRY, O. H., ROSEBROUGH, N. J., FARR, A. L., and RANDALL, R. J. 1951. Protein measurement with Folin phenol reagent. J. Biol. Chem. 193:265–275.

NADKARNI, B. B., HUNT, B., and HEGGTVEIT, H. A. 1972. Early ultrastructural and biochemical changes in the myopathic hamster heart. *In* E. Bajusz and G. Rona (eds.), Recent Advances in Studies on Cardiac Structure and Metabolism. Vol. 1: Myocardiology, pp. 251–261. University Park Press, Baltimore.

NAYLER, W. G., and MERRILLEES, N. C. 1964. Some observations on the fine structure and metabolic activity of normal and glycerinated ventricular muscle of the toad. J. Cell. Biol. 22:533–550.

ONISHI, S., BAJUSZ, E., BÜCHNER, F., and RICKERS, K. 1970. Herzmuskelhypertrophie bei erbbedigter Myopathie des syrischen Hamsters nach elektronenmikroskopischen Untersuchungen. Beitr. Pathol. Anat. 140:119–141.

SAWANT, P. L., SHIBKO, S., KUMTA, U. S., and TAPPEL, A. L. 1964. Isolation of rat-liver lysosomes and their general properties. Biochim. Biophy. Acta 85:82–92.

SOSA-LUCERO, J. C., de la IGLESIA, F. A., LUMB, G., BERGER, J. M., and BENCOSME, S. 1969. Subcellular distribution of catecholamines and specific granules in rat heart. Lab. Invest. 21:19–26.

WADA, A., YONEDA, H., SHIBATA, S., INUI, Y., and ONISHI, S. 1975. Morphological and biochemical studies on the heart of the cardiomyopathic Syrian hamster. *In* A. Fleckenstein and G. Rona (eds.), Recent Advances in Studies on Cardiac Structure and Metabolism. Vol. 6: Pathophysiology and Morphology of Myocardial Cell Alterations, pp. 275–282. University Park Press, Baltimore.

WADA, A., YONEDA, H. SHIBATA, N., INUI, Y., FUSHIMI, H., TAKEMURA, K., and

ONISHI, S. 1976. Tissue-cultured heart cells from the cardiomyopathic hamster. J. Mol. Cell. Cardiol. 8:619–626.

Mailing address:
Akeia Wada, M.D.,
The Center for Adult Diseases, Osaka,
3–3, Nakamichi 1-chome, Higashinari, Osaka 537 (Japan).

Author Index

Subject Index